Acute & Chronic Wounds

NURSING MANAGEMENT

SECOND EDITION

RUTH A. BRYANT, RN, MS, CWOCN
Partner, Bryant Rolstad Consultants, LLC;
Program Director
Saint Mary's University
Wound Ostomy Continence Nursing Education Program
Minneapolis, Minnesota

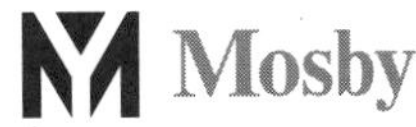

A Harcourt Health Sciences Company

St. Louis London Philadelphia Sydney Toronto

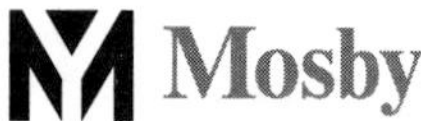

A Harcourt Health Sciences Company

Vice-President, Nursing Editorial Director: Sally Schrefer
Executive Editor: N. Darlene Como
Developmental Editor: Barbara Watts
Project Manager: Catherine Jackson
Senior Production Editor: Jeff Patterson
Designer: Judi Lang

SECOND EDITION

Mosby, Inc.
A Harcourt Health Sciences Company
11830 Westline Industrial Drive
St. Louis, Missouri 63146

Printed in the United States of America

ISBN 1-55664-410-8

00 01 02 03 04 GW/FF 9 8 7 6 5 4 3 2 1

Contributors

Barbara W. Barr, BSN, RN, CWOCN
Corporate Quality Assurance Nurse
Blue Ridge Nursing Homes, Inc.
Tucker, Georgia

Monica Beshara, BSN, RN, CWOCN
Staff Nurse
Wound Treatment Center
WellStar Cobb Hospital
Austell, Georgia

Craig L. Broussard, MSN, RN, CNS
Corporate Wound Care Nurse
Integrated Wound Care Systems
Pt. Arthur, Texas

Diane M. Cooper, PhD, RN, FAAN
Director, Wound Healing Research
Clinical Affairs
ORTHO-MCNEIL PHARMACEUTICAL, INC
Raritan, New Jersey

Dorothy B. Doughty, MN, RN, FNP, CWOCN
Director, Emory University Wound, Ostomy, Continence Nursing Education Center
Atlanta, Georgia

Rita A. Frantz, PhD, RN, FAAN, CWCN
Professor College of Nursing
University of Iowa
Iowa City, Iowa

Michael L. Gimbel, MD
Surgery Resident
University of Pittsburgh Medical Center
Pittsburgh, Pennsylvania

Margaret T. Goldberg, MSN, RN, CWOCN
Consultant
Wound Treatment Center
Delray Medical Center
Delray Beach, Florida

Mark S. Granick, MD
Professor and Chief Plastic Surgery
MCP-Hahnemann School of Medicine;
Medical Director, Comprehensive Wound Healing Center at
Roxborough Memorial Hospital
Philadelphia, Pennsylvania

Ann H. Harris, MSN, RN, CS
Wound Consultant
Spring Lake, Michigan

Gayle Jameson, BSN, RN, CWOCN, CWS
Nurse Manager
Wound, Ostomy, Continence Nursing
WellStar Health System
Marietta, Georgia

Bruce A. Kraemer, MD
Associate Professor, Plastic and Reconstructive Surgery
Barnes-Jewish Hospital Plaza
St. Louis, Missouri

Diane Krasner, PhD, RN, CETN, CWS
Wound Care Consultant and Adjunct Associate Professor
Johns Hopkins University School of Nursing
Baltimore, Maryland

Margaret McGinn-Byer, RN, CWOCN, OCN
E.T. Nurse – Outreach Services Coordinator
Fox Chase Cancer Center
Philadelphia, Pennsylvania

Laurie L. McNichol, MSN, RNCS, CWOCN, GNP
Clinical Program Coordinator
Advanced Home Care
Greensboro, North Carolina

Susan Mendez-Eastman, RN, CWCN, CPSN
Nebraska Health System Center for Wound Healing
Clarkson Hospital
Omaha, Nebraska

Donald J. Morris, MD
Chief, Section of Plastic Surgery
Carney Hospital
Dorchester, Massachusetts

Lisa G. Ovington, PhD, CWS
President, Ovington & Associates;
Instructor, University of Miami
Department of Dermatology and Cutaneous Surgery
Dania Beach, Florida

Barbara Pieper, PhD, RN, CS, CETN, FAAN
Associate Professor/Nurse Practitioner
Grosse Pointe Park, Michigan

Janet M. Ramundo, MSN, RN, CWOCN, FNP
Assistant Program Director
Emory University
Wound Ostomy Continence Nursing Education Program
Atlanta, Georgia

Bonnie Sue Rolstad, BA, RN, CWOCN
Partner, Bryant Rolstad Consultants, LLC
Minneapolis, Minnesota;
Saint Mary's University of Minnesota
Wound Ostomy Continence Nursing Education Program
Minneapolis, Minnesota;
Advisory Editorial Board, Ostomy/Wound Management

Gregory S. Schultz, PhD
Professor, Institute for Wound Research
Department of Obstetrics and Gynecology
University of Florida
Gainesville, Florida

Nancy A. Stotts, RN, EdD
Professor, University of California San Francisco
San Francisco, California

Nancy Tomaselli, MSN, RN, CS, CRNP, CWOCN
WOC Nurse/Nurse Practitioner Private Practice
Premier Health Solutions
Cherry Hill, New Jersey

JoAnn D. Waldrop, MN, RN, CWOCN
Assistant Director
Emory University Wound, Ostomy, Continence Nursing Education Center
Atlanta, Georgia

Judy A. Wells, MN, RN, GNP.C, CWOCN
Assistant Director
Emory University Wound, Ostomy, Continence Nursing Education Center
Atlanta, Georgia

Judith M. West RN, DNS
Research Coordinator, Department of Surgery
University of California San Francisco
Wound Healing Lab/Clinic
San Francisco, California

Laurel A. Wiersema-Bryant, MSN, RN, CS
Clinical Nurse Specialist/Adult Nurse Practitioner
Barnes-Jewish Hospital, a Member of BJC Health System
St. Louis, Missouri

Ruth E. Wilson, MSN, RN, CETN
Clinical Nurse Specialist
Inpatient Surgery
Memorial Health, University Medical Center
Savannah, Georgia

Kristy Wright, MBA, RN, FAAN, CHE, ET
President/CEO
VNA Services and Foundation,
Western Pennsylvania
Butler, Pennsylvania

Annette B. Wysocki, PhD, RN, C
Chief, Wound Healing;
Director, Division of Intramural Research,
National Institute of Nursing Research,
National Institutes of Health
Bethesda, Maryland

Reviewers

Chapter 15

Karen Huskey, RN, BSN, CGRN, CWOCN
Patient Education Department
Memorial Hospital
Chattanooga, Tennessee

Chapter 16

Joseph G. Kusiak, MD, FACS
Chief, Plastic and Reconstructive Surgery
Fox Chase Cancer Center
Philadelphia, Pennsylvania

Nancy L. Tomaselli, MSN, RN, CS, CRNP, CWOCN
WOC Nurse/Nurse Practitioner Private Practice
Premier Health Solutions
Cherry Hill, New Jersey

Dedicated to my children

Michael Edward Confer
and
Charles Orman Confer

Preface

Many changes have occurred in the science of wound management since the first edition of *Acute and Chronic Wounds: Nursing Management* was published. Skin and wound care is a much more common consideration in the day-to-day care of patients, whether the patient is in acute care, long-term care, home care, the operating room, or the outpatient clinic. Staff awareness of pressure ulcer risk assessment, primary interventions (i.e., prevention), basic wound assessment, and documentation has been emphasized through the adoption of the AHCPR (now AHRQ) Pressure Ulcer Prevention and Detection guideline as well as through the interventions of many wound care nurses. The pathophysiology of, and risk factors associated with, venous ulcerations and neuropathic foot ulcers have been more clearly delineated and described. Diagnostic tools for distinguishing wound etiology and determining the extent of the underlying pathology are better understood and more commonly utilized during the assessment phase.

Refinements in wound measurement, wound evaluation, and correlation with healing have been reported. Specific to venous ulcers, many advances concerning wound measurement and the ability to predict healing have been made. For example, Kantor and Margolis (1998) have reported the correlation of simple wound measurements (length, width, and length × width) with planimetric area. Furthermore, by using a new measure of healing (the mean-adjusted healing rate), complete healing of a venous ulcer can be predicted at the end of 3 weeks of appropriate therapy (Tallman et al, 1997). Margolis, Berlin, and Strom (1999) found that the failure of a venous ulcer to heal within 24 weeks of limb-compression therapy was associated with several risk factors: initial area of the wound, duration of the wound at time of evaluation, a history of venous ligation or venous stripping, a history of hip or knee replacement surgery, an ankle-brachial index (ABI) of less than 0.80, and more than 50% of the wound covered in fibrin. Although additional studies are needed to confirm these findings, it is exciting to realize that information such as this will provide the ability to predict healing and formulate appropriate treatment decisions (Skene et al, 1992).

Relative to topical wound management, during the 1990s, growth factor technology, combination wound dressings (i.e., hydrocolloid dressings combined with an alginate component), and adjuvant technology such as negative pressure wound management were introduced. Wound care continues to be provided in acute care settings and has become an essential service provided by long-term care facilities as well as home care agencies. Furthermore, the management of wounds is well accepted to require the integrative services of multiple health care disciplines. Although the wound care nurse has a specific interest and focus in the prevention and management of wounds, he or she will not be effective working in isolation; a team approach is critical.

As the many changes in the science of wound management have evolved, so has the role of the wound care nurse. Today the wound care nurse manages and cares for wound patients who have increasingly complex problems. Extensive knowledge and skills are required. To accurately determine wound etiology and risk factors, the wound care nurse must conduct a thorough and extensive physical examination. In collaboration with the patient's health care team, the wound care nurse must process and interpret the patient's data (results of relevant laboratory, radiologic tests, medical history, etc.) so that an appropriate plan of care can be developed and instituted. The wound care nurse must be familiar with the scientific review of the literature so that the care plan developed is state-of-the-art, is appropriate, and has a high probability of success. An ability to provide strong leadership and collaborative consultation with a variety of discipline's is essential to the delivery of effective and timely wound management.

Today's wound care nurse must also function as a change agent, constantly reviewing the literature to identify and introduce opportunities to challenge or improve individual patient care and programs. Concurrently the wound care nurse must operate from an outcomes management perspective, incorporating an understanding of desirable outcomes, data collection techniques, and statistical analysis into their daily operations. Only then can improvements to the process be made and efficient effective patient care identified.

This textbook is a resource for nurses with a range of interests in wound care, with diverse educational preparation, and with work experience. For the generalist nurse or the nurse who specializes in another aspect of nursing, this textbook can be a reference when seeking to answer specific questions. For the nurse interested in the specialty of wound management, this book must be read cover to cover and should serve as the textbook that launches such a career.

Given all the transitions that have occurred in wound care during the past 10 years, the practice of wound care is destined to become increasingly complex. To adequately prepare the wound care nurse to meet the expectations of this complex specialty, the educational preparation of the wound care nurse in the future will undoubtedly require graduate study (Hamric, 2000). With this educational foundation, the wound care nurse will be positioned to create either a specialty-based practice or an advanced practice nurse practice (Beitz, 2000; Bryant, 1993; Doughty, 2000). Our patients deserve it.

REFERENCES

Beitz JM: Specialty practice, advanced practice, and WOC nursing: current professional issues and future opportunities, *J Wound Ostomy Continence Nurs* 27(1):55, 2000.

Bryant R: ET nursing: advanced practice, specialty practice-or both? *J ET Nurse* 20:229, 1993.

Doughty D: Integrating advanced practice and WOC nursing education, *J Wound Ostomy Continence Nurs* 27(1):65, 2000.

Hamric AB: WOC nursing and the evolution to advanced nursing practice, *J Wound Ostomy Continence Nurs* 27(1):46, 2000.

Kantor J, Margolis DJ: Efficacy and prognostic value of simple wound measurements, *Arch Dermatol* 134(12):1571, 1998.

Margolis DJ, Berlin JA, Strom BL: Risk factors associated with the failure of a venous leg ulcer to heal, *Arch Dermatol* 135(8):920, 1999.

Skene AI et al: Venous leg ulcers: a prognostic index to predict time to healing, *Brit Med J* 305:1119, 1992.

Tallman P et al: Initial rate of healing predicts complete healing of venous ulcers, *Arch Dermatol* 133(10):1232, 1997.

Acknowledgements

Many people have encouraged me along my journey to complete this second edition. I owe my sincere gratitude to my partner Bonnie Sue Rolstad for her patience and advice during this project. I also want to thank all of the contributors for their professional dedication to wound management as evidenced not only through their excellent careers but also through their commitment to writing. This edition is in print in large part because of the prodding, warm encouragement, and support that I received from Barb Watts at Mosby. Thank you, Barb! Finally, I would like to thank my husband, Dennis Confer, for his daily doses of love and support, particularly during this endeavor.

Contents

CHAPTER 1

Anatomy and Physiology of Skin and Soft Tissue

ANNETE B. WYSOCKI

OBJECTIVES

1. Explain the importance of normal skin integrity.
2. Describe the size, thickness, function, vascular supply, and cellular composition of the major layers of the skin.
3. List the key structures and functions of the layers of the epidermis.
4. Discuss the significance of the following structures and cells: rete ridges, keratinocytes, melanocytes, basement membrane zone, tropocollagen.
5. Distinguish between the composition of the papillary dermis and that of the reticular dermis.
6. Describe the six major functions of the skin.
7. Identify three ways in which the skin protects against pathogenic invasion.
8. Describe the role of the following cells in providing the skin immune system: Langerhans' cells, tissue macrophages, and mast cells.
9. Explain the relationship between skin pigmentation and protection against ultraviolet radiation.
10. Identify the two mechanisms by which the skin provides thermoregulation.
11. Compare and contrast the structural and cellular development of the skin in the premature infant (between 23 to 32 weeks' gestation), full-term neonate, adolescent, and adult.
12. Describe at least two effects that the following have on the skin: hydration, sun, nutrition, soaps, and medications.

The skin is the one organ of the body that is constantly exposed to a changing environment. Maintaining its integrity is a complex process, and assaults from surgical incisions, injuries, or burns can lead to life-threatening consequences without appropriate treatment.

Human skin is divided into two primary layers—epidermis (outermost layer) and dermis (innermost layer) (Figure 1-1). These two layers are separated by a structure called the *basement membrane*. Beneath the dermis is a layer of loose connective tissue called the *hypodermis*. Major functions of the skin are protection, immunity, thermoregulation, sensation, metabolism, and communication (Jacob, Francone, and Lossow, 1982; Millington and Wilkinson, 1983; Woodburne and Burkel, 1988).

The skin of the average adult covers approximately 3000 square inches, or an area almost equivalent to 2 square meters. From birth to maturity the skin covering will undergo a sevenfold expansion. It weighs about 6 pounds, is the largest organ, and receives one third of the body's circulating blood volume. The skin forms a protective barrier from the external environment while maintaining a homeostatic internal environment. Epidermal appendages—nails, hair follicles, sweat or sebaceous glands—which are lined with epidermal cells, are also present in the skin. During the healing of partial-thickness wounds, these epidermal cells migrate to resurface the wound. This organ is capable of self-regeneration and can withstand limited mechanical and chemical assaults. The skin varies in thickness from 0.5 mm in the tympanic membrane to 6 mm in the soles of the feet and the palms of the hands. Variations are attributable to differences in the thickness of the skin layers covering underlying organs, bones, muscle, and cartilage.

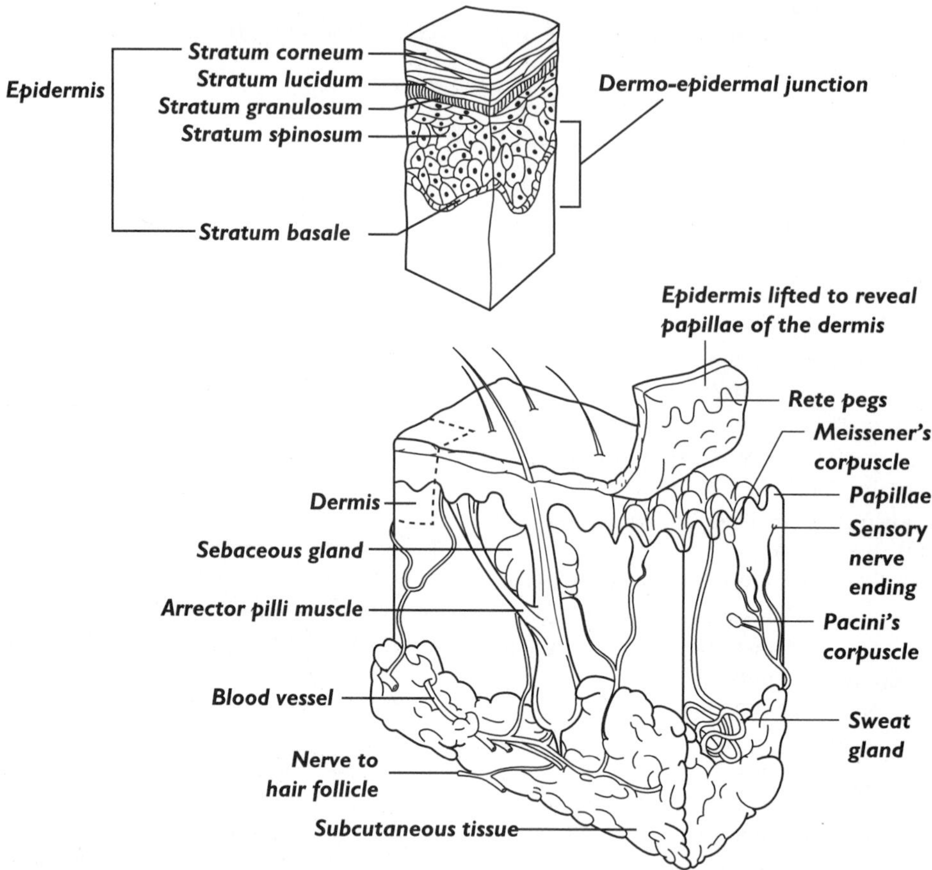

Figure 1-1 Schema of anatomy of skin and subcutaneous tissue. (From Hooper BJ, Goldman MP: *Primary dermatologic care*, St Louis, 1999, Mosby.)

SKIN LAYERS

Epidermis

The epidermis, the outermost skin layer, is avascular and is derived from embryonic ectoderm. This layer is relatively uniform in thickness over the body and is between 75 and 150 μm, except for the soles and palms where thickness is between 0.4 and 0.6 mm. The epidermal layer is constantly being renewed with a turnover time ranging from 26 to 42 days. Complete epidermal renewal occurs between 45 and 75 days, or about every 2 months (Odland, 1991). The epidermal layer is composed of stratified squamous epithelial cells, or keratinocytes, and is divided into five layers (see Figure 1-1). These layers, beginning from the outermost to the innermost, are the stratum corneum, stratum lucidum, stratum granulosum, stratum spinosum, and stratum basale (stratum germinativum, or simply, basal layer).

Stratum Corneum. The stratum corneum, or horny layer, is the top layer and is composed of dead keratinized cells. These squames, or corneocytes, are the cells that are abraded by the daily mechanical and chemical trauma of hand-washing, scratching, bathing, exercising, and changing of clothes. The stratum corneum is composed of layers of thin, stacked, pancake-appearing, anucleate cells. These cells are filled with about 80% keratin, a tough, fibrous, insoluble protein; hence they are called *keratinocytes.* Keratinocytes are initially formed in the basal layer and undergo the process of differentiation. The normal stratum corneum is composed of completely differentiated keratinocytes. Keratin is resistant to changes in temperature or pH and to chemical digestion by trypsin and pepsin. This same protein is found in hair and nails; in these structures keratin is referred to as "hard" keratin compared with the "soft" keratin of the skin (Jacob, Francone, and Lossow, 1982; Solomons, 1983).

Stratum Lucidum. The stratum lucidum is the layer directly below the stratum corneum. This layer is found in areas where the epidermis is thicker, such as the palms of the hands or soles of the feet, and where it is prominent but absent from thinner skin, such as the eyelids. This layer can be one to five cells thick and is transparent. Cell boundaries are often difficult to identify in histologic sections under a light microscope. The stratum lucidum is a transitional layer where active lysosomal enzymes degrade the nucleus and cellular organelles before moving into the stratum corneum (Jacob, Francone, and Lossow, 1982; Wysocki, 1995).

Stratum Granulosum. The stratum granulosum, or granular layer, is beneath the stratum lucidum when present; otherwise it lies beneath the stratum corneum. This layer is one to five cells thick and is so named because of the granules present in the keratinocytes of this layer. The cells of the stratum granulosum have not yet been compressed into a flattened layer and are diamond shaped. The structures contained in these cells are keratohyalin granules, which become intensely stained with the appropriate acid and basic dyes. The protein contained in these granules helps to organize the keratin filaments in the intracellular space. Cells in this layer still have active nuclei (Millington and Wilkinson, 1983; Wheater, Burkitt, and Daniels, 1987).

Stratum Spinosum. The stratum spinosum is the next layer below the stratum granulosum. This layer is often described as the prickly layer because cytoplasmic structures in these cells take on this morphology. Generally the cells of this layer are polyhedral in shape. A prominent feature of the prickle layer is desmosomes, a type of cell-cell junction. Cells in this layer begin to synthesize involucrin, a soluble precursor of the cornified envelopes (Millington and Wilkinson, 1983).

Stratum Basale, or Stratum Germinativum. The stratum basale, or stratum germinativum, is the innermost epidermal layer. It is often referred to simply as the basal layer and can be seen in Figure 1-1. It is a single layer of mitotically active cells called *basal keratinocytes*, or *basal cells*. These active cells respond to several factors, such as extracellular matrix, growth factors, hormones, and vitamins.

Once cells leave the basal layer they begin an upward migration, which can take 2 to 3 weeks. After leaving the basal layer the cells begin the process of differentiation. All layers of the epidermis consist of peaks and valleys. This arrangement is more dramatic in the basal layer. In fact, the epidermal protrusions of the basal layer that point downward into the dermis are called *rete ridges*, or *rete pegs*. Rete ridges are partly responsible for anchoring the epidermis, thus providing structural integrity. Basal cells in the base of the rete ridges have an increased proliferative capacity compared with cells at the top of the ridges (Briggamann, 1982).

Also distributed in this layer are melanocytes, the cells responsible for skin pigmentation. These are dendritic cells arising from the neural crest that synthesize melanin. In normal skin the number of melanocytes present is nearly the same regardless of skin color. There is approximately one melanocyte for every 36 basal cells. The primary difference between light- and dark-skinned individuals is the size and distribution of the melanosomes, the structures containing the melanin pigment, and the activity of the melanocytes. Carotene or carotenoids are responsible for imparting the yellow hue to the skin of some individuals (Jacob, Francone, and Lossow, 1982; Sams, 1990; Solomons, 1983).

Basement Membrane Zone

The basement membrane zone (BMZ), or epidermal-dermal junction, is the area that separates the epidermis from the dermis. Closer examination of the BMZ in the past decade has revealed it to be more complex than previously believed. The BMZ is subdivided into two distinct zones—lamina lucida and lamina densa. The lamina lucida is so named because it is an electron-translucent zone compared with the electron-dense zone of the lamina densa. The major proteins found in the BMZ are fibronectin, an adhesive glycoprotein; laminin, also a glycoprotein; type IV collagen, a non–fiber-forming collagen; and heparan sulfate proteoglycan, a glycosaminoglycan that probably acts as a type of ground substance. A lesser amount of type VII collagen has also been detected. The BMZ anchors the epidermis to the dermis and is the layer that is affected in blister formation. During wound healing the BMZ is disrupted and must be reformed (Sams, 1990).

Dermis

The dermis, or corium, is the thickest tissue layer of the skin. Compared with the cellular epidermal layer, the dermis is sparsely populated primarily by fibroblast cells and is vascularized and innervated. The dermal layer is derived from the middle embryonic germ layer, the mesoderm. Dermal thickness ranges from 2 to 4 mm but on average is 2 mm. Variations in dermal thickness account for differences in total skin thickness that have been measured throughout the body. The dermis of the back is thicker than the dermis covering the scalp, forehead, abdomen, thigh, wrist, and palm.

The major proteins found in the dermis are collagen and elastin. The other category of proteins found occupying the space between collagen and elastin fibers is referred to as the *ground substance.* This category of proteins is largely composed of proteoglycans (PGs) and glycosaminoglycans (GAGs). Included in this category of proteins are chondroitin sulfates and dermatan sulfate (ersican, decorin, biglycan), heparan and heparan sulfate proteoglycans (syndecan, perlecan), and chondroitin-6 sulfate proteoglycans. Although these proteins only account for about 0.2% of the dry weight of the dermis, these large molecules are capable of binding up to 1000 times their volume. Thus PGs and GAGs play a role in regulating the water-binding capacity of the dermis that can determine dermal volume and compressibility. This material can bind growth factors and provide cellular linkages with other matrix materials (Haake and Holbrook, 1999). Fibroblasts are the cells distributed in this layer that synthesize and secrete these proteins. The dermis is a matrix supporting the epidermis and can be divided into two areas—papillary dermis and reticular dermis (Figure 1-2).

Papillary Dermis. The papillary dermis lies immediately below the BMZ and forms interdigitating structures with the rete ridges of the epidermis called *dermal papillae.* The dermal papillae contain capillary loops (see Figure 1-2), which supply the necessary oxygen and nutrients to the overlying epidermis via the BMZ. The collagen fibers contained in the papillary dermis are much smaller in diameter and form smaller, wavy, cablelike structures compared with the reticular dermis. This portion of the dermis also contains small elastic fibers and has a greater proportion of ground substance than the reticular dermis.

Reticular Dermis. The reticular dermis is the area below the papillary dermis and forms the base of the dermis. The collagen fibers in this layer are thicker in diameter and form larger cablelike structures. There is no clear separation of papillary and reticular dermis because the collagen fibers change in size gradually between the two layers. Thicker elastic fibers are found in the reticular dermis but substantially less ground substance is present. A complex of cutaneous blood vessels is also found in this part of the dermis.

Dermal Proteins

Collagen. Collagen is the major structural protein found in the dermis and is secreted by dermal fibroblasts as tropocollagen. After additional extracellular processing, mature collagen fibers are formed. Normal human dermis is primarily composed of type I collagen, a fiber-forming collagen. Type I collagen represents about 77% to 85% of the collagen present, and type III collagen, also a fiber-forming collagen, represents the remaining 15% to 23% (Gay and Miller, 1978). Type V and VI collagen are also found in small amounts. Collagen is the protein that gives the skin its tensile strength. Chemically processed collagen from bovine sources results in leather handbags valued for their strength and long life. The primary constituents of collagen are proline, glycine, hydroxyproline and hydroxylysine.

Elastin. Elastin, another protein found in the dermis, provides the skin with its elastic recoil. This

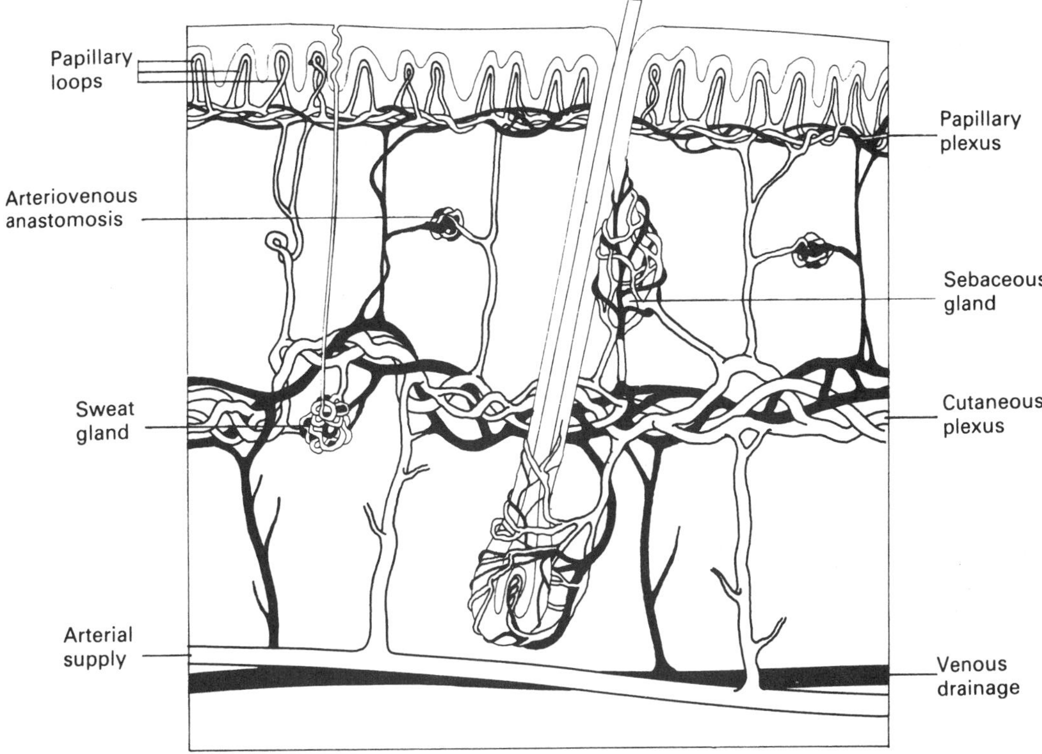

Figure 1-2 Blood circulation in the skin with papillary loops, which supply oxygen and nutrients to the epidermis, and dermal cutaneous plexuses, which arise from the deeper blood supply located in the hypodermis. (From Wheater PR, Burkett HG, Daniels VG: *Functional histology: a text and colour atlas*, ed 2, Edinburgh, 1987, Churchill Livingstone.)

prevents the skin from being permanently reshaped. Elastin is a fiber-forming protein like collagen and has a high amount of proline and glycine. However, unlike collagen, elastin lacks large amounts of hydroxyproline. Elastin fibers form structures similar to a spring or coil that allow this protein to be stretched and, when released, to return to its inherent configuration. It accounts for less than 2% of the skin's dry weight (Millington and Wilkinson, 1983; Sams, 1990; Wysocki, 1995).

Other cells found in the dermis are mast cells, macrophages, and lymphocytes. All of these cells are involved with immune surveillance of the skin, often referred to as the skin immune system (SIS).

Hypodermis

Hypodermis, or superficial fascia, forms a subcutaneous layer below the dermis. This is an adipose layer containing a subdermal plexus of blood vessels giving rise to the cutaneous plexus in the dermis, which in turn gives rise to the papillary plexus and loops of the papillary dermis (see Figure 1-2). The hypodermis attaches the dermis to underlying structures. This layer provides insulation for the body, a ready reserve of energy, and additional cushioning, and it also adds to the mobility of the skin over underlying structures (Haake and Holbrook, 1999). In certain pathologic disease states such as Werner's syndrome and scleroderma, this layer is largely absent.

SKIN FUNCTIONS

Protection

The skin provides protection against aqueous, chemical, and mechanical assaults; bacterial and viral pathogens; and ultraviolet radiation (UVR). It also prevents excessive loss of fluids and electrolytes to maintain the homeostatic environment. The effectiveness of the skin in preventing excessive fluid loss can be seen in burn patients; patients with burns involving 30% of their body can lose up to 4.1 liters of fluid compared with 710 ml for a normal adult (Rudowski, 1976). Protection against mechanical assaults is mainly provided by the tough fibroelastic tissue of the dermis, collagen, and elastin. Collagen, the most abundant protein in mammals, represents 25% of total weight (Stryer, 1995) and provides tensile strength, which makes the skin resistant to tearing forces. Elastin is distributed with collagen but in smaller amounts. Large concentrations of elastin are present in blood vessels, especially the aortic arch near the heart.

Protection Against Pathogens. Protection against aqueous, chemical, bacterial, and viral pathogens is provided by the stratum corneum, secretions from the sebaceous glands, and the skin immune system. The primary line of defense against all of these agents is an intact stratum corneum (Roth and James, 1988). As mentioned previously, the insoluble protein keratin found in the horny layer provides good resistance. In addition the constant shedding of squames from the stratum corneum prevents the entrenchment of microorganisms.

Sebum, a lipid-rich oily substance secreted by the sebaceous glands onto the skin surface, usually via hair follicles and shafts, provides an acidic coating with a pH ranging from 4 to 6.8 (Spince and Mason, 1987) and a mean pH of 5.5 (Roth and James, 1988). This acidity and natural antibacterial substances found in sebum retard the growth of microorganisms. These glands are stimulated by sex hormones (androgens) and become very active during adolescence. Sebum, along with keratin, provides resistance to aqueous and chemical solutions. When sebaceous glands occur in association with hair follicles, they are called a *pilosebaceous unit*. Sebaceous glands are not found on palms or soles and occur in areas that lack hair, such as the lips.

Resistance to pathogenic microorganisms is also provided by normal skin flora through bacterial interference (Weinberg and Swartz, 1987). Conceptually, there are two categories of skin flora—resident (the bacteria normally found on a person) and transient (bacteria that are not normally found on a person and are usually shed by daily hygienic practices, such as bathing and hand washing). Resident bacteria are found on exposed skin; moist areas such as the axilla, perineum, and toe webs; and covered skin. Bacterial microcolonies are found in hair follicles and at the edges of squames as halos in the upper loose surface layers. The following species of bacteria are found in human skin: *Staphylococcus, Micrococcus, Peptococcus, Corynebacterium, Brevibacterium, Proprionibacterium, Streptococcus, Neisseria*, and *Acinetobacter*. The yeast *Pityrosporum* and the mite *Demodex* are also found. Not all species are found on any one individual, but most carry at least five of these genera. Normal viral flora are not known to exist (Noble, 1983).

Protection Against Ultraviolet Radiation. Protection against ultraviolet radiation is provided by skin pigmentation, which results from synthesis of the pigment melanin. Harmful effects are primarily attributable to the long-wave form of UVR, or UVA, which ranges spectrally from 320 to 400 nm (Council on Scientific Affairs, 1989). The shorter the waves, the more dangerous they become. UVC is effectively blocked by an intact ozone layer. With holes appearing in the ozone layer there is concern over the effects that this may have on skin diseases caused by UVR. Because of the increased synthesis, amount, and distribution of melanin in dark skin, these individuals are better protected against skin cancer. Melanin is distributed in all layers of the epidermis in dark skin in contrast to light skin (Spince and Mason, 1987). Exposure to UVR can lead to skin cancer, sunburn (first- or second-degree burns), compromised immunity, and long-term skin damage.

Skin Immune System

The SIS also provides protection against invading microorganisms and antigens. The cells of the skin that provide immune protection are the Langerhans' cells, an antigen-presenting cell found in the epidermis; tissue macrophages, which ingest and digest bacteria and other substances; and mast cells, which contain histamine (released in inflammatory reactions). Both macrophages and mast cells are found in the dermis (Auger, 1989; Benyon, 1989; Wolff and Stingl, 1983).

Tissue macrophages are derived from monocytes, which are derived from bone marrow precursor cells. Macrophages are among the most important cells of the skin immune system because they are versatile. Once these monocytes migrate into the tissue they differentiate and become macrophages. Cells in the dermis that are not completely differentiated are difficult to distinguish, and much effort has been made to recognize the various cells in the dermis in the last decade. Macrophages, in addition to their antibacterial activity, can process and present antigen to immunocompetent lymphoid cells; are tumoricidal; and can secrete growth factors, cytokines, and other immunomodulatory molecules. Macrophages are involved in coagulation, atherogenesis, wound healing, and tissue remodeling (Haake and Holbrook, 1999).

Mast cells are usually found distributed in the papillary dermis; around epidermal appendages, blood vessels, and nerves found in the subpapillary plexus; and in subcutaneous fat. These cells are distributed in connective tissue throughout the body in places where there is an interface of an organ with the environment. Mast cells contain or secrete on demand a host of proteins. Thus mast cells are the primary effector cells in an allergic reaction. They are also involved in the presence of subacute and chronic inflammatory disease. As a part of the SIS, mast cells play a role in protection against parasites; stimulate chemotaxis; promote phagocytosis; are involved in the activation and proliferation of eosinophils; are capable of altering vasotension and vascular permeability; and can promote connective tissue repair and angiogenesis. Their role in tumor surveillance awaits further study (Haake and Holbrook, 1999).

Thermoregulation

Thermoregulation of the body is provided by the skin, which acts as a barrier between the outside and inside environments to maintain body temperature. The two primary thermoregulatory mechanisms are circulation and sweating. Blood vessels can either dilate to dissipate heat or constrict to shunt heat to underlying body organs. When dilated, these vessels have an increased blood flow and release heat by conduction, convection, radiation, and evaporation. Vasoconstriction is often accompanied by actions of the arrector pili muscle attached to hair follicles, which results in the hair standing vertically. In mammals that depend on hair for warmth, this action fluffs up the fur to increase thermal capacity. The bulge around the hair shaft that is visible when this occurs is commonly referred to as *goose bumps*. In humans, shivering is more important for maintaining body temperature when the outside environment is cold than the vertical orientation of hair (Jacob, Francone, and Lossow, 1982; Sams, 1990). In cold weather the "core" body temperature encompasses a smaller zone, whereas in warm weather the "core" is expanded. Clinically it has been estimated that for each 1° C (1.8° F) increase in fever there is a 13% increase in a patient's fluid and calorie needs. At rest the trunk, viscera, and brain account for 70% of heat production but are only 36% of body mass. However, during exercise, muscle and skin account for 90% of heat production while representing 56% of body mass (Wenger, 1999).

Sweating occurs when there is an increase in the activity of the sweat glands. It has been estimated that there are about two million sweat glands. Sweat glands are of two types—eccrine and apocrine. Eccrine glands arise from epidermal invagination and are found abundantly on the palms of the hand and soles of the feet. These glands are largely under control of the nervous system, responding to temperature differences and emotional stimulation. Muscular activity also influences their secretory activity. The sweat glands, located in the dermis as a coil, secrete fluid consisting of sodium chloride, urea, sulfates, and phosphates (Solomons, 1983; Spince and Mason, 1987). Thermoregulatory control occurs as a result of cooling when fluid is evaporated from the skin surface, since such evaporation requires heat. The odor associated with sweat is largely a result of bacterial action.

Apocrine sweat glands are usually found in association with hair follicles but do not play a significant role in thermoregulation. These coiled tubular glands are present in the axilla and anogenital area;

modifications of these glands are found in the ear and secrete ear wax, or cerumen (Spince and Mason, 1987).

Sensation

Nerve receptors located in the skin are sensitive to pain, touch, temperature, and pressure. When stimulated, these receptors transmit impulses to the cerebral cortex where they are interpreted. Combinations of these four basic types of sensations result in burning, tickling, and itching (Jacob, Francone, and Lossow, 1982). These sensations are propagated by unmyelinated free nerve endings, Merkel's cells, Meissner's corpuscles, Krause's end bulbs, Ruffini's terminals, and Pacini's corpuscles. Identification of particular responses with specific nerve structures has not been successful. In part, the reason is that some receptors seem to respond to a variety of stimuli. However, it is known that Meissner's corpuscles are involved in touch reception; Pacini's corpuscles (see Figure 1-1) respond to pressure, coarse touch, vibration, and tension; and free nerve endings respond to touch, pain, and temperature (Wheater, Burkitt, and Daniels, 1987).

Skin sensation is a part of the body's integrative response to protect itself from the surrounding environment. Sensation assists with the skins regulatory function and can signal sweating, shivering, weight shifts (Alterescu and Alterescu, 1988), laughter, and scratching.

Sensation also moderates psychobiologic phenomena made famous by Harlow, who demonstrated the preference of young animals for warm objects and those that provided better tactile sensitivity. In addition, early studies by Spitz (1947) point to the importance of touch in mediating social interactions with children and infants. Deprivation of touch can lead to psychomotor retardation and an increased risk of death (Ottenbacher et al, 1987). Other studies on touch indicate that it may be a factor in the development of atherosclerotic lesions in animals. In studies examining the effect of stroking, handling, talking, and playing with rabbits, investigators (Nerem, Levesque, and Cornhill, 1980) found a 60% reduction in aortic atherosclerotic lesions in treated animals compared with controls, even though both groups were fed the same cholesterol-containing diet and had similar blood pressures, heart rates, and serum cholesterol levels.

Metabolism

Synthesis of vitamin D occurs in the skin in the presence of sunlight. Ultraviolet radiation converts a sterol (7-dehydrocholesterol) to cholecalciferol (vitamin D). Vitamin D participates in calcium and phosphate metabolism and is important in the mineralization of bone. Because vitamin D is synthesized in the skin but then transmitted to other parts of the body, it is considered an active hormone when converted to calcitriol (1,25-dihydroxycholecalciferol) (Lehninger, 1982; Stryer, 1995).

Communication

In addition to its biologic, structural, functional, and physiologic functions, human skin also functions as an organ of communication and identification. The skin over the face is especially important for identification of a person and plays a role in internal and external assessments of beauty. Injury to the skin can result in not only functional and physiologic consequences, but also changes in body image. Scarring from trauma, surgery, or incisions can lead to changes in clothing choices, avoidance of public exposure, and a decrease in self-esteem. Research (Shuster et al, 1978) indicates that with increased scarring from facial acne, the self-image is progressively reduced. Adolescents are especially sensitive to physical appearance (Bernstein, 1976). As an organ of communication, facial skin along with underlying muscles is capable of expressions such as smiling, frowning, and pouting. The sensation of touching can also convey feelings of comfort, concern, friendship, and love.

FACTORS ALTERING SKIN CHARACTERISTICS

Age

Age is an important factor in altering skin characteristics. More recently the scarless healing of fetal tissue has come under more intense investigation (Longaker et al, 1990; Siebert et al, 1990). It has been found that wounds heal without scarring in fetal lambs up until 120 days of gestation. Collagen deposition in fetal wounds occurs more rapidly and in a normal dermal pattern (Longaker et al, 1990). In addition, an important difference between fetal and adult skin is the amount of hyaluronic acid, a glycosaminoglycan. In the laboratory setting, topical application of hyaluronic acid has been associated with a reduction in scar formation in postnatal wounds. This glycosaminoglycan is associated with collagen, and it has been proposed that a hyaluronic acid-collagen-protein complex plays a role in fetal scarless healing (Siebert et al, 1990). Transforming growth factor beta-1 (TGF-β1) is the other modulator of scarless healing in fetal wounds. Fetal wounds usually contain less TGF-β1 compared with adult wounds (Roberts and Sporn, 1996). In addition, differential patterns of expression of the various isoforms of TGF-β also affect the relative amount of scarring in fetal versus adult wounds.

At birth the skin and nails are thinner than those in an adult but will gradually increase in thickness with aging. Formation of the epidermal and dermal layers occurs within the first 2 weeks of embryonic development. Epidermal development is complete by the end of the second trimester, and at birth epidermal thickness is almost that of adult skin, although newborn skin is not as effective as adult skin in providing an effective barrier to transcutaneous water loss. On the other hand, development of the dermis lags behind and does not take on the characteristics of adult dermis until after birth.

The ratio of type I to III collagen is similar to the fetal ratios. Soluble collagen is about 24%, compared with 1% in the adult. This persists until about 6 months of age. The newborn dermis is about 60% as thick as that found in an adult, and as expected, the dermal fibers are significantly finer. Newborn dermis contains a much higher cellular component compared with mature adult skin. The epidermal-dermal junction remains flat until the beginning of the third trimester, and at birth the rete ridges are only weakly developed, thus making premature and newborn skin subject to tearing or blistering. At birth the capillary beds do not have a mature adult pattern and are still disorganized. An adult pattern of capillary loops occurs at about 14 to 17 weeks after skin growth slows (Holbrook, 1991).

Immature skin, or skin from premature infants between 23 or 24 weeks' up to 32 weeks' gestation, requires special attention compared with that of infants beyond 32 weeks. In particular, before 28 weeks' gestation the skin is thin and poorly keratinized and functions weakly as a barrier. An article appearing in *Lancet* (Immature skin, 1989) has characterized the skin of infants born at the limits of viability as more suitable to an "aquatic environment" than to atmospheric conditions. Transepidermal water loss is high, and application of tape strips the outer immature epidermal layer that can leave behind raw damaged skin prone to infection and occasional scarring. At 24 weeks' gestation, transepidermal water loss can be 10 times greater per unit area compared with an infant born at term (Rutter, 1988). In addition, premature infants have high evaporative heat losses resulting in increased risk for hypothermia.

Because premature infants have a greater surface-area-to-volume ratio compared with full-term infants, they are at an increased risk for skin complications. These infants may also have alterations in metabolism, excretion, distribution, and protein binding of chemical agents, placing them at increased risk for local or systemic toxicity from soaps, lotions, or other topical agents (Weston and Lane, 1999). Other dangers are percutaneous absorption of topical agents, including antiseptics. Hemorrhagic necrosis of the dermis from alcohol absorption has been reported if the alcohol does not quickly evaporate and is sometimes mistaken for bruising. The use of topical antibiotic sprays containing neomycin should be avoided since it is an ototoxic aminoglycoside. Thus water-based topical antiseptics are preferred but should be used sparingly. Cleaning should be done with care using normal saline or water. Chlorhexidine, a commonly used antiseptic, is not known to have any adverse effects, but it is probably absorbed from the skin and should be used judiciously. Likewise iodine has been reported to be absorbed, leading to goiter and hypothyroidism (Rutter, 1988). If required, moisturizing creams or ointments may be applied to dry, flaking, or fissured skin, and the best agents appear to be those with little or no preservatives since these offer the greatest benefit with decreased risk (Weston and Lane, 1999).

Interestingly, exposure of the premature infant's skin to air seems to accelerate skin maturation and occurs in about 2 weeks after birth. Similar findings using an animal model support these observations. Interventions that seem to be helpful during this 2-week period are the avoidance of tape to the skin with the use of a self-adherent wrap like Coban (roller gauze), which is taped without direct skin contact, or stockinette material (Bryant, 1988). Raising the humidity of the air close to the skin surface in the incubator or use of a waterproof blanket appears useful. The use of surface probes should be minimized, if possible. It has been reported that the use of polyurethane film dressings, such as Tegaderm or Opsite, have several advantages. This dressing material results in a 50% reduction in transepidermal water loss, allows the attachment of temperature and electrocardiogram (ECG) electrodes, resulting in the achievement of normal readings, and can provide a surface that can be taped. Polyurethane film dressings provide air exchange but prevent bacterial invasion and have good release characteristics that eliminate or minimize skin damage by stripping when removed. Karaya gum ECG electrodes also seem to be beneficial by reducing pain and epidermal damage when removed and can be repositioned for ultrasound or radiographic examinations. Polyurethane film dressings can hinder gas transfer, and PO_2 and PCO_2 readings are not accurate. A spray-on dressing appears to eliminate this problem. Further studies of the use of polyurethane film dressings is warranted (Immature skin, 1989).

The next period of change occurs in adolescence when hormonal stimulation results in increased activity of sebaceous glands and hair follicles. Sebaceous glands increase their secretory rate, and hair follicles, giving rise to secondary sexual characteristics, become activated. From adolescence to adulthood there is a gradual change in skin characteristics. By the time the skin reaches mature adulthood, several changes become apparent. The dermis decreases in thickness by about 20%, whereas the epidermis remains relatively unchanged. Epidermal turnover time is increased; this means that wound healing may take longer. For instance, in young adults, epidermal turnover takes about 21 days, but by 35 years of age this turnover time is doubled. Barrier function is reduced, and such reduction may increase the risk of irritation. The number of active melanocytes per unit body surface area decreases with aging, which means that protection against UVR is diminished. Skin dryness is also associated with aging and an increase in wrinkles. Sensory receptors are diminished in capacity, meaning that the skin is more likely to be burned or traumatized without perception. Vitamin D production is decreased and may be a factor in osteomalacia.

With aging there is a decrease in the number of Langerhans' cells, which affects the immunocompetence of the skin and can lead to an increased risk of skin cancer and infection by invading microorganisms. There is also a decrease in mast cells and melanocytes. The inflammatory response is decreased, and such a decrease may alter allergic reactions and healing. A decrease in the number of sweat glands, diminished vascularity, and a reduction in the amount of subcutaneous fat compromise the thermoregulatory capacity of the skin. Epidermal-dermal junction changes, such as the flattening of the prominent dermal papillae and of the rete ridges, alter junctional integrity. Consequently, the skin is more easily torn in response to mechanical trauma, especially shearing forces. Because the epidermal rete pegs flatten, the unique microenvironment of the basal keratinocytes changes; it is thought that this explains the decrease in epidermal proliferative capacity with aging (Lavker, Zheng, Dong, 1986).

Skin elasticity decreases with age and is related to a combination of aging and solar damage. Microscopic analysis of collagen and elastin fibers reveals that these are more compact with a loss of ground substance from the spaces between these cablelike structures. Collagen fibers appear to be unwinding while elastin fibers appear to be lysing. The degradation of elastin can be detected at about

30 years of age but becomes marked at 70 years of age (Braverman, 1986). There is also a marked reduction in vascular beds in the vertical capillary loops in the dermal papillae. It is thought that this leads to atrophy of the hair bulbs, sweat glands, and sebaceous glands. Because the hypodermis also becomes thinner, mature individuals are more prone to pressure necrosis (Gilchrest, 1989).

Changes in hair color and hair follicles also accompany aging. Age-related changes in active melanocytes result in gray hair. About 50% of the body's hair will be gray by the age of 50 in about 50% of the population. This change is accompanied by a reduction in the number of hair follicles and a decrease in the diameter of the hair. The rate of hair growth is also decreased (Silverberg and Silverberg, 1989).

The density of skin melanocytes is relatively constant until about 40 years of age. By about 45 years of age, skin melanocytes have decreased in density to approximately half that seen between 30 and 39 years of age (Nordlund, 1986). It is thought that loss of skin melanocytes contributes to an increase in the formation of skin cancers. Other overt changes are wrinkling and sagging, which occur as a result of loss of underlying tissue in addition to changes seen in collagen and elastin.

Changes in thermoregulatory capacity occur with age, and older individuals are more prone to hypothermia and heat stroke. This has been attributed to changes in blood capillaries and eccrine sweat glands. In healthy older individuals, sweating may be decreased by up to 70% (Gilchrest, 1991). Sebum secretion also declines with age. In addition to these changes, pain perception is dulled, and there is reduced skin reactivity upon exposure to irritants. Cutaneous immune function also changes with aging as seen by a reduction in Langerhans' cell density. Skin damaged by sun exposure, or actinically damaged skin, has been found to have a 50% reduction of Langerhans' cell density compared with sun-protected skin (Sauder, 1986). Reduction in immunocompetence of the skin is thought to contribute in part to skin cancer in the elderly.

Other factors that may contribute to the development of skin cancer in aged individuals are cumulative exposure to carcinogens, diminished DNA repair capacity, decreased melanocyte density, and alterations in dermal matrix (Lin and Carter, 1986). Not surprisingly, wound healing in older individuals is delayed compared with that of younger individuals.

Sun

Excessive exposure to UVR can have harmful effects that accelerate aging of the skin. For this reason the condition associated with UVR-damaged skin is referred to as *photoaging*. Dermatologically it is called *dermatoheliosis*. Obvious clinical signs of photodamaged skin are dryness, tough leathery texture, wrinkling (as a result of collagen and elastin degeneration), and irregular pigmentation (from changes in melanin distribution) (Silverberg and Silverberg, 1989). Excessive exposure to UVR increases the risk of developing skin cancers such as basal or squamous cell carcinoma and malignant melanoma. Damage to the DNA of skin cells leads to transformation of cells and cancer (Council on Scientific Affairs, 1989). Changes also occur in epidermal and dermal cells; epidermal cells become thickened, fibroblasts become more numerous, and dermal vessels become dilated and tortuous. Langerhans' cells are reduced in number by about 50%, thereby diminishing the immunocompetence of the skin (Lober and Fenske, 1990).

Immediate short-term exposure to UVR can lead to sunburn. This type of red sunburn is the result of a vasodilatory response that increases blood volume. Whether an individual will become sunburned depends on the extent of skin pigmentation. Naturally, those with the least pigmentation are more prone to sunburn and the harmful long-term effects of UVR. Severe short-term exposure of unprotected, lightly pigmented skin can lead to blistering (a second-degree burn).

There is an association between melanoma and sunburn: if a patient has had more than six serious sunburns, then he or she is at an increased risk for melanoma (Green et al, 1985). Exposure to UVR and the rise of malignant melanomas has led to the development of more effective sun-blocking agents. Over time the incidence of malignant melanoma has increased from 1/1500 people in

1930 to 1/250 in 1980. By the year 2000 the incidence is expected to be 1/150 (Potts, 1990). Sunscreens should be used on a regular basis, be applied at least 30 minutes before exposure, and have a sun protection factor (SPF) ranging from 15 to 30 (Pathak et al, 1999). Individuals with moderately pigmented skin require about 3 to 5 times more exposure to UVR to induce sunburn inflammation compared with Caucasians, and for individuals with darker skin 10 times more exposure is required (McGregor and Hawk, 1999).

Hydration

Adequate skin hydration is normally provided by sebum secretion and an intact stratum corneum with its keratinized cells. Several factors can affect skin hydration. Among these are relative humidity, removal of sebum, and age. Each of these factors increases water loss from the skin, leading to dryness and scaling. Application of emollients to the skin replaces the barrier function of lost sebum or decreased evaporative water loss when the relative humidity is low. Retention of water in the epidermal layers after application of a lotion leads to swelling of the skin, which is perceived as smoothness and softness.

Often various products are promoted with claims of superiority over others without adequate in vitro, in vivo, or clinical data. The superiority of oil baths over water baths was found to be only marginal (Stender, Blichmann, and Serup, 1990). Twenty minutes after both kinds of bath, skin hydration was increased when measured by water evaporation and electrical conductance and capacitance. A small but significantly greater amount of water was bound in the skin after the oil bath, whereas no change was seen in evaporation, conductance, or capacitance. Thus increases in water-holding capacity of the skin after an oil bath may not be of importance. On the other hand, a difference was found in skin-surface lipids, which lasted at least 3 hours. This effect is comparable with application of a traditional moisturizing lotion. The authors of this study conclude that because daily use of bath oil is not practical, application of moisturizing lotions may be more advantageous and that the beneficial effects of bath oils are related to lipidization of the skin surface (Stender, Blichmann, and Serup, 1990).

Soaps

Washing or bathing with an alkaline soap reduces the thickness and number of cell layers in the stratum corneum (White, Jenkinson, and Lloyd, 1987). Generally, soap emulsifies the lipid coating of the skin and removes it along with resident and transient bacteria. Excessive use of soap or detergents can interfere with the water-holding capacity of the skin and may impair bacterial resistance. Use of alkaline soaps increases skin pH, which may change bacterial resistance. The time for recovery to normal skin pH of 5.5 depends on the length of exposure. Ordinary washing requires 45 minutes to restore skin pH, whereas prolonged exposure can require 19 hours (Bettley, 1960). Other agents that can lead to delipidization or dehydration of skin are alcohol and acetone.

Nutrition

Normal healthy skin integrity can be maintained by an adequate dietary intake of protein, carbohydrate, fats, vitamins, and minerals. Under normal conditions in healthy individuals, increased nutrition is not beneficial if there is adequate dietary intake. If the skin is damaged, increased dietary intake of some substances such as vitamin C for collagen formation may be beneficial. A healthy diet of protein breaks down to supply the necessary amino acids for protein synthesis. Fats are broken down into essential fatty acids, which can then be used by cells to form their lipid bilayer. Carbohydrates are digested to supply energy for cell metabolism. Vitamins C, D, and A; the B vitamins pyridoxine and riboflavin; the mineral elements iron, zinc, and copper; and many others are needed to maintain a normal healthy skin. Adequate dietary intake can be ensured by ingestion of amounts consistent with the recommended daily allowances (RDA) (Roe, 1986).

Medications

Various medications affect the skin. Some of the best studied are the corticosteroids, which are known to interfere with epidermal regeneration and collagen synthesis (Ehrlich and Hunt, 1968; Pollack, 1982). Photosensitive and phototoxic reactions are also known to occur from medications. Some categories of medications that can affect the skin are antibacterials, antihypertensives, analgesics, tricyclic antidepressants, antihistamines, antineoplastic agents, antipsychotic drugs, diuretics, hypoglycemic agents, sunscreens, and oral contraceptives (Potts, 1990). Skin flora can be changed by the use of antibacterials, orally administered steroids, and hormones. Analgesics, antihistamines, and nonsteroidal antiinflammatory drugs (NSAIDs) can alter inflammatory reactions. Thus whenever drugs are prescribed and skin reactions occur, medications should always be examined to check whether they are responsible.

SUMMARY

As the body's largest organ, the skin serves several complex functions: protection, thermoregulation, sensation, metabolism, and communication. Numerous factors influence the skin's ability to adequately provide these functions, such as age, UVR exposure, hydration, medications, nutrition, and soaps. The skin's integrity can also be jeopardized by many of these factors.

Wound management and skin care must be grounded in a comprehensive knowledge base of the structure and function of the skin. After reviewing this chapter, the nurse should closely scrutinize many of the skin-care practices and bathing routines that are subconsciously engrained in day to day patient care activities that may compromise the function and integrity of the skin.

SELF-ASSESSMENT EXERCISE

1. Explain why maintenance of skin integrity is vital to health and life.
2. List the key layers of the skin.
3. Explain why the cells of the stratum corneum are also called *keratinocytes*.
4. The reproductive layer of the epidermis is known as the:
   a. Stratum lucidum
   b. Stratum granulosum
   c. Stratum germinativum, or basal layer
   d. Stratum spinosum, or prickly layer
5. Describe the significance of rete ridges.
6. The epidermis receives its vascular nourishment from the:
   a. Basement membrane
   b. Papillary dermis
   c. Reticular dermis
   d. Stratum germinativum
7. Describe the purpose and key constituents of the two dermal proteins.
8. List the six major functions of the skin.
9. Identify at least two mechanisms by which the skin protects against pathogenic invasion.
10. Which of the following components of the skin immune system are derived from bone marrow precursor cells?
    a. Mast cells
    b. Fibroblasts
    c. Macrophages
    d. Langerhans' cells
11. Which of the following can be synthesized in the skin?
    a. Vitamin E
    b. Vitamin K
    c. Vitamin D
    d. Vitamin A
12. List characteristics of premature skin and newborn skin.
13. Identify changes in the skin that occur in adolescence and in adulthood.
14. Excessive exposure to ultraviolet radiation creates all of the following skin changes EXCEPT:
    a. Irregular pigmentation
    b. Increased number of Langerhans' cells
    c. Malignant melanoma
    d. Wrinkling
15. True or False: Excessive use of soaps or detergents may impair the bacterial resistance of the skin.
16. Which of the following is known to interfere with epidermal regeneration and collagen synthesis?
    a. Antibiotics
    b. Oral contraceptives
    c. Steroids
    d. Antihypertensives

REFERENCES

Alterescu V, Alterescu K: Etiology and treatment of pressure ulcers, *Decubitus* 1(1):28, 1988.

Auger MJ: Mononuclear phagocytes, *Br Med J* 298:546, 1989.

Benyon RC: The human skin mast cell, *Clin Exp Allergy* 19:375, 1989.

Bernstein NR: Appearance: concepts of perception and disfigurement (Chapter 1); Body and face images: personality and self-representation (Chapter 2); Disfigurement and personality development (Chapter 3). In Bernstein NR: *Emotional care of the facially burned and disfigured*, Boston, 1976, Little, Brown & Co.

Bettley FR: Some effects of soap on the skin, *Br Med J* 1:1675, 1960.

Braverman IM: Elastic fiber and microvascular abnormalities in aging skin. In Gilchrest BA, editor: The aging skin, *Dermatol Clin* 4:391, 1986.

Briggamann RA: Epidermal-dermal interaction in adult skin, *J Invest Dermatol* 88:569, 1982.

Bryant RA: Saving the skin from tape injuries, *Am J Nurs* 88(2):189, 1988.

Council on Scientific Affairs: Harmful effects of ultraviolet radiation, *JAMA* 262:380, 1989.

Ehrlich HP, Hunt TK: Effects of cortisone and vitamin A on wound healing, *Ann Surg* 167:324, 1968.

Gay S, Miller S: *Collagen in the physiology and pathology of connective tissue*, Stuttgart, Germany, 1978, Gustav Fischer Verlag.

Gilchrest BA: Physiology and pathophysiology of aging skin. In Goldsmith LA, editor: *Physiology, biochemistry, and molecular biology of the skin*, ed 2, New York, 1991, Oxford University Press.

Gilchrest BA: Skin aging and photoaging, *J Am Acad Dermatol* 21:610, 1989.

Green et al: Sunburn and malignant melanoma, *Br J Cancer* 51:393, 1985

Haake AR, Holbrook K: The structure and development of skin. In Freedberg IM et al, editors: *Fitzpatrick's dermatology in general medicine*, ed 5, New York, 1999, McGraw-Hill.

Holbrook KA: Structure and function of the developing human skin. In Goldsmith LA, editor: *Physiology, biochemistry, and molecular biology of the skin*, ed 2, New York, 1991, Oxford University Press.

Immature skin, *Lancet* 2(8672):1138, 1989.

Jacob SW, Francone CA, Lossow WJ: *Structure and function in man*, ed 5, Philadelphia, 1982, W.B. Saunders.

Lavker RM, Zheng P, Dong G: Morphology of aged skin. In Gilchrest BA, editor: The aging skin, *Dermatol Clin* 4:379, 1986.

Lehninger AL: *Principles of biochemistry*, New York, 1982, Worth Publishers.

Lin AN, Carter DM: Skin cancer in the elderly, *Dermatol Clin* 4(3):467, 1986.

Lober CW, Fenske NA: Photoaging and the skin: differentiation and clinical response, *Geriatrics* 45:36, 1990.

Longaker MT et al: Studies in fetal wound healing. Part VI. Second and early third trimester fetal wounds demonstrate rapid collagen deposition without scar formation, *J Pediatr Surg* 25:63, 1990.

McGregor JM, Hawk JLM: Acute effects of ultraviolet radiation on the skin (Chapter 134). In Freedberg IM et al, editors: *Fitzpatrick's dermatology in general medicine*, ed 5, New York, 1999, McGraw-Hill.

Millington PF, Wilkinson R: *Skin*, Cambridge, England, 1983, Cambridge University Press.

Nerem RM, Levesque MJ, Cornhill JF: Social environment as a factor in diet-induced atherosclerosis, *Science* 208:1475, 1980.

Noble WC: *Microbial skin disease: its epidemiology*, London, 1983, Edward Arnold.

Nordlund JJ: The lives of pigment cells. In Gilchrest BA, editor: The aging skin, *Dermatol Clin* 4:407, 1986.

Odland GF: Structure of the skin. In Goldsmith LA, editor: *Physiology, biochemistry, and molecular biology of the skin*, ed 2, New York, 1991, Oxford University Press.

Ottenbacher KJ et al: The effectiveness of tactile stimulation as a form of early intervention: a quantitative evaluation, *J Dev Behav Pediatr* 8:68, 1987.

Pathak MA et al: Sun-protective agents: formulations, effects, and side effects (Chapter 248). In Freedberg IM et al, editors: *Fitzpatrick's dermatology in general medicine*, ed 5, New York, 1999, McGraw-Hill.

Pollack SV: Systemic medications and wound healing, *Int J Dermatol* 21:489, 1982.

Potts JF: Sunlight, sunburn, and sunscreens, *Postgrad Med* 87:52, 1990.

Roberts AB, Sporn MB: Transforming growth factor-β. In Clark RAF, editor: *The molecular and cellular biology of wound repair*, ed 2, New York, 1996, Plenum Press.

Roe DA: *Nutrition and the skin*, New York, 1986, Alan R. Liss.

Roth RR, James WD: Microbial ecology of the skin, *Annu Rev Microbiol* 42:441, 1988.

Rudowski W: *Burn therapy and research*, Baltimore, 1976, Johns Hopkins University Press.

Rutter N: The immature skin, *Br Med Bull* 44:957, 1988.

Sams WM: Structure and function of the skin. In Sams WM, Lynch PJ, editors: *Principles and practice of dermatology*, New York, 1990, Churchill Livingstone.

Sauder DN: Effect of age on epidermal immune function. In Gilchrest BA, editor: The aging skin, *Dermatol Clin* 4:447, 1986.

Shuster S et al: The effect of skin disease on self image, *Br J Dermatol* 90(suppl 16):18, 1978.

Siebert JW et al: Fetal wound healing: a biochemical study of scarless healing, *Plast Reconstr Surg* 85:495, 1990.

Silverberg N, Silverberg L: Aging and the skin, *Postgrad Med* 86:131, 1989.

Solomons B: *Lecture notes on dermatology*, ed 5, Oxford, 1983, Blackwell Scientific Publications.

Spince AP, Mason EB: *Human anatomy and physiology*, Menlo Park, Calif, 1987, The Benjamin/Cummings Publishing Company.

Spitz R: An inquiry into the genesis of psychiatric conditions in early childhood. In Nagera H: *Psychoanalytical studies of the child*, vol 2, London, 1947, International.

Stender IM, Blichmann C, Serup J: Effects of oil and water baths on the hydration state of the epidermis, *Clin Exp Dermatol* 15:206, 1990.

Stryer L: *Biochemistry*, ed 4, New York, 1995, WH Freeman & Co.

Weinberg AN, Swartz MN: General considerations of bacterial diseases. In Fitzpatrick TB et al, editors: *Dermatology in general medicine: textbook and atlas*, New York, 1987, McGraw-Hill.

Wenger CB: Thermoregulation. In Freedberg IM et al, editors: *Fitzpatrick's dermatology in general medicine*, ed 5, New York, 1999, McGraw-Hill.

Weston WL, Lane AT: Neonatal dermatology. In Freedberg IM et al, editors: *Fitzpatrick's dermatology in general medicine*, ed 5, New York, 1999, McGraw-Hill.

Wheater PR, Burkitt HG, Daniels VG: *Functional histology*, ed 2, Edinburgh, 1987, Churchill Livingstone.

White MI, Jenkinson DM, Lloyd DH: The effect of washing on the thickness of the stratum corneum in normal and atopic individuals, *Br J Dermatol* 116:525, 1987.

Wolff K, Stingl G: The Langerhans' cell, *J Invest Dermatol* 80:17S, 1983.

Woodburne RT, Burkel WE: *Essentials of human anatomy*, New York, 1988, Oxford University Press.

Wysocki AB: A review of the skin and its appendages, *Adv Wound Care* 8:53, 1995.

CHAPTER

2 Wound-Healing Physiology

JOANN WALDROP & DOROTHY DOUGHTY

OBJECTIVES

1. Discriminate among the following types of wound-healing techniques: primary intention, secondary intention, and tertiary intention.
2. Distinguish between tissue repair and tissue regeneration.
3. Distinguish between partial-thickness wound repair and full-thickness wound repair, addressing the key components, phases, usual time frames, and wound appearance.
4. Explain the physiologic basis for enhanced wound repair in a moist environment.
5. For the following cells, describe when they enter the wound-repair cycle, the approximate duration of their presence, the stimulus for their arrival to the wound site, and their primary function: platelets, polymorphonuclear leukocytes, macrophages, and fibroblasts.
6. Describe the effects of at least seven cofactors (conditions or treatments) on the wound-healing process.
7. Correlate the role of at least three growth factors with the process of tissue repair.
8. Distinguish between acute wounds and chronic wounds in terms of the molecular environment.

Nurses play a vital role in wound management. They are responsible for dressing and monitoring acute wounds, such as surgical incisions, and are frequently asked to establish management protocols for chronic wounds, such as pressure ulcers or vascular ulcers. Nursing interventions can either enhance or delay the wound-healing process; thus nurses must be knowledgeable regarding the wound-healing process and the implications for wound management.

For centuries wound healing was regarded as a mysterious process, with wound management based on practitioner preference as opposed to scientific principles. Recent research has contributed much information regarding the wound-healing process and the factors that facilitate this process. Today nurses must base their care on research findings and must remain abreast of new findings if they are to provide appropriate wound care. In this chapter the normal process of wound healing is reviewed and the implications for wound management are discussed.

PHYSIOLOGY OF WOUND HEALING

The ability to repair tissue damage is an important survival tool for any living organism. Regardless of the type or severity of the injury, there are only two mechanisms by which repair occurs—*regeneration,* or replacement of the damaged or lost tissue with more of the same, or *connective tissue repair*, in which the damaged or lost tissue is replaced by scar formation. Regeneration is obviously the preferred mechanism of repair since it maintains normal function and appearance. Connective tissue repair is a less satisfactory alternative and is used only when the tissues involved are incapable of regeneration. Many invertebrate and amphibian species have the ability to regenerate entire limbs; however, humans have limited capacity for regeneration and most wounds require connective tissue repair (Calvin, 1998; Mast and Schultz, 1996).

The mechanism of repair for any specific wound is determined by the tissue layer or layers involved and their capacity for regeneration. Wounds that are confined to the epidermal and superficial dermal layers (partial-thickness wounds) heal by regeneration because epithelial, endothelial, and connective tissue can be reproduced. In contrast, wounds extending through the dermis (full-thickness wounds) heal by scar formation because most of the deeper structures (hair follicles, sweat glands, sebaceous glands, subcutaneous tissue, and muscle) do not regenerate (Martin, 1997; Mast and Schultz, 1996). Skeletal muscle may regenerate if innervation and vascularization are maintained or reestablished and if reproductive muscle cells are present in the remaining muscle. Unfortunately, most wounds involving muscle loss fail to meet these criteria and therefore heal by scar formation. Traumatic bone injuries, such as fractures, heal by regeneration. The presence of chronic or necrotic processes, however, usually require resection of the involved bone to eliminate infection and promote healing. The epidermis overlying a wound healed by connective-tissue repair actually retains the ability to regenerate hairs; however, it no longer receives "hair-production" signals because the source of those signals (normal dermis) has been lost (Martin, 1997).

The standard repair mechanism for human soft tissue wounds is connective tissue (scar) formation; the one exception is repair of soft tissue wounds in the fetus, which is typically "scarless" (Martin, 1997). This finding has sparked considerable interest and research into the phenomenon of fetal repair with the hope of altering the healing environment of human wounds to match that of the fetus and thereby restore the ability to heal without scar in humans.

Types of Wound Healing

Wound healing occurs by primary, secondary, or tertiary (delayed primary) intention. (Spotnitz, Falstrom, and Rodeheaver, 1997). This classification system is based on the ideal of primary surgical closure for all wounds. Primary closure minimizes the volume of connective tissue deposition required for wound repair and restores the epithelial barrier to infection (Figure 2-1, *A*). Approximated surgical incisions are therefore said to heal by *primary intention*; they usually heal quickly, with minimal scar formation, as long as infection and secondary breakdown are prevented. Unfortunately, there are several types of wounds that cannot be safely managed with primary closure because of contamination or severe edema (wounds that must be managed by delayed closure or allowed to heal by scar formation).

Wounds that are left open and allowed to heal by scar formation are classified as healing by *secondary intention* (Figure 2-1, *B*). These wounds heal more slowly because of the volume of connective tissue required to fill the defect, and because they lack the epidermal barrier to microorganisms, they are more subject to infection. Chronic wounds such as pressure ulcers and vascular ulcers typically heal by secondary intention (Calvin, 1998).

Wounds managed with delayed closure are classified as healing by *tertiary intention*, or *delayed primary closure* (Figure 2-1, *C*). This is an approach generally required for abdominal incisions complicated by massive infection.

Wound-Healing Process

Wound healing is best understood as a cascade of events. Injury sets into motion a series of physiologic responses that are coordinated and sequenced and that, under normal circumstances, invariably result in repair (Figure 2-2). Wounds that proceed normally through the repair process from injury to healing are typically referred to as *acute wounds*; wounds that are indolent and that fail to heal in a timely and orderly manner are considered *chronic wounds* (Eaglstein and Falanga, 1997). Current understanding of wound repair is based on acute wound healing models. In this section the repair process for partial- and full-thickness acute wounds is discussed. Differences in the wound-repair process and the wound environment that typify chronic wounds as well as implications for management are discussed later in this chapter.

Partial-Thickness Wound Repair. Partial-thickness wounds are shallow wounds involving epidermal loss and possibly partial loss of the dermal layer (Plate 1). These wounds are moist and painful because of the loss of the epidermal covering and resultant exposure of the nerve endings. When the wound involves loss of the epidermis with exposure of the basement membrane, the

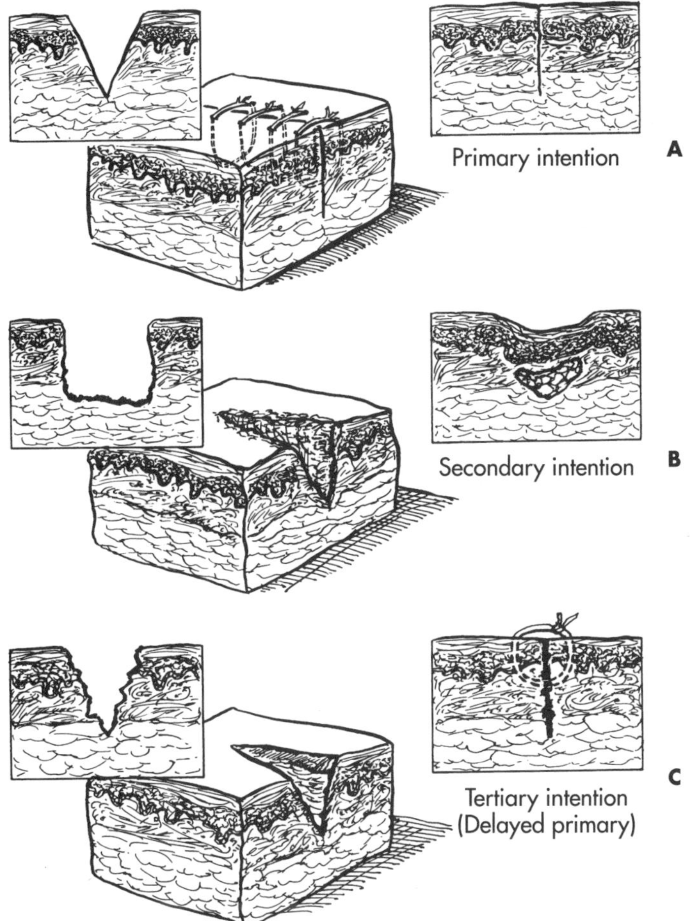

Figure 2-1 **A,** Wound healing by primary intention, such as with a surgical incision (*left*). Wound edges are pulled together and approximated with sutures, staples, or adhesive tapes, and healing occurs mainly by connective tissue deposition. **B,** Wound healing by secondary intention. Wound edges are not approximated, and healing occurs by granulation tissue formation and contraction of the wound edges. **C,** Wound healing by tertiary (delayed primary) intention. Wound is kept open for several days. The superficial wound edges are then approximated, and the center of the wound heals by granulation tissue formation. (From Trott AT: *Wounds and lacerations*, ed 2, St Louis, 1997, Mosby.)

wound base appears bright pink or red. In the presence of partial dermal loss, the wound base usually appears pale pink with distinct red "islets." These "islets" represent the basement membrane of the epidermis, which projects deep into the dermis to line the epidermal appendages. These islands of epidermal basement membrane are important in partial-thickness wound healing because all epidermal cells are capable of regeneration and each islet will serve as a source of new epithelium (Winter, 1979).

The major components of partial-thickness repair include an initial inflammatory response to injury, epithelial proliferation and migration (resurfacing), and reestablishment and differentiation of the epidermal layers to restore the protective

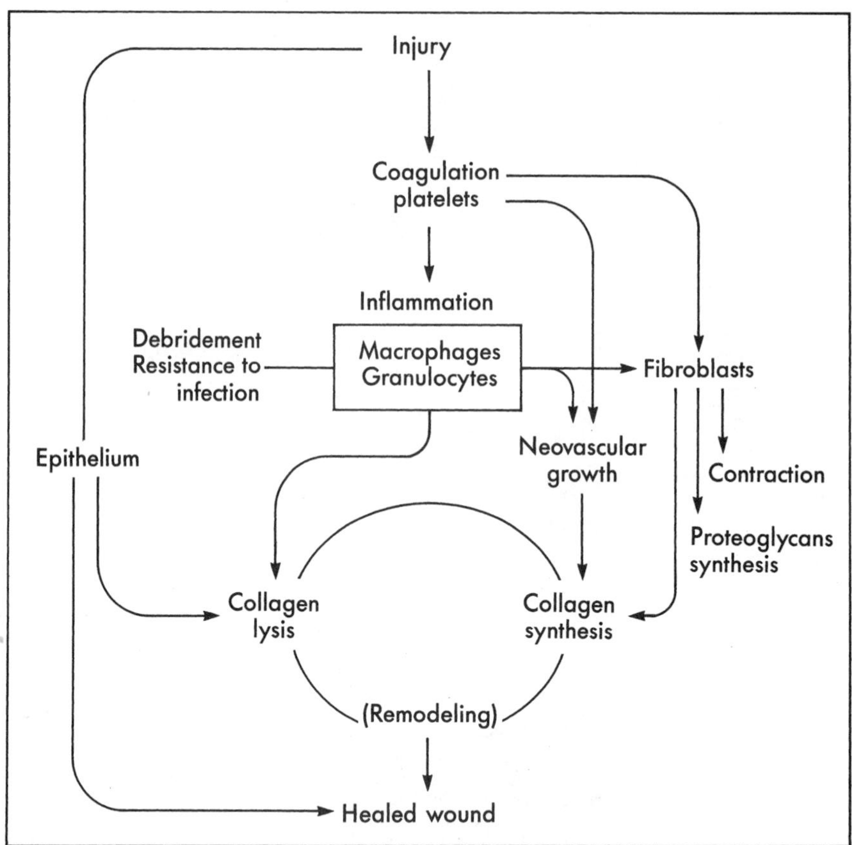

Figure 2-2 Schema demonstrating that coagulation triggers the wound-healing cascade. (From Levenson S, Seiffer E, Van Winkle E Jr: Nutrition. In Hunt TK, Dunphy JE, editors: *Fundamentals of wound management*, New York, 1979, Appleton-Century-Crofts.)

function of the skin (Martin, 1997; Winter, 1979). If the wound involves dermal loss, connective tissue repair will proceed concurrently with epithelial repair.

Epidermal repair. Tissue trauma triggers an acute inflammatory response. Erythema and edema in the injured area result, and a serous exudate containing leukocytes is produced. When this exudate is allowed to dry on the wound surface, a scab will form. In partial-thickness wounds the inflammatory response is limited, typically subsiding in less than 24 hours (Winter, 1979).

Epidermal cells stimulated by growth factors proliferate and begin migration across the wound bed within 12 to 24 hours after injury (Rohovsky and D'Amore, 1997; Waldorf and Fewkes, 1995). In a moist wound this migration may begin as early as 8 hours after wounding. Soon after epithelial migration begins, a proliferative burst occurs within the epithelial cells just proximal to the area of injury, providing new epithelial cells to replace those that were lost (Martin, 1997). Peak epithelial proliferation occurs within 24 to 72 hours after injury (Waldorf and Fewkes, 1995). The new epidermis originates from the epidermal cells at the wound margins and from epidermal cells lining the epidermal appendages; thus the wound rapidly resurfaces.

Wounds left open to air will usually completely resurface within 6 to 7 days, whereas wounds that are kept moist will resurface more rapidly (within

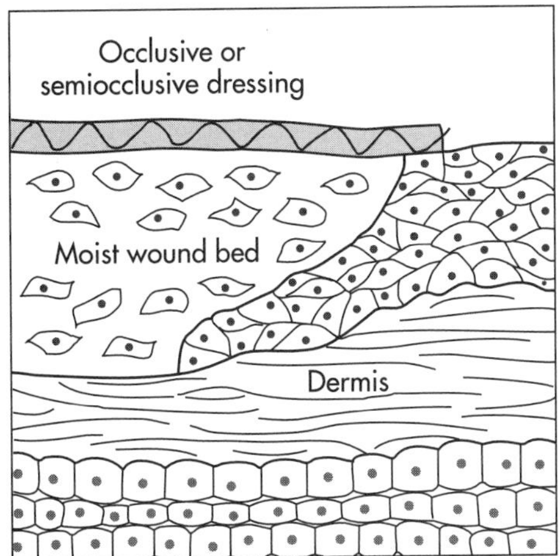

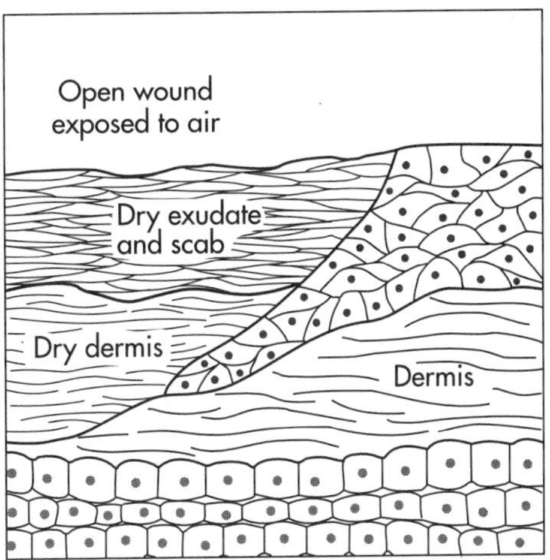

Figure 2-3 Diagram of migration of epidermal cells in moist environment and dry environment.

4 days) (Field and Kerstein, 1994; Winter, 1979). This difference is because epidermal cells can only migrate across a moist surface. In a dry wound the epidermal cells must tunnel down to a moist level and secrete proteolytic enzymes to lift the scab away from the wound surface before migration can occur (Figure 2-3).

Epithelial migration is a complex sequence of events that is mediated by a chemotactic gradient of growth factors (Garrett, 1997; Waldorf and Fewkes, 1995). To migrate, the epidermal cells must break free of cellular attachments to one another and to the basement membrane; they then undergo cytoskeletal alterations that support lateral movement. The cells at the advancing edge of epithelium flatten and form protrusions, or pseudopods, that attach to the wound bed and help pull the cell across the wound surface. It is postulated that the cells move in a "leapfrog" pattern, where a single cell moves only two or three cell lengths and then stops, allowing consecutive cells to "climb over." This process is repeated until the wound surface is reepithelialized (Figure 2-4).

Initially, the new epithelium is only a few cells thick and must undergo stratification and differentiation before it can resume its normal functions. As epidermal cells of opposing wound borders meet, lateral migration stops (contact inhibition). At this point, the cells resume upward migration and differentiation, which reestablishes the normal epidermal thickness (Garrett, 1997; Winter, 1979). The normal anchors to adjacent epidermal cells and the basement membrane, known as *hemidesmosomes*, are also reestablished.

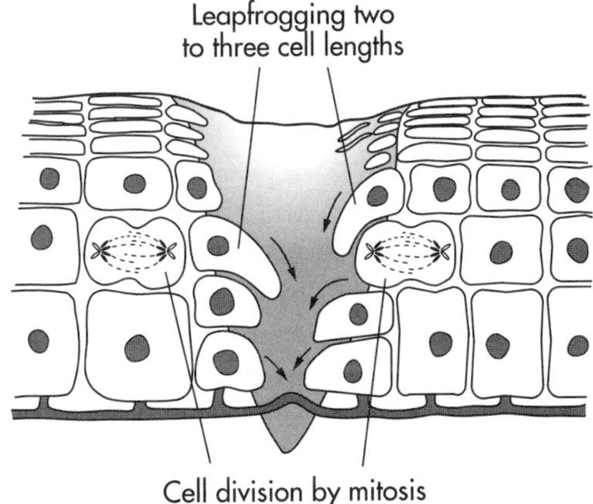

Figure 2-4 Illustration of epidermal cell migration via development of pseudopod and "leapfrogging."

The new epidermis appears pink and dry. As the epidermal cells resume their normal functions, the epidermis gradually repigments to match the individual's normal skin tone. This has clinical relevance in that the wound is not completely healed until repigmentation has occurred. Until that time, the new epithelium is fragile and requires continued protection.

Dermal repair. In wounds involving both dermal and epidermal loss, dermal repair proceeds concurrently with reepithelialization. On the fifth day after injury, a layer of fluid collects under the new epidermal cells, separating the epidermis from the dermal tissue. New blood vessels begin to sprout, and fibroblasts become plentiful by about 7 days after injury. Collagen fibers are visible in the wound bed by the ninth day, and collagen synthesis continues, producing new connective tissue, until about 10 to 15 days after injury. This new connective tissue grows upward into the fluid layer. At the same time, the flat epidermis falls down around the new vessels and collagen fibers, recreating ridges at the dermal-epidermal junction. The new connective tissue gradually contracts, bringing the epidermis close to the dermis (Winter, 1979). When the wound is kept moist, connective tissue repair begins 2 to 3 days after the injury (about 3 days earlier than when the wound is left open to air) because new connective tissue forms only in the presence of cytokine-rich exudate. Connective tissue deposition is delayed when a wound is left open to air because a moist environment is not established until the epidermis has migrated across the wound bed, lifting the scab and providing protection from dehydration (Waldorf and Fewkes, 1995; Winter, 1979).

Full-Thickness Wound Repair. Full-thickness wounds, by definition, involve total loss of the epidermal and dermal layers, extending at least to the subcutaneous tissue layer and possibly as deep as the fascia-muscle layer and the bone. Full-thickness wounds that are not closed typically present as craters; the tissue layers involved and the patient's body build determine depth (Plate 2). Full-thickness lesions may be complicated by necrosis and/or infection and are frequently associated with extensive tissue damage, such as sinus tract formation or undermining.

There are several processes involved in full-thickness repair, but they are commonly conceptualized as three phases—inflammatory, proliferative, and remodeling. There is considerable overlap among the phases, and the cells involved in one phase produce the chemical stimuli that serve to move the wound into the next phase. Thus normal repair is a complex and well-orchestrated series of events (Figure 2-5).

Inflammatory phase. The inflammatory phase represents the body's initial response to an acute injury. The goals are to control cellular injury and blood loss and to establish a clean wound bed in preparation for repair. The two key events during this phase are hemostasis and inflammation (Waldorf and Fewkes, 1995).

Hemostasis. Acute wounds extending to the dermis or beyond cause disruption of blood vessels and exposure of subendothelial collagen to platelets. In addition, injured cells in the wound area release clotting factors. The result is platelet aggregation and activation of both the intrinsic and extrinsic coagulation pathways, which produces fibrin clot formation. Hemostasis is further supported by a brief period of vasoconstriction mediated by platelets. Clot formation serves to seal the disrupted vessels so that blood loss is controlled. The clot also provides a temporary bacterial barrier and an interim matrix that serves as a scaffolding for migrating cells (Waldorf and Fewkes, 1995; Witte and Barbul,1997).

Key to the wound healing process is the subsequent breakdown of platelets releasing a potent "cocktail" of growth factors from the α-granules of the platelets. These growth factors attract the cells and substances required for initiation of the repair process. Thus hemostasis, which is the body's normal response to tissue injury, actually initiates the entire wound-healing cascade. The importance of hemostasis to wound healing is underscored by the finding that inadequate clot formation is associated with impaired wound healing (Waldorf and Fewkes, 1995; Witte and Barbul, 1997).

Inflammation. Tissue injury and the activation of clotting factors stimulate the release of vasoactive substances, such as prostaglandins and histamine, causing local vasodilation and increased capillary permeability (Steed, 1997; Waldorf and Fewkes, 1995). The resulting vasocongestion and leakage of serous fluid into the wound bed is manifested at the wound site as erythema, edema,

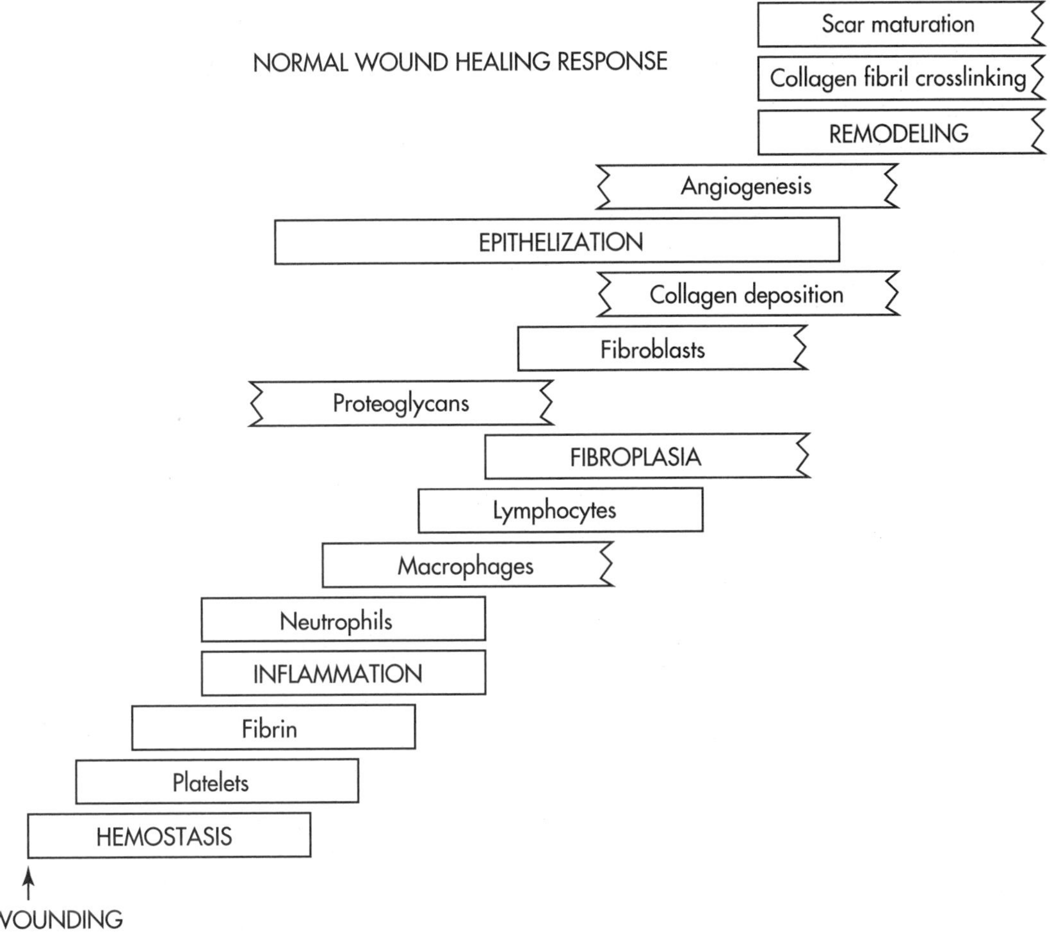

Figure 2-5 Sequence of events in wound healing. (From Mast BA: The skin. In Cohen IK, Diegelmann RF, Lindblad WJ, editors: *Wound healing: biochemical and clinical aspects*, Philadelphia, 1992, W.B. Saunders.)

warmth, and the production of varying amounts of exudate.

Chemoattractants produced by the degranulated platelets, activated clotting factors, fibrin breakdown products, and bacterial proteins attract neutrophils and monocytes to the wound bed (Martin, 1997; Waldorf and Fewkes, 1995). Polymorphonuclear leukocytes (PMNs) are the first cells to arrive at the wound site, may be seen in the wound bed as early as 2 minutes after injury, and serve to provide the initial barrier to bacterial invasion. These neutrophils dominate the scene for the first 2 to 3 days, phagocytizing bacteria and foreign debris. They also release growth factors that serve to attract additional leukocytes to the wound site; later these growth factors will trigger activation of fibroblasts and keratinocytes.

Neutrophils begin to disappear through the process of apoptosis about 3 days after injury (Steed, 1997). Monocytes, which have been present since initial injury, become phagocytic and are now referred to as *macrophages*. The function of the macrophage is to continue to phagocytize bacteria and debris, ingest the dead neutrophils, and synthesize nitric oxide, which has antimicrobial effects that are further enhanced by the hypoxic wound environment (Witte and Barbul, 1997). Macrophages also release a large number of potent growth factors that attract fibroblasts, epithelial cells, and vascular endothelial cells to the wound bed. Although both leukocytes and macrophages act as the body's defenders to eliminate bacteria and foreign material, it is the macrophage that actually regulates the entire wound-repair process. Studies indicate that wounds can heal without neutrophils, especially if there is no bacterial contamination; however, elimination of macrophages severely inhibits or even prevents wound repair (Steed, 1997; Waldorf and Fewkes, 1995).

An important aspect of the inflammatory phase of wound repair is the complex regulation of events that terminates in leukocyte migration into the wound bed because it typifies the regulatory phenomena that occur throughout the sequence of normal repair. There are at least four categories of regulatory factors that contribute to leukocyte migration—vasoactive substances; chemoattractants, cell adhesion molecules, and enzymes. *Vasoactive substances* are released by damaged cells and trigger local vasodilation and increased permeability. *Chemoattractants* are released by the degranulating platelets and other products resulting from clot dissolution. Together, vasoactive substances and chemoattractants provide a powerful signal to attract leukocytes to the area of injury. *Cell adhesion molecules* (intravascular selectins) are produced within the capillary bed and pull circulating leukocytes out of the bloodstream and lay them against the vessel wall. This action allows for diapedesis (the migration of large cells such as platelets and neutrophils through the walls of the blood vessels) into the wound bed. Once in the wound bed, neutrophils express adhesion molecules known as integrins that help them bind to the extracellular matrix of the wound bed. To enhance diapedesis and in response to the activiated neutrophils, *enzymes* such as elastase and collagenase are released (Martin, 1997; Waldorf and Fewkes, 1995).

The result of the inflammatory phase of wound healing is control of bleeding and establishment of a clean wound bed. In a clean acute wound the inflammatory phase lasts approximately 3 days. However, when wounds are complicated by necrosis and/or infection, the inflammatory phase is prolonged and wound healing is delayed.

Proliferative phase. The second phase of full-thickness wound healing is the proliferative phase. During this phase, vascular integrity is restored, the soft tissue defect is filled with new connective tissue, and the wound surface is covered with new epithelium. The key components of the proliferative phase are neoangiogenesis, matrix deposition/collagen synthesis, and epithelialization, and contraction, which serves to reduce the size of the defect (Martin, 1997; Witte and Barbul, 1997).

The processes that occur during the proliferative phase are interdependent. New capillary networks must be established to provide the oxygen and nutrients needed for synthesis of collagen and other connective tissues. Conversely, these fragile new capillary networks require the support of collagen fibers. Thus collagen synthesis and angiogenesis occur simultaneously in a codependent fashion to create granulation tissue and to fill open spaces. Granulation tissue is composed primarily of capillary loops; fibroblasts, inflammatory cells, and matrix proteins are also present.

Neoangiogenesis. Neoangiogenesis is stimulated by a combination of angiogenic growth factors and the hypoxic gradient that exists between the center of the wound and the vascularized tissue at the periphery. Endothelial cells in the venules adjacent to the wound bed initiate new capillary production by projecting pseudopods into the wound bed. Endothelial cells also produce enzymes that break down the extracellular matrix. This creates tissue defects that facilitate the formation of capillary "sprouts," or hollow tubes that form the basis of capillary plexuses (Figure 2-6). Capillary production is followed by the formation of arterioles to create a new vascular network so that perfusion to the wound bed is reestablished. Finally, extracellular matrix components (ECM) are deposited to create a new basement membrane within the capillaries. Angiogenesis is regulated by a complex interplay between the hypoxic environment, numerous growth factors, and additional cytokines such as interleukins and interferons (Rohovsky and D'Amore, 1997).

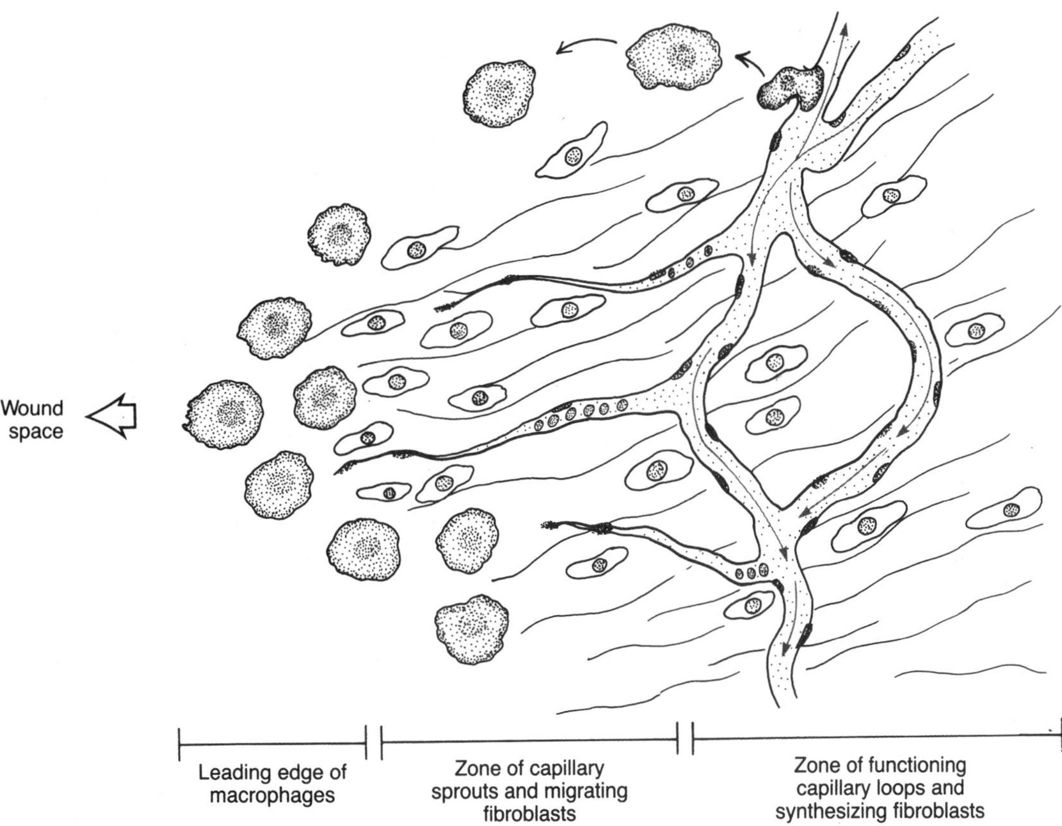

Figure 2-6 Advancing module of reparative tissue during proliferative and remodeling phases. (From Whalen GF, Zetter BR: Angiogenesis. In Cohen IK, Dieglemann RF, Lindblad WJ, editors: *Wound healing: biochemical and clinical aspects*, Philadelphia, 1992, W.B. Saunders.)

Matrix deposition/collagen synthesis. The formation of this new collagen is commonly referred to as *collagen synthesis*, terminology that is a significant oversimplification of the actual process. In reality the formation of scar tissue involves multiple phases and the synthesis of many connective tissue substances. As noted in the discussion of the inflammatory phase of repair, clot formation provides an initial fibrin matrix to support cell migration. A matrix material composed primarily of fibronectin and hyaluronic acid subsequently replaces this structure. Because these substances promote cell migration and proliferation, this matrix material serves primarily to stimulate and support continued matrix formation. This "support" matrix is in turn replaced by a matrix of collagen, GAGs, PGs, and elastin. As this matrix matures, collagen becomes the predominant protein. The early collagen is known as Type III collagen, comprises 30% of granulation tissue, and does not contribute to the wound's tensile strength. The healing wound exhibits only 20% of its final strength around 3 weeks after injury. As the collagen matures, Type III collagen is converted to Type I collagen, the type normally found in dermal tissue. However, even the final form of collagen does not exhibit the normal basket-weave pattern of the collagen in unwounded dermis. Rather, the fibers of "repair collagen" are aligned parallel to the stress lines of the wound (Waldorf and Fewkes, 1995; Witte and Barbul, 1997).

Fibroblasts are responsible for synthesis of collagen and other connective tissue substances and are therefore critical to the repair process. Fibroblasts migrate into the wound bed from the surrounding tissues in response to cytokines, growth factors produced by platelets (PDGF), activated neutrophils, and activated macrophages. They begin to appear toward the end of the inflammatory phase and persist throughout the remodeling phase. After migration into the wound bed, fibroblasts are stimulated by growth factors present in the wound bed to proliferate and are converted by cytokines derived from macrophages into "wound fibroblasts." These wound fibroblasts differ from typical dermal fibroblasts in that they exhibit decreased proliferative behavior but increased collagen synthesis and wound contraction (Witte and Barbul, 1997). In summary, fibroblasts are attracted to the wound bed, encouraged to reproduce, and finally directed to produce connective tissue, a well-ordered sequential process controlled by various concentrations and combinations of growth factors.

Collagen synthesis follows the established process for synthesis of any protein. The collagen molecule is characterized by a Gly-X-Y repeating sequence; the molecule undergoes a series of intracellular modifications and is then secreted into the extracellular environment as the triple helix procollagen. Enzymes in the extracellular matrix cleave the propeptide ends, which renders the molecule less soluble. The procollagen strands are then formed into fibrils, and the fibrils are cross-linked, further reducing their vulnerability to breakdown. This series of reactions is partially dependent on the enzyme lysyl oxidase. The collagen fibers gradually thicken and assume a parallel orientation, which is accompanied by increased tensile strength (Witte and Barbul, 1997; Steed, 1997).

In wounds healing by primary intention, such as sutured incisions, collagen synthesis usually peaks at about the fifth day, although collagen production continues for weeks or months (Arlein and Caldwell, 1997). Only a small amount of collagen is needed to mend the defect in sutured incisions, and collagen synthesis occurs concurrently with epidermal migration. Although the granulation tissue is not visible in these wounds, by day 5 it is possible to palpate a "healing ridge" just under the intact suture line, which is produced by the newly formed collagen. Absence of this healing ridge indicates impaired healing and increased risk for dehiscence (Hunt and Van Winkle, 1997).

In wounds healing by secondary intention, the proliferative phase is typically prolonged because of the increased volume of connective tissue that must be produced to fill the defect. In these wounds, granulation tissue is visible. Healthy granulation tissue presents as a red, vascular, granular wound bed (Plate 3). This appearance is attributable to the numerous capillary loops in combination with collagen fibers. This extremely vascular granulation tissue actually matures into a relatively avascular scar, because once the repair process is complete, the need for oxygen and nutrients is reduced and many of the vessels regress (Waldorf and Fewkes, 1995).

Each phase of collagen production has specific oxygen and nutrient requirements. Thus the patient's ability to heal is directly related to his or her vascular and nutritional status.

Contraction. Contraction is a phenomenon that occurs only in open wounds; skin and tissue around the defect are mobilized in response to forces generated within the newly formed connective tissue. Contraction can significantly reduce healing time because it reduces the amount of matrix that must be produced to fill the defect (Calvin, 1998). There are conflicting theories regarding the mechanism by which contraction occurs (Berry et al, 1998; Martin, 1997; Rohovsky and D'Amore, 1997; Witte and Barbul, 1997). Traditionally, contraction has been thought to be mediated by myofibroblasts (i.e., modified fibroblasts) that express α-smooth muscle actin and that are capable of generating strong contractile forces that act to "pull" the opposing edges of the wound together. This theory is supported by the finding that although wound contraction begins before myofibroblasts are evident in the wound bed, myofibroblasts disappear from the wound once contraction is complete. A second theory suggests that the wound fibroblasts act in concert to reorganize and "shrink" the matrix. This is supported by the finding that fibroblasts added to a collagen lattice are actively moving and are capable of inducing contraction. A third theory is that the newly produced collagen fibers are compacted by cellular forces, which produces a "pulling" force on the surrounding tissues.

The degree of contraction occurring within a wound is determined by the mobility of the surrounding tissue. Sacral and abdominal wounds are located in areas where the surrounding tissue is quite mobile and can contract easily, whereas a wound on the extremity or overlying a bony prominence has limited potential for contraction. Contraction is considered undesirable in some wounds because it can cause cosmetic deformities or flexion contractures of joints (Berry et al, 1998; Ehrlich, 1998).

Epithelialization. The final component of the proliferative phase is epithelialization, which is the migration, proliferation, and differentiation of epithelial cells from the wound edges to resurface the defect. In wounds with minimal tissue loss, such as surgical incisions, epithelial migration occurs concurrently with collagen synthesis (Martin, 1997; Steed, 1997; Waldorf and Fewkes, 1995). In open wounds, epithelialization is delayed until a bed of granulation tissue is established since epithelial cell migration can only proceed over a moist, vascular wound surface and is impeded by a dry or necrotic wound surface (Winter, 1979). Because full-thickness wounds involve loss of the deep dermis and epidermal appendages (along with their epithelial lining), epithelialization in these wounds proceeds from the periphery of the wound inward in a centripetal fashion (Calvin, 1998; Martin, 1997; Waldorf and Fewkes, 1995).

Mitosis of the bordering epithelial cells and alteration of their normal characteristics to permit lateral migration constitutes epithelialization. Specifically, the normal attachments between the epithelial cells and basement membrane are dissolved so that epithelial cells migrate across the open wound bed, guided by collagen in the underlying wound matrix. There are several theories regarding the specific mechanism by which epithelial cell migration occurs: 1) formation of pseudopods and single-cell migration, 2) a "leapfrogging" mechanism whereby the leading cell migrates two or three lengths and then stops so that the cells behind it crawl over, and 3) the "tractor-tread" theory (attachment of the migrating epidermal cell to the underlying wound bed via adhesion molecules) (Waldorf and Fewkes, 1995). However the cells migrate, it is known that lateral migration continues until the defect is covered, at which time the cells resume upward migration and differentiation until the epidermis regains its normal thickness and stratification. Since the underlying dermis has been replaced by granulation tissue, the normal dermal papillae are generally absent.

Epithelial migration requires an "open" proliferative wound edge; "closed" wound edges (also known as *epibole*) are sometimes seen in chronic wounds as a result of a "rolling under" of the border epidermis (Figure 2-7). In these wounds, an open edge must be reestablished, either via surgical excision or chemical cauterization, for epithelial migration to occur.

Remodeling phase. The final phase in full-thickness wound healing is the maturation, or remodeling phase, which continues for up to 1 year or longer. The simultaneous processes of wound matrix breakdown and synthesis of new matrix components characterize the remodeling phase. Fibroblasts regulate these dual processes through the synthesis of extracellular matrix components and the production of matrix metalloproteinases (MMPs), which degrade the matrix (Mast and Schultz, 1996). During this process the scar tissue gains strength. However, the tensile strength of scar tissue is never more than 80% of the tensile strength in nonwounded tissue.

An imbalance between the dual processes of matrix synthesis and matrix breakdown can complicate wound healing. For example, hypertrophic scarring and keloid formation are believed to be caused by an excess of matrix synthesis as compared with matrix degradation. On the other hand, hypoxia or malnutrition significantly reduces the rate of collagen synthesis and may result in wound breakdown. Figure 2-8 provides a schematic overview of the processes involved in normal wound healing.

REGULATION OF WOUND HEALING

Wound healing represents a cascade of overlapping events regulated by a complex interplay among growth factors, cytokines, MMPs and TIMPs (tissue inhibitors of matrix metalloproteinases), and

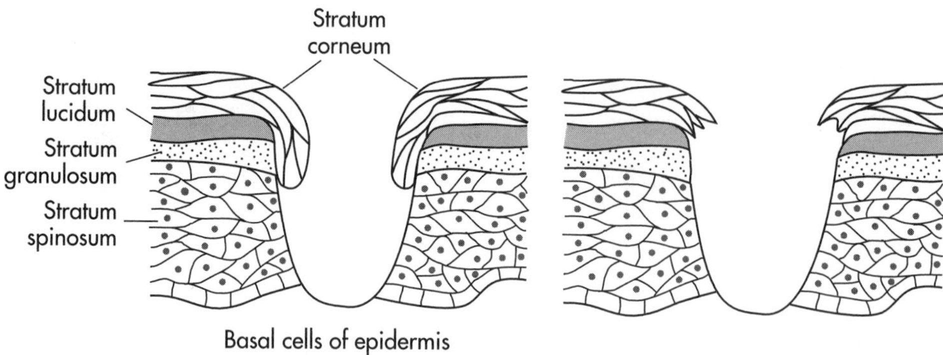

Figure 2-7 Schematic depiction of closed wound edges (*left*) in which epidermis of wound edges has rolled under so that epithelial cells cannot migrate. Open wound edges (*right*) from which epithelial cells can migrate.

hormones. The effect of these regulatory factors is further influenced by systemic factors such as the host's nutritional status. This section provides a brief review of the major categories of wound-healing regulators and the mechanisms governing their collective effects on the repair process.

Growth Factors

Growth factors are polypeptides that control the growth and differentiation of cells. They act much like hormones, binding to specific cell receptors to alter the cell's function. Growth factors attract needed cells to the wound bed and stimulate cell division and specific cellular activities. They may act on distant cells (endocrine stimulation), act on neighboring cells (paracrine stimulation) or "act back" on themselves (autocrine stimulation) (Figure 2-9). Multiple growth factors either directly or indirectly regulate all phases of wound repair (Schultz and Mast, 1998; Steed, 1997). For example, the repair process is initiated by platelet degranulation and the release of PDGF (platelet-derived growth factor). Two important functions of PDGF include chemoattraction of macrophages and fibroblasts and stimulation of collagen synthesis. Macrophages, present throughout most of the repair process, are another significant source of growth factors and synthesize most of the growth factors critical to repair. As research continues into the identification and effects of the various growth factors, their importance to wound repair becomes even more clear. Currently there is an emphasis on commercial production of various growth factors based on the hope that exogenous application of these factors will be able to stimulate repair in chronic wounds. Table 2-1 summarizes the effect of the key growth factors in the wound-repair process. A more in-depth discussion of the regulation of wound repair by growth factors is found in Chapter 19.

Cytokines

The term *cytokine* was originally used to reference a variety of substances known to affect cellular function, including growth factors. Currently the term is used more specifically to indicate substances *other than* growth factors that contribute to the regulation of cellular function and wound repair. Most cytokines are produced by macrophages. They work with one another along with growth factors and other regulatory substances to "fine tune" wound-repair processes. Examples of cytokines that affect wound repair include interleukin-1 (IL-1), tumor necrosis factor-α (TNF-α), and the interferons.

MMPs and TIMPs

MMPs include three enzymatic compounds capable of connective tissue degradation:

1. *Collagenases.* Provide for initial breakdown of Type 1 collagen.
2. *Gelatinases.* Further degrade Type 1 collagen

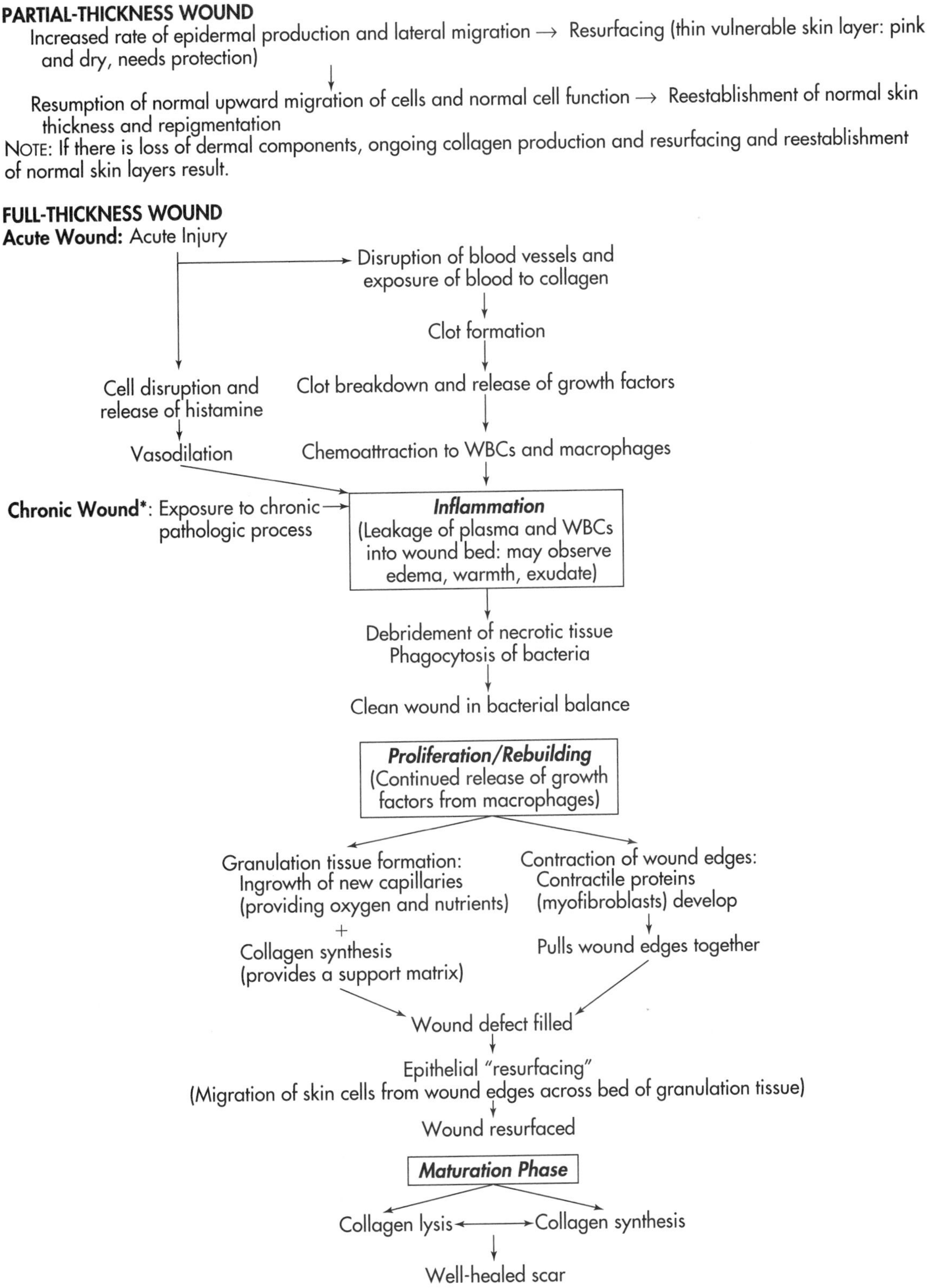

PARTIAL-THICKNESS WOUND

Increased rate of epidermal production and lateral migration → Resurfacing (thin vulnerable skin layer: pink and dry, needs protection)

↓

Resumption of normal upward migration of cells and normal cell function → Reestablishment of normal skin thickness and repigmentation

NOTE: If there is loss of dermal components, ongoing collagen production and resurfacing and reestablishment of normal skin layers result.

FULL-THICKNESS WOUND

Acute Wound: Acute Injury

→ Disruption of blood vessels and exposure of blood to collagen

↓

Clot formation

↓

Clot breakdown and release of growth factors

↓

Chemoattraction to WBCs and macrophages

↓ (to Inflammation)

→ Cell disruption and release of histamine

↓

Vasodilation → (to Inflammation)

Chronic Wound*: Exposure to chronic pathologic process → (to Inflammation)

Inflammation
(Leakage of plasma and WBCs into wound bed: may observe edema, warmth, exudate)

↓

Debridement of necrotic tissue
Phagocytosis of bacteria

↓

Clean wound in bacterial balance

Proliferation/Rebuilding
(Continued release of growth factors from macrophages)

→ Granulation tissue formation:
Ingrowth of new capillaries (providing oxygen and nutrients)
+
Collagen synthesis (provides a support matrix)

→ Contraction of wound edges:
Contractile proteins (myofibroblasts) develop
↓
Pulls wound edges together

→ Wound defect filled

↓

Epithelial "resurfacing"
(Migration of skin cells from wound edges across bed of granulation tissue)

↓

Wound resurfaced

Maturation Phase

Collagen lysis ↔ Collagen synthesis

↓

Well-healed scar

Figure 2-8 Key events in wound healing. *Note that chronic wounds do not undergo hemostasis.

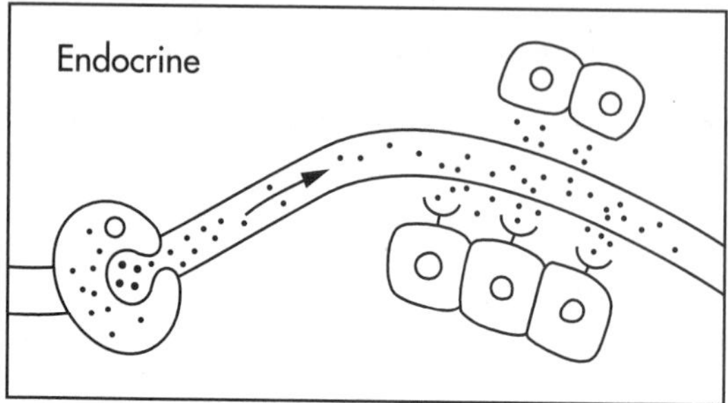

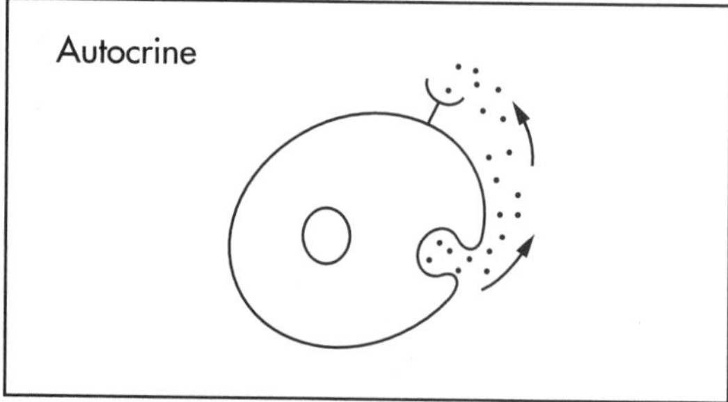

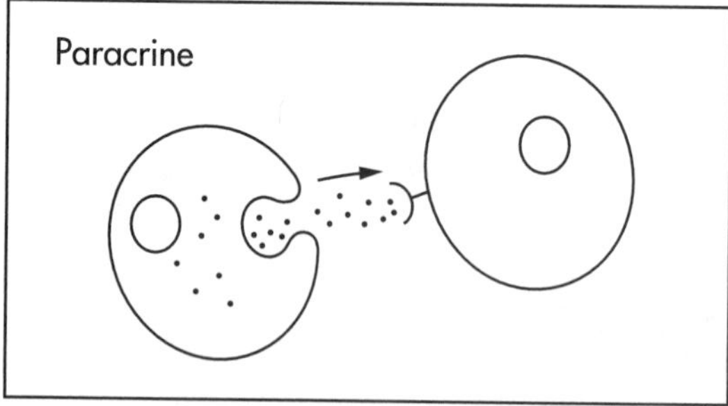

Figure 2-9 Mechanisms of growth factor activity.

and break down Type IV collagen, which is found in basement membranes
3. *Stromelysins*. Break down collagens and proteoglycans.

During the inflammatory phase, MMPs contribute to diapedesis of inflammatory cells by breaking down the basement membrane within blood vessels and degrade damaged extracellular matrix. During the proliferative phase, MMPs contribute to neoangiogenesis by facilitating the ingrowth of new capillaries. During the maturation phase, MMPs provide for remodeling of the extracellular matrix to increase tensile strength. MMPs are produced by neutrophils, macrophages, fibroblasts, and endothelial cells in response to growth factors, cytokines, and TIMPs (Tarnuzzer and Schultz, 1996).

TIMPs are produced by cells within the wound and are also found in serum. TIMPs bind to MMPs, rendering the MMP inactive. The production of MMPs and TIMPs is coordinated to achieve the desired outcome in the repair process (Tarnuzzer and Schultz, 1996).

Hormones

Endocrine hormones may also contribute to the regulation of wound healing. Specific situations in which altered hormone levels negatively affect wound repair include estrogen deficiency, insulin deficiency, and excess levels of cortisol (Schultz and Mast, 1998).

Interplay of Regulatory Factors

Cells involved in wound healing exhibit variable responses to regulatory substances. Factors such as the concentration and combination of the various regulatory substances, specificity of the cellular receptors, and effects of cell activation determine the specific response of the cell.

Concentration and Combination of Regulatory Substances. Cytokines and growth factors may affect the same target cell differently, depending on the concentration and combination of the regulatory factors and on the wound milieu. For example, PDGF acts as a chemoattractant for fibroblasts at low levels, whereas higher levels stimulate fibroblast proliferation (Martin, 1997; Witte and Barbul, 1997). Similarly, fibroblasts cultured in a fibrin-fibronectin gel respond to PDGF by upregulating the integrin receptors that support diapedesis and cell migration, whereas fibroblasts cultured in a collagen gel respond to the same growth factor by synthesizing collagen. This is consistent with the wound milieu and fibroblast activity during the inflammatory and proliferative phases of wound repair. During the inflammatory phase the wound matrix is composed of fibrin and fibronectin and the release of PDGF serves as a chemoattractant to fibroblasts. In contrast, a collagen-based matrix and ongoing collagen synthesis characterize the proliferative phase by the fibroblasts (Schultz and Mast, 1998).

TABLE 2-1 Effects of Key Growth Factors in the Wound-Repair Process

FACTOR	MAJOR SOURCE	MAJOR EFFECTS
Platelet-derived growth factor (PDGF)	Platelets Fibroblasts Endothelial cells	Chemoattraction Mitogen Protein synthesis
Insulin-like growth factors (IGF-1, IGF-2)	Platelets Fibroblasts	Mitogen
Epidermal growth factors	Platelets	Epithelial cell synthesis
Transforming growth factor-beta (TGF-β)	Platelets Keratinocytes	Chemoattraction for inflammatory cells Cell growth Associated with fibrosis and scarring
Transforming growth factor-alpha (TGF-α)	Macrophages Keratinocytes Fibroblasts	Mitogen Regulator of inflammation
Basic-fibroblast growth factors (bFGF)	Fibroblasts Endothelial cells	Angiogenesis Chemoattraction
Vascular endothelial growth factor/vascular permeability factor (VEGF/VPF)	Macrophages Endothelial cells	Angiogenesis Chemoattraction
Keratinocyte growth factor (KGF)	Fibroblasts	Activation of monocytes Chemoattraction/mitogen for epithelial cells

Specificity of Receptors. Although all cells within the wound bed are exposed to the same mix of regulatory substances, only selected cells respond. In addition, different cells may exhibit different responses to the same regulatory substance because the regulatory substances exert their effects primarily through binding with cell receptors. Therefore only cells with the specific receptor sites respond to the regulatory substance, and the effects of receptor binding vary based on cell type. For example, PDGF stimulates migration of some cells and mitosis in others, yet some cells are completely unaffected by PDGF (Martin, 1997; Witte and Barbul, 1997). Furthermore, studies indicate that the fibroblasts and keratinocytes in elderly individuals have a decreased number of receptor sites, which may explain why elderly patients tend to exhibit a diminished response to some regulatory substances (Gerstein et al, 1993).

Cell Activation. The effects of cell activation further affect the complexity of the response to regulatory substances. All cells involved in wound repair must undergo activation. A cell is "activated" when a regulatory substance binds to a specific receptor site and causes the cell to undergo a change in structure or function. For example, receptor binding may cause the cell to express a new surface antigen, which then alters the cell's activity and response to regulatory substances. Activated macrophages and fibroblasts commonly produce additional cytokines, further altering the wound environment (Witte and Barbul, 1997).

The biology of wound healing is extremely complex; however, recent research has provided new insights that may eventually allow the nurse to manage both acute and chronic wounds in a manner that consistently optimizes outcomes.

ACUTE VERSUS CHRONIC WOUNDS

Assuming a relatively healthy host, the acute wound will heal fairly quickly because of a cascade of growth factors and cellular stimulants that tend to keep the acute wound on the "healing track." In clinical practice, however, nurses are frequently dealing with chronic wounds, such as pressure ulcers, vascular ulcers, and neuropathic wounds, that behave differently from acute wounds, such as incisions.

Acute wounds begin with an injury that disrupts blood vessels and initiates clotting. The resulting clot breakdown causes the release of the growth factors that initiate the wound-healing cascade. In chronic wounds, however, there is usually no clot formation and no clot breakdown. The absence of these triggering events may help to explain the static nature of chronic wounds. In addition, chronic wounds frequently occur in compromised patients who are less able to heal. The effects of specific host factors on wound healing are discussed in the next section.

Over the past decade, extensive research analyzing the cellular, biochemical, and molecular components of acute and chronic wounds has significantly expanded understanding of the detailed complexities of normal wound healing and the pathophysiologic mechanisms of chronic wounds. In comparing acute and chronic wounds, several significant differences have been noted that may explain why chronic wounds fail to heal.

The nature of the injury differs between acute and chronic wounds. Acute wounds usually begin with a sudden, solitary insult and proceed to heal in an orderly manner. In contrast, an underlying pathologic process, such as vascular insufficiency, which produces repeated and prolonged insults to the tissues, usually causes chronic wounds. Thus the process of clot formation, which subsequently signals a cascade of events, is sidestepped. In addition, local tissue ischemia, necrotic tissue, heavy bacterial contamination, and tissue breakdown are typical of chronic wounds. These are factors that prolong the inflammatory phase of wound healing and stimulate macrophage and neutrophil migration into the wound bed (Tarnuzzer et al, 1997). In fact, a vicious cycle is created whereby inflammatory cells release proinflammatory cytokines, and the fragments from the breakdown of these products act as chemoattractants, which attracts additional inflammatory mediators that cause further tissue damage (Figure 2-10).

Another difference between the acute and chronic wound is the alteration in the molecular environment of the chronic wound. An imbalance in the concentration and combination of cytokines, proteases, protease inhibitors, and growth factors occurs, as well as a decrease in their responsiveness.

Inflammatory cells (macrophage and neutrophil) normally release proinflammatory cytokines such as TNF-α and IL-1β. The presence of these proinflammatory cytokines (e.g., TNF-α, IL-1β, and IL-6) in the wound does not impair reparative cellular functions as long as these cytokines are in normal concentrations. In acute wounds the levels of inflammatory cytokines are tightly controlled by the presence of antagonists so that the ratio of antagonists to inflammatory cytokines is in favor of inhibition. However, in chronic wounds the ratio of antagonists to inflammatory cytokines is only slightly in favor of inhibition. When compared with acute wounds, samples of chronic wound fluid contain up to a 100-fold increase of TNF-α and IL-1β, as well as a significant increase in the level of IL-6 (Mast and Schultz, 1996; Schultz and Mast, 1998; Tarnuzzer and Schultz, 1996; Tarnuzzer et al, 1997). Levels of inflammatory cytokines have been reported to decrease 2 weeks after chronic ulcers begin to heal (Harris et al, 1995). Consequently, levels of inflammatory cytokines are more tightly regulated in acute wounds than in chronic wounds.

Another peculiarity of the molecular environment of chronic wounds is that chronic wounds have elevated protease levels and deficient protease inhibitor (TIMPs) levels as compared with acute wounds (Schultz and Mast, 1998; Wysocki, Staiano-Coico, and Grinnell, 1993; Vaalamo et al, 1996). The synthesis of MMPs and suppression of TIMP is stimulated by proinflammatory cytokines (TNF-α and IL-1β) (Mast and Schultz, 1996; Tarnuzzer et al, 1997). MMPs play an important role in all phases of wound healing by promoting cell migration, breaking down damaged extracellular matrix, and remodeling. However, an imbalance between the levels of protease (MMP) and protease inhibitors (TIMPs) can be detrimental since excessive MMP activity can result in increased degradation of fibronectin and various growth factors. A high level of TIMP-collagenase complexes within the wound bed is indicative of elevated protease activity (Yager et al, 1996). Normal controlled fluctuations of MMPs are seen in healing wounds as compared with the prolonged elevations that are characteristic of chronic wounds. It is the prolonged elevations in protease levels that are associated with excess degradation of collagen and

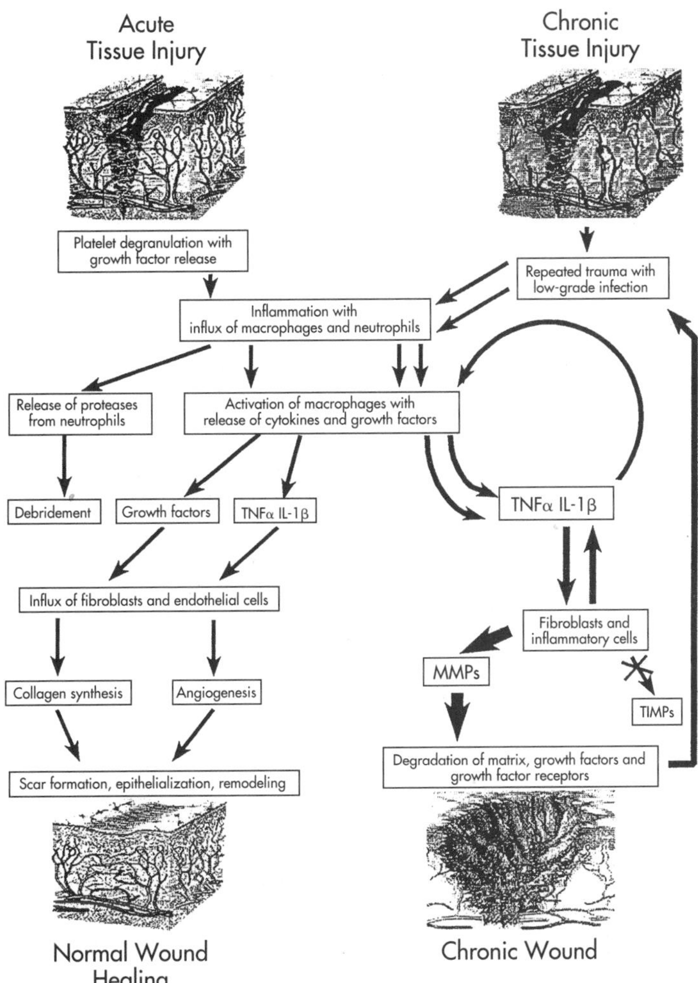

Figure 2-10 Diagrammatic representation of the pathophysiologic "vicious cycle" characteristic of chronic wounds. Prolonged inflammation and elevated levels of proinflammatory cytokines stimulate protease synthesis, which degrades ECM and stimulates additional secretion of inflammatory cytokines. (From Mast BA, Schultz GS: Interactions of cytokines, growth factors and proteases in acute and chronic wounds, *Wound Repair Regen* 4(4):411, 1996).

growth factors (Tarnuzzer et al, 1997). After chronic wounds begin to heal, a decline in MMP levels is noted (Bullen et al, 1995). In addition, patients with chronic wounds treated with a protease inhibitor (e.g., Galardin) demonstrate a significant reduction in matrix degradation within 24 hours.

The molecular environment of a chronic wound also contains abnormal levels of growth factors. Levels of TGF-α, TGF-β, and IGF-I are elevated, whereas EGF levels are decreased (Tarnuzzer and Schultz, 1996). MMPs may contribute to some of this since MMPs degrade growth factors and their receptors as well as other vital components of the extracellular matrix.

Thus far, an environmental milieu that favors prolonged inflammation and degradation of components critical to normal wound healing has been described. The activity and response of the wound matrix cells to cytokines, growth factors, and proteases is also influenced by the age of the chronic wound (Schultz and Mast, 1998). Fibroblasts from chronic venous ulcers of greater than 3 years' duration respond more slowly and poorly to the growth factor PDGF than chronic venous ulcers of less than 3 years' duration. Similarly, although acute wound fluid stimulates DNA synthesis of skin fibroblasts, keratinocytes, and vascular endothelial cells, cells exposed to chronic wound fluid exhibit no DNA synthesis. This is a reflection of the detrimental effect of chronic wound fluid on healing.

In summary, differences in the molecular environment of acute and chronic wounds stem both from the nature of the injury and from the cellular events that follow. In general, healing wounds are characterized by high mitotic activity, therapeutic levels of inflammatory cytokines, low levels of proteases, and mitotically competent cells. On the contrary, chronic wounds exhibit low mitotic activity, excessive levels of inflammatory cytokines, high levels of proteases, and senescent or mitotically incompetent cells.

FACTORS AFFECTING THE REPAIR PROCESS

Wound healing is a systemic process and is therefore significantly affected by systemic conditions. Consequently, the nurse must assess the patient in terms of systemic support for wound repair and intervene accordingly.

Tissue Perfusion and Oxygenation

Oxygen fuels the cellular functions essential to the repair process; therefore the ability to perfuse the tissues with adequate amounts of oxygenated blood is critical to wound healing. Although the negative effects of ischemia on wound repair are well known, the specific oxygen level required for the support of healing is not clear. Oxygen tension in normal tissue is approximately 40 mm Hg, and clinicians have used cut-off values between 10 and 40 mm Hg to predict the potential for wound healing in patients with arterial insufficiency (Padberg et al, 1996; Waldorf and Fewkes, 1995). Current evidence suggests that tissue oxygen requirements vary based on the specific stage of repair. Fibroblast proliferation and bacterial resistance require oxygen tensions greater than 30 mm Hg, whereas keratinocyte mitosis and collagen synthesis can proceed as long as the tissue oxygen levels are between 15 and 30 mm Hg. Some phases of wound repair occur best in hypoxic conditions. Cell migration and angiogenesis continue at tissue oxygen levels of less than 10 mm Hg (Waldorf and Fewkes, 1995).

Obviously, tissue oxygen levels are dependent both on perfusion status and on oxygenation of the blood. However, because wounds remove only 1 ml of oxygen per each 100 ml of blood perfusing the tissues, compromised perfusion is more likely to jeopardize wound healing than compromised oxygenation secondary to pulmonary conditions (Waldorf and Fewkes, 1995). Therefore tissues that are adequately perfused are usually able to heal even if the blood is poorly oxygenated or the patient is anemic. In fact, anemia usually does not significantly affect repair unless the hematocrit drops below 20%. Cigarette smoking is particularly deleterious to wound repair because it affects perfusion and oxygenation. The gas phase of cigarette smoke is carbon monoxide, which binds to hemoglobin and reduces the hemoglobin's ability to transport oxygen. The particulate phase of cigarette smoke is nicotine, which causes vasoconstriction and increased coagulability.

Chronic tissue hypoxia has been associated with impaired collagen synthesis and reduced tissue resistance to infection. Because collagen synthesis requires fairly high levels of oxygen, poorly perfused wounds typically fail to produce connective tissue of adequate tensile strength (Padberg et al, 1996). Basic fibroblast growth factor and transforming growth factor-β have been studied to assess the possible benefits of angiogenic growth factors in the management of ischemic wounds (Quirinia and Viidik, 1998; Wu and Mustoe, 1995).

Although leukocytes can migrate and ingest bacteria in hypoxic environments, their ability to kill bacteria is largely oxygen dependent. The critical tissue oxygen level for bacterial control is 30 mm Hg (Waldorf and Fewkes, 1995).

Acute and chronic illnesses that compromise pulmonary or cardiovascular function, such as hypotension, hypovolemia, trauma, sepsis, or impaired cardiac function, precipitate hypoxia and compromise perfusion and oxygenation. Likewise, disease states that result in damage to the capillary basement membrane, such as radiation, diabetic angiopathy, and peripheral vascular disease, also restrict tissue perfusion. Thus interventions to support wound healing must address both tissue perfusion and oxygenation. Fundamental nursing interventions such as adequate hydration, warmth, and pain control are important steps toward optimizing the healing environment (Cooper, 1990). Nasal oxygen and management of edema are also beneficial. Referrals for further evaluation and management of vascular status as well as hyperbaric oxygen treatments may also be warranted.

Nutritional Status

Nutritional status is as critical to wound repair as perfusion (Brylinsky, 1995). Nutrients provide the raw materials needed for the multitude of cellular activities that constitute wound healing. Adequate nutrition is critically important to maintain a competent immune system and therefore prevent an infection. Protein, calories, vitamin C, vitamin A, and zinc are important components to supplement and monitor; the amino acids arginine and glutamine may also be important to supplement (Breslow et al, 1993; Flanigan, 1997; Kiy, 1997; Pories et al, 1967; Taylor et al, 1974; Ter Riet, Kessels, and Knipschild, 1995; Schaffer and Barbul, 1997; Thomas, 1997; Ziegler et al, 1997). Additional information concerning the role of the various nutrients in the wound healing process and the daily requirement levels are available in Chapter 3.

Infection

A third factor affecting wound repair is the presence or absence of infection. Wound infection prolongs the inflammatory phase, delays collagen synthesis, prevents epithelialization, and increases the production of proinflammatory cytokines, which may lead to additional tissue destruction. Infection is a common cause of wound chronicity and requires prompt aggressive treatment. Bacterial contamination necessitates treatment when the wound is stagnant for more than 2 weeks after appropriate therapy and when B-hemolytic streptococcus is present (Carlson, 1997; Robson, 1997; Waldorf and Fewkes, 1995). Issues pertaining to infection are addressed further in Chapters 4 and 8.

Diabetes Mellitus

Impaired wound healing in patients with diabetes mellitus has been well established. Diabetes mellitus represents a significant problem in the United States since approximately 16 million Americans have diabetes. Studies indicate that wound repair in patients with diabetes mellitus is characterized by reduced collagen synthesis and deposition, decreased wound-breaking strength, and impaired leukocyte function (Bitar, 1997; Bitar, 1998; Bitar and Labbad, 1996; Pierre et al, 1998; Schaffer et al, 1997; Waldorf and Fewkes, 1995). These differences in wound repair may be partially explained by increased levels of proteases (gelatinase), decreased levels of growth factors (IGF-1 and TGF-B) and altered levels of insulin (Bitar and Labbad, 1996). Insulin therapy and exogenous growth factors have been shown to increase collagen deposition and improve tensile strength (Bitar, 1997; Bitar, 1998; Bitar and Labbad, 1996; Schaffer et al, 1997). Patients with diabetes also experience impaired leukocyte chemotaxis, impaired phagocytosis, a decrease in the number of macrophages in the wound matrix, and impaired perfusion as a result of vascular changes (Bitar, 1997; Waldorf and Fewkes, 1995). Many of the adverse effects of diabetes are at least partially related to glycemic control; therefore the management of diabetic patients with wounds should include strict glycemic control as well as measures to maximize tissue perfusion and reduce repetitive trauma. (A more detailed discussion of pathophysiologic changes in patients with diabetes is provided in Chapter 13.)

Corticosteroids

Administration of corticosteroids or the hypercortisolemia produced during periods of stress affects wound healing through several mechanisms: suppression of inflammation, antimitotic effects on keratinocytes and fibroblasts, decreased synthesis of extracellular matrix components, and delayed epithelialization (Anstead, 1998; Bitar, 1998; Waldorf and Fewkes, 1995).

High levels of cortisol or exogenous steroids inhibit leukocyte and macrophage migration, which increases the wound's vulnerability to infection and interrupts the inflammatory phase of the healing cascade. Reduced migration of macrophages is particularly significant since it is the macrophage that produces the chemoattractants and growth factors that drive collagen synthesis and wound contraction (Anstead, 1998; Bitar, 1998; Ehrlich and Hunt, 1968; Ehrlich and Hunt, 1969).

One way in which steroids exert their powerful antiinflammatory effect is by stabilization of lysosomal membranes. Lysosomes are cellular structures that normally are activated to facilitate the breakdown of phagocytized material within the macrophage. This breakdown process is critical to macrophage function. In addition to providing for bacterial control and wound cleanup, this process produces lactate as a byproduct, which stimulates collagen synthesis and angiogenesis. Stabilization of lysosomal membranes by high levels of cortisol renders the lysosomes inactive. Dose equivalents of less than 10 mg of prednisone a day do not exert adverse effects; however, 10 to 30 mg per day have been noted to affect tensile strength and to greatly increase the risk of infection. Doses greater than 40 mg of prednisone a day have definite deleterious effects on wound healing (Anstead, 1998; Waldorf and Fewkes, 1995).

Vitamin A and anabolic steroids can partially counteract the effects of corticosteroids. Anabolic agents stimulate cellular proliferation and regulation of gene transcription, which tends to "offset" the negative effects of elevated cortisol levels on these processes (Anstead, 1998; Erlich and Hunt, 1968). The mechanism by which vitamin A works is not fully understood (Ulland and Caldwell, 1997). It is believed that vitamin A works by labilizing, or breaking down, lysosomal membranes, which restores the normal inflammatory response. Although vitamin A is effective in steroid-impaired wound healing, it does not enhance healing beyond the normal rate. Furthermore, there is inconclusive evidence of any beneficial effects in the absence of corticosteriods (Anstead, 1998; Erlich and Hunt, 1969; Hunt et al, 1969).

Vitamin A can be taken systemically or applied topically. Topical preparations are generally preferred to systemic administration because there is less risk of reversing the desired therapeutic effect of the steroid therapy. A dose of 25,000 IU is recommended for oral administration and 25,000 to 100,000 IU for topical therapy. Vitamin A should be used with caution in patients with preexisting liver disease because of decreased toxicity thresholds (Anstead, 1998).

Age

The aging process produces many changes in the skin and underlying tissues that render a person more susceptible to injury and less able to heal. Aging affects all phases of wound healing. A decline in the number of mast cells and compromised macrophage function lead to a delayed or decreased inflammatory response, limited mitogenic responses of keratinocytes and fibroblasts to the wound environment, reduced collagen synthesis, reduced quality of collagen, and slower epithelialization (Ashcroft, Horan, and Ferguson, 1998; Desai, 1997; Gerstein et al, 1993; van de Kerhoff et al, 1994; Yaar, 1997). Aging is also associated with concomitant medical conditions and polypharmaceutical use, factors that may adversely affect healing. Aging is inevitable, so it is critical to maximize healing in the older patient by providing optimal systemic and topical support and eliminating any correctable impediments.

Stress

Stress, both psychologic and physiologic, has been implicated as a potential cofactor in impaired wound healing because of its effects on 1) serum levels of corticosteroids, which directly affect immune function, and 2) the sympathetic nervous system (Kiecolt-Glaser et al, 1995; Padgett, Marucha, and Sheridan, 1998; Stotts and Wipke-Tevis, 1996). Sympathetic stimulation causes a release of vasoactive substances, such as catecholamines, and vasoconstriction results, which may impair perfusion to the wound bed. Animal and human studies have investigated the effects of elevated serum corticosterones on cellular functions critical to wound repair. Stress was indeed positively related to hypercortisolemia and delayed wound healing as compared with controls. Cellular analysis revealed a delayed onset of cellular infiltration into the wound bed, indicating a lag in the initiation of inflammation (Padgett, Marucha, and Sheridan, 1998). This may be attributed to lower levels of IL-1β, a proinflammatory cytokine that chemoattracts neutrophils and macrophages to the wound site. Most studies related to the effects of stress on wound repair were performed on acute wounds; further research is needed to replicate these findings in chronic wounds. However, it is evident that comprehensive wound management must include interventions to reduce physiologic or psychologic stress; specific strategies include measures such as environmental control (e.g., noise reduction and temperature control), pain control, use of guided imagery, music therapy, patient education, and counseling.

Immunosuppression

Any disease process or medication that suppresses the immune system can alter healing. This is attributable primarily to impairment of the inflammatory process. An impaired immune system is less able to initiate chemotaxis and the release of proinflammatory cytokines, such as lymphokines, from the T-lymphocytes. Lymphokines are particularly important because they regulate chemoattraction of macrophages, destruction of target cells, and promotion of cellular proliferation (Schaffer and Barbul, 1998). Thus immunosuppression can retard wound healing and increase susceptibility to infection.

Other Factors Affecting Wound Repair

In addition to the specific conditions noted previously, any systemic condition that adversely affects health status can negatively affect wound healing. Renal and hepatic disease, malignancy, and sepsis are among these conditions. Hematopoietic abnormalities can impair wound healing because red blood cells are needed for oxygen transport and platelets are necessary for hemostasis and initiation of the wound-healing cascade.

In addition to systemic factors, local factors such as wound bed desiccation, hypothermia, and/or heavy bacterial colonization can affect the repair process. Thus to maximize wound healing, the nurse must maintain a holistic perspective and strive to enhance the patient's overall health status in addition to providing appropriate local wound care.

SUMMARY

In summary, wound healing is a complex series of events. It is normally initiated by an injury that leads to clot formation and platelet degranulation, controlled by a myriad of growth factors and other cytokines, and affected significantly by systemic factors such as perfusion, nutritional status, and steroid levels. Effective management of any wound requires an understanding of the normal repair process and the factors that may interfere with normal repair, including knowledge that serves as the basis for comprehensive assessment of the wound and the patient and selection of interventions designed to optimize the process of healing.

SELF-ASSESSMENT EXERCISE

1. Explain why wounds confined to the epidermal and dermal layers heal by regeneration, whereas wounds extending through the dermal layer into the subcutaneous tissue or fascia or muscle layer must heal by scar formation.
2. Explain what is meant by primary, secondary, and tertiary intentions.
3. Identify the major components of partial-thickness repair.
4. Explain why epidermal resurfacing and dermal repair proceed more rapidly when the wound surface is kept moist.
5. Summarize the activities that occur in the three key phases of full-thickness wound repair (in order).
6. Which of the following cells appear to be the principal mediators for full-thickness wound repair?
   a. Endothelial cells and macrophages
   b. Neutrophils and platelets
   c. Fibroblasts and neutrophils
   d. Platelets and macrophages
7. Describe the inflammatory phase of full-thickness wound repair to include key events, mediating cells, result, and wound appearance.
8. Differentiate between the terms *granulation* and *epithelialization*.

9. Explain the significance of the fibroblast in wound healing.
10. Explain how both hypoxia and oxygenation are critical to the repair process.
11. Contraction plays an important role in wound healing for:
    a. Wounds healing by primary intention
    b. Wounds healing by secondary intention
    c. Superficial abrasions
    d. Partial-thickness wounds
12. Explain why large wounds healing by secondary intention may require skin grafting, whereas large partial-thickness wounds will epithelialize.
13. Identify the two components of the maturation phase and the desired outcome.
14. Summarize the effects of two factors that contribute to the indolent nature of chronic wounds as compared with acute wounds.
15. List at least six factors that affect wound healing.
16. A significant source of growth factors is the:
    a. Endothelial cell
    b. Fibroblast
    c. Monocyte
    d. Macrophage
17. The molecular environment of a chronic wound is characterized by:
    a. Tight regulations of levels of inflammatory cytokines
    b. Increased levels of proteases
    c. Increased levels of protease inhibitors
    d. Excessive collagen synthesis

REFERENCES

Anstead G: Steroids, retinoids, and wound healing, *Adv Wound Care* 11:277, 1998.

Arlein S, Caldwell M: Endogenous growth factors and nutrients in the healing wound. In Ziegler T, Pierce G, Herndon D, editors: *Growth factors and wound healing: basic science and clinical applications*, Norwell, Mass, 1997, Springer.

Ashcroft G, Horan M, Ferguson M: Aging alters the inflammatory and endothelial cell adhesion molecule profiles during human cutaneous wound healing, *Lab Invest* 78(1):47, 1998.

Berry D et al: Human wound contraction: collagen organization, fibroblasts, and myofibroblasts, *Plast Reconstr Surg* 102:124, 1998.

Bitar M: Glucocorticoid dynamics and impaired wound healing in diabetes mellitus, *Am J Pathol* 152:547, 1998.

Bitar M: Insulin-like growth factor-1 reverses diabetes-induced wound healing impairment in rats, *Horm Metab Res* 29:83, 1997.

Bitar M, Labbad Z: Transforming growth factor-β and insulin-like growth factor –1 in relation to diabetes-induced impairment of wound healing, *J Surg Res* 61(1):113, 1996.

Breslow R et al: The importance of dietary protein in healing pressure ulcers, *J Am Geriatr Soc* 41:357, 1993.

Brylinsky C: Nutrition and wound healing: an overview, *Ostomy Wound Manage* 41(10):14, 1995.

Bullen E et al: Tissue inhibitor of metalloproteinases-1 is decreased and activated gelatinases are increased in chronic wounds, *J Invest Dermatol* 104:236, 1995.

Calvin M: Cutaneous wound repair, *Wounds* 10(1):12, 1998.

Carlson M: Acute wound failure, *Surg Clin North Am* 77(3):607, 1997.

Cooper D: Optimizing the wound environment, *Nurs Clin North Am* 25:165, 1990.

Desai H: Ageing and wounds. Part 2. Healing in old age, *J Wound Care* 6(5):237, 1997.

Eaglstein W, Falanga V: Chronic wounds, *Surg Clin North Am* 77(3):689, 1997.

Ehrlich P: The physiology of wound healing: a summary of normal and abnormal wound healing processes, *Adv Wound Care* 11(7):326, 1998.

Ehrlich P, Hunt T: Effects of cortisone and Vitamin A on wound healing, *Ann Surg* 167(3):324, 1968.

Ehrlich P, Hunt T: The effects of cortisone and anabolic steroids on the tensile strength of healing wounds, *Ann Surg* 170(2):203,1969.

Field C, Kerstein M: Overview of wound healing in a moist environment, *Am J Surg* 167(1AS):2S, 1994.

Flanigan K: Nutritional aspects of wound healing, *Adv Wound Care* 10(3):48, 1997.

Garrett B: The proliferation and movement of cells during reepithelialization, *J Wound Care* 6(4):174, 1997.

Gerstein A et al: Wound healing and aging, *Dermatol Clin* 11(4):749, 1993.

Harris I et al: Cytokine and protease levels in healing and non-healing chronic venous leg ulcers, *Exp Dermatol* 4(3):42, 1995.

Hunt TK et al: Effect of vitamin A on reversing the inhibitory effect of cortisone on healing of open wounds in animals and man, *Ann Surg* 170(4):633, 1969.

Hunt TK, Van Winkle W Jr: Normal repair. In Hunt TK, Dunphy JE, editors: *Fundamentals of wound management*, New York, 1997, Appleton-Century-Crofts.

Kiecolt-Glaser J et al: Slowing of wound healing by psychological stress, *Lancet* 346(8984):1194, 1995.

Kiy A: Nutrition in wound healing: a biopsychosocial perspective, *Nurs Clin North Am* 32(4):849, 1997.

Levenson S, Seiffer E, Van Winkle E Jr: Nutrition. In Hunt TK, Dunphy JE, editors: *Fundamentals of wound management*, New York, 1979, Appleton-Century-Crofts

Martin P: Wound healing: aiming for perfect skin regeneration, *Science* 276(4):75, 1997.

Mast BA: The skin. In Cohen IK, Diegelmann RF, Lindblad WJ, editors: *Wound healing: biochemical and clinical aspects*, Philadelphia, 1992, W.B. Saunders.

Mast BA, Schultz G: Interactions of cytokines, growth factors, and proteases in acute and chronic wounds, *Wound Repair Regen* 4(4):411, 1996.

Padberg R et al: Transcutaneous oxygen ($TcPO_2$) estimates probability of healing in the ischemic extremity, *J Surg Res* 60(2):365, 1996.

Padgett D, Marucha P, Sheridan J: Restraint stress slows cutaneous wound healing in mice, *Brain Behav Immun* 12:64, 1998.

Pierre E et al: Effects of insulin on wound healing, *J Traum Inj Infect Crit Care* 44:342, 1998.

Pories W et al: Acceleration of healing with zinc sulfate, *Ann Surg* 165(3):432, 1967.

Quirina A, Viidik A: The effect of recombinant basic fibroblast growth factor (bFGF) in fibrin adhesive vehicle on the healing of ischaemic and normal incisional skin wounds, *Scand J Plast Reconstr Surg Hand Surg* 32:9, 1998.

Robson M: Wound infection: A failure of wound healing caused by an imbalance of bacteria, *Surg Clin North Am* 77(3):637, 1997.

Rohovsky S, D'Amore P: Growth factors and angiogenesis in wound healing. In Ziegler T, Pierce G, Herndon D, editors: *Growth factors and wound healing: basic science and clinical applications*, Norwell, Mass, 1997, Springer.

Schaffer M, Barbul A: Lymphocyte function in wound healing and following injury, *Br J Surg* 85:444, 1998.

Schaffer M, Barbul A: Use of exogenous amino acids in wound healing. In Ziegler T, Pierce G, Herndon D, editors: *Growth factors and wound healing: basic science and clinical applications*, Norwell, Mass, 1997, Springer.

Schaffer M et al: Diabetes-impaired healing and reduced wound nitric oxide synthesis: a possible pathophysiologic correlation, *Surgery* 121:513, 1997.

Schultz G, Mast B: Molecular analysis of the environment of healing and chronic wounds: cytokines, proteases, and growth factors, *Wounds* 10(suppl F):1F, 1998.

Spotnitz W, Falstrom J, Rodeheaver G: The role of sutures and fibrin sealant in wound healing, *Surg Clin North Am* 77(3):651, 1997.

Steed D: The role of growth factors in wound healing, *Surg Clin North Am* 77(3):575, 1997.

Stotts N, Wipke-Tevis D: Co-factors in impaired wound healing, *Ostomy Wound Manage* 42(2):44, 1996.

Tarnuzzer R et al: Epidermal growth factor in wound healing: a model for the molecular pathogenesis of chronic wounds. In Ziegler T, Pierce G, Herndon D, editors: *Growth factors and wound healing: basic science and clinical applications*, Norwell, Mass, 1997, Springer.

Tarnuzzer R, Schultz G: Biochemical analysis of acute and chronic wound environments, *Wound Repair Regen* 4:321, 1996.

Taylor T et al: Ascorbic acid supplementation in the treatment of pressure sores, *Lancet* 2(7880):544, 1974.

Ter Riet G, Kessels A, Knipschild P: Randomized clinical trial of ascorbic acid in the treatment of pressure ulcers, *J Clin Epidemiol* 48(12):453, 1995.

Thomas D: Specific nutritional factors in wound healing, *Adv Wound Care* 10(4):40, 1997.

Trott AT: *Wounds and lacerations*, ed 2, St Louis, 1997, Mosby

Ulland A, Caldwell M: Vitamin A-growth factor interactions in wound healing. In Ziegler T, Pierce G, Herndon D, editors: *Growth factors and wound healing: basic science and clinical applications*, Norwell, Mass, 1997, Springer.

Vaalamo M et al: Patterns of matrix metalloproteinase and TIMP-1 expression in chronic and normally healing human cutaneous wounds, *Br J Dermatol* 135(1):52, 1996.

van de Kerkhof P et al: Age-related changes in wound healing, *Clin Exp Dermatol* 19:369, 1994.

Waldorf H, Fewkes J: Wound healing, *Adv Dermatol* (10):77, 1995.

Whalen GF, Zetter BR: Angiogenesis. In Cohen IK, Dieglemann RF, Lindblad WJ, editors: *Wound healing: biochemical and clinical aspects*, Philadelphia, 1992, W.B. Saunders.

Winter G: Epidermal regeneration studied in the domestic pig. In Hunt T, Dunphy J, editors: *Fundamentals of wound management*, New York, 1979, Appleton-Century-Crofts.

Witte M, Barbul A: General principles of wound healing, *Surg Clin North Am* 77(3):509, 1997.

Wu L, Mustoe T: Effect of ischemia on growth factor enhancement of incisional wound healing, *Surgery* 117(5):570, 1995.

Wysocki A, Staiano-Coico L, Grinnell F: Wound fluid from chronic leg ulcers contains elevated levels of metalloproteinases MMP-2 and MMP-9, *J Invest Dermatol* 101:64, 1993.

Yaar M: Molecular mechanisms of skin aging, *Adv Dermatol* 10:64, 1997.

Yager D et al: Wound fluids from human pressure ulcers contain elevated matrix metalloproteinase levels and activity compared to surgical wound fluid, *J Invest Dermatol* 107:743, 1996.

Ziegler T et al: Interactions between nutrients and growth factors in cellular anabolism and tissue repair. In Ziegler T, Pierce G, Herndon D, editors: *Growth factors and wound healing: basic science and clinical applications*, Norwell, Mass, 1997, Springer.

CHAPTER 3

Nutritional Assessment and Support

NANCY A. STOTTS

OBJECTIVES

1. Identify the effects of injury on metabolic needs.
2. Define *malnutrition.*
3. Compare and contrast the causes and signs of marasmus, kwashiorkor, and mixed marasmus-kwashiorkor
4. Identify four factors that contribute to obesity being a risk factor for impaired healing.
5. Link the clinical manifestations and phases of starvation.
6. Identify the factors in the patient's history that would predispose him or her to malnutrition.
7. Describe the major physical findings of malnutrition.
8. Identify the laboratory work consistent with malnutrition.
9. Identify the nutrients needed for repair and their role in wound healing.
10. Propose parameters to monitor nutritional status during nutritional support.

Nutritional assessment and support of the patient with a wound, persons at-risk for pressure ulcers, and those who will undergo surgery are based on the appreciation that nutrition is fundamental to normal cellular integrity and tissue repair. Malnutrition is associated with delayed healing, infection, slowed recovery from illness, and increased morbidity and mortality (Bergstrom and Braden, 1992; Dempsey, Mullen, and Buzby, 1988; Detsky et al, 1987; Seltzer et al, 1979; Seltzer et al, 1981). Identification of those at-risk as well as those experiencing malnutrition is the basis for timely intervention that can mitigate the negative effects of malnutrition and support healing.

INJURY AND NUTRIENT NEED

Effects of Injury on Metabolic Need

With injury, there is an increased metabolic rate that results in an increase in caloric need. The degree of hypermetabolism is directly related to the severity of injury (Box 3-1). The caloric needs are increased, and at the same time the need for protein is increased disproportionally. The hypermetabolic demands decrease gradually, and if no additional insult occurs, the metabolic needs return to baseline within 10 to 14 days of the acute injury (Stanek, 1994; Stotts and Friesen, 1982). This is seen in the surgical patient who undergoes coronary artery bypass surgery and has an uncomplicated postoperative course.

Often with chronic wounds, there is a secondary insult that occurs, and this causes the metabolic needs to rise. This can be seen during infection in chronic wounds. In addition, with chronic wounds there may be exudative losses from the wound that increase the nutrient requirements. An example of this problem is seen in patients with venous ulcers (Wipke-Tevis and Stotts, 1998).

Inadequate Intake in Persons with Wounds

In healthy persons who are wounded, inadequate intake for a brief period of up to 5 to 7 days is usually not a major problem. During this time, these patients experience a combination of hypermetabolism and starvation. The hypermetabolic response is a physiologic response to injury and results in increased energy needs. At the same time, these patients usually have inadequate intake that results in them using their body substrate to meet their metabolic needs. They usually have a brief but rapid decrease in weight. When they return to their normal diet, they regain the lost weight.

Malnutrition

When inadequate intake in healthy people persists for more than 5 to 7 days and when patients with depleted nutrient stores are injured, malnutrition may develop. Malnutrition is undernutrition or overnutrition that is caused by a deficit or excess of nutrients in the diet, inability to absorb nutrients, or inability to metabolize substrates needed for normal function. Malnutrition is a major health problem in hospitalized patients and those with acute and chronic illness. The prevalence of malnutrition in hospitalized patients is between 10% and 50% (Daley and Bistrian, 1994). Some patients are admitted to the hospital with malnutrition, and others develop it during hospitalization.

The type of malnutrition that occurs depends on the dietary deficiencies. Table 3-1 outlines the characteristics of the classic types of malnutrition (Pinchcofsky-Devin, 1997). These are important for diagnostic purposes and may alter the treatment plan. From a nursing perspective, understanding the processes that take place during starvation is important because it allows the nurse to appreciate why specific assessment parameters are used and specific nutrients are prescribed.

BOX 3-1 Increase in Energy Requirements with Injury

Elective surgery	±10%
Multiple fractures	10% to 25%
Major infection	20% to 50%
Burns	50% to 125%

Phases of Starvation

When intravenous intake is inadequate, glycogen stored in the liver is used for energy. Normally the glycogen stores are exhausted in less than 24 hours and the energy needed for cellular activities is formed by the catabolism of muscle. There are no protein stores in the body, so when protein is used for gluconeogenesis, functional tissue is destroyed. Concomitantly, catecholamines are released and stimulate the breakdown of body fat and protein, and weight loss is rapid. The weight loss occurs from both the breakdown of protein and the osmotic diuresis that occurs as the byproducts of protein metabolism are excreted in the urine (Table 3-2). This phase, sometimes called *brief starvation*, continues for several days (Barton, 1994; Stanek, 1994; Stotts and Friesen, 1982).

If intake still is less than the individual's metabolic needs, compensatory processes take place that allow fat to become the primary energy source and for protein to be used at a much slower rate. Important compensations are that the brain can use ketones from fat metabolism for energy, the muscle releases less protein, and the kidney recy-

TABLE 3-1 Cause and Manifestations of Marasmus, Kwashiorkor, and Marasmus-Kwashiorkor

TYPE OF MALNUTRITION	CAUSE	MANIFESTATIONS
Marasmus	Inadequate protein and calories	Gradual weight loss Visceral protein levels are preserved Immune function is well preserved
Kwashiorkor	Inadequate protein with adequate carbohydrate and fat	Rapid onset with loss of visceral protein Skeletal muscle mass is well preserved
Marasmus-Kwashiorkor	Inadequate protein and calories	Acute onset Common in hospitalized patients Low visceral protein Presents with rapid weight loss, fat and muscle wasting

cles the end products of protein metabolism for glucose. Because fat has more than twice as many calories per gram of tissue than protein (9 calories compared with 4 calories), weight loss is slowed. Protein is converted to glucose for use by only a few tissues (e.g., RBCs, fibroblasts, renal medulla). During this time, changes in fat stores are gradual, as are declines in muscle stores. Serum measures reflecting protein status are slow to change during this phase, although they do gradually decline. Clinical manifestations that reflect the body's adaptation to starvation are listed in Table 3-2 (Barton, 1994; Stanek, 1994; Stotts and Friesen, 1982).

When fat stores are depleted, the body moves into premorbid starvation, where protein again is the primary energy source. Rapid depletion occurs, skeletal muscle size rapidly decreases, and serum protein levels fall (Barton, 1994; Stanek, 1994; Stotts and Friesen, 1982). Table 3-2 lists signs and symptoms of this phase. If treatment is not prompt, death will ensue.

TABLE 3-2 Manifestations of Starvation

TYPE OF STARVATION	MANIFESTATIONS
Brief	Increased nitrogen in urine Increased urine output Rapid weight loss Decreased muscle mass Low normal glucose and insulin levels
Prolonged	Slow weight loss Slow loss of muscle mass Increased urinary ammonia Decreased urinary nitrogen Metabolic acidosis, usually compensated
Premorbid	Cachectic appearance Rapid weight loss Decreased midarm muscle circumference Increased creatinine/height index Increased urinary urea Decreased serum albumin Decreased transferrin Decreased lymphocyte count Anergy to recall antigens

Adapted from Stotts NA, Friesen L: Understanding starvation in the critically ill patient, *Heart Lung* 11(5):469, 1982.

Overnutrition as Malnutrition

On the other end of the continuum of malnutrition is overnutrition, most commonly seen as obesity. Obese patients may develop wound-healing problems because of several obesity-related issues (Gallagher, 1997). Often persons who are obese have concomitant medical problems that include diabetes, hypertension, and poor oxygenation from pulmonary restrictive disease as a result of their obesity. Fat tissue is not as well perfused as is muscular tissue, so obese people are at risk for delayed healing and infection. Mobility also may be a problem, and they may develop pneumonia or deep venous thrombosis secondary to immobility. Caloric need for repair is directly related to weight, so obese patients need greater calories for maintenance than with persons of normal weight. On the other hand, given equal health, obese persons' ability to tolerate prolonged starvation is better than a person of normal weight because of their greater fat stores. Obese patients with wounds need exogenous nutrients to heal, so a weight-loss diet is not recommended.

Needs for Healing

Nutrition is critical to healing. With injury, more calories and substrates are needed for healing when compared with the uninjured state. Protein needs are especially increased (Flanigan, 1997). Table 3-3 lists the nutrients needed and their role in repair.

Deficiencies in any of the nutrients may result in impaired or delayed healing. The specific alteration, in part, may vary depending on the defect (e.g., protein is needed for antibody formation).

Nutrients are critical for synthesis of tissue. Normally, dietary intake provides the building blocks for repair and tissue replacement. Most diets are a combination of protein, carbohydrate, fat, vitamins, and minerals, so deficiencies of individual nutrients are uncommon. However, often patients

TABLE 3-3 Nutrients and Their Role in Wound Healing

NUTRIENT	ROLE IN HEALING
Protein	Fibroplasia, neogenesis, collagen formation, wound remodeling; maintenance of integrity of immune system
Carbohydrates	Energy supply, protein sparing
Fat	Cell walls, intracellular organelles, fat-soluble vitamins
Vitamin A	Epithelialization, wound closure, inflammatory response
B vitamins	Synthesis of protein, fat and carbohydrate
Vitamin C	Collagen synthesis, capillary wall integrity, fibroblast function, immunologic function
Vitamin D	Calcium metabolism for building and maintaining bone
Vitamin E	Unknown
Vitamin K	Coagulation
Copper	Cross-linking of collagen
Iron	Collagen formation
Magnesium	Protein synthesis
Zinc	Collagen formation and protein synthesis

are unable or unwilling to ingest a balanced diet and a multivitamin.

Good nutrition should include protein, fat, and carbohydrates. Vitamin C, iron, zinc, and copper are needed for collagen formation. Vitamin A and multivitamins are required because of their role as coenzymes (Flanigan, 1997). No single nutrient has been shown to accelerate healing. Adequate quantities of the various nutrients are critical to support healing. Normally the dietician does an individual evaluation and makes a dietary recommendation.

NUTRITIONAL ASSESSMENT

Initial nutritional assessment provides baseline data regarding a person's nutritional status. Subsequent assessments reflect changes in status and effects of interventions. The assessment identifies the presence of or risk for malnutrition or specific nutrient deficiencies. The data derived provide the basis for developing a nutritional plan.

Nutritional assessment is most effectively performed by a multidisciplinary team composed of dieticians, nurses, pharmacists, and doctors. Depending on the setting, the nurse may be the initial person to do the nutritional assessment. Especially in home care, the nurse may be the only professional to see a patient unless other specific needs are identified. In the home care setting, the wound care nurse might consider a prepackaged approach to nutritional assessment such as the Nutritional Screening Initiative, which was developed for use with geriatric patients (deGroot et al, 1998). This tool includes a nutritional screening that can be performed at regular intervals, as well as a comprehensive assessment that includes nutritional assessment, functional assessment, and evaluation for depression. This comprehensive approach allows the home care wound nurse to quantify the nature of the nutritional problem and mobilize resources that are appropriate to meet the specific needs. Regardless of who performs the assessment or whether a prepackaged approach is used, it is critical that the nutritional assessment be completed soon after the patient is admitted to the service. The components of a nutritional assessment include the patient history, physical examination, and laboratory data.

Patient History

The history and physical examination are the oldest and probably the most widely used evaluations of nutritional status. Most information about a patient is derived from the history, and it gives focus to the physical examination and laboratory work.

The history provides a chronologic picture of the person's nutritional health. Initially, the person's chief complaint and present illnesses are elicited. General health, major adult illnesses, and childhood illnesses are elicited. Prior surgery, functional limitations, and emotional status all are evaluated as related to nutrient intake. The social history is important, including personal history, home conditions, and environment. The history concludes with a review of systems (Seidel et al, 1999).

Conditions or diseases that have produced alterations in ingestion, digestion, absorption, and metabolism are elicited with the history. The following are common conditions that raise the nurse's suspicion that malnutrition is present or may be a risk factor:

- Conditions that cause hypermetabolism
- Treatment with immunosuppressive drugs
- Weight loss
- Changes in appetite
- Food intolerances
- Dietary restrictions
- Lack of teeth or poorly fitting dentures
- Inability to feed oneself
- Altered smell or taste
- Need to restrict intake for tests

Issues related to obtaining and preparing food also may affect intake. These include limited income, environment at mealtime, social isolation, inability to purchase and prepare meals, and educational level. Specific information obtained by history includes usual weight, weight changes, change in the pattern or variety of food ingested, changes in appetite, and signs and symptoms of related problems (e.g., nausea, vomiting, anorexia, diarrhea).

No single physical finding is diagnostic of malnutrition. Table 3-4 lists examples of signs and symptoms associated with specific nutritional alterations (e.g., coarse hair, thin skin). These are not specific, so the examiner must consider explanations other than nutritional alterations for the findings, such as the following:

- Disease process, medication side effect, or a metabolic alteration that may account for the signs and symptoms

TABLE 3-4 Examples of Physical Findings Seen with Nutritional Deficiencies

	SIGNS AND SYMPTOMS	RELATED NUTRITIONAL DEFICIENCY
Skin manifestations	Dermatitis	Protein, calories, zinc, vitamin A
	Petechiae	Vitamin C
Muscles	Weakness	Protein, calories
	Weight loss, wasting	Protein, calories
Mouth	Glossitis	Riboflavin, niacin
	Bleeding	Vitamins A, C, K

- Effect of age on expected findings
- Half-lives of nutrients suspected as being deficient

Yet physical findings often are used to confirm suspicions raised with the history or the laboratory work. For those at risk or with early malnutrition, the physical findings for malnutrition may be subtle or absent because some signs do not appear until the malnutrition becomes advanced. With overt malnutrition, anthropometric changes often are key findings. The additional challenge is that many signs of malnutrition may have nonnutritional causes. In addition, obese patients are especially difficult to evaluate because their weight may mask the skeletal muscle wasting of malnutrition.

Anthropometric measures are easy to perform and are pivotal in the evaluation of nutritional status. Areas addressed include weight, midarm muscle circumference, skin-fold measures, and head circumference.

Weight is a cornerstone in the diagnosis of malnutrition and can be used alone or in relation to height or frame size (Pinchcofsky-Devin, 1997; Stotts and Bergstrom, 1997). A loss of 5% of usual weight, weight less than 90% of ideal body weight, or a decrease of 10 pounds in a brief period are all signs of actual or potential nutritional problems. One of the ongoing issues in using weight to measure nutritional status is what value to use for comparison (i.e., ideal weight, usual weight). Data indicate that the appropriate value may vary by population (Beck and Ovesen, 1998). Until a decision has been made as to what is optimal, each institution should set its own standard to enhance continuity of care.

Weight for height is often examined. Recent tables for interpretation of these parameters are based on the National Research Council data on weight and height, the dietary guidelines, and the body mass index (BMI). The BMI is calculated by dividing weight in kilograms by height in meters squared and most often is used to determine whether people are undernourished or obese. It also is a predictor of morbidity and mortality (Gallagher, 1997; Pinchcofsky-Devin, 1997; Stotts and Bergstrom, 1997).

Arm muscle circumference and skin-fold measurement were initially employed in underdeveloped countries using only very basic instruments to evaluate the nutritional status of the population (Jeliffe, 1966). There are standards in the United States for specific age groups and for a limited number of minority populations (Frisancho, 1984; Gray and Gray, 1979; Marshall et al, 1999). Although performed by primarily by dieticians, it is important for the nurse to understand what the tests measure to be able to appreciate the meaning of the findings to the patient's status.

Mid-upper arm circumference (MAC) is a measure of muscle mass, bone, and skin. It is used to calculate midarm muscle circumference (MAMC) as a measure of lean body mass (Stotts and Bergstrom, 1997). The MAC itself is meaningful only as part of the calculation of MAMC. A decrease in arm muscle mass occurs with muscle disease and nutritional deficiencies. Severe depletion is present when the person is in the lowest fifth percentile on established tables, and those in the sixth to tweny-fifth percentiles are moderately depleted.

Fat stores are measured with skin-fold measures. A skin-fold caliper (Lange, Holtain, Harpenden) is used to evaluate skin-fold thickness (SFT). Several sites are available (e.g., scapula, waist, triceps), but the triceps site is the most frequently used. Fat stores do not change rapidly, thus SFT is not a sensitive measure of malnutrition. Depletion occurs with chronic malnutrition and severe hypermetabolism (Pinchcofsky-Devin, 1997).

Head circumference is used in children to evaluate their growth. Measurements are compared with tables of norms, allowing head size to be classified in percentiles. Chronic undernutrition results in a delay in growth of the head, and its identification and treatment are important so that permanent damage does not occur (Mascarenhas, Zemel, and Stallings, 1998).

Laboratory Data

Biochemical parameters reflect the end product of ingestion, digestion, absorption, and metabolism of nutrients. Biochemical measures are a simple approach that offers a minimally invasive strategy to evaluate nutritional status.

Serum proteins are biochemical indicators of malnutrition (Stotts and Bergstrom, 1997). They are synthesized by the liver and vary primarily in their rate of turnover. Table 3-5 lists the serum protein measures frequently used to evaluate protein status. For all of them, hydration status is important in their validity, with dehydration producing falsely elevated serum levels and overhydration producing false negatives values. It should be noted that posture and circadian rhythm also can affect hydration and the accuracy of the values.

Serum albumin is probably the most frequently measured of these laboratory parameters. Albumin has a long half-life (18 to 20 days), is not sensitive to rapid changes in nutritional status, and falls late in prolonged and premorbid starvation (Pinchcofsky-Devin, 1997; Stotts and Bergstrom, 1997). It is not an appropriate measure to use to diagnose either recent or mild to moderate malnutri-

TABLE 3-5 Normal and Decreased Levels of Albumin, Transferrin, and Prealbumin

VISCERAL PROTEIN	NORMAL	MALNUTRITION
Serum albumin	3.5-5.5 g/dl	<3.5 g/dl
Transferrin	200-400 mg/dl	<100 mg/dl
Prealbumin	15-25 mg/dl	<15 mg/dl

tion. Decreased albumin levels have long been associated with increased morbidity and mortality in medical-surgical patients (Seltzer et al, 1979) and intensive care patients (Seltzer et al, 1981).

Transferrin, another frequently used measure of protein status, has a shorter half-life (8 to 10 days) and a smaller body pool. Its major function is to transport iron, and usually about one third of the body's transferrin is bound to iron (Pinchcofsky-Devin, 1997). Transferrin is affected by many factors other than protein-calorie malnutrition, so it is not sufficiently sensitive or specific to be a meaningful measure. For example, a deficiency of iron as is frequently seen with protein-calorie malnutrition stimulates hepatic synthesis, so very high levels result. At the other extreme, inflammatory states, liver disease, and some anemias result in depressed transferrin levels (Stotts and Bergstrom, 1997).

Prealbumin is a plasma protein with a short half-life (2 days). It is also known as thyroxin-binding prealbumin and transthyretin (Stotts and Bergstrom, 1997). It transports a portion of thyroxine and vitamin A. Because of its short half-life, prealbumin decreases quickly when protein or calorie intake is decreased. In contrast, it responds quickly when exogenous nutrients are provided. Prealbumin is an excellent measure of nutritional status because it reflects not only what has been ingested but also what has been able to be absorbed, digested, and metabolized. On the other hand, prealbumin is sensitive to the inflammatory response and decreases rapidly with a decrease in protein synthesis.

Less commonly measured is retinol-binding protein, a plasma protein with a very short half-life (12 hours) and very low serum levels. It also participates in the transport of vitamin A, and its response follows that of prealbumin. Although it has a theoretic advantage over other plasma proteins by virtue of its short half-life, its low normal values and the technical difficulties in measurement have not demonstrated its superiority over other measures of nutrient status (Stotts and Bergstrom, 1997).

Creatinine is another measure of protein status that has been used for more than 20 years in nutritional support settings to evaluate lean body mass. Creatinine is complex because it requires normal renal function and urinary output, the ability to accurately collect a 24-hour urine, adequate hydration, and that the patient not be on prolonged periods of bed rest and not have a recent high-protein meal. Normally nutritional status with creatinine is evaluated using a 24-hour urine creatinine excretion divided by normal creatinine for height, producing a creatinine height index (CHI). Age-specific tables are used to interpret the findings.

Another measure, 3-Methylhistidine is a measure of skeletal muscle breakdown. Its excretion is seen as a sensitive measure of catabolism; however, because there is a large pool of 3-Methylhistidine outside of skeletal muscle, it is not a specific test. Criteria for its use, collection, and processing are similar to that for creatinine.

Basic to the discussion of protein status is the concept of nitrogen balance. The concept is that nitrogen turnover is in balance (i.e., intake and loss from the body are carefully regulated and closely approximate each other under normal nutritional circumstances). Anabolism and repair require positive nitrogen balance. Negative nitrogen balance is a reflection of catabolism (Flanigan, 1997).

The immune system is very sensitive to protein status because protein is a major constituent of immune system components such as antibodies and lymphocytes. Consequently, gross tests of immune function, such as total lymphocyte count (TLC), also reflect protein status. Lymphocytes constitute a variable percentage of the circulating white blood cells and are reported in a white blood cell differential. The TLC is calculated by multiplying the percentage of lymphocytes by the white cell count. The normal level is 1500 to 3000 cells per mm^3. Below normal levels may be a reflection of malnutrition; however, TLC may also be depressed by chemotherapy, autoimmune diseases, stress, and infection, including HIV (Flanigan, 1997; Stotts and Bergstrom, 1997).

NUTRITIONAL SUPPORT

Referral for Definitive Nutritional Support

The nurse who identifies a patient at risk for or with existing malnutrition needs to work with the health care team to see that appropriate nutrients are provided. Depending on the system, the appropriate action is for the nurse to refer the patient to the dietician, notify the physician of the findings, or call the nutritional support team so that appropriate nutritional support can be prescribed.

Nutrient Needs

Nutritional support therapy should provide a balanced intake of necessary nutrients based on the person's energy and protein requirements. Because a person's nutritional needs are dependent on many variables (such as age, sex, height, weight, presence of severe wasting or obesity, current disease state, severity of illness, and the presence and severity of a wound), it may be an oversimplification to give a range of calories and protein that a patient with wounds will require. However, it is useful to remember that a healthy person requires approximately 0.8 g of protein per kilogram per 24 hours (the presence of a wound will increase these protein requirements). In general, a patient with wounds needs adequate calories and increased amounts of protein (1.25 to 2.0 g/kg/24 hr). Daily vitamin and mineral needs also are increased to 1600 to 2000 retinol equivalents of vitamin A, 100 to 1000 mg of vitamin C, 15 to 30 mg of zinc, 200% of the RDA of the B vitamins, and 20 to 30 mg of iron (Flanigan, 1997).

Nutritional Support for Patients with Wounds

Nutritional support for patients with wounds is the same as support for those with specialized nutritional needs. The preferred route of support is orally, and whenever possible, the gastrointestinal tract should be used for feeding. If the patient's intake is not adequate with oral feeding, then one of the various approaches to the gastrointestinal tract used for tube feedings is selected to supplement or supplant the oral feeding. When the gastrointestinal tract cannot be used, parenteral nutrition is the route of choice. Further information on management of persons using nutritional support is available in several textbooks (Black and Matassarin-Jacobs, 1997).

SUMMARY

Nutritional assessment and support play an important role in wound healing. All patients with wounds should have their nutritional status evaluated. A thorough nutritional assessment should reveal the risk for or presence of malnutrition and provide the necessary information to develop an individualized nutritional plan of care. The nutritional status should be evaluated at baseline and at regular intervals for determination of the effectiveness of the nutritional plan.

CASE STUDY

KH is a 48-year-old paraplegic who has developed a Stage IV pressure ulcer on the sacrum. The opening is 4 × 2 cm, and it is 4 cm deep with undermining 2 cm in all directions. This large ulcer is full of yellow-gray slough that is malodorous and highly exudative. The skin surrounding the wound is intact. He does not have signs of sepsis. He is admitted to acute care for treatment of the wound and possible flap surgery.

His history indicates that he was injured in a fall 8 years ago. He lives independently and works as an accountant. He has managed well until his only sister and primary support person was diagnosed with cancer 8 weeks ago. She had surgery and radiation therapy. He has been spending time after work providing care for her four young children and assisting the family. This has required him to be in his wheelchair about 5 additional hours per day, and he is quite concerned about her prognosis.

KH is 5 feet 9 inches tall and usually weighs 160 pounds. His current weight is 147, having lost 10 pounds in the last month. He says that all of his energy is going to help is sister. He has not been following his usual pressure-relief program and has had no appetite. His albumin is 3.2 g/dl. His CBC is within normal limits.

A consultation with the dietician results in him receiving a special diet high in protein (2 g/kg/day), iron, vitamin C, and zinc. The 3-day dietary record shows that he consumes less than 50% of the recommended intake. Prealbumin drawn at the end of the 3 days of oral support reveals a level of 12 mg/dl. His weight is 144 pounds. Nasogastric (NG) feedings are started, and within 3 days he has reached the dietician's goal of needed calories and protein. GI evaluation is negative. His sister finishes her radiation therapy, and her prognosis is positive. His oral intake increases.

Local wound care has cleaned up the wound, and there is granulation tissue in its base. It is larger now than on admission (4 × 4 × 6) and the decision is made to discharge the patient and reevaluate him in 1 month as to the need for the flap. The nutritional plan is to leave the NG tube in place, increasing his oral intake and reducing his NG feedings until he can maintain intake by the oral route.

SELF-ASSESSMENT EXERCISE

1. Generally speaking, major penetrating traumatic injuries with associated wounds result in:
   a. Increased metabolic rate for 10 to 14 days after injury
   b. Decreased metabolic rate to help conserve energy for the first 2 to 5 days after injury
   c. Decreased metabolic rate for 48 hours, and then increased for the following 10 to 14 days
   d. Unknown metabolic consequences (cannot be determined without more information)
2. After injury, the nutrient that is most in demand is:
   a. Vitamin C
   b. Zinc
   c. Fat
   d. Protein
   e. None of the above
3. FD is a 65-year-old male who is retired and lives alone. He is healthy except for a venous ulcer on his high leg, and he needs a "water pill for his high blood pressure." He does not eat breakfast or lunch but goes to the local restaurant every evening for dinner. Over the past 3 months he has lost 15 pounds. Your initial suspicion is that he has:
   a. Marasmus
   b. Kwashiorkor
   c. Marasmus-kwashiorkor
   d. Chronic dehydration
4. All of the following statements describe why obesity is a risk factor for poor healing EXCEPT:
   a. Fat is more poorly perfused than lean tissue
   b. Many obese persons are diabetics
   c. Obese persons are often hypotensive
   d. Abdominal fat pushes on the diaphragm
5. Your 86-year-old patient had surgery 2 days ago for a below-the-knee amputation after arterial emboli and gangrene of the right foot. Preoperatively he was relatively healthy, having normal serum proteins, CBC, and height for weight. He is receiving a 5% Dextrose solution at 25 ml/hr. Symptoms of brief starvation that you expect are:
   a. Slow weight loss and low albumin
   b. Slow weight loss and normal albumin
   c. Rapid weight loss and low albumin
   d. Rapid weight loss and normal albumin
6. The factor in the history and physical examination that most often contributes to malnutrition is:
   a. Low albumin
   b. Decreased triceps skin-fold
   c. Low income
   d. Positive nitrogen balance
7. Physical findings of premorbid starvation include:
   a. Low serum albumin
   b. Decreased triceps skin-fold
   c. Increased BMI
   d. Positive nitrogen balance
8. Which of the following findings is consistent with brief starvation?
   a. Decreased albumin
   b. Decreased triceps skin-fold
   c. Positive nitrogen balance
   d. Glossitis
9. Essential factors in collagen formation are:
   a. Vitamin A, vitamin C, copper
   b. Vitamin C, zinc, iron
   c. Vitamin K, vitamin B, zinc
   d. Vitamin E, iron, copper
10. Anabolism over the last 2 to 3 days of feeding with either enteral or parenteral nutrition is best evaluated with:
    a. Weight change
    b. Serum albumin
    c. Transferrin
    d. BMI
    e. Prealbumin.

REFERENCES

Barton RG: Nutrition support in critical illness, *Nutr Clin Pract* 9(4):127, 1994.

Beck AM, Ovesen L: At which body mass index and degree of weight loss should hospitalized elderly patients be considered at nutritional risk? *Clin Nutr* 17(5):195, 1998.

Bergstrom N, Braden B: A prospective study of pressure sore risk among institutionalized elderly, *J Am Geriatr Soc* 40:747, 1992.

Black JM, Matassarin-Jacobs E: *Medical-surgical nursing: clinical management for continuity of care,* ed 5, Philadelphia, 1997, W.B. Saunders.

Daley BJ, Bistrian: Nutritional assessment. In Zologa GP, editor: *Nutrition in critical care,* St Louis, 1994, Mosby.

deGroot LC et al: Evaluating DETERMINE Your Nutritional Health Checklist and the Mini Nutritional Assessment tool to identify nutritional problems in elderly Europeans, *Eur J Clin Nutr* 52(12): 877, 1998.

Dempsey DT, Mullen JL, Buzby GP: The link between nutritional status and clinical outcome: can nutritional intervention modify it? *Am J Clin Nutr* 47(2 suppl):352, 1988.

Detsky AS et al: Predicting nutrition-associated complications for patients undergoing gastrointestinal surgery, *J Parenter Enteral Nutr* 11:440, 1987.

Flanigan KH: Nutritional aspects of wound healing, *Adv Wound Care* 10(2):48, 1997.

Frisancho AR: New standards of weight and body composition by frame size and height for assessment of nutritional status of adults and the elderly, *Am J Clin Nutr* 40:808, 1984.

Gallagher SM: Morbid obesity: a chronic disease with an impact on wounds and related problems, *Ostomy Wound Manage* 43(5):18, 1997.

Gray GE, Gray LK: Validity of anthropometric norms used in the assessment of hospitalized patients, *J Parenter Enteral Nutr* 3:366, 1979.

Jeliffe DB: Direct nutritional assessment of human groups. In *The assessment of nutritional status of the community,* Geneva, Switzerland, 1966, World Health Organization Monograph No. 53.

Marshall JA et al: Indicators of nutritional risk in a rural elderly Hispanic and non-Hispanic white population: San Luis Valley Health and Aging Study, *J Am Diet Assoc* 99(3):315, 1999.

Mascarenhas MR, Zemel B, Stallings VA: Nutritional assessment in pediatrics, *Nutrition* 14(1):105, 1998.

Pinchcofsky-Devin G: Nutritional assessment and intervention. In Krasner D, Kane D, editors: *Wound care,* ed 2, Wayne, Penn, 1997, Health Management Publications.

Seidel HM et al: *Mosby's guide to physical assessment,* ed 4, St Louis, 1999, Mosby.

Seltzer MH et al: Instant nutritional assessment, *J Parenter Enteral Nutr* 3(3):157, 1979.

Seltzer MH et al: Instant nutritional assessment in the intensive care unit, *J Parenter Enteral Nutr* 5(1):70, 1981.

Stanek GS: Metabolic and nutritional management of the trauma patient. In Cardona VD et al, editors: *Trauma nursing: from resuscitation through rehabilitation.* ed 2, Philadelphia, 1994, W.B. Saunders.

Stotts NA, Bergstrom N: Measuring dietary intake and nutritional outcomes. In Frank-Stromborg M, Olsen SJ, editors: *Instruments for health-care research,* ed 2, Sudbury, Mass, 1997, Jones and Bartlett.

Stotts NA, Friesen L: Understanding starvation in the critically ill patient, *Heart Lung* 11(5):469, 1982.

Wipke-Tevis DD, Stotts NA: Nutrition, tissue oxygen, and healing of venous leg ulcers, *J Vasc Nurs* 16(3):48, 1998.

CHAPTER 4

Assessment, Measurement, and Evaluation: Their Pivotal Roles in Wound Healing

DIANE M. COOPER

OBJECTIVES

1. Describe four methods of categorizing wound evaluation instruments, and include two examples of each category.
2. Define each stage in the staging system for pressure ulcers.
3. Differentiate between partial and full thickness.
4. Correlate wound pathology with the most appropriate measures of wound healing.
5. Describe the procedure, advantages, and disadvantages of at least three techniques of two-dimensional and three-dimensional wound measurements.
6. Briefly describe the potential indications for using the Wound Characteristics Instrument (WCI), Pressure Ulcer Scale for Healing (PUSH) tool, and Pressure Sore Status Tool (PSST).
7. List the key macroscopic indices of healing.

BACKGROUND

"What cannot be measured, cannot be managed" (Woods et al, 1996). These words sum up current thinking about wound assessment and evaluation. As with monitoring blood pressure, temperature, and pulse rate, those attending to wounds should never observe, care for, or chart about a wound without some objective criteria by which to reflect its present status. Accurate and regular assessments of the patient's wound and the relevant systemic parameters related to healing are the critical underpinnings of any wound care plan. These assessments drive treatment decisions (e.g., type and effectiveness of treatment plan, adequacy of debridement, and frequency of dressing changes). Such wound assessments also provide the baseline data against which one could predict and subsequently evaluate the status and quality of repair that has occurred at any point in time.

Unfortunately, many clinicians do not perform regular systematic wound assessments. If assessments are performed, they are largely subjective or employ approaches that lack reliability (i.e., there is no consistency between clinicians when repeated over time) and validity (i.e., they do not measure what they propose to measure). As a result, the ability to track or monitor tissue healing objectively has been hampered greatly up to this time. The ability to retrospectively evaluate wound treatments and the outcomes of therapies has been and continues to be thwarted because objective criteria are absent from the patient record. Thus thousands of hours of sincere effort and therapies have gone unidentified and unsupported because, in general, "wounds" have been relegated either undeserving or too difficult to measure.

The responsibility for this state of affairs does not, however, lay with clinicians. Despite the fact that during their student years they are taught many complex approaches to assessing other physiologic phenomena, measuring and assessing wounds are not among them. Many reasons account for this, including the fact that most wound-healing studies occur in the laboratory where tissue culture or animal models are the focus. These studies often employ measurement approaches that are meaningless or do not transfer to the human situation. Well-designed clinical trials on humans are a more recent occurrence, and through them the dilemma of how to measure human healing accurately has emerged as a subject warranting considerable attention. This and other current trends in the health care arena may finally result in healing being taken seriously and measured in ways that are useful and can be relied upon.

Certainly some valid and reliable instruments for use in the measurement of human healing have been identified, but in many cases they have yet to be modified for easy and ready use in the everyday clinical and home care setting. Although appropriate for clinical research, any complicated method that is dependent upon technology will not be convenient or readily accessible to most clinicians (Kantor and Margolis, 1998). In other words, in the clinical situation, if a nurse or physician does not have a readily usable and available tool at hand, which they are reasonably assured will provide useful data, measurement is unlikely to occur. Because of this, often only the "serious" wound is measured and the results plotted. Other wounds are left to subjective assessments with little objective criteria supporting whether a therapy is effective or ineffective.

The changing economics of health care impose additional motivation for systematizing the measurement of wound healing. Without objective criteria of the status or progress of repair, it is difficult for some treatments to be justified and for reimbursement to be appropriately assigned. Thus pressure is being applied increasingly from both the scientific and reimbursement sides of health care to make assessment and evaluation an inherent and mandatory part of wound care.

In an effort to address some of these issues, this chapter does the following:

1. Discusses advances in current thinking regarding approaches to wound measurement based on the physiologic processes inherent to wound healing and wound type
2. Describes some of the approaches available for wound measurement based on wound type, specific wound-healing process, and setting in which the measurement is to be taken
3. Discusses several of the more generic characteristics of the open wound that clinicians most frequently describe
4. Discusses several novel concepts regarding wound assessment that take into consideration financial and emotional considerations related to healing
5. Discusses the potential effects of emerging consensus on the science of repair, algorithms for treatment, and reimbursement
6. Proposes challenges for the future regarding evaluation of healing

MEASUREMENT: PHYSIOLOGIC PROCESSES, WOUND TYPE, OR BOTH

In the past, measurement was described primarily by the type of tools available or whether the goal was to 1) predict the occurrence of a wound, 2) classify wounds, 3) measure an existing wound, or 4) assess an existing wound. Selected aspects of this categorization still apply, but in the ensuing years some evolution in wound measurement has occurred. Two or three "camps" have emerged, which focus on evaluating healing based on an understanding of the selected process one desires to measure or based on a knowledge of the predominance of these processes in the healing patterns of the specific wound type being assessed. A third approach is to assess wounds at the molecular level and subsequently categorize them.

Wound-Repair Processes

Most recent articles on wound repair point out that *healing* is not a generic term but rather a phenomena made up of multiple processes, each of which must function properly for healing to result (Robson, 1997). These processes include inflammation, epithelization, angiogenesis, granulation (or deposition of extracellular matrix), tissue formation, and contraction. Not all of these are amenable to measurement at the macroscopic level. Table 4-1 lists ways to measure selected processes. Given this approach, it is important to know the specific process being measured for the results to be of value. Measuring anything simply for the sake of obtaining a value without knowing the meaningfulness of the measure is a waste of time. One would not use a blood pressure cuff to assess temperature or a thermometer to measure blood pressure. With wound healing, there must be a focus on the distinct processes being measured while knowing their relevance to process and to this particular

TABLE 4-1 Approaches to Physical Measurement of Parameters of Healing Based on Wound Repair Processes

PROCESS	TOOL	DIMENSIONS
Granulation tissue formation (deposition of extracellular matrix)	Saline instillation	3
	Geltrate mold	3
	Kundin gauge	3
	L × W × D	3
Contraction	All of the above	3
	Acetate tracing	2
	Photograph	2
Epithelization	Ruler	2
	Acetate tracing	2

wound type. Specific measurement tools and knowledge of how to use them correctly become increasingly important. Plotting these measures over time reveals the pattern of the attribute being measured. In this way the time expended performing the measure becomes meaningful. If one is measuring contraction in a full-thickness wound and the results from a three-dimensional tool being used do not reveal a decline in the values obtained, the therapy being used or the status of the wound should be questioned. In this way, measurement is linked to outcomes and therapy follows objective criteria.

Linking Predominant Processes and Wound Types

Robson (1997) has taken the notion of wound repair processes one step further by linking them with the predominant processes occurring in selected wound types. Selected processes amenable to measurement at the macroscopic level include deposition of extracellular matrix, contraction, and epithelialization.

Pressure Ulcer. Focusing on the pressure ulcer, Robson (1997) demonstrates that it heals primarily by the "processes of angiogenesis, deposition of extracellular matrix, and contraction." This means that the pressure ulcer fills in with new tissue and contracts over time. Contraction occurs to such an extent that, when healed, only a small strip of epithelium is usually apparent where once there was a cavernous wound. The process of epithelization is minimal; new tissue formation and contraction account for most of what occurs during the healing process in this wound type. The pressure ulcer, because of its usual location on the body and the type of tissue involved, contracts a great deal and is followed by a relatively small amount of epithelial migration. Because of the size of many pressure ulcers, it would be counterproductive for them not to contract but instead to reveal a large surface area covered by a thin layer of epithelial cells prone to repeated shearing and reinjury.

When measuring a pressure ulcer, it is important to focus on the emergence of new tissue in the base of the wound and on contraction. A tool aimed at evaluating three dimensions is most appropriate. In this way one can gather information about both the amount of new tissue being produced and the amount of contraction occurring.

Venous Ulcer. The venous ulcer, another full-thickness wound, heals predominantly by epithelization and less so by contraction. In the case of a healed venous ulcer, often an outline of where the ulcer once existed can be traced on the intact skin. Unlike the pressure ulcer, this occurrence in the venous stasis ulcer reflects the relatively minimal contraction that has taken place. This difference in the predominant processes occurring between the pressure ulcer and the venous ulcer is greatly influenced by the usual position of each wound type on the body. In the case of the venous ulcer, the relative lack of depth of the tissue and the stability of the adjacent structures that hold the skin more taut influence the amount of flexibility present during the healing process, thereby reducing the extent of contraction. In the venous ulcer it becomes important for the clinician to focus on epithelization and on the various aspects of the process of epithelization.

Epithelization can be divided into keratinocyte proliferation, migration, and differentiation. Recent studies propose that migration and differentiation may be more important than proliferation, because without differentiation, cells will not move (migrate) and establish a new surface able to withstand shearing forces and other such injury. Two-dimensional approaches for measurement of the venous ulcer log the ingrowth of new epithelium as it makes its way across the surface of the wound to reestablish an intact surface. Accurately measuring the depth of this wound type is all but impossible and does not reflect an understanding of the predominant healing process taking place. Even if the depth could be measured initially, as healing occurs, the reliability of the measurement of this parameter becomes increasingly questionable.

Diabetic Foot Ulcer. The diabetic foot ulcer appears to heal by a more equal distribution of three processes: deposition of extracellular matrix, contraction, and epithelization. Both two- and three-dimensional tools can be used to assess progress in healing. A growing body of data reveals that the "typical" diabetic foot ulcer measures about 10 centimeters or less (planimetry) in area and occurs on the plantar surface of the foot (most often the forefoot). Because of its size, this wound type also does not usually allow one to accurately measure wound depth. Because of the lack of reliability, other approaches to evaluate healing must be used, the most useful of which are two-dimensional. In this wound type, acetate tracings can be used more reliably to infer both deposition of extracellular matrix and contraction.

Using this framework of linking predominant processes with wound type, one could selectively use the tools listed in Table 4-1 but choose them now based on a knowledge of the predominant processes occurring in each of these three chronic wound types. Thus use of saline instillation or a Geltrate mold to measure deposition of extracellular matrix and contraction in a pressure ulcer would be a meaningful intervention, whereas measuring depth in a venous ulcer would deny understanding of the predominant process occurring in that full-thickness wound type. Because of the limited number of clinically useful measurement tools currently available, not all wounds are amenable to a focused measurement of all processes as with the diabetic foot ulcer.

Wound Milieu

At the molecular level, some investigators would state that it is more important to know about the cellular milieu and the wound microenvironment. In knowing about the levels of various substances (e.g., endogenous growth factors, proteinases, or inhibitors of proteinases), one is able to predict whether the wound is spiraling further into chronicity or moving toward acuteness and healing. At present, most measures of such substances occur in wound-healing laboratories. It will be some time before measurement techniques can be adapted for the clinical and home care setting that will tell the clinician quickly the status of the microenvironment of the wound. Approaches such as developing a "dip stick" for the wound have been discussed, but these appear to be theoretic at this time. In the meantime, certain physiological parameters (i.e., oxygen status, tissue bacterial levels) that are known to influence the microenvironment can be measured. Greater attention to the accurate assessment of these parameters helps to support more timely healing and greater effectiveness of treatments.

EXTENT OF PATHOLOGY AND POTENTIAL FOR HEALING

It is essential to measure the physical dimensions of the wound on initial inspection and throughout the course of repair. Assessment of other parameters that reveal information about the extent of pathology and the potential for wound healing must be included also to bring as much information as possible to the selection of treatment options (Table 4-2). In the case of chronic wounds, information continues to be reported that sheds light on the mechanisms responsible for specific chronic wound types. With that information comes sup-

TABLE 4-2 Physiologic Parameters that Determine Potential for Wound Healing

PARAMETER	APPROACH
Oxygen status	Transcutaneous oxygen
Bacterial status	Tissue biopsy
Vessel compliance	Ankle-brachial index

port for focused measurement of physiologic processes, which, if compromised, could alter how a wound is treated.

Processes

Some of the processes that can be measured in a wound are tissue oxygenation, bacterial status, blood flow and vessel compliance, and extent of neuropathy. As with all diagnostic tests, however, a good understanding of the underlying pathophysiologic process is necessary to use the test appropriately and to interpret the results accurately.

Tissue Oxygenation. Tissue oxygenation is a valuable reflection of a wound's ability to heal and reflects the mechanisms underlying the specific wound type. An example of the importance of understanding the underlying specific wound type is evident in a recent paper questioning the usefulness of assessing the transcutaneous oxygen in most patients with pressure ulcers. Measurements of transcutaneous oxygen ($TcPo_2$) were taken on 61 patients enrolled in a clinical trial evaluating sequential cytokine therapy. One of the inclusion criteria for entry into the study was the presence of a minimum of 30 mm Hg of oxygen at the ulcer rim. None of the patients had an oxygen of 30 mm Hg or less, and the mean and the median on day zero was 46 mm Hg, demonstrating that "truncal pressure ulcers are neither hypoxic nor ischemic." The investigators, although acknowledging that the pressure ulcer most often arises as a result of ischemia, question the usefulness of measuring $TcPo_2$ in the "typical" truncal pressure ulcer (Ochs et al, 1999).

In other words, once the pressure is relieved, the tissue surrounding it is usually not inherently ischemic. Thus a series of interventions aimed at relieving pressure usually promotes healing of these often debilitating wounds. On the other hand, the use of $TcPo_2$ to establish the level of amputation has been written about widely and has been responsible for unnecessary repeated surgical procedures for revisions of those amputations. The measurement of $TcPo_2$ can reveal much about the perfusion to the limb and, in the case of chronic wounds, often clearly predicts whether local therapy alone will be sufficient or whether a vascular procedure is warranted to ensure restoration of structural integrity.

Numerous articles are written on this technique, although the equipment necessary to carry out the assessment of $TcPo_2$ is expensive and the ability to carry out the test with any accuracy involves a steep learning curve. Tests of $TcPo_2$ are most often conducted in a research environment or in specialized laboratories. This does not discredit the importance of this test; if properly conducted, the information that it provides can add enormously to the full assessment of the wounded patient's potential for healing. Tissue oxygenation is discussed further in Chapter 9.

Bacterial Status. Bacterial burden and oxygen status can be considered different sides of the same coin where wound chronicity is concerned. Few clinicians would argue that bacteria are not a deterrent to healing. How bacterial levels in wounds are measured, however, is an area of clinical medicine where little is formally taught in school and opinion and tradition take precedence over scientific data.

This is not a sterile environment; therefore a certain number of bacteria are inevitable in any wound, be it an acute surgical incision or a chronic open ulcer. Given an intact immune system, the human body can usually phagocytize the bacteria present and, in the case of healing, move the process forward to wound closure. When tissue bacterial levels exceed 100,000 colony forming units (cfu) per gram of tissue, however, the body's ability dwindles and infection occurs. Because of the virulence of the organism, the same is true if the *Streptococcus* species is present in even small numbers (i.e., 1 per field). With increasing resistance to antibiotics, overtreatment or nontargeted treatment is discouraged.

Knowledgeable measurement of the number of bacteria and the specific organisms present in excess is the only sound way to approach the possibility of treating bacterial invasion. This is best accomplished by performing a punch biopsy for quantitative and qualitative bacteriology (Robson and Heggers, 1991). Although not performed in every laboratory, it is a relatively simple test and one for which clinicians should encourage adoption wherever possible. Continuing the use of swab cultures of the surface of the wound, which are correlated with the actual organisms present only about 29% of the time, becomes a questionable practice and a reason for unnecessary treatment of many so-called "infections."

Blood Flow and Vessel Compliance. Doppler ultrasound can be used to measure the extent of blood flow in both the veins and the arteries. This procedure, known as the *ankle-brachial index* (ABI), assists in determining the extent of disease within the vessels and can help in the selection of appropriate treatment (e.g., whether compression would be helpful or injurious). To carry this procedure out, an appropriately sized blood pressure cuff is placed above the brachial artery and, after placing the Doppler probe over the vessel, the cuff is inflated until the sound disappears. Slowly deflating the cuff, the clinician waits for the first sound to appear. This number is recorded and referred to as the *brachial systolic pressure.* Subsequently the same procedure is carried out over the ankle, with the Doppler probe placed over the dorsalis pedis or the posterior tibialis artery. The resultant number is referred to as the *ankle systolic pressure.* Once these two numbers are obtained, the ankle reading is divided by the brachial reading. Standards vary, but normal is usually considered to be greater than 0.9, and ischemic (or indices usually seen in arterial disease) is less than 0.5. Mixed disease can range between 0.5 to 0.7 for arterial/venous and 0.7 to 0.8 for mixed venous/arterial. Because of calcification, these readings can be elevated in individuals with diabetes, arteriosclerosis, and atherosclerosis. Frequently they can be greater than 1 and are not of predictive value.

Neuropathy. Approximately 80% of individuals with diabetic foot ulcers acquire them as a result of neuropathy; however, assessment of this dimension of the potential for such wounds is seldom a routine practice. The 5.07 monofilament is very discriminating and useful in the clinical setting. This single filament is a simple and inexpensive tool that offers a quick way to determine loss of protective sensation.

Although use of this technique is increasing, lack of it in many physical examinations exemplifies the difference between the routine assessment of a patient for hypertension (by performing various checks of the vascular system) and the physical assessment of a patient with diabetes who is at risk for a soft tissue wound on the foot (by evaluating the extent of neuropathy). If the patient can easily feel the 5.07 monofilament (equivalent to 10 grams of force), he or she most likely requires no direct intervention. On the other hand, if the individual cannot feel the 5.07 monofilament, a thorough workup is in order, including assessment of gait, footwear, and so forth.

WOUND PARAMETERS VIEWED GENERICALLY

Waltz, Strickland, and Lenz (1991) define *measurement* as "the process of assigning numbers to objects to represent the kind (qualitative) and/or amount (quantitative) of an attribute or characteristic possessed by those objects." Thus in the case of wound healing, both qualitative (e.g., exudate, epithelial migration, oxygenation) and quantitative (e.g., the amount of exudate, percentage of epithelial migration, and mm Hg of oxygen) attributes can be described. This definition makes measurement of healing sound like a rather straightforward activity. In the case of wound healing, however, with the exception of a few parameters, measurement is not that easy (Bates-Jensen, 1997; Cooper, 1990c; Gilman, 1990; Robson et al, 1992; Tallman et al, 1997; van Rijswijk and the Multi-Center Leg Ulcer Study Group, 1993; van Rijswijk and Polansky, 1994; Xakellis and Frantz, 1997).

The problem in measuring wound healing is in deciding what to measure. Researchers still struggle with clear answers regarding what best reflects healing. Furthermore, there is increasing discussion about whether the same parameters should be measured in various wound types (e.g., the chronic wound vs. the acute or the diabetic foot ulcer vs. a pressure ulcer vs. the venous ulcer). It is unclear as to which attributes or constellation of attributes of healing described thus far are most predictable of positive or negative outcomes.

The longer and more intently one cares for human wounds, the more complex the concept of "wound" becomes. Because wounds are complex phenomena, there is no single approach to wound evaluation for all wound types. Actually, few pathologic conditions are evaluated with a single instrument or parameter. The more intricate the process (e.g., congestive heart failure), the more clinicians rely on several measures (e.g., radiologic examination, physical examination, pulse characteristics, treadmill tests, hematocrit) to capture accurately a full description of the extent of the condition.

In recognition of the complexity of the healing process and the uniqueness of various types of wounds, evaluation of wound status and healing, historically viewed as basic and easy to accomplish, is now being exposed for its inherent difficulty and demand for rigor. Therefore the clinician should be familiar with the strengths and limitations of several methods currently available to assess wound status. In addition, the clinician must develop an appreciation for the need to use a combination of evaluative modalities that allow one to assess wound status accurately and infer the quality of repair in relation to the normal healing trajectory.

Unfortunately, reliable and valid instruments to clinically measure the reparative process are currently lacking. Ideally, such instruments should be clinically useful, be theoretically based, and provide a mechanism that systematically and objectively monitors the status of tissue healing. This lack of valid wound healing assessment tools can be attributed to several factors; three in particular are relevant for nursing:

1. The importance of nursing interventions in supporting wound healing has been clearly articulated. Levine (1967, 1971, 1973, 1989) describes healing activities as being "central" to nursing practice. This recognition has facilitated an active approach to wound management by nurses. Before this heightened awareness of the effects of nursing interventions on wound repair, the inadequacy of wound evaluation was not fully appreciated. Nurses are now struggling with the need for terms and tools to accurately evaluate wounds and the healing process (Bates-Jensen, 1994; Bates-Jensen, 1995; Cooper, 1990a, 1990b).
2. Despite the recent explosion in scientific or basic science-related knowledge regarding the intricacies of the healing process, little agreement exists, even among noted authorities, about which indices of wound healing are most appropriate to evaluate clinically.
3. Many clinicians lack adequate knowledge regarding the science of instrument development, particularly those that are valid, reliable, and clinically useful (Waltz, Strickland, and Lenz, 1991).

Despite this set of circumstances, there are several ways to cluster currently available approaches to the evaluation of tissue repair: invasive and noninvasive instruments, research-appropriate instruments, clinically "user-friendly" approaches, instruments that provide readily usable information, and those that require skillful interpretation of the data obtained. However, the clinically based practitioner needs readily usable tools to measure the complex wound repair process. Furthermore, these tools need to provide theoretically based information so that appropriate and timely interventions can be derived. Therefore the remainder of this chapter will focus on the clinically useful yet noninvasive approaches to the assessment of wound status.

Present vs. Past in Measurement of Wound Healing

Approaches to the measurement of wound healing are divided into four categories: 1) prediction of wound development, 2) classification of existing wound, 3) measurement of existing wound, and 4) assessment of wound status (Table 4-3). This model for addressing wound measurement reveals one perspective, but clinicians have moved beyond these categories and the science of tissue repair has

TABLE 4-3 Noninvasive Instruments for Clinical Evaluation of Wound Status and Healing

CATEGORY	INSTRUMENT	GOAL
Prediction	Norton Scale	Pressure ulcer risk
	Gosnell Scale	Pressure ulcer risk
	Braden Scale	Pressure ulcer risk
	SENIC	Risk of postoperative Infection
	SWIPS-R	Risk of sternal wound infection
Classification	Red-Yellow-Black	Describes wound status
	Wound Severity Score	Describes wound status
	Wells Incisional Category	Grades incision
	Staging	Level of tissue damage
	Burn Area	Amount of skin surface damaged
Measurement	Linear	Area of wound and contraction
	Photography	Area of wound and contraction
	Wound Tracings	Area of wound and contraction
	Planimetry	Area of wound and contraction
	Kundin Wound Gauge	Area of wound and contraction
	Molds	Area of wound and contraction
	Foam	Area of wound and contraction
	Water Instillation	Area of wound and contraction
Assessment	Red-Yellow-Black	Describes surface tissue status
	Wound Assessment Inventory	Assesses inflammation
	Wound Characteristics Instrument	Assesses essential wound characteristics
	Pressure Ulcer Scale for Healing	Assesses essential wound characteristics
	Pressure Sore Status Tool	Assesses essential wound characteristics
	Sussman Wound Healing Tool	Assesses essential wound characteristics

offered new insights in approaching wound measurement. However, a brief review of the four categories follows.

Prediction of Wound Development. Instruments have been developed to determine a patient's risk for developing a wound, specifically a pressure ulcer. Such tools, including the Norton scale (Norton, 1989; Norton, McLaren, and Exton-Smith, 1962; Waterlow, Vernon, and Gilchrist, 1996), the Gosnell scale (Gosnell, 1973, 1989), and the Braden scale (Bergstrom, Demuth, and Braden, 1987b; Bergstrom et al, 1987a; Braden and Bergstrom, 1989), are discussed in detail in Chapter 11 and printed in Appendix B. Although more commonly associated with risk assessment, many of the parameters measured by these tools are pertinent to impaired wound healing and can therefore provide data regarding a patient's healing potential. A patient's risk for developing a surgical wound infection can also be anticipated with instruments as described by Haley and colleagues (1985). Sternal wound infections can be predicted using the Sternal Wound Infection Prediction Scale-R (SWIPS-R) (Hussey, Leeper, and Hynan, 1998).

Classification of Wounds. Several methods exist to classify wounds (Cuzzell, 1988; Fylling, 1989; Knighton et al, 1986; NPUAP, 1989, 1999; Percoraro and Reiber, 1990; Wells, Newsom, and Rowlands, 1983). Such classification can be done according to the involved tissue layers or the color of the wound bed. Another classification system has been devel-

TABLE 4-4 Classification System for the Diabetic Foot with or without a Wound

LEVEL	NAME	CHARACTERISTICS
0	Minimal pathology present	Patient has diabetes mellitus Sensorium intact (Semmes-Weinstein 5.07 wire detectable or vibratory perception threshold < 25 volts) ABI >0.80 mm Hg Foot deformity may be present No history of ulceration
1	Insensate foot	Above criteria with following modifications: Sensorium absent No history of diabetic neuropathic osteoarthropathy (Charcot's joint) No foot deformity
2	Insensate foot with deformity	Same as with 1 except now: Foot deformity present
3	Demonstrated pathology	Same as with 2 except now: History of neuropathic ulceration History of Charcot's joint
4a	Neuropathic ulceration	Patient has diabetes mellitus Sensorium may or may not be intact ABI >0.80 mm Hg and toe systolic pressure >45 mm Hg Foot deformity normally present Noninfected neuropathic ulceration No acute diabetic neuropathic osteoarthropathy (Charcot's joint)
4b	Acute Charcot's joint	Sensorium absent ABI and toe systolic as for 4a Noninfected neuropathic ulceration may be present Charcot's joint present
5	Infected diabetic foot	Patient has diabetes mellitus Sensorium may or may not be intact Infected wound Charcot's joint may be present
6	Dysvascular foot	Patient has diabetes mellitus Sensorium may or may not be intact ABI <0.80 mm Hg or toe systolic pressure of <45 mm Hg Ulceration may be present

Data from Armstrong DG, Lavery LA, Harkless LB: Treatment-based classification system for assessment and care of diabetic feet, *Ostomy Wound Manage* 42(8):50, 1996.

oped to classify the diabetic foot with or without a wound (Table 4-4) (Armstrong et al, 1996). Unfortunately, many inconsistencies exist in the terminology of the classification systems, creating confusion among practitioners. Validity and reliability data are also lacking for most of these tools.

Tissue layers

Staging. Shea (1975) first described a method for classifying wounds according to tissue layers, which has subsequently undergone revision (Glugla and Mulder, 1990; Knighton et al, 1986; Lavery, Armstrong, and Harkless, 1997; NPUAP,

BOX 4-1 Pressure Ulcer Staging Systems*

Stage 1

An observable, pressure-related alteration of intact skin whose indicators, as compared with the adjacent or opposite area on the body, may include changes in one of more of the following: skin temperature (warmth or coolness), tissue consistency (firm or boggy feel) and sensation (pain, itching). The ulcer appears as a defined area of persistent redness in lightly pigmented skin, whereas in darker skin tones the ulcer may appear with persistent red, blue, or purple hues.

Stage 2

Partial-thickness skin loss involving epidermis, dermis, or both. The ulcer is superficial and presents clinically as an abrasion, blister, or shallow crater.

Stage 3

Full-thickness skin loss involving damage or necrosis of subcutaneous tissue, which may extend down to but not through underlying fascia. The ulcer presents clinically as a deep crater with or without undermining of adjacent tissue.

Stage 4

Full-thickness skin loss with extensive destruction, tissue necrosis, or damage to muscle bone or supporting structures (such as tendon, joint capsule).

NOTE: If the wound involves necrotic tissue, staging cannot be confirmed until the wound base is viable.

*Intervention may prevent progression, or a stage 1 lesion may be the first clinical indicator of deep tissue damage, which is irreversible.

1989, 1999; Percoraro and Reiber, 1990; WOCN, 1992) Consequently, confusion currently exists about staging systems between institutions and clinicians. Some of these instruments are designed for specific ulcers, such as pressure or diabetic ulcers.

The Wound Ostomy Continence Nurses Society (WOCN, 1992) and the National Pressure Ulcer Advisory Panel (NPUAP, 1989, 1999) have advanced a four-stage classification scheme as described in Box 4-1. Although this system was designed for use with pressure-induced ulcers, it is frequently used with wounds of any etiology. Such use should be questioned until these instruments have undergone reliability and validity testing in wounds other than pressure ulcers.

The staging or classification systems for the diabetic foot include additional factors in conjunction with level of tissue involvement when assigning a stage. Factors included in these classification systems are history of previous ulceration, presence of bony deformity, presence and severity of ischemia, and presence and severity of infection (Tables 4-5 and 4-6).

Accurate staging requires knowledge of the anatomy of skin and deeper tissue layers, the ability to recognize these tissues, and the ability to differentiate between them. Careful evaluation of the wound bed facilitates accurate staging. Staging wounds is a complex skill that takes time to develop. It is often easier, more accurate, and more reliable for novice clinicians to describe the wound according to other macroscopic observations while learning to recognize the specific tissue layers delineated in the pressure ulcer staging system.

Although staging terms describe the type of tissue involved, additional important wound characteristics are not revealed, such as depth of the wound, topography of the wound, exudate, condition of the wound bed, and condition of the surrounding skin. Furthermore, because the staging system is based on recognition of the predominant wound bed tissue such as dermis, epidermis, muscle, or tendon, a wound that is healing optimally may manifest tissue that is difficult to classify. Therefore it is unclear how to stage a healing wound where granulation tissue has filled the wound bed. Also, because the staging system is

TABLE 4-5 Wagner Grading System for Vascular Wounds on Extremities

GRADE	CHARACTERISTICS
0	Preulcerative lesion Healed ulcers Presence of bony deformity
1	Superficial ulcer without subcutaneous tissue involvement
2	Penetration through the subcutaneous tissue; may expose bone, tendon, ligament, or joint capsule
3	Osteitis, abscess, or osteomyelitis
4	Gangrene of digit
5	Gangrene of foot requiring disarticulation

From Wagner FW: The dysvascular foot: a system for diagnosis and treatment, *Foot Ankle* 2:64, 1981.

TABLE 4-6 University of Texas Health Sciences Center, San Antonio, Diabetic Wound Classification System

STAGE	GRADE 0	GRADE I	GRADE II	GRADE III
A	Preulcerative or post-ulcerative lesion completely healed	Superficial wound, not involving tendon, capsule or bone	Wound penetrating to tendon or capsule	Wound penetrating to bone or joint
B	Preulcerative or post-ulcerative lesion completely epithelialized with infection	Superfical wound, not involving tendon, capsule or bone with infection	Wound penetrating to tendon or capsule with infection	Wound penetrating to bone or joint with infection
C	Preulcerative or post-ulcerative lesion completely epithelialized with ischemia	Superficial wound, not involving tendon, capsule or bone with ischemia	Wound penetrating to tendon or capsule with ischemia	Wound penetrating to bone or joint with ischemia
D	Preulcerative or post-ulcerative lesion completely epithelialized with infection and ischemia	Superficial wound, not involving tendon, capsule or bone with infection and ischemia	Wound penetrating to tendon or capsule with infection and ischemia	Wound penetrating to bone or joint with infection and ischemia

From Lavery LA, Armstrong DG, Harkless LB: Classification of diabetic foot ulcerations, *J Foot Ankle Surg* 35(6):528, 1996.

based on the ability to assess the type of tissue in the wound bed, a wound bed covered with necrotic tissue cannot be accurately staged. In such situations, staging must be deferred. Despite these flaws, staging tissue layers provide 1) increased uniformity of language and 2) a beginning basis for evaluation of protocols. Nurses need to adopt agreed-upon terms and discontinue use of many differing categories. Reliability and validity studies are also needed for these staging systems. The practice of reverse staging where the wound is described as progressing from a stage 3 to a stage 2 to a stage 1 is incorrect. The staging system is to be used to describe the wound in its most severe state, and once accurately described, these descriptor levels endure, even in the presence of healing. Therefore a stage 3 pressure ulcer that appears to be granulating and resurfacing is described as a healing stage 3 pressure ulcer.

Partial thickness versus full thickness. The terms *partial thickness* and *full thickness* can also be used to describe the extent of tissue damage. These terms pertain strictly to the amount of true skin injured. For example, a full-thickness wound indicates that the epidermis and dermis into the subcutaneous tissue or beyond have been damaged; tissue loss extends below the dermis (Plate 2). Wound repair then will occur by neovascularization, fibroplasia, contraction, and then epithelial migration from the wound edges. A partial-thickness wound is confined to the skin layers; damage does not penetrate below the dermis and may be limited to the epidermal layers only. These wounds heal primarily by reepithelialization (Plate 1).

Unfortunately, *partial thickness* and *full thickness* are imprecise terms when describing the specific type of tissue present in the wound bed and thus the extent of the wound. For example, a full-thickness wound may expose subcutaneous tissue, muscle, tendon, or bone. Furthermore these terms fail to convey the depth of the wound, the condition of the surrounding skin, presence of exudate, and the topography. Partial-thickness and full-thickness terminology is more commonly used in burn therapy (see Chapter 10).

Color. The Red-Yellow-Black (RYB) (Cuzzell, 1988) color concept is another suggested wound classification method. This technique directs the clinician to assess the surface of the open wound (regardless of origin) and to categorize it as falling within one of the three color categories. The red wound is viewed as healthy, whereas the black wound is worrisome. The yellow wound lies somewhere in between, with the goal of therapy being the removal of the yellow surface and exposure of the underlying healthy red tissue. This system was developed originally by industry and has not undergone testing for reliability and validity.

Although the system is useful in that it offers clinicians clear categories by which to classify wounds, directs them to look at wounds more closely, and focuses them toward a system of treatment, it also has the potential of oversimplifying the complexity of the healing process. To encourage clinicians to think that healing can be evaluated by a single variable is, in many ways, to trivialize the healing process.

Additionally, because of the ease with which clinicians can assess wounds using this system, it erroneously allows some to believe they have fully assessed a wound as a result of making a single observation. The conclusion that all red wounds are healthy should be rejected; healthy and unhealthy shades of red exist. The RYB system should not be considered to be an adequate evaluation of the status of a wound. However, incorporation of the color concept into a system where other essential manifestations of wound healing are present could be of value in wound assessment.

Measurement of Wounds. Many current approaches to wound evaluation commonly focus on wound measurement and may involve either two-dimensional or three-dimensional measurements. Each approach has its own advantages and disadvantages; some are more realistic in the laboratory setting than in the clinical setting (Gilman, 1990; Harding, 1995).

Two-dimensional measurement. In clinical practice, the two-dimensional measurement is one of the simplest and most widely used approaches to wound measurement. Linear measurements (e.g., length and width), wound tracings, and wound photographs are examples of commonly used two-dimensional measurements. Unfortunately, these types of measurements used in isolation do not provide information about the depth of a wound. Planimetry may be used with wound tracings or wound photographs to more precisely document the surface area of shallow wounds and wounds with depth. Software programs have been developed specifically for use in rapidly translating a wound perimeter tracing into the wound area.

Planimetry. Wound surface area can be calculated by multiplying length times width (L X W). However, this calculation overestimates the actual wound surface area because it is based on a rectangle. Consequently, more accurate calculations of the wound surface area can be obtained from planimetry. Planimetry is a method in which the complete graph squares that are contained within a wound tracing or photograph on metric graph paper are counted. This technique involves measuring *only* the area that falls within the wound perimeter. Thus an area calculated using planimetry is expressed in square centimeters (cm^2) and would always be less than the area determined by multiplying length and width. Planimetry is particularly useful for large or irregularly shaped wounds (Liskay, Mion, and Davis, 1993). Counting graph squares that fall within the area of the wound is an inexpensive but time-consuming portable technique that has demonstrated high reliability (Ferrell, Artinian, and Sessing, 1995). Computer-aided planimeters have expedited the tedious manual process. Such technology is understandably expensive, and the process is still somewhat time consuming, requiring a protracted learning curve (Harding, 1995).

Either approach for planimetry (manual or computer assisted), however precise, hardly seems realistic for use by the bedside clinician. Although planimetry is generally accurate when used on flat wounds, it ceases to provide a complete picture of the wound in the case of full-thickness or deep wounds. Because of the time and precision involved, it is not surprising that researchers have employed this method more than practicing clinicians.

Linear measurements. Increasingly, clinicians have begun to routinely record the size of the wound or extent of tissue injury by measuring the involved area. Although in most cases these measurements are imprecise, linear measurements provide an objective basis for evaluating the overall dimensions of a wound. Paper or plastic rulers can be used and are commercially available. Measurements, recorded in centimeters or millimeters, should describe the length and width of an open wound and the extent of ecchymosis or erythema surrounding the wound. Such measurements are inexpensive, readily available, and easily accomplished by most clinicians and cause little discomfort to the patient.

To strengthen the value and accuracy of linear measurements, one should take measurements in a consistent manner and record them in such a way that communicates the specific aspects of the wound used as landmarks. For example, numerical readings may be accompanied by arrows to clearly indicate the direction of the measurements relative to the position of the wound on the body; north-south measurements can be indicated by an arrow drawn vertically (↑), and measurements for the east-west axis can be depicted by horizontal arrows (→). Such an approach decreases confusion and allows the measurement to be repeated with some degree of consistency.

Although linear measurements provide greater objectivity than subjective appraisals of wound size, they are problematic (Gorin et al, 1996). Because the perimeter of open wounds is often irregular, it can be difficult to determine the best position on the wound surface from which to obtain the readings. Furthermore, two-dimensional measurements are unable to account for variations in irregular wounds or wounds with depth and are essentially meaningless. The rigor with which the measurement is obtained influences the results (Langemo et al, 1998), and the reliability of such measures is low. However, when repeated over time, linear measurements of wounds without depth provide gross information regarding the trend of the wound-repair process.

Wound tracings. Another approach to open wound measurement is tracing the external surface or perimeter of the wound using transparent paper or transparent acetate and a marking pen. This approach received attention as early as 1937 when Lecomte du Nouy (1937), using this technique, defined the "index of cicatrization" (i.e., the index of scar tissue formation) after taking serial tracings of hundreds of wounds. As with rulers, the use of a transparent medium to record the external shape of the wound is inexpensive and easily accomplished and produces minimal discomfort for the patient. Both tracing and linear appraisal of a wound should be obtained at the time of the dressing change.

Numerous wound-care products are now packaged in transparent wrappings, making such tracing material readily accessible. Some manufacturers have incorporated rulers or concentric circles on their packaging to facilitate both tracings and linear measurements. The sterile side of such packaging can be placed over the wound, and the perimeter can be easily traced.

Although obtaining such measurements is certainly better than not, the consistency with which these measurements are taken affects reliability of the measurements. Some wounds may be difficult to trace because of their position on the body, and measurements obtained with the patient lying in different positions or by the use of different landmarks cannot be considered reliable. Clinicians may experience difficulty in determining what constitutes the wound edge. Most often the tracing should be taken where the "raw" tissue meets the intact skin.

Wound tracings can be used to generate two-dimensional measurements but can also be used to calculate the surface area of the wound. Unfortunately, when Bohannon and Pfaller (1983) studied the practicality and accuracy of various techniques to determine the area of a wound, they concluded that "the greatest source of error in tracing wounds may be in the tracing itself rather than the determination of the area traced." Therefore it is imperative to use rigor and precision when tracing the wound to increase the reliability of the measures.

More often, however, wound tracings are used as a pattern against which subsequent tracings can be compared; this is best accomplished if each pattern is dated. In this way, multiple clinicians have a rough, visual estimate of the size of the external wound opening and can determine if the size or shape of the wound is changing.

Wound photography. Wound photographs can be used with linear measurements to provide a two-dimensional approach that facilitates both wound measurement and wound assessment. Whether pictures of a wound are taken with a conventional camera or with a Polaroid, the resulting image provides a template against which changes in wound status can be observed and compared. The use of such pictures can reveal much about the course of healing over time: the relative size of the wound, the color of the tissue, the amount of exudate, and the condition of the surrounding skin. Serial photographs should be taken from the same distance, or even better from the same f-stop on the camera so that changes in the course of healing become apparent. In this way changes can be evaluated quickly, even by clinicians who are less familiar with the patient.

Photographs that can be viewed in a timely manner are superior to those that require a lapse before developing. However, the quality of the image from a Polaroid camera may not be ideal. Additionally, the camera may not adequately capture the three-dimensional wound, thus leaving the clinician in doubt about the depth of the wound, the character of the exudate, or the topography of the wound.

The color of tissue within the wound or exudate on the surface of the wound can also be greatly modified as a consequence of the color image processing, resolution, and calibration (Berriss and Sangwine, 1997). It is not unusual for a wound photograph to reflect an image vastly different in color from that of the actual wound. For this and other reasons, wound photographs, although helpful in some situations, may not prove reliable. Additionally, in most clinical settings, an expensive camera and a person skilled in its use may not be a realistic approach for bedside clinicians.

Stereophotogrammetry. By combining the video camera and a software package, the wound image can be captured on videotape and the image downloaded to a computer. Using a computer mouse, the length, width, and area of the wound is traced, and the software program calculates the wound area, length, and width. Specific areas of interest such as the necrotic tissue can also be calculated by tracing the area. Color images of wound can be stored, printed, and monitored sequentially for changes. Stereophotogrammetry is noninvasive and has a high reliability (Bulstrode, Goode, and Scott, 1986; Frantz and Johnson, 1992). In one study of nursing students and staff nurses, stereophotogrammetry was the most accurate and least biased for two-dimensional wound measurements (Langemo et al, 1998).

Three-dimensional measurement. Two-dimensional measurements are relatively simple to use; however, they do not accurately describe wounds with depth. Accurate measurement of full-thickness wounds requires a three-dimensional approach. Such approaches include linear measurements, wound molds, foam dressings, and fluid instillation.

Linear measurements. To obtain the three dimensions of the wound, one must measure the depth of the wound in addition to the length and width. The most common method of obtaining wound depth is by insertion of a cotton-tipped applicator into the wound bed and placement of a mark on the applicator to indicate the level of the skin. This mark is often simply the examiner's thumb and index finger, but it may also be an ink mark. The cotton-tipped applicator is then held against a metric ruler to determine the depth of the wound. Although this technique is inherently imprecise (particularly with irregularly shaped wound beds), serial measurements provide a trend of measurements that one can only hope will reflect a tendency toward healing.

Aware of the lack of clinically useful ways to measure "irregular structures on the human body with or without depth," Kundin (1985, 1989) developed the Kundin Wound Gauge (Figure 4-1). This instrument, composed of three rulers placed at right angles, provides the clinician with a user-friendly device by which the length, width, and

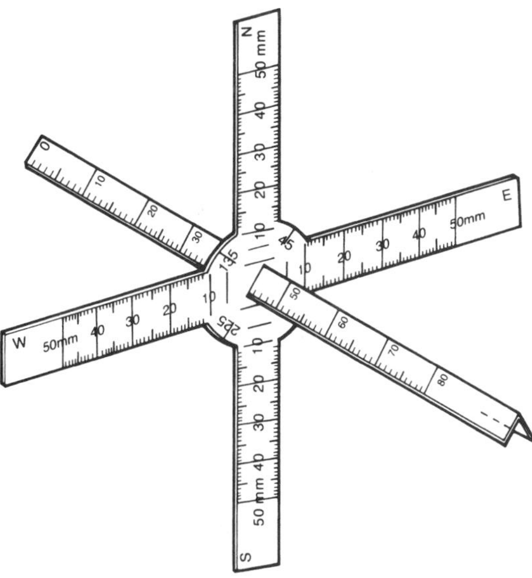

Figure 4-1 Kundin Wound Gauge. (Courtesy Pacific Technologies and Development Corporation, San Mateo, Calif.)

depth (in the case of "crater" wounds) of the wound is measured. By then using a specific mathematic formula or formulas, one can ascertain the area of a surface lesion or the volume of wounds with depth.

Although clinically useful, this instrument presents problems with reliability when used by different clinicians. To obtain and compare serial measures, it is essential that the instrument be consistently placed over the same location of the open wound bed. Such placement can be challenging in the presence of a wound with a greatly irregular base or when the readings are being collected by different clinicians. Furthermore, if it is used correctly, attempts to account for the extent of undermining in a pressure ulcer, for example, must be consistent between clinicians.

Thomas and Wysocki (1990) demonstrated that, although the Kundin gauge was equally reliable to photographs and acetate tracings in the evaluation of small wounds, it consistently produced data that indicated underestimation of wound area in larger and irregularly shaped wounds. Unfortunately, it is these wounds that are most in need of accurate measurement. These investigators showed that when photographs, acetate tracings, and the Kundin gauge were compared, the three measurements were highly correlated ($r = 0.93$), although correlation between acetate and photographs were the highest ($r = 0.99$). However, Thomas and Wysocki's findings were obtained by using two nurses specifically trained to use these instruments and to identify wound landmarks. The reliability of such measurement devices when used by multiple nurses with varying skill levels is not known but would probably be lower.

An additional concern with the use of the wound gauge as a clinical measurement tool is cost. Each gauge costs approximately $2.00 and should not be reused. In these times of cost containment, a financial outlay of this magnitude to monitor a patient's wound over time may be unacceptable.

Wound molds. In 1966, Pories and colleagues reported the use of molds to assess the volume of open wounds. Studying eight servicemen undergoing excision of pilonidal cysts, the investigators instilled alginate (a substance used to make dental impressions) into the open wounds each day after surgery to monitor the course of healing. Once placed in the wound, the initially liquid medium thickens and can then be removed easily from the wound and subsequently placed in a liquid beaker (or weighed). By calculating the amount of fluid displaced (or the actual weight) over a series of molds, the status of the wound repair process can be assessed.

Other investigators have used this wound mold approach to evaluate healing, particularly in pressure ulcers (Resch et al, 1988). The ability of several trained individuals to instill this material in the same manner has been reported to be high. Standard deviations in one report, however, ranged between 5% and 16% when three groups of hospital staff repeatedly measured a set of six different wound models. The molds did, however, perform better than saline instillation where deviations of 9% to 18% of the actual volume occurred. The authors pointed out that, in addition to being difficult to perform, molding was a time-consuming process (Plassmann, 1994).

Reports indicate that placement of molding medium in wounds does not appear to injure granulating wounds, nor has it been reported to cause patient discomfort. Additionally, properly stored wound molds (in air-sealed bags to avoid desiccation and wrapped in clorox-moistened gauze to prevent bacterial growth) provide some "permanence" of the reflection of the course of healing, a quality that few other approaches to wound evaluation possess. Realistically, however, it is difficult to imagine that the instillation of the mold medium would be practical in most clinical settings as an everyday method of evaluating wounds by bedside clinicians.

Structured light. This noninvasive approach to three-dimensional measurement is based on structured light. The wound is illuminated with a set of parallel lights via a projector. A camera connected to a computer then picks up the image. Integrating the intersecting points, the computer produces a three-dimensional representation by triangulation. In the same study cited previously, this approach produced more reliable results than either fluid instillation or wound molds with a standard deviation of 3% to 15%. This method is, however, "not applicable for undermined, very deep and very large wounds." It is also costly and, at this point, not useful in the everyday clinical setting (Plassmann, 1994).

Foam dressings. More recently, various dressing materials (e.g., silicone elastomer, Silastic) that serve not only to provide local wound care therapy but also to provide information about progress in healing have been described (Gledhill and Waterfall, 1983; Hughes, 1983; Wood, Williams, and Hughes, 1977). These dressings have not been approved for use in the United States. This approach should afford another source of information about wound volume. If these dressings could be retained and reviewed serially, then like the alginate molds they could provide more objective evidence of the course of the healing process. In addition to ease of application, these materials could be particularly beneficial when monitoring wound healing in patients in the community.

Fluid instillation. Another way to measure wound volume, although imprecise, is to instill a known quantity of solution (such as sterile water or saline) into the wound cavity, allowing it to fill to the perimeter. The fluid is then extracted by syringe or suction, and the amount is recorded. When carried out serially, with the patient in the same position each time that the measurement is taken, changes in the size of the wound cavity can be determined. This approach appears more feasible in the clinical setting than the use of alginate molds. Problems can arise, however, in situations where, because of the position of the wound on the body, instillation and brief retention of the fluid in the wound crater are difficult to accomplish.

Summary. Several two- and three-dimensional methods for wound measurement exist. Although linear measurements are the most commonly employed clinically, reliability is lacking. Because such measurements are frequently used as indices of progression in healing or as reflections of the effectiveness of a particular therapy, caution should be exercised in accepting all readings as accurate. Clinicians must use accuracy and precision when obtaining measurements. Furthermore, wound landmarks from which the measurements are obtained must be clearly documented and communicated to subsequent caregivers.

In addition to measurement of the length, width, and depth of wounds, there are several techniques that can be used to calculate the area of the wound. Such calculations can be done from linear measurements or wound photographs with linear measurements or using wound molds, foam dressings, or fluid instillation. Acetate tracings of the wound perimeter are reportedly more accurate in determining actual wound area than either wound photographs or calculations with the Kundin three-dimensional wound gauge.

Assessment of Wound Status. Although most clinicians can easily identify a healed or unhealed wound, many have difficulty delineating the subtle changes within a wound that indicate that healing is occurring (the status of the wound). Detailing the minute changes that occur in the healing process has been viewed as being of marginal importance. However, with the changes in health care and an increasing number of chronic wounds, knowledge of macroscopic changes in a wound becomes more valued. The ability to assess the status of the wound over time and to monitor its progress relative to known markers becomes desirable. Assessment of wound status can serve as a barometer of the wound's health status (Cooper, 1990d). These markers, however, are not randomly selected but are theory-based macroscopic reflections of the wound. Over time the collection of numerous wound status reports can serve to reveal the actual course of healing. Instruments currently used for assessment of wound status can be classified according to those that assess closed wounds and open wounds.

Closed wounds. Two instruments are designed specifically to assess incisional wounds or wounds closed by primary intention: the ASEPSIS (Byrne, Napier, and Cuschieri, 1988; Wilson et al, 1986) and the Wound Assessment Inventory (WAI) (Holden-Lund, 1988). When measures are repeated over time, a trend in the healing process is revealed. Each of these approaches to wound assessment has undergone varying degrees of testing for reliability and validity and should be thoroughly evaluated before use with patients.

Open wounds. Four instruments have been described for use in the assessment of open wounds or wounds healing by secondary intention: the Wound Characteristics Instrument (WCI) (Cooper, 1990e), the Pressure Sore Status Tool (PSST) (Bates-Jensen, 1994; Bates-Jensen, Vredevoe, and Brecht, 1992), the Pressure Ulcer Scale for Healing (PUSH) (NPUAP, 1998), and the Sussman Wound Healing Tool (SWHT) (Sussman and Swanson, 1997). Not all of these instruments report reliability and validity scores. Two instruments, the PUSH and PSST, are specific to the pressure ulcer. The WCI asks the clinician to assess the essential characteristics of postsurgical wounds not at a single point in time, but serially so that trends and patterns in the status of the wound may be identified.

Wound Characteristics Instrument. The WCI (Cooper, 1990e, 1991), a criterion-referenced measurement, is a 17-item rating scale designed for use by clinicians evaluating the macroscopic (visible to the naked eye) characteristics of open, soft tissue, postsurgical wounds. Two sample items from the WCI are provided in Figure 4-2. In addition to encouraging the use of a common vocabulary among clinicians when open wounds are being discussed, this instrument directs the clinician to complete a wound assessment in a systematic manner. A systematic and consistent wound evaluation technique is essential to capture the subtle changes within a wound that can be otherwise easily overlooked.

The clinician using the WCI is directed to assess essential components or generic characteristics within the specific regions of the wound. For example, Plates 4 and 5 demonstrate the contrast in the presence of epithelial tissue at the rim of two wounds. These observations are then ranked along a continuum from the optimal to the worst manifestations of that state.

The WCI underwent reliability testing and both content and construct validity testing. Content validity scores by surgeon experts indicated a high level of agreement regarding the structural and generic characteristics of the open wound with an average congruency percentage at 90%. Construct validity and reliability testing by registered nurses indicated a range of difficulty scores among the items. Before use in the clinical setting,

Instructions: Circle the ONE NUMBER that best approximates your assessment of the wound:

Tissue-Floor of the Wound

Floor-tissue shine

(5)	(4)	(3)	(2)	(1)
(Glistening)		(Semi-glossy)		(Dull)

Floor-tissue moisture

(1)	(2)	(3)	(4)	(5)
(Dry)		(Moist)		(Wet)

Floor-tissue color

(5)	(4)	(3)	(2)	(1)
(Beefy red)		(Pink)		(Yellowish-brown)

Edge or Rim of the Wound (position of the wound where the open tissue meets the normal hair bearing skin)

Extension of external skin over the wound

(5)	(4)	(3)	(2)	(1)
(Appropriate to wound and moving inward)		(Undercut)	(Gnarled)	(No new growth apparent)

Color of majority of edge of the wound

(5)	(4)	(3)	(2)	(1)
(Dull, pale pink)				(No edge apparent)

Amount of new edge surrounding the wound

(=75% around the edge)	(5)
(>50%, but <75% around the edge)	(4)
(>25%, but <50% around the edge)	(3)
(Between 1% and 25% around the edge)	(2)
(No new edge apparent)	(1)

Figure 4-2 Two sample items from the Wound Characteristics Instrument. (Copyright Diane M. Cooper, 1990.)

the instrument requires further assessment of its validity and reliability.

Pressure Sore Status Tool. The PSST is a paper-and-pencil test that addresses 15 macroscopic wound characteristics (Figure 4-3). Specific definitions are provided for each characteristic. Individual items are scored on a modified Likert scale (1 = best for that characteristic; 5 = worst). Individual items are summed, and a total score is calculated, which provides a measure of overall wound status. The range of scores is from 13 to 65.

A benefit of the PSST is that it allows for tracking over time of each item or wound characteristic as well as the total score. Thus each item can be monitored for improvement or deterioration. In this way, the PSST can be used to evaluate the effectiveness of specific interventions or short-term outcomes, such as to manage wound infection or to debride the wound (Bates-Jensen, 1995).

The mean overall content validity of the PSST with a nine-member expert judge panel was 0.91. The mean interrater reliability coefficient was 0.915 when used with wound care specialists in an acute care hospital; intrarater reliability was 0.975. The interrater reliability of the PSST in long-term care with LPNs, RNs and PTs who had no experience in wound care yielded a mean of 0.78; intrarater reliability for this group was 0.89, and agreement with an expert was 0.82 (Bates-Jensen, 1995; Bates-Jensen, Vredevoe, and Brecht, 1992).

Pressure Ulcer Healing Scale (PUSH). The PUSH was developed by the NPUAP (Stotts and Rodeheaver, 1997) to monitor pressure ulcer healing overtime. Typical of the instrument-development process, the first draft of PUSH has been revised (Version 3.0) (Figure 4-4). The PUSH tool is designed to monitor three critical parameters that are considered the most indicative of healing: size (length and width), exudate, and tissue type. Each parameter has at least four sublevels. The subscore for each parameter is totaled, and the total score is calculated and ranges from 0 to 17. Assessment of additional parameters remains essential to determine the specific plans for the patient and the treatment plan (NPUAP, 1999). Reliability and validity for this instrument as yet is unavailable, although publication of current findings is planned (Stotts, 1999; Stotts and Rodeheaver, 1997; Thomas et al, 1997).

Sussman Wound Healing Tool. The SWHT is an instrument developed to track physical therapy technologies used for wound healing (Sussman and Swanson, 1997). This device contains 10 variables that address wound attributes and 9 variables that address wound dimensions and extent of tissue damage. Reliability and validity measures for the SWHT have not been reported (Sussman and Bates-Jensen, 1998; Sussman and Swanson, 1997).

Summary of tools. Several tools are available to enable the clinician to predict the development of wounds, classify existing wounds, measure existing wounds, and assess the status of a wound. Unfortunately, these methods have undergone varying degrees of rigorous testing and vary in reliability and validity. When selecting a tool, the clinician must first determine the parameters to be assessed. Once this determination is made, a decision can be made regarding which tool is most appropriate for the situation. When considering appropriateness, it is important to recall reliability and validity measures. In addition, reliability and validity are never "established" for any measuring device or instrument (Fawcett, 1999). Therefore the clinician should select a tool in which the reliability and validity has been supported previously in a similar population and then assess its reliability for the specific application before assuming that the scores generated are valid (Strickland, 1995). The clinician must keep in mind that it is unrealistic to expect one instrument to be an adequate gauge of wound status. One tool will not capture all the information necessary to adequately describe and evaluate the dynamic nature of a wound. For example, wounds that are classified as stage 3, or full thickness, often require additional descriptions of wound parameters. Such macroscopic indices of healing are discussed in the next section.

MACROSCOPIC INDICES OF HEALING

Several wound parameters that serve as a macroscopic index of healing can be assessed clinically with the naked eye (Box 4-2, p. 76). The parameters that are presented are those that 1) are based on current understanding of wound-healing physiology, 2) have a range of manifestations, and 3) have the potential of being manipulated by the clinician. Each parameter

(Text continued on p. 76)

PRESSURE SORE STATUS TOOL

Instructions for use

General guidelines:

Fill out the attached rating sheet to assess a pressure sore's status after reading the definitions and methods of assessment described below. Evaluate once a week and whenever a change occurs in the wound. Rate according to each item by picking the response that best describes the wound and entering that score in the item score column for the appropriate date. When you have rated the pressure sore on all items, determine the total score by adding together the 13 item scores. The *higher* the total score, the more severe the pressure sore status. Plot total score on the Pressure Sore Status Continuum to determine progress.

Specific instructions:

1. SIZE: Use ruler to measure the longest and widest aspect of the wound surface in centimeters; multiply length × width.

2. DEPTH: Pick the depth, thickness, most appropriate to the wound using these additional descriptions:

1 = Tissues damaged but no break in skin surface.
2 = Superficial, abrasion, blister, or shallow crater. Even with, and/or elevated above, skin surface (e.g., hyperplasia).
3 = Deep crater with or without undermining of adjacent tissue.
4 = Visualization of tissue layers not possible due to necrosis.
5 = Supporting structures include tendon, joint capsule.

3. EDGES: Use this guide:

Indistinct, diffuse	=	Unable to clearly distinguish wound outline.
Attached	=	Even or flush with wound base; *no* sides or walls present; flat.
Not attached	=	Sides or walls *are* present; floor or base of wound is deeper than edge.
Rolled under, thickened	=	Soft to firm and flexible to touch.
Hyperkeratosis	=	Callous-like tissue formation around wound and at edges.
Fibrotic, scarred	=	Hard, rigid to touch.

4. UNDERMINING: Assess by inserting a cotton-tipped applicator under the wound edge; advance it as far as it will go without using undue force; raise the tip of the applicator so it may be seen or felt on the surface of the skin; mark the surface with a pen; measure the distance from the mark on the skin to the edge of the wound. Continue process around the wound. Then use a transparent metric measuring guide with concentric circles divided into four (25%) pie-shaped quadrants to help determine percent of wound involved.

5. NECROTIC TISSUE TYPE: Pick the type of necrotic tissue that is *predominant* in the wound according to color, consistency, and adherence using this guide:

White/gray, nonviable tissue	=	May appear prior to wound opening; skin surface is white or gray.
Nonadherent, yellow slough	=	Thin, mucinous substance; scatterd throughout wound bed; easily separated from wound tissue.
Loosely adherent, yellow slough	=	Thick, stringy, clumps of debris; attached to wound tissue.
Adherent, soft, black eschar	=	Soggy tissue; strongly attached to tissue in center or base of wound.
Firmly adherent, hard/black eschar	=	Firm, crusty tissue; strongly attached to wound base *and* edges (like a hard scab).

6. NECROTIC TISSUE AMOUNT: Use a transparent metric measuring guide with concentric circles divided into four (25%) pie-shaped quadrants to help determine percent of wound involved.

7. EXUDATE TYPE: Some dressings interact with wound drainage to produce a gel or trap liquid. Before assessing exudate type, gently cleanse wound with normal saline or water. Pick the exudate type that is *predominant* in the wound according to color and consistency, using this guide:

Bloody	=	Thin, bright red.
Serosanguineous	=	Thin, watery, pale red to pink.
Serous	=	Thin, watery, clear.
Purulent	=	Thin or thick, opaque tan to yellow.
Foul purulent	=	Thick, opaque yellow to green with offensive odor.

Figure 4-3 Pressure Sore Status Tool (PSST). (Copyright Barbara Bates-Jensen, 1990.)

PRESSURE SORE STATUS TOOL (continued)

Instructions for use

8. **EXUDATE AMOUNT:** Use a transparent metric measuring guide with concentric circles divided into four (25%) pie-shaped quadrants to determine percent of dressing involved with exudate. Use this guide:

None	=	Wound tissues dry.
Scant	=	Wound tissues moist; no measurable exudate.
Small	=	Wound tissues wet; moisture evenly distributed in wound; drainage involves ≤25% of dressing.
Moderate	=	Wound tissues saturated; drainage may or may not be evenly distributed in wound; drainage involves >25% to ≤75% of dressing.
Large	=	Wound tissues bathed in fluid; drainage freely expressed; may or may not be evenly distributed in wound; drainage involves >75% of dressing.

9. **SKIN COLOR SURROUNDING WOUND:** Assess tissues within 4 cm of wound edge. Dark-skinned persons show the colors "bright red" and "dark red" as a deepening of normal ethnic skin color or a purple hue. As healing occurs in dark-skinned persons, the new skin is pink and may never darken.

10. **PERIPHERAL TISSUE EDEMA:** Assess tissues within 4 cm of wound edge. Nonpitting edema appears as skin that is shiny and taut. Identify pitting edema by firmly pressing a finger down into the tissues and waiting for 5 seconds; on release of pressure, tissues fail to resume previous position and an indentation appears. Crepitus is accumulation of air or gas in tissues. Use a transparent metric measuring guide to determine how far edema extends beyond wound.

11. **PERIPHERAL TISSUE INDURATION:** Assess tissues within 4 cm of wound edge. Induration is abnormal firmness of tissues with margins. Assess by gently pinching the tissues. Induration results in an inability to pinch the tissues. Use a transparent metric measuring guide with concentric circles divided into four (25%) pie-shaped quadrants to determine percent of wound and area involved.

12. **GRANULATION TISSUE:** Granulation tissue is the growth of small blood vessels and connective tissue to fill in full-thickness wounds. Tissue is healthy when bright, beefy red, shiny and granular with a velvety appearance. Poor vascular supply appears as pale pink or blanched to dull, dusky red color.

13. **EPITHELIALIZATION:** Epithelialization is the process of epidermal resurfacing and appears as pink or red skin. In partial-thickness wounds it occurs throughout the wound bed as well as from the wound edges. In full-thickness wounds it can occur from the edges only. Use a transparent metric measuring guide with concentric circles divided into four (25%) pie-shaped quadrants to help determine percent of wound involved and to measure the distance the epithelial tissue extends into the wound.

Figure 4-3, cont'd.

PRESSURE SORE STATUS TOOL (continued)

NAME: ______________________________

Complete the rating sheet to assess pressure sore status. Evaluate each item by picking the response that best describes the wound and entering the score in the item score column for the appropriate date.

LOCATION: Anatomic site. Circle, identify right **(R)** or left **(L)** and use "**X**" to mark site on body diagrams:

_________ Sacrum & coccyx _________ Lateral ankle
_________ Trochanter _________ Medial ankle
_________ Ischial tuberosity _________ Heel _________ Other site

SHAPE: Overall wound pattern; assess by observing perimeter and depth. Circle and *date* appropriate description:

_________ Irregular _________ Linear or elongated
_________ Round/oval _________ Bowl/boat
_________ Square/rectangle _________ Butterfly _________ Other shape

Item	Assessment	Date	Date	Date
		Score	Score	Score
1. SIZE	1 = Length × width <4 sq cm 2 = Length × width 4-16 sq cm 3 = Length × width 16.1-36 sq cm 4 = Length × width 36.1-80 sq cm 5 = Length × width >80 sq cm			
2. DEPTH	1 = Nonblanchable erythema on intact skin 2 = Partial-thickness skin loss involving epidermis &/or dermis 3 = Full-thickness skin loss involving damage or necrosis of subcutaneous tissue; may extend down to but not through underlying fascia; &/or mixed partial- & full-thickness &/or tissue layers obscured by granulation tissue 4 = Obscured by necrosis 5 = Full-thickness skin loss with extensive destruction, tissue necrosis, or damage to muscle, bone, or supporting structures			
3. EDGES	1 = Indistinct, diffuse, none clearly visible 2 = Distinct, outline clearly visible, attached, even with wound base 3 = Well defined, not attached to wound base 4 = Well defined, not attached to base, rolled under, thickened 5 = Well defined, fibrotic, scarred or hyperkeratotic			
4. UNDERMINING	1 = Undermining <2 cm in any area 2 = Undermining 2-4 cm involving <50% wound margins 3 = Undermining 2-4 cm involving >50% wound margins 4 = Undermining >4 cm in any area 5 = Tunneling &/or sinus tract formation			
5. NECROTIC TISSUE TYPE	1 = None visible 2 = White/gray nonviable tissue &/or nonadherent yellow slough 3 = Loosely adherent yellow slough 4 = Adherent, soft, black eschar 5 = Firmly adherent, hard, black eschar			
6. NECROTIC TISSUE AMOUNT	1 = None visible 2 = <25% of wound bed covered 3 = 25% to 50% of wound covered 4 = >50% to <75% of wound covered 5 = 75% to 100% of wound covered			
7. EXUDATE TYPE	1 = None or bloody 2 = Serosanguineous: thin, watery, pale red/pink 3 = Serous: thin, watery, clear 4 = Purulent: thin or thick, opaque, tan/yellow 5 = Foul purulent: thick, opaque, yellow/green with odor			

Figure 4-3, cont'd.

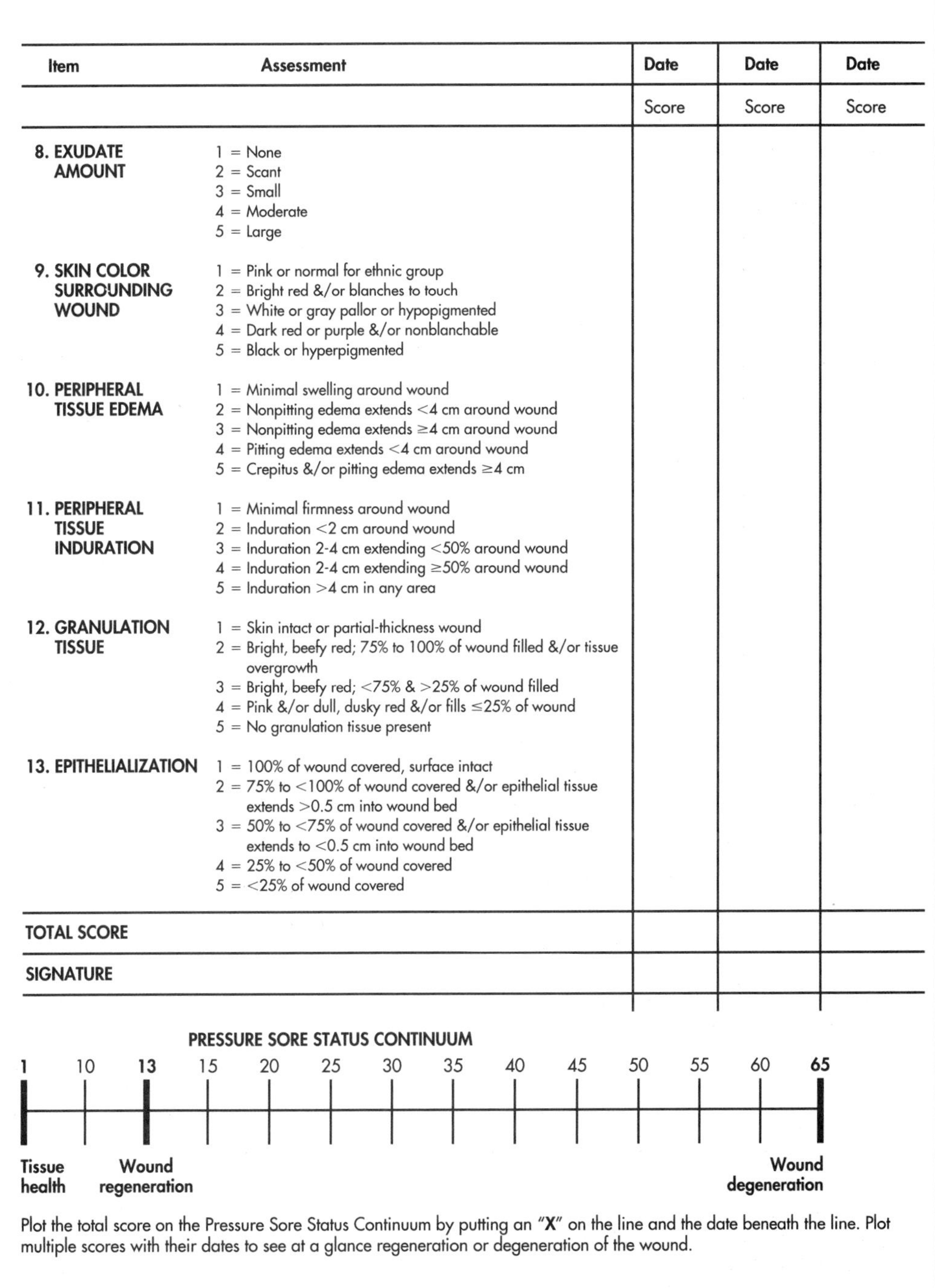

Item	Assessment	Date	Date	Date
		Score	Score	Score
8. EXUDATE AMOUNT	1 = None 2 = Scant 3 = Small 4 = Moderate 5 = Large			
9. SKIN COLOR SURROUNDING WOUND	1 = Pink or normal for ethnic group 2 = Bright red &/or blanches to touch 3 = White or gray pallor or hypopigmented 4 = Dark red or purple &/or nonblanchable 5 = Black or hyperpigmented			
10. PERIPHERAL TISSUE EDEMA	1 = Minimal swelling around wound 2 = Nonpitting edema extends <4 cm around wound 3 = Nonpitting edema extends ≥4 cm around wound 4 = Pitting edema extends <4 cm around wound 5 = Crepitus &/or pitting edema extends ≥4 cm			
11. PERIPHERAL TISSUE INDURATION	1 = Minimal firmness around wound 2 = Induration <2 cm around wound 3 = Induration 2-4 cm extending <50% around wound 4 = Induration 2-4 cm extending ≥50% around wound 5 = Induration >4 cm in any area			
12. GRANULATION TISSUE	1 = Skin intact or partial-thickness wound 2 = Bright, beefy red; 75% to 100% of wound filled &/or tissue overgrowth 3 = Bright, beefy red; <75% & >25% of wound filled 4 = Pink &/or dull, dusky red &/or fills ≤25% of wound 5 = No granulation tissue present			
13. EPITHELIALIZATION	1 = 100% of wound covered, surface intact 2 = 75% to <100% of wound covered &/or epithelial tissue extends >0.5 cm into wound bed 3 = 50% to <75% of wound covered &/or epithelial tissue extends to <0.5 cm into wound bed 4 = 25% to <50% of wound covered 5 = <25% of wound covered			
TOTAL SCORE				
SIGNATURE				

PRESSURE SORE STATUS CONTINUUM

1 10 **13** 15 20 25 30 35 40 45 50 55 60 **65**

Tissue health — **Wound regeneration** — **Wound degeneration**

Plot the total score on the Pressure Sore Status Continuum by putting an "**X**" on the line and the date beneath the line. Plot multiple scores with their dates to see at a glance regeneration or degeneration of the wound.

Figure 4-3, cont'd.

PUSH Tool 3.0

Patient Name: ______________________________ Patient ID#: ______________

Ulcer Location: ______________________________ Date: ______________

DIRECTIONS:
Observe and measure the pressure ulcer. Categorize the ulcer with respect to surface area, exudate, and type of wound tissue. Record a sub-score for each of these ulcer characteristics. Add the sub-scores to obtain the total score. A comparison of total scores measured over time provides an indication of the improvement or deterioration in pressure ulcer healing.

Length	0 0 cm²	1 <0.3 cm²	2 0.3-0.6 cm²	3 0.7-1.0 cm²	4 1.1-2.0 cm²	5 2.1-3.0 cm²	
× **Width**		6 3.1-4.0 cm²	7 4.1-8.0 cm²	8 8.1-12.0 cm²	9 12.1-24.0 cm²	10 >24.0 cm²	**Sub-score**
Exudate Amount	0 None	1 Light	2 Moderate	3 Heavy			**Sub-score**
Tissue Type	0 Closed	1 Epithelial Tissue	2 Granulation Tissue	3 Slough	4 Necrotic Tissue		**Sub-score**
							Total Score

Length × Width: Measure the greatest length (head to toe) and the greatest width (side to side) using a centimeter ruler. Multiply these two measurements (length width) to obtain an estimate of surface area in square centimeters (cm²). Caveat: Do not guess! Always use a centimeter ruler and always use the same method each time the ulcer is measured.

Exudate Amount: Estimate the amount of exudate (drainage) present after removal of the dressing and before applying any topical agent to the ulcer. Estimate the exudate (drainage) as none, light, moderate, or heavy.

Tissue Type: This refers to the types of tissue that are present in the wound (ulcer) bed. Score as a "4" if there is any necrotic tissue present. Score as a "3" if there is any amount of slough present and necrotic tissue is absent. Score as a "2" if the wound is clean and contains granulation tissue. A superficial wound that is reepithelializing is scored as a "1". When the wound is closed, score as a "0".

4 - Necrotic Tissue (Eschar): black, brown, or tan tissue that adheres firmly to the wound bed or ulcer edges and may be either firmer or softer than surrounding skin.
3 - Slough: yellow or white tissue that adheres to the ulcer bed in strings or thick clumps, or is mucinous.
2 - Granulation Tissue: pink or beefy red tissue with a shiny, moist, granular appearance.
1 - Epithelial Tissue: for superficial ulcers, new pink or shiny tissue (skin) that grows in from the edges or as islands on the ulcer surface.
0 - Closed/Resurfaced: the wound is completely covered with epithelium (new skin).

Figure 4-4 Pressure Ulcer Healing Scale (PUSH). Unmodified Version 3.0. (Copyright 1998 National Pressure Ulcer Advisory Panel. Reprint permission granted. Further reprint requests should be directed to National Pressure Ulcer Advisory Panel, 11250 Roger Bacon Drive, Suite 8, Reston, VA 20190-5205.)

PRESSURE ULCER HEALING CHART

(use a separate page for each pressure ulcer)

Patient Name: ______________________ Patient ID#: ______________

Ulcer Location: ______________________ Date: ______________

Directions: Observe and measure pressure ulcers at regular intervals using the PUSH Tool. Date and record PUSH Sub-scale and Total Scores on the Pressure Ulcer Healing Record below.

	PRESSURE ULCER HEALING RECORD												
DATE													
Length × Width													
Exudate Amount													
Tissue Type													
Total Score													

Graph the PUSH Total Score on the Pressure Ulcer Healing Graph below.

PUSH Total Score	PRESSURE ULCER HEALING GRAPH												
17													
16													
15													
14													
13													
12													
11													
10													
9													
8													
7													
6													
5													
4													
3													
2													
1													
Healed 0													
DATE													

Figure 4-4, cont'd.

BOX 4-2 Macroscopic Indices of Wound Healing

Anatomic location of wound
Dimensions and depth of wound (in centimeters)
Extent of tissue loss (stage of wound)
Characteristics of wound base
- Type of tissue
- Percentage of wound containing each type of tissue observed

Presence or absence of undermining or sinus tract formation
Exudate (volume and color)
Condition of surrounding skin
Presence or absence of new epithelium at the rim

gains clinical significance when described with precision. Because a discussion of assessment of wounds closed by primary intention is presented in Chapter 9, only those pertaining to wounds healing by secondary intention are discussed in this chapter.

Size

Determing the size of the wound is a basic assessment parameter; its significance is demonstrated by the inclusion of this parameter in many evaluation tools and in clinical practice. Although the clinician cannot directly control the size of a wound, ensuring that the patient's nutritional needs are met will influence the quality of healing and the ability of the open wound to contract, hence affecting the size of the wound. Nursing interventions that support the delivery of nutrients (such as oxygen, vitamins, and micronutrients) to the wound help the wound to decrease in size and heal (Pinchkofsky-Devin, 1990; West, 1990; Whitney, 1990). For example, the fibroblast requires nutrients to synthesize hydroxyproline and collagen. As collagen remodels in the third stage of healing, wound contraction continues. In a starved environment this will not proceed effectively, and contraction will be thwarted.

Evaluating the size (or area) of a wound is one of the first local measurements that the clinician should obtain and should be repeated at intervals. Wound-size determinations are recorded in centimeters or millimeters and include the length, width, and depth of the wound. Irregularly shaped wounds may require several measurements of each dimension to adequately capture the size of the wound. Locations from which measurements are obtained can be indicated with an ink mark on the surrounding intact skin or recorded in the care plan.

Area measurement provides overall gross changes in size as an indicator of healing. Unfortunately, size measurement has several reliability problems (Bates-Jensen, 1995):

1. Variations in the clinicians ability to define wound edge cannot be controlled.
2. Change in size occurs with debridement, yet the wound is better as necrotic tissue is removed.
3. Measuring the area is an imprecise method of measuring depth.

Extent of Tissue Involvement

The larger or deeper the wound, the greater the potential for secondary problems (such as infections) and prolonged healing. Any injury involving vessel interruption institutes the healing trajectory and elicits a systemic response. Therefore assessing a wound to determine the extent of tissue involvement is an essential aspect of wound evaluation. The extent of tissue damage guides the selection of interventions appropriate to restore tissue integrity and also provides some information about the length of time that the healing process may require.

Several methods are available to describe the extent of tissue damage. These include partial thickness, full thickness, and with pressure ulcers, staging (see Box 4-1). In the case of burn wound, the classical estimation of area of the burn can be used (Lund and Browder, 1944). A specific ulcer grading system for vascular wounds on the extremities has also been described (Glugla and Mulder, 1990) (see Table 4-5). Increasingly, these systems are being related to algorithms, or plans of care. However, such protocols need to be researched to determine effectiveness, a process that will require sound methods of assessing and measuring wound-healing progress.

Presence of Undermining or Tracts

Full-thickness wounds must be carefully evaluated for evidence of undermining or sinus tract formation as demonstrated in Plate 4. Undermining involves a large proportion of wound edge, whereas tracts are limited to a small edge and extend in one direction for a considerable length (Bates-Jensen, 1995). Undermining most often occurs with pressure-induced ulcers that are complicated by shear force, whereas tracts occur in dehisced wounds and ulcers caused by a combination of neuropathy and arterial insufficiency. Undermining is a result of subcutaneous fat necrosis, and the amount of undermining is directly related to the severity of necrosis.

Location and extent of undermining or sinus tracts must be accurately documented so that progress in wound healing and effectiveness at eliminating or reducing the cause can be evaluated. For example, extension of tissue damage by continued shear is evidenced by enlargement of the undermined area. Gentle probing of the wound bed with a cotton-tipped applicator reveals undermined tissue or tracts.

Anatomic Location

The anatomic location of the wound or skin damage should also be documented. Descriptors are used to convey which bony prominence the lesion lies over or the specific body locations. For example, a pressure ulcer may develop on the right calcaneous or left ischial tuberosity, a shear injury may be located in the gluteal fold, and a venous ulcer may develop on the medial aspect of the right lower leg.

Location is significant not only because of the need to communicate accurately with colleagues, but also because location influences healing potential. The closer the wound is to the upper region of the body, the greater the likelihood of healing. Extremity wounds in the elderly, therefore, are often slow to heal, not only because of underlying conditions that thwart healing, but also because they are distant from the upper body regions.

Type of Tissue in Wound Bed

The type of tissue that can be present in the wound bed can range from viable tissue to nonviable tissue. Viable tissue (e.g., granulation, epithelialization, muscle, subcutaneous tissue) must be distinguished from nonviable tissue. These terms are defined in the Figure 4-3 and in the Glossary. The distinction between tissue types is most commonly made by observation of the color of the tissue in the wound. Unfortunately, this requires skill because slough, fibrinous exudate, and pus can all be misinterpreted. Fibrinous exudate can be distinguished from slough in that fibrinous exudate is not firmly attached to the wound base and can be lifted (Tong, 1999).

The presence of nonviable tissue (or necrotic tissue) in the wound is cause for concern because it is often associated with altered tissue oxygenation, wound desiccation, or increased bacterial burden. Color, consistency, and adherence of the necrotic tissue to the wound bed should be noted. Clinical appearance of necrotic tissue correlates with level and type of tissue death (Table 4-7).

Because wound healing is greatly compromised in the midst of necrotic tissue (Hohn, 1980), prompt removal of necrotic tissue from wounds must be a common goal of the multidisciplinary health care team. A recent article by Steed and colleagues (1996) reports the effectiveness of debridement in the healing of chronic diabetic foot ulcers. In a retrospective analysis of percentage of times that debridement occurred in a multicenter double-blind, placebo-controlled, randomized trial, the results showed that the greater the percentage of office visits at which the patient was debrided, the greater the potential for healing. Debridement options are discussed further in Chapter 7.

TABLE 4-7 Correlation of Necrotic Tissue Type with Level of Tissue Disease

TYPE OF NECROTIC TISSUE	LEVEL OF TISSUE DAMAGE
Stringy, yellow slough	Subcutaneous fat tissue dies
Thicker yellow slough and more tenacious	Muscle degenerates
Hard black eschar	Full-thickness destruction

Color

Color, as discussed previously, is another important index of healing. Typically, clean granular wounds are described as being red; yellow, tan, and black may be used to describe the presence of necrotic tissue or desiccated tissue, such as tendon. In reality, these colors are inadequate in truly reflecting the many colors that can accompany a wound. For example, a wound may be pink, as shown in Plate 3, pale red as shown in Plate 6, or intensely red as shown in Plates 5 and 10. This range of the color red portrays the continuum of healing from optimal to suboptimal. The WCI is an attempt to capture the range of color states that reflect optimal to worst healing within and surrounding the wound. Therefore it is important to closely observe and precisely describe the color of the wound tissue, wound exudate, and changes in the skin surrounding the wound.

Terminology should be standardized to accurately describe optimal and suboptimal wound colors. For example, healthy granulation tissue is characteristically described as "beefy, red, and shiny" (Plate 5). Deviations from this optimal state should be described carefully and correlated with conditions that may account for the abnormality.

Suboptimal wound colors may be an indication of physiologic abnormalities, such as those in the patient's fluid status, serum hemoglobin level, or nutritional status as shown in Plate 6 (Maibach and Rovee, 1971; Rodeheaver, 1989). Fluid status, as reflected by hematocrit, indicates adequacy of tissue hydration and tissue oxygenation potential. Both hydration and oxygenation affect new vessel formation, which can be inferred macroscopically in the color and sheen of granulation tissue. Likewise, vitamin and mineral intake (specifically vitamin C and iron) affect collagen synthesis, new vessel formation, capillary stability, and hemoglobin formation and are therefore potentially reflected in tissue color.

Exudate

Exudate within the wound should be assessed for volume, color, consistency, and odor. The type and color of exudate depends on wound moisture and organisms present. Exudate characteristics also vary with the type of wound present (e.g., a venous ulcer may produce more exudate than an arterial ulcer). Odor and color of exudate offer information that may be indicative of a wound infection. Extremely odorous, purulent exudate is frequently suggestive of an anaerobic infection. Excessive exudate production uses energy in a patient who typically has limited resources.

Edge of Open Wound

The edge, or rim, of the open wound should be assessed as an integral part of wound evaluation. Plate 3 reveals the presence of new epithelial tissue at the wound edge. This is in contrast to the absence of epithelial tissue at the wound edge as shown in Plate 4. New epithelial tissue will not grow into a wound covered with necrotic debris or deprived of oxygen. Instead, these wounds demonstrate persistently gnarled edges with little to no evidence of new tissue growth at the wound rim. The clinician should observe closely for the appearance of new tissue at the wound edges. Unfortunately, assessment of the edge of the open wound is commonly overlooked and unappreciated. This situation underscores the need for a systematic approach to evaluate key landmarks within the open wound and the need for formal instruction regarding the structural components of the open wound (Cooper, 1990e).

Interventions that can facilitate the appearance of new tissue at the rim of the wound are similar to those that influence the size of the wound: improved nutrition, supporting wound (tissue) oxygenation, and effective removal of necrotic tissue. Appropriate use of dressings that incorporate the principles of moist healing can also greatly facilitate epithelial migration (Alverez, Rozint, and Wiseman, 1989; Winter and Scales, 1963).

Presence of Foreign Bodies

The presence of foreign bodies (such as suture material) within an open wound should be assessed. Although routine in the care of an acute wound, suture material always presents a challenge to the healing process. The integrity of an approximated incision is threatened when an excessive number of sutures is used, when sutures are placed under tension, and when sutures are knotted numerous times. Timely removal of any foreign body in the wound closed by primary or secondary intention can enhance wound repair and conserve the patient's energy.

Condition of Surrounding Skin

Evaluation of the skin adjacent to the wound should also be a part of wound assessment because it reveals much about the patient's age, health status, and at times, medications that they may be taking, such as steroids. Assessment of the skin surrounding a wound may provide an indication of the adequacy of the wound dressing's ability to absorb and contain exudate. Maceration of surrounding skin occurs when exudate pools onto intact skin for prolonged periods of time or when gauze is inappropriately applied and overlaps onto intact skin. The following assessments of the skin surrounding the wound are essential: discoloration: erythema or paleness, hematoma formation, interruptions in integrity (such as denudement, erosion, papules, pustules), edema, maceration, or desiccation. In people with darker skin, erythema is difficult to assess; these areas may appear purple or have a deepening of the natural skin color. The surrounding skin should also be palpated for the presence or absence of induration, which may be an indication of deeper tissue damage. These assessments must be routine and regular.

Duration of Wound

Although seldom regarded a priority, the time since wounding, or "age" of the wound, is a macroscopic parameter that deserves careful consideration. Given a clear understanding of healing, the 7-day-old surgical wound that shows no signs of inflammation is worrisome for different reasons than those for the venous ulcer that has persisted for several years. Both wounds are out of synchronization and need to be evaluated in light of what mechanisms might have altered the normal course of the healing trajectory. The fact that the surgical incision closed by primary intention is most likely to dehisce from 5 to 12 days after surgery, or that a healing ridge should be apparent by approximately 7 days after surgery, can be evaluated knowledgeably only when the time span since wounding is used as a guidepost. Postoperatively, surgical patients should be observed for the presence or absence of such key time-related manifestations of optimal healing. With changing practices such as early discharge to home, astute wound assessments become increasingly important for home care nurses and long-term care nurses.

DOCUMENTATION GUIDELINES

The nurse who provides wound care requires a thorough understanding of the normal physiologic process, evaluation of underlying conditions that might alter the optimal course, coordination of an outcome-driven plan used knowledgeably, and consistent evaluation of those outcomes at regularly prescribed intervals. Thus the importance of documentation and frequent evaluation becomes evident. Evaluation of outcomes and consistency of care are possible only when observations and interventions are documented. In the open soft tissue wound, documentation of macroscopic indices of wound healing is a nursing responsibility (see Box 4-2).

One wound assessment tool cannot provide all of these data. A combination of many tools is often necessary for a comprehensive and accurate reflection of the status of the wound and the healing trend. For example, the classification system of staging should be used in combination with descriptive terminology to capture the color and size of the wound and type of tissue in the wound bed. Regular and routine wound evaluations collected at intervals over time should provide the information necessary to reflect the healing status of the wound. From this, the effectiveness of the plan of care (topical and systemic) can be evaluated and revised as needed.

It is difficult to stipulate the appropriate frequency for wound assessment because no research to provide this information has been reported. Multiple variables influence the manner in which different types of wounds heal. Furthermore, healing will vary from one person to another. Given these constraints, it becomes necessary to suggest frequency intervals for wound assessment based strictly on clinical experience. Acute wound situations (such as a wound infection or recent dehiscence) require close monitoring; thus assessments may be conducted as often as every 2 to 4 hours.

Although chronicity in a wound is not a reason to be less vigilant, assessments may be conducted less frequently. For example, in the acute care setting, wound assessments may be documented with every dressing change but do not need to exceed once per day. In the home care and long-term care settings, weekly wound assessments may be more practical and informative in terms of identifying a trend in the wound-repair process. When assessment and measurement trends fail to indicate a movement toward healing in the wound, reevaluation of the treatment plan, treatment goals, causative factors, and institution of new therapies are warranted and essential.

RECOMMENDATIONS FOR MORE ACCURATE WOUND ASSESSMENT

Because so little has been documented about specific macroscopic indices of healing, it is imperative for clinicians to accept the responsibility and challenge to work at systematically recording and testing visible observations believed to reflect optimal and suboptimal healing. This is a particularly important activity given the increasing number of wound-care products that flood the market, the potential for enhancing or accelerating healing with substances containing growth factors, the trend toward earlier patient discharge, and the advancing age of the population.

Nurses are critical participants in the process of developing a systematic approach for evaluating the healing wound. Unfortunately, many issues have delayed the development of such tools, and most of those are issues that nursing can control. To facilitate the development of a systematic approach to evaluating wound healing, five conditions seem necessary:

1. Nurses must recognize the value and merit of the process of observation as an assessment methodology. Although in the early days of health care observation was considered one of the finest forms of patient assessment, in recent times observation has been relegated to a position of lesser value. Instruments and machines are now viewed as superior, more objective, and of greater value.
2. Nurses must document and describe the manner in which the wound is observed and exactly what is observed. Restoration of stature to observational activities is incomplete if nurses fail to share or communicate these observations. This provides the database needed from which a consensus on terminology can be derived; hence the components of an evaluation instrument become apparent.
3. Nurses must acknowledge the difference between simply measuring the dimensions of a wound and the more complex process of assessing the status of the wound's multiple components and healing status. It is the experienced nurse who recognizes that wound assessment is a process that involves critical thinking skills and correlation of observations to potential causes. Wound assessment requires a comprehensive examination of the wound. The nurse must examine the wound not only for current observations but also in comparison to past observations. These observations are then pondered in light of the patient's indicators for healing potential (i.e., health status, nutritional status, and perfusion). Attention to detail is imperative. No existing tests or methods duplicate the data that a careful wound assessment provides. The limitations of linear wound measurements or serial tracings alone become apparent; these methods present an incomplete picture for certain wound types. To accurately describe the diabetic wound, for example, it must be assessed using additional parameters that complement linear measurement. As the second condition is fulfilled, correlations of wound measurements with healing will emerge and it will become possible to predict healing based on select wound attributes.
4. The terms used to describe wounds must be standardized. By adopting a common vocabu-

lary, an accurate description of the wound can be reliably conveyed to individuals and groups, such as institutions. Furthermore, testing of wound therapies is facilitated because the observations can now be clearly shared and understood between all involved health care providers. Although an organized vocabulary is yet to emerge, numerous terms have been defined and should be critiqued and adopted as appropriate (Boarini, Bryant, and Zink, 1987; Cooper, 1990e; NPUAP, 1989; WOCN, 1992). For example, as a result of a consensus panel conference, the NPUAP recommends that *pressure ulcer* be the term that clinicians use when referring to lesions otherwise known as *bedsores, pressure sores,* and *decubitus ulcers.* Such a recommendation greatly streamlines clinical vocabulary and begins to standardize the way clinicians speak about wounds. Clinicians interested in rectifying the confusion surrounding wounds should adopt the language suggested by this panel and other panels (Lazarus et al, 1994) as a first step toward order.

5. Nurses must employ clinically useful evaluation tools with demonstrated reliability and validity. Support should be provided to those researchers who have developed clinically useful wound-evaluation tools. Continuing to use ill-defined methods of assessing patients when sound instruments exist perpetuates the problem. Selected tools are more appropriate for certain types of wounds. Therefore nurses must describe and isolate the various tools available and critique them carefully for their merits or drawbacks in particular healing situations.

SUMMARY

In 1973 Levine stated that "every healing process, regardless of its nature, occurs over a period of time. The success of the ultimate healing depends in large measure on what happens to the individual during that time. The nurse is the person on the health team who shares the most time with the patient, and thus no worker can influence the success of the healing process more than the nurse. Nursing processes of every kind are dedicated to the promotion of healing." Despite the emphasis on the "wound" throughout this chapter, there needs to be an increased realization that evaluating wounds as if they exist separately from the patient is not only inadequate but also inconsistent with the practice of nursing. Wound evaluation is patient evaluation. With the increased realization of the complexity of healing comes the obligation to know as much as possible about the healing milieu (physiologic, psychologic, biochemical, etc.). Careful accurate wound assessments are critical and guide decisions for wound care. However, providing care to the wound in isolation or evaluating the wound in isolation belies the fundamental holism of nursing (Levine, 1967; Levine, 1971).

SELF-ASSESSMENT EXERCISE

1. Distinguish between measurement of an existing wound and assessment of the wound status.
2. Which of the following methods is an example of categorizing a wound by classification?
   a. Linear measurements
   b. Photographs
   c. Staging
   d. Wound molds
3. Blisters are an example of which stage of tissue loss?
   a. Stage 1
   b. Stage 2
   c. Stage 3
   d. Stage 4
4. Define *partial thickness* and *full thickness.*
5. Describe three limitations associated with using only linear measurements to evaluate the wound and to assess wound status.
6. List the 11 macroscopic indices of wound healing that should be assessed and recorded.
7. Describe the following terms:
   a. Nonviable
   b. Eschar
   c. Granulation
   d. Epithelialization

REFERENCES

Alvarez O, Rozint J, Wiseman D: Moist environment for healing: matching the dressing to the wound, *Wounds* 1(1):35, 1989.

Armstrong DG, Lavery LA, Harkless LB: Treatment-based classification system for assessment and care of diabetic feet, *Ostomy Wound Manage* 42(8):50, 1996.

Bates-Jensen BM: Indices to include in wound healing assessment, *Adv Wound Care* 8(4):28, 1995.

Bates-Jensen BM: The pressure sore status tool a few thousand assessments later, *Adv Wound Care* 109(5):65, 1997

Bates-Jensen BM: The pressure sore status tool: an outcome measure for pressure sores, *Top Geriatr Rehabil* 9(4):17,1994.

Bates-Jensen BM, Vredevoe DL, Brecht ML: Validity and reliability of the pressure sore status tool, *Decubitus* 5(6):20, 1992.

Bergstrom N, Demuth PJ, Braden B: A clinical trial of the Braden scale for predicting pressure sore risk, *Nurs Clin North Am* 22:417, 1987b.

Bergstrom N et al: The Braden scale for predicting pressure sore risk, *Nurs Res* 36:205, 1987a.

Berris WP, Sangwine SJ: Automatic quantitative analysis of healing skin wounds using colour digital image processing. Available on-line at www.smtl.co.uk/*World-Wide-Wounds*/1997/july/Berris/Berris.html, July, 1997.

Boarini JH, Bryant R, Zink M: *Achieving autolysis with transparent dressings*, St Paul, Minn, 1987, Medical-Surgical Division: 3M Health Care.

Bohannon RW, Pfaller BA: Documentation of wound surface area from tracings of wound perimeters, *Phys Ther* 63:1622, 1983.

Braden BJ, Bergstrom N: Clinical utility of the Braden scale for predicting pressure sore risk, *Decubitus* 2(3):44, 1989.

Bulstrode DJ, Goode AW, Scott PJ: Stereophotogrammetry for measuring rates of cutaneous healing: a comparison with conventional techniques, *Clin Sci* 71:437, 1986.

Byrne DJ, Napier A, Cuschieri A: Validation of the ASEPSIS method of wound scoring in patients undergoing general surgical operation, *J R Coll Surg Edinb* 33:154, 1988.

Cooper DM: Challenge of open wound assessment in the home setting, *Progressions* 2(3):11, 1990c.

Cooper DM: Clinical assessment/measurement of healing: evolution and status, *Clin Materials* 8:263, 1991.

Cooper DM: *Development and testing of an instrument to assess the visual characteristics of open, soft tissue wounds, doctoral dissertation*, Philadelphia, 1990e, University of Pennsylvania.

Cooper DM: Human wound assessment: status report and implications for clinicians, *AACN Clin Issues Crit Care Nurs* 1(3):533, 1990d.

Cooper DM: Optimizing wound healing: a practice within nursing's domain, *Nurs Clin North Am* 25:165, 1990a.

Cooper DM: Preface, *Nurs Clin North Am* 25:163, 1990b.

Cuzzell J: The new RYB color code, *Am J Nurs* 88:1342, 1988.

Fawcett J: *The relationship of theory and research*, ed 3, Philadelphia, 1999, F.A. Davis.

Ferrell BA, Artinian BM, Sessing D: The Sessing scale for assessment of pressure ulcer healing, *J Am Geriatr Soc* 43:37, 1995.

Frantz RA, Johnson DA: Stereophotogrammetry and computerized image analysis: a 3-dimensional method of measuring wound healing, *Wounds* 4:58, 1992.

Fylling CP: A comprehensive wound management protocol including topical growth factors, *Wounds* 1:79, 1989.

Gilman TH: Parameter for measurement of wound closure, *Wounds* 2(3):95, 1990.

Gledhill T, Waterfall WE: Silastic foam: a new material for dressing wounds, *Can Med Assoc J* 128:685, 1983.

Glugla M, Mulder GD: The diabetic foot: medical management of foot ulcers. In Krasner D, editor: *Chronic wound care: a clinical source book for healthcare professionals*, King of Prussia, Penn, 1990, Health Management Publications.

Gorin B et al: The influence of wound geometry on the measurement of wound healing rates in clinical trials, *J Vasc Surg* 23(3):524, 1996.

Gosnell DJ: An assessment tool to identify pressure sores, *Nurs Res* 22:55, 1973.

Gosnell DJ: Pressure sore risk assessment. Part II. Analysis of risk factors, *Decubitus* 2:40, 1989.

Haley RW et al: Identifying patients at high risk of surgical wound infection, *Am J Epidemiol* 121:206, 1985.

Harding KG: Methods for assessing change in ulcer status, *Adv Wound Care* 8(4), 1995.

Hohn DC: Host resistance to infection: established and emerging concepts. In Hunt TK, editor: *Wound healing and wound infection: theory and surgical practice*, New York, 1980, Appleton-Century-Crofts.

Holden-Lund C: Effects of relaxation with guided imagery on surgical stress and wound healing, *Res Nurs Health* 11:235, 1988.

Hughes LE: Wound measurement, *Can J Surg* 26:210, 1983.

Hussey LC, Leeper B, Hynan LS: Development of the sternal wound infection prediction scale, *Heart Lung* 27:326, 1998.

Kantor J, Margolis DJ: Efficacy and prognostic value of simple wound measurements, *Arch Dermatol* 134(12):1571, 1998.

Knighton DR et al: Classification and treatment of chronic nonhealing wounds, *Ann Surg* 204:322, 1986.

Kundin JI: A new way to size up a wound, *Am J Nurs* 89:206, 1989.

Kundin JI: Designing and developing a new measuring instrument, *Perioperative Nurs Q* 1:40, 1985.

Langemo DK et al: Two-dimensional wound measurement: comparison of four techniques, *Adv Wound Care* 11:337, 1998.

Lavery LA, Armstrong DG, Harkless LB: Classification of diabetic foot wounds, *Ostomy Wound Manage* 43:44, 1997.

Lazarus GS et al: Definition and guidelines for assessment of wounds and evaluation of healing, *Arch Dermatol* 130:489, 1994.

Lecomte du Nouy P: *Biological time*, New York, 1937, The Macmillan Company.

Levine ME: Holistic nursing, *Nurs Clin North Am* 6:253, 1971.

Levine ME: *Introduction to clinical nursing*, Philadelphia, 1973, FA Davis.

Levine ME: The four conservation principles of nursing, *Nurs Forum* 2:22, 1967.

Levine ME: The four conservation principles twenty years later. In Riehl-Sisca JP, editor: *Conceptual models for nursing practice*, ed 3, Norwalk, Conn, 1989, Appleton & Lange.

Liskay AM, Mion LC, Davis BR: Comparison of two devices for wound measurement, *Dermatol Nurs* 5:434, 1993.

Lund CC, Browder NC: Estimation of areas of burns, *Surg Gynecol Obstet* 79:352, 1944.

Maibach H, Rovee D, editors: *Epidermal wound healing*, St Louis, 1971, Mosby.

National Pressure Ulcer Advisory Panel: National Consensus Conference, Washington, DC, 1998, NPUAP.

National Pressure Ulcer Advisory Panel: *Stage I assessment in darkly pigmented skin*. Available on-line at www.npuap.org/positn4.htm, August, 1999.

Norton D: Calculating the risk: reflections on the Norton scale, *Decubitus* 2(3):24, 1989.

Norton D, McLaren R, Exton-Smith IN: *An investigation of geriatric nursing problems in hospital*, London, 1962, National Corporation for the Care of Old People.

Ochs DE et al: Truncal pressure ulcers are neither hypoxic nor ischemic and should respond to exogenous growth factor therapy, *Wounds* 11(5):110, 1999

Percoraro RE, Reiber GE: Classification of wounds in diabetic amputees, *Wounds* 2:65, 1990.

Pinchkofsky-Devin G: Nutritional assessment and intervention. In Krasner D, editor: *Chronic wound care*, King of Prussia, Penn, 1990, Health Management Publications.

Plassman P, Melhuish JM, Harding KG: Methods of measuring wound size: a comparative study, *Ostomy Wound Manage* 40(7):50, 1996.

Pories WJ et al: The measurement of human wound healing, *Surgery* 59:821, 1966.

Resch CS et al: Pressure sore volume measurement, *Am J Geriatr Soc* 36:444, 1988.

Robson MC: Wound infection: a failure of wound healing caused by an unbalance of bacteria, *Surg Clin North Am* 77(33):637, 1997.

Robson MC et al: The safety and effect of topically applied recombinant basic fibroblast growth factor on the healing of chronic pressure sores, *Ann Surg* 216:401, 1992.

Robson MC, Heggers JP: *Quantitative bacteriology: its role in the armamentarium of the surgeon*, Boca Raton, Fla, 1991, CRC Press.

Rodeheaver G: Controversies in topical wound management, *Wounds* 1(1):19, 1989.

Shea JD: Pressure sores: classification and management, *Clin Orthop* 112:89, 1975.

Steed DL et al: Effect of extensive debridement and treatment on the healing of diabetic foot ulcers, *J Am Coll Surg* 183:61, 1996

Stotts NA: Personal communication, October 22, 1999.

Stotts NA, Rodeheaver GT: Revision of the PUSH Tool using an expanded database, *Adv Wound Care* 10(5):107, 1997.

Strickland OL: Can reliability and validity be established? *J Nurs Manage* 3(2):91, 1995.

Sussman C, Bates-Jensen BM: Tools to measure wound healing, In Sussman C, Bates-Jensen BM, editors: *Wound care*, Gaithersberg, Md, 1998, Aspen.

Sussman C, Swanson G: Utility of the Sussman Wound Healing Tool in predicting wound healing outcomes in physical therapy, *Adv Wound Care* 10(5):74, 1997.

Tallman P et al: Initial rate of healing predicts complete healing of venous ulcers, *Arch Dermatol* 133:1231, 1997.

Thomas AC, Wysocki AB: The healing wound: a comparison of three clinically useful methods of measurement, *Decubitus* 3:18, 1990.

Thomas DR et al: Pressure ulcer scale for healing: derivation and validation of the PUSH tool, *Adv Wound Care* 10(5):96, 1997.

Tong A: The identification and treatment of slough, *J Wound Care* 8(7):338, 1999.

van Rijswijk L, Multi-Center Leg Ulcer Study Group: Full-thickness leg ulcers: patient demographics and predictors of healing, *J Fam Pract* 36:625, 1993.

van Rijswijk L, Polansky M: Predictors of time to healing deep pressure ulcers, *Ostomy Wound Manage* 40(8):40, 1994.

Waltz CF, Strickland OL, Lenz ER: *Measurement in nursing research*. Philadelphia, 1991, FA Davis.

Waterlow J, Vernon MJ, Gilchrist B: The Norton score and pressure sore prevention, *J Wound Care* 5(2):93, 1996.

Wells FC, Newsom SWB, Rowlands C: Wound infection in cardiothoracic surgery, *Lancet* 1:1209, 1983.

West JM: Wound healing in the surgical patient: influence of the perioperative stress response on perfusion, *AACN Clin Issues Crit Care Nurs* 1:595, 1990.

Whitney JD: The influence of tissue oxygen and perfusion on wound healing, *AACN Clin Issues Crit Care Nurs* 1:578, 1990.

Wilson AP et al: A scoring method (ASEPSIS) for postoperative wound infections for use in clinical trials of antibiotic prophylaxis, *Lancet* 1(8476):311, 1986.

Winter GD, Scales JT: Effect of air-drying and dressings on the surface of a wound, *Nature* 197:91, 1963.

Wood RA, Williams RH, Hughes LE: Foam elastomer dressing in the management of open granulating wounds: experience with 250 patients, *Br J Surg* 64:554, 1977.

Woods FM et al: Current difficulties and the possible future directions in scar assessment, *Burns* 22(6):455, 1996.

Wound Ostomy Continence Nurses Society: *Guidelines for management: dermal wounds: pressure ulcers*, revised ed, Laguna Beach, Calif, 1992, WOCN.

Xakellis GC, Frantz RA: Pressure ulcer healing: what is it? what influences it? how is it measured? *Adv Wound Care* 10(5):20, 1997.

CHAPTER 5

Principles of Wound Management

BONNIE SUE ROLSTAD, LIZA G. OVINGTON, & ANN HARRIS

OBJECTIVES

1. Discuss the implementation of wound-care principles in an integrated health care system.
2. Identify three principles of wound management and an intervention model that demonstrates an organization of thinking for clinical practice.
3. Describe how the holistic approach affects local wound management.
4. Identify four parameters of a physiologic wound environment.
5. Differentiate between the immune states and respective approaches to treatment of bacterial colonization and bacterial infection.
6. Identify at least five objectives in local wound management.
7. Define the following terms related to wound dressing materials: *occlusive*, *semiocclusive*, *moisture-retentive*, *biologic dressings*, *synthetic dressings*, *skin substitutes*, and *growth factors*.
8. Identify general and specific wound-care dressing performance parameters.
9. Demonstrate the correlation between needs of the wound and dressing selection.
10. Define *cost-effectiveness* in relation to local wound management.

This chapter presents principles of wound management and integrates wound-care advances in basic sciences and developments in biotechnology into clinical practice in order to present a physiologic approach to local wound management. Controlled clinical trials are cited if available. However, much research is needed to support and improve clinical practice. If clinical studies are not available, expert opinion and case studies are used.

EXPECTED OUTCOME: GOAL FOR WOUND

The expected outcome or goal for the wound is usually *healing* but is dependent upon the condition of the host and numerous other factors. Another goal may be *delayed healing* in a patient who is immune compromised. In the terminally ill patient the goal may be *maintenance* or *symptom control* (Rolstad and Harris, 1997). Goals for the wound should be established early and guide decision making at each patient contact so that local wound-care decisions are realistic and appropriate for the patient's situation. Modification of the goal for the wound may be necessary if the patient's condition changes. When the goal is maintenance or symptom control, expensive technologic treatment modalities and biologic dressings may be impractical. Unobtrusive care may be the priority in these cases. Additional potential goals include saving a life, limb preservation, and pain control (Hollinworth, 1995; Krasner and Kane, 1997).

Interim outcomes can also be established for the wound. These short-term markers assist the patient and clinician with recognizing wound improvement and serve to confirm that the patient's wound-healing response is following an appropriate trajectory. Examples are listed in Box 5-1. It should be noted that outcome measures and time frames are not standardized; these are examples only and should be modified before being applied to a specific clinical situation.

BOX 5-1 Examples of Interim Outcomes for Wound Management

- Resolution in extent of erythema surrounding the wound by 1 week
- 50% reduction in wound dimensions or depth of sinus tract in 2 weeks
- Reduction in volume of exudate
- 25% reduction in amount of necrotic tissue (or eschar) by 1 week
- Decrease in pain intensity during dressing change

PATIENT ASSESSMENT

Before establishing the goal for the wound, a thorough patient assessment relative to the wound and the patient's ability to heal the wound must be obtained. Identification of wound etiology and the presence of cofactors that affect the healing response is necessary. Information should be obtained about the patient's health history, wound history, current and proposed care setting, living situation, caregiver status, financial situation, reimbursement issues, transportation concerns, work situation, and other individual issues (Pieper and DiNardo, 1998; van Rijswijk, 1997).

Since reimbursement varies based on settings and insurance programs, the nurse needs to be aware of the type of insurance coverage the patient has and which products are reimbursed. When the patient needs to pay out-of-pocket for wound-care supplies, the risk of noncompliance with wound care is increased. Therefore treatment decisions should be made while keeping in mind what is financially reasonable for the patient to enhance their ability to comply with therapy (Turnbull, 1995).

PRINCIPLES OF WOUND MANAGEMENT

Wounds do not occur in isolation from the total patient. Consequently, the principles of effective wound management (Box 5-2) must incorporate a holistic approach to the patient. Failure to address any one of these principles jeopardizes care and may result in an unhealed wound, complications, or recurrence.

Principle 1: Control or Eliminate Causative Factors

The first treatment principle is elimination of causative factors, thus assessment focuses initially on determination of wound origin. This applies primarily to chronic wounds. The cause of acute wounds is usually known and irreversible, such as surgical incisions or accidental injuries. A chronic wound has been referred to as a *symptom* because unlike the acute wound there are frequently numerous factors related to etiology as well as contributing factors (or cofactors) precipitating the current wound. Addressing the cause of the wound and cofactors must occur simultaneous with local wound care.

In addition to evaluating the patient's general risk factors (such as overall health, mobility, sensory status, nutritional status, and continence status), the nurse should assess for specific indicators related to the cause of the wound. These may be derived from wound location or wound characteristics. Additional indicators that may reveal the origin of the wound are listed in Table 6-2 on p. 130. Diagnostic tests may also be required to clearly establish the wound etiology and cofactors.

Having identified causative factors, steps must be taken to eliminate or control these factors. This may involve the following:

- Selection of an appropriate support surface for reduction of pressure, shear, friction, or moisture
- Implementation of a turning schedule
- Implementation of measures to reduce shear and friction, such as use of a turn sheet or trapeze, socks or heel protectors, a knee gatch when head is elevated, and light dusting of powder or cornstarch on sheets
- Incontinence management, such as bowel training or prompted voiding programs, external collection devices, and skin care
- Use of compression therapy to reduce venous hypertension
- Measures to promote blood flow to ischemic areas, such as hydration, elimination of nicotine and caffeine, and avoidance of cold
- Rigorous monitoring of blood glucose level, avoidance of sources of potential trauma such as foot soaks and chemical callous removers, and offloading techniques such as orthotics

BOX 5-2 Wound Management Principles

1. Control or eliminate causative factors:
   a. Pressure
   b. Shear
   c. Friction
   d. Moisture
   e. Circulatory impairment
   f. Neuropathy
2. Provide systemic support to reduce existing and potential cofactors:
   a. Nutritional and fluid support
   b. Control of systemic conditions affecting wound healing
3. Maintain physiologic local wound environment
   a. Prevent and manage infection
   b. Cleanse wound
   c. Remove nonviable tissue (debridement)
   d. Manage exudate
   e. Eliminate dead space
   f. Control odor
   g. Protect wound

The importance of these familiar nursing interventions cannot be emphasized too strongly. *Failure to address causative factors and cofactors will result in a nonhealing wound, despite appropriate systemic and topical therapy.* There is no dressing available that can compensate for an uncorrected pathologic condition (Bolton et al, 1990).

Principle 2: Provide Systemic Support of Patient to Reduce Existing and Potential Cofactors

The complex phenomenon of repair occurs only in the presence of adequate oxygen, growth factors, cytokines, and nutrients and in the absence of deterrents. Thus nursing assessment must include evaluation of the patient's cardiovascular and pulmonary function, nutritional and fluid status, and concommitant conditions that affect the wound-healing process. Assessment factors may include the following:

- Cardiovascular and pulmonary function, such as blood pressure, pulse and respiratory rates, distal pulses, capillary refill, presence of absence of edema, pallor, temperature changes, and PO_2 (WOCN, 1993)
- Nutritional and fluid status, such as actual weight as compared with ideal weight; laboratory indicators of visceral protein status such as albumin, transferrin, and prealbumin; current total intake of calories and protein to include oral, enteral, and parenteral routes; clinical indicators of malnutrition such as joint edema, sparse hair, dry skin, and lethargy (WOCN, 1993)
- Conditions or factors known to deter wound healing, such as diabetes, steroid administration, and immunosuppression (WOCN, 1993)

Having assessed the patient for evidence of systemic support for wound healing, the nurse must intervene to correct any deficiencies. This may involve the following:

- Measures to support tissue oxygenation, such as hydration, elevation of edematous extremities, and administration of nasal oxygen to the patient with low PO_2.
- Measures to correct nutritional deficiencies, such as dietary or nutritional support consultation; provision of oral, enteral, or parenteral support; and provision of vitamin and mineral supplements.
- Measures to control wound-healing deterrents, such as blood glucose control and administration of vitamin A for the patient on steroids.

Principle 3: Maintain a Physiologic Local Wound Environment

A critical aspect of local wound care lies in the third principle, that of maintaining a physiologic local wound environment for optimal healing by using appropriate topical therapy. Examination of the phrase *physiologic wound environment*, in terms of the definitions of the individual words, yields the following (*Merriam-Webster's Medical Desk Dictionary*, 1993):

- *Physiologic* means "characteristic of an organism's healthy or normal functioning."
- *Wound* refers to "an injury to the body consisting of a laceration or breaking of the skin."
- *Environment* refers to "the complex physical, chemical, and biotic factors that act upon an organism and ultimately determine its form and survival."

Based on this information, an operational definition of a *physiologic wound environment* can be

TABLE 5-1 Physiologic Wound Environment: Key Factors and Characteristics

FACTORS	PROCESS	OBJECTIVE OF PROCESS	CLINICAL APPLICATION
Physical	Tissue hydration	Maintain cell viability	Appropriate use of moisture-retentive, absorptive, or hydrating dressings
	Temperature control	Maintain optimum function of phagocytic and mitotic activity	Cover wound, use solutions that are at body temperature
Chemical	pH level (acidity)	Optimize chemical processes of healing	Consider acidity and alkalinity of chemicals placed into the wound, avoid mixing of topical agents without indication
Biotic	Adequate perfusion	Provide oxygen and nutrients to sustain tissue viability	Avoid excessive or sustained pressure in or around the wound
	Control of microorganisms	Avoid colonization, infection	Minimize necrotic tissues, use appropriate cleansing techniques and solutions, use appropriate technique in applying and removing dressings

stated as "those physical, chemical, and biotic (living) factors that are characteristic of healthy skin in the absence of a break or compromise." This definition is relatively concise but can benefit from further explanation. In the realm of science, *physical factors* or properties are usually measurable quantities that describe a substance as it is in its most common or normal state. *Chemical factors* or properties describe or affect the ability of a substance to undergo change via chemical reactions (Hess, 1984). *Biotic properties* describe the conditions required for viability of a substance. The substance under discussion in this case is a wound or break in the skin, and the *physiologic* state of a wound is nonwounded or healthy skin. The following sections examine more closely the purpose and clinical relevance of these three factors (Table 5-1).

Physical Factors of a Physiologic Wound Environment. Physical factors of a physiologic wound environment may be thought of as properties that characterize a healthy body. Two common physical properties reflective of health are body temperature and hydration levels. The normal anatomy and physiology of the skin are discussed in detail in Chapter 1. This discussion focuses on the fact that all of the cellular and chemical components of the dermis and epidermis have distinct functions that can only be carried out under specific levels and ranges of hydration and temperature, the physical factors of a "physiologic wound environment."

Tissue hydration

Normal function. *Hydration* refers to a contained amount of water. Water, vital in most of the body's cellular biochemical processes, is the primary constituent of blood and serves to transport nutrients and oxygen to cells and remove metabolic wastes. The human body is more than 65% water; the primary means of maintaining this level of moisture is located in the epidermis (Spruitt, 1972). The stratum corneum prevents loss of excessive amounts of water in the form of vapor to the external environment. Given time, water will readily evaporate at temperatures lower than its boiling point of 212° F. Normal body temperatures of 98.6° F would facilitate evaporative loss of water from tissue cells if not for the moisture barrier properties of the stratum corneum.

An early study of transepidermal water loss (TWL) in humans documented that the TWL, through intact skin on the backs of adult males, averaged 0.18 mg of moisture vapor per square centimeter of skin per hour ($mg/cm^2/hr$). Target areas on the skin were then sequentially tape-stripped to remove the stratum corneum completely and create a glistening area, indicating that the basal layer had been reached. Subsequent TWL measurements of the areas without the stratum corneum averaged 32.81 mg/cm^2/hr (Rovee et al, 1972). In the absence of the stratum corneum, water loss from the skin increased by almost 200-fold. Because TWL through intact skin varies slightly by location on the body, this magnitude of difference may not be observed uniformly; however, investigators have reported differences in TWL of intact versus damaged skin at other anatomic sites, ranging from 50- to 100-fold (Bothwell et al, 1972).

Clinical applications. Hydration levels of healthy skin are maintained by an intact stratum corneum. In a wound, where the stratum corneum has been removed or compromised, tissues or cells are subject to increased loss of water vapor and may desiccate and eventually die. A physiologic wound environment would consequently be a local environment in which tissue hydration levels and therefore viability were maintained by something other than the stratum corneum.

Currently there is an abundance of wound dressings that can function as an exogenous barrier to water vapor loss from a wound. The dressing materials are usually comprised of synthetic or natural polymers, and their barrier ability can be characterized by a measurement known as *moisture vapor transmission rate* (MVTR). MVTR and TWL are similar quantities in that both refer to the quantity of water vapor that passes through a substance. In general, MVTR is measured in units of weight of moisture vapor per area of material per time period. MVTR is usually reported as g/m^2/day but could also be reported as mg/cm^2/hr or other combinations. When comparing MVTRs of different dressing materials, it is important to make sure that the unit of measure is the same.

Several terms are used to refer to dressings that provide some level of barrier to moisture vapor loss from a wound, including semiocclusive, occlusive, moisture retentive, synthetic, and advanced. Semiocclusive and occlusive are often used interchangeably, although they have different meanings. *Occlusive* implies that no liquids or gases (e.g., moisture vapor, oxygen, and carbon dioxide) can be transmitted through the dressing material, whereas *semiocclusive* means that no liquids, but variable levels of gases, are transmitted. An example of an occlusive material is polyethylene (e.g., Saran Wrap), which transmits no gases, either odors or moisture vapor. An example of a semiocclusive material is a transparent film (polyurethane) used for wound care, which transmit variable levels of moisture vapor as well as other gases. Early versions of hydrocolloids were described as being fully occlusive. Today most hydrocolloids are backed with a semiocclusive film layer, which renders them semiocclusive. Most wound dressings are actually semiocclusive rather than occlusive.

Moisture retentive is a more general term that refers to any dressing that is able to consistently retain moisture at the wound site by interfering with the natural evaporative loss of moisture vapor; therefore any semiocclusive dressing is by definition moisture retentive. Providing moisture is not the same thing as retaining moisture over time. Saline-moistened gauze may be used to provide moisture to a wound if changed or remoistened frequently; however, it cannot keep the wound continually moist on its own and is not considered moisture retentive. Semiocclusive dressings, such as films, foams, and hydrocolloids, are able to keep a wound moist, even when no additional moisture is supplied, by "catching" and retaining moisture vapor that is being lost by the wound on a continual basis. *Synthetic* is a term used to describe dressings that are composed of man-made materials, such as polymers, as opposed to materials from nature, such as cotton. The term *advanced* is the most general term and is used relative to "nonadvanced" dressings such as gauze, which has been used for centuries. The term *advanced dressings* usually refers to any of the newer, semiocclusive dressings.

It is tempting to think that the ideal wound dressing should exactly mimic the barrier function of healthy intact skin and therefore have an MVTR close to the value of the TWL of intact skin. The average TWL value of intact skin on the back (0.18 mg/cm^2/hr) from the previously described study can be mathematically converted to an MVTR of 43.2 g/m^2/day. However, many dressing materials have MVTR values much greater than this. For example, many film dressings have MVTRs ranging from 400 to 800 $g/m^2/day$, and it may appear from these numbers that they would therefore allow tissue desiccation. In practice, desiccation is rare in wounds treated with film dressings because of the greater level of moisture vapor lost from *damaged* tissue. The average TWL value of tape-stripped skin is 32.81 $mg/cm^2/hr$, which converts to an MVTR value of 7874 $g/m^2/day$. Tape stripping creates a very superficial wound, and many wounds lose larger amounts of moisture vapor depending on their nature and extent. Film dressings transmit less moisture vapor than the average wound loses and thus facilitate tissue moisture as opposed to desiccation. In general, if the dressing material transmits less moisture vapor than the wound loses, then the wound will remain moist. If the dressing material transmits more moisture vapor than the wound loses, then the wound may dry out.

The ability of saline-moistened gauze dressings to keep a wound from drying out depends on the drainage level of the wound and the frequency with which the gauze is changed or moistened. It is possible to prolong the loss of moisture from saline-moistened gauze by incorporating petrolatum-impregnated gauze as an upper layer of the dressing. Because petrolatum is hydrophobic, it will not absorb and transmit moisture from the moistened materials beneath it, and the life of the saline-moistened gauze is prolonged.

In reality, wounds usually lose more than just water *vapor*; they lose *liquid* water in the form of wound drainage. When drainage levels are high, simple transmission of vapor will not dissipate adequate moisture to maintain *physiologic* tissue hydration. If the moisture vapor transmitted by a dressing is significantly less than the moisture being lost by the wound in vapor and liquid form, then drainage accumulates and remains in contact with the wound and surrounding skin. Tissues may subsequently become wet and periwound skin macerated. Healthy tissues in the wound are moist but not wet and not dry. To manage high drainage levels, a dressing must also have a liquid absorptive capacity in addition to vapor transmission ability. The process of absorption physically moves drainage away from the wound's surface and edges and into the dressing material. At the other end of the hydration spectrum, wound tissue that is already dry may need to be actively rehydrated using dressing materials that donate water to the tissue.

A physiologic wound environment relative to tissue hydration involves promoting and maintaining moist—not wet, not dry—tissue using exogenous materials that function to maintain adequate moisture, absorb excess liquid moisture, or donate moisture under certain circumstances to desiccated tissues. Wounds may have variable hydration needs based on the type of wound and the phase of healing. It is unlikely that a single type of dressing will be appropriate for all types of wounds or even for a single wound throughout the course of its healing.

Temperature

Normal function. Stable body temperature is critical for warm-blooded animals. All cellular functions are affected by temperature, including chemical reactions (e.g., metabolism, enzymatic catalysis, protein synthesis, and oxidation) and processes (e.g., phagocytosis, mitosis, and locomotion). Most reactions and processes occur at rates directly proportional to temperature; the operative range of body temperature for optimal cellular function in humans is narrow (97.5° F [36.4° C] to 99° F [37.2° C]). Above or below this range the cellular reaction or process may be impaired or even shut down.

Clinical application. The temperature of wound tissues should remain as close as possible to normal. However, in the case of an open wound, local cooling can occur as a result of moisture vapor loss from the exposed tissues and as a result of using refrigerated solutions for irrigation.

Local hypothermia can impair both the healing process and the immune response; it can lead to increased risks of infection by causing vasoconstriction and by increasing hemoglobin's affinity for oxygen, both of which result in a decreased availability of oxygen to phagocytes. The consequence of hypothermia on phagocytes includes decreased phagocytic activity, decreased production of reactive oxygen products (Clardy, Edwards, and Gay, 1985), and impaired ability to migrate (Akriotis and Biggar, 1985; Wenisch et al, 1996). Reduced mitotic activity and decreased production of growth factors IL-1 beta and IL-2 have been reported when surgical patients experience a reduction in core body temperature of 1° C (Beilin et al, 1998). IL-1 beta is associated with chemoattraction of neutrophils, monocytes, and lymphocytes and with stimulation of collagen synthesis (Falanga, 1993), whereas IL-2 is associated with regulation of the microbicidal activity of monocytes (Wahl and Wahl, 1992). The reduced oxygen tension resulting from hypothermia-induced vasoconstriction can impair collagen deposition and decrease the strength of the healing wound (Kurz, Sessler, and Lenhardt, 1996).

Wound management practices such as wound cleansing or irrigation with refrigerated solutions can induce hypothermia. One study in 420 patients found that local tissue temperatures were reduced for up to 40 minutes after wound cleansing. It was further demonstrated that mitosis and leukocyte activities were decreased for up to 3 hours after cleansing (Thomas, 1990).

Topical wound dressings that reduce moisture loss from wounded tissues can diminish local cooling and avoid potential effects of local hypothermia. Local tissue temperatures of air-exposed wounds in pigs have been measured at 69.8° F (21° C) (Thomas, 1990). When the wounds were dressed with gauze, films, and foams, the tissue temperatures were 77° to 80.6° F (25° to 27° C), 86° to 89.6° F (30° to 32° C), and 91.4° to 95° F (33° to 35° C), respectively. These data suggest that dressing materials have differential thermal insulating properties that parallel their MVTR or ability to lessen evaporative cooling because of moisture vapor loss. The inherent insulating properties of occlusive and semiocclusive wound dressings may be important contributors to their beneficial effects on wound healing.

Chemical Factors of the Physiologic Environment. Chemical factors of a physiologic wound environment refer to characteristics (such as pH) that affect the ability of cells and other substances in healthy tissues of the skin to carry out biochemical reactions. In technical terms, pH is a number that indicates the relative concentration of hydrogen ions in an aqueous solution compared with the hydrogen ion concentration of pure water.

pH

Normal function. The pH of the external surface of the skin is normally slightly acidic, ranging from 4.2 to 5.6 (Rothman, 1954) and plays an important role in preventing bacterial penetration or colonization. Secretions from sweat glands and sebaceous glands are responsible for this surface acidity. The pH of the blood is essentially neutral (7.4), and any significant acidic or alkaline change can have health effects such as lowered perfusion, arrhythmia, and hypoventilation.

Clinical application. When the skin is broken and the resulting wound is exposed to air, the tissues lose not only water vapor but also carbon dioxide and may become mildly alkaline as a consequence of local respiratory alkalosis (Hermans, 1990). This change in pH may in some instances predispose the wound to bacterial infection. In practice, the pH of the fluids and exposed tissues of a wound may vary depending on what exogenous substances (e.g., dressings or topical agents) have been added to the wound surface (Chen, Rogers, and Lydon, 1992).

The chemical constituents of a dressing material or adhesive may affect wound fluid pH beneath different types of semiocclusive and occlusive dressings. Wound fluid pH beneath a transparent film dressing and a hydrocolloid dressing has been measured at 7.1 and 6.1, respectively. Bacterial pathogens such as *Escherichia coli, Staphylococcus aureus,* and *Pseudomonas aeruginosa* isolated from the wound fluids were subsequently grown in vitro at a pH of 5.5 and 7.4 (Varghese et al, 1998). Growth rates at 8 hours were decreased for the lower pH environment, suggesting that a mildly acidic wound environment (pH 5.8 to 6.6) may be of benefit in resisting infection. Such a wound environment may also have a beneficial effect on epithelialization (Wiseman, Rovee, and Alvarez, 1992). However, if the pH value is too low, various cellular functions may decline or stop; the cells themselves may also die under conditions of very low or very high pH. Acetic acid, with a pH of 2.4 (1M solution), is an effective antiseptic in controlling bacteria, especially anaerobes, but is also toxic to endogenous cells such as fibroblasts and white blood cells.

The presence of urine, stool, or fistula drainage in a wound may also have effects on the local pH and healing. Appropriate dressing materials that repel exogenous contaminants are important to protect the wound. Wound pH should also be considered when using topical enzymatic debriding agents. Most enzymes have a pH activity profile, meaning that they are active over a certain range of pH but may exhibit optimal function only at a specific pH (Lehninger, 1975). For example, trypsin has a pH activity profile ranging from around 6 to 10, but activity peaks at 8. Papain has an enzymatic profile ranging from around 4 to 9 but has equal activity at all pH levels. Nurses should also be cautious of mixing different topical agents together for use in a wound because ingredients in one agent may interact with the ingredients in another. For example, the enzymatic activity of collagenase is adversely affected by certain detergents and heavy metal ions such as mercury and silver, which are used in some antiseptics, and is inactivated by povidone iodine. If the use of collagenase enzyme were combined with the use of a new transparent film that releases silver ions, the silver ions would inactivate the enzyme, resulting in no enzymatic debridement and little or no antibacterial effect of the silver. Similarly, certain foams are degraded by hydrogen peroxide, and the two should not be used sequentially. It is of vital importance to thoroughly read product package inserts and instructions for use when two products are being used together or sequentially in the same wound.

Biotic Factors of a Physiologic Environment. Biotic factors are conditions that sustain life, specifically the viability of the cells of the skin or wound. Fuel in the form of oxygen and food and the control of microflora are essential for optimal cellular function. Oxygen and nutrients are supplied to the local wound environment by the blood; therefore an adequate blood supply is a biotic condition. Cellular and organism viability can be threatened by invasion of bacterial pathogens; therefore control of microflora is a biotic condition.

Adequate perfusion

Normal function. Blood carries oxygen and nutrients to all of the tissues of the body and removes carbon dioxide and waste products through an intricate system of arteries, veins, and capillaries. If the blood supply to an area of tissue is compromised or cut off, ischemic damage ensues that can result in tissue death if it is not remedied.

Clinical application. Unrelieved external pressure is an example of a condition that can decrease blood supply by shutting down capillaries. Nurses should make sure that dressings or devices used in wound management (e.g., compression bandages and wound packing materials) do not create areas of unrelieved pressure in or around the wound (Thomas, 1994).

When blood supply to a wound is compromised and cannot be remedied through revascularization, a moist wound environment may not be indicated. Without oxygen and nutrients from the blood, the tissue in the area of the wound cannot proliferate and cannot mount a defense against bacteria, and the risk of gangrene may be potentiated. In the presence of necrotic tissue and no underlying blood supply, semiocclusive dressings should not be used. Depending on the level of ischemia, it may be most appropriate to use dry dressings.

Control of Microorganisms

Normal function. Healthy skin has a multifaceted system to control bacteria, beginning with the acid mantle of the stratum corneum. If the stratum corneum is compromised, cellular defenses such as white blood cells, monocytes, and macrophages are impaired or overwhelmed and local or systemic infection may occur.

Clinical application. Strategies for preventing wound infection include appropriate wound cleansing, removal of nonviable tissue, appropriate use of dressings, and adherence to universal precautions.

Wound cleansing is an area of controversy in wound management, both in terms of cleansing products and techniques. There are three distinct

BOX 5-3 Microbiologic States of the Wound

Wound contamination. An unavoidable state; the presence of bacteria on the wound surface without proliferation.

Wound colonization. Both the presence and proliferation of the bacterial organisms, which may invade necrotic tissue. Colonization elicits no response from the host.

Infection. Represents the invasion of the bacteria into healthy tissues where they continue to proliferate and elicit a reaction from the host (e.g., erythema, pain, warmth, swelling, and changes in exudate and odor).

microbiologic states possible in a wound—contamination, colonization, and infection—that are defined in Box 5-3 (Gilchrist, 1997). Since bacteria cannot invade healthy tissue unless they first adhere or attach (Mertz and Ovington, 1993), wound-cleansing techniques that physically remove surface bacteria serve a preventive role. The physical removal of bacteria does not necessarily require the use of an antiseptic agent. Normal saline is an effective cleansing agent when delivered to the wound site with adequate force to agitate and wash away bacteria. Irrigation is a common method of delivering the wound cleansing solution to the wound surface. Studies have shown that there is an optimal effective range of irrigation pressures that ensure adequate removal of bacteria (Rodeheaver et al, 1975). Pressures below 4 pounds per square inch (psi) are not sufficient to remove bacteria, and pressures above 15 psi risk driving the bacteria into the tissue rather than off of the surface. One easy way to ensure an irrigation pressure within this range is to use a 35 ml syringe and a 19-gauge needle, or angiocatheter (to avoid risk of needlestick).

Many studies have documented that the use of antiseptics (such as povidone iodine, Dakin's, acetic acid, or hydrogen peroxide) in open wounds is not only cytotoxic to bacteria but also to white blood cells and vital wound healing cells such as fibroblasts. This is because their primary mechanism of action is to destroy cell walls regardless of the identity of the cell. All of the aforementioned antiseptics have been shown to damage endogenous wound cells, and their preventive use in open wounds should be weighed in light of this (Doughty 1994; Hellewell et al, 1997; Hess, 1990; Lineweaver et al, 1985). In addition to the absence of clinical benefit, antiseptics may also encourage the development of resistant organisms (Nwomeh, Yager, and Cohen, 1998).

Often, commercial wound-cleansing solutions contain antimicrobial ingredients or other chemicals that can cause damage to wound cells. A recent evaluation of 10 commercial wound cleansers (both antimicrobial and nonantimicrobial) revealed that all inhibited the viability and phagocytic activity of polymorphonuclear leukocytes unless diluted 10- to 1000-fold (Hellewell et al, 1997). An earlier evaluation of commercial cleansers on the market in 1993 reported similar results (Foresman et al, 1993). The FDA does not regulate wound cleansers. The FDA designation of "wound cleansers" is intended primarily as a category of products to be used for minor, acute injuries as opposed to solutions for repeated use in chronic wounds.

The most effective action that can be undertaken to prevent wound infection is to keep the wound free of nonviable tissue that serves as the nutritional source for bacterial proliferation. The development of nonviable or necrotic tissue in the form of slough or eschar may potentially be avoided by the use of dressings that prevent viable tissue from desiccating. Necrotic tissue must be removed by some form of debridement for optimal healing to proceed (see Chapter 7).

Semiocclusive dressings reduce the incidence of wound infections by more than 50% as compared with traditional gauze dressings (Hutchinson, 1989, 1993). This supports the theory that semiocclusive dressings optimize the phagocytic efficiency of endogenous leukocytes by maintaining a moist wound environment, reduce airborne dispersal of bacteria during dressing changes (Lawrence, Lilly, and Kidson, 1992), and in many cases provide a mechanical barrier to the entry of exogenous bacteria (Mertz and Ovington, 1993). One study found that bacteria can penetrate up to 64 layers of gauze (Lawrence, 1994).

Bacterial bioburden in the wound may also be affected by the techniques used to apply and remove dressings and topical agents. Recent clinical guidelines for the treatment of pressure ulcers have advocated the use of clean dressings and clean technique over sterile ones, albeit it with the caveat "until research proves otherwise." There is not much evidence that sterile versus clean techniques has a significant effect on wound healing outcomes (Bergstrom et al, 1994). There also appears to be a lack of agreement among nurses as to what constitutes sterile technique versus nonsterile technique (Faller, 1997).

Some experts advocate a no-touch technique to ensure that the bioburden of the wound is not increased beyond its normal state. No-touch technique mandates the use of sterile materials and equipment for direct contact with the wound surface and clean materials and equipment otherwise (Krasner and Kennedy, 1994).

Principles of body substance isolation and universal precautions for the caregiver should be routinely followed during wound-care practices (Crow, 1997). Handwashing is the most effective and most frequently overlooked precaution (Pittet et al, 1999). Caregivers should wash their hands 1) before and after patient contact, 2) after contact with a source of microorganisms (body fluid and substances, mucous membranes, broken skin, or inanimate objects that are likely to be contaminated), and 3) after removing gloves. An easily overlooked opportunity for handwashing is between care of a dirty and clean body site; an analogy could be made to the removal of the dirty wound dressing and application of a new dressing. Although it has not been researched specifically, it is best to change gloves once the old dressing is removed so that a clean pair of gloves is worn while applying the new wound dressing. This is even more important in light of studies that suggest that at least 25% of the population and almost 40% of health care workers have nasal colonization by *Staphylococcus aureus* (Crow, 1997), the most prevalent wound pathogen (Raz et al, 1996).

MAINTENANCE OF A PHYSIOLOGIC LOCAL WOUND ENVIRONMENT

Topical wound management, the focus of this chapter, largely influences the physiologic local wound environment. A physiologic local wound environment incorporates factors that mimic healthy skin—promotes adequate moisture levels, normal temperature, and pH and does not interfere with local blood supply or control of microflora. These various physical, chemical, and biotic conditions create a milieu that is conducive to a successful and expedient journey from skin compromise to skin repair and restoration of function. Based on the need to create and support a physiologic local wound environment, seven objectives for local wound management become apparent (Table 5-2). Maintenance of a physiologic local wound environment is translated into clinical practice by considering characteristics of the wound, product performance parameters, and patient-related individualization.

Wound Characteristics

The essential question that guides decision-making in local wound care is "What does the wound need to achieve a physiologic environment?" The answer is derived from a careful and accurate assessment and documentation of the wound status (van Rijswijk, 1997; van Rijswijk and Braden, 1999). Additionally, serial assessments indicate how the wound is responding to the treatment and progressing toward the planned goal. Several wound characteristics are influential when selecting topical therapy (Box 5-4).

Etiology. The cause of the wound directly affects wound dressing treatment choices. For example, ulceration resulting from venous insufficiency requires compression and exudate management. Arterial ulcers (after revascularization) are generally nonexudative and as a result require dressings that provide moisture. Neuropathic ulcers commonly have tunnels, whereas pressure ulcers may have undermining; both require dressings to fill the defect or dead space.

TABLE 5-2 Objectives for Local Wound Care and Implications

OBJECTIVES	IMPLICATIONS
Prevent and manage infection	Sterile vs. nonsterile technique, cleaning vs. disinfection, debridement
Cleanse wound	Solutions, irrigation pressures and methods, antiseptics, antibiotics
Remove nonviable tissue (debridement)	Methods, effects on infection, effects on healing
Manage exudate	Role of MVTR, absorption, hydration
Eliminate dead space	Wound-packing materials and methods
Control odor	Dressings, dressing changes, debridement, and products
Protect wound and periwound skin	Minimization of tissue disturbance, protection of the wound base and periwound skin, protection from exogenous substances

BOX 5-4 Wound Assessment Parameters that Influence Topical Dressing Selection

- Etiology
- Location of the wound
- Extent of tissue loss (stage)
- Phase of healing
- Wound size
- Presence of undermining, sinus tracts, or tunnels
- Condition of wound bed
- Condition of wound edges
- Volume of exudate
- Condition of periwound skin
- Infection
- Odor
- Extent of pain

Location of the Wound. Wound location, particularly the wound in areas that are difficult to manage, affect significantly the type of dressing selected. Digit dressings are useful for the toes and fingers. Dressings with a contour, such as a sacral shape, are more effective than square- or rectangular-shaped dressings at the sacrum, coccyx, and heel. Elbows can pose application challenges, and flexible, conformable dressing materials are needed. Wounds in locations exposed to friction and shear from sheets, clothing, or braces require thin adhesive dressings with smooth backings.

Extent of Tissue Loss (Stage). The extent of tissue loss influences wound dressing selection in that wound fillers or wound packing dressings will be needed to fill the dead space created by the tissue loss. The shallower wound may require granules, beads, or pastes, whereas deeper wounds often require alginates, gauze, or hydrofibers.

Phase of Healing. Within the three phases of healing, the needs of the wound differ. Some nurses use the phase of the wound as the basis for dressing selection (Table 5-3). For example, wounds in the maturation stage are closed, and collagen remodeling is occurring. These wounds require protection from mechanical and chemical trauma as tensile strength increases (Barr, 1995).

Wound Size. Wound size affects the selection of both dressing size and material. For example, a wafer or pad product form may be selected to cover the wound and extend at least 2.5 cm (1 inch) onto periwound skin to adequately secure the dressing. Wounds with depth require dressing materials to fill the defect (e.g., pastes, impregnated gauze, alginates, hydrofiber, hydropolymer) (Walsh, 1996). Secondary dressings (used to secure or cover primary dressings) are required to secure wound fillers. Wound size is also an index for evaluation of the effectiveness of the treatment plan and appropriateness of topical therapy.

Presence of Undermining, Sinus Tracts, or Tunnels. The presence of these wound architectures indicates more complex wound management

TABLE 5-3 Dressing Selection Based on Phase of Wound Healing

PHASE AND WOUND DESCRIPTION	CLINICAL WOUND NEEDS	APPROACH AND DRESSINGS
Inflammatory phase		
Necrotic tissue	Debridement	Autolysis alone or in combination with other methods of debridement Moisture-retentive dressings such as alginates, hydrogels, impregnated gauzes, hydrocolloids Enzyme debridement with gauze
Dry wound	Hydrate	Film, hydrogels
Moderate to heavy exudate	Absorption	Hydrocolloid, foam, absorbent impregnated gauze, alginate, hydrofiber, superabsorbent
May exhibit depth	Packing	*Shallow*: powder, paste, alginate *Deep*: impregnated gauze, alginate, cavity foam or sheet foam, strip packing
Erythema, warmth, edema, tenderness, pain	Managing infection	*Local*: antimicrobial dressings *Systemic*: systemic antibiotics/antimicrobial dressings or moisture-retentive dressings
Open wound	Protection	Film, hydrocolloid, foam, composite
Periwound skin	Protection	Skin sealant, barrier ointment
Granulation phase (proliferative)		
Red, granulating wound	Protection	Film, hydrocolloid, foam, composite
Minimal to moderate exudate	Absorption	*Minimal*: thin hydrocolloid, thin foam, absorbent powder/film, absorbent paste/composite *Moderate*: hydrocolloid, foam, alginate/film
May exhibit depth	Packing	*Shallow*: powder, paste, alginate *Deep*: impregnated gauze, alginate, cavity foam or sheet foam, strip packing
Periwound skin	Protection	Skin sealant, barrier ointment
Remodeling/maturation phase		
Pink, resurfacing wound	Protection	Film, thin or traditional hydrocolloid, thin or traditional foam, composite

and increased healing time. A packing material and secondary dressing are usually indicated. The dressing material selected should be retrievable upon dressing change, and the amount of product selected should loosely fill the defect (e.g., absorbent or hydrating impregnated gauze strip or sponge). An antimicrobial product may be indicated to control bacterial burden.

Condition of Wound Bed. This parameter has been used as a basis for decision making and dressing selection in wound care in the form of the Red-Yellow-Black (RYB) classification system (Table 5-4). Granulation is inferred by the red classification; this wound bed requires a dressing that will maintain a moist wound surface. Yellow and black typify necrotic tissue (slough and eschar, respectively). Dressings used in the presence of a yellow or black wound bed must facilitate debridement. Unfortunately, the presence of tendon, ligament, and/or bone in the wound bed, com-

TABLE 5-4 Dressing Selection Based on the Red-Yellow-Black System

WOUND BASE TISSUE AND LEVEL OF EXUDATE	PHASE OF HEALING	LOCAL WOUND CARE OBJECTIVES	DRESSING ALTERNATIVES	
			SHALLOW WOUND	DEEP WOUND
Red				
None	Maturation (scar)	Maintain intact skin	Film, thin foam or hydrocolloid, skin sealant	N/A
Minimal	Inflammatory or proliferative	Maintain a moist environment Provide minimal absorption or minimal hydration Protect periwound skin Fill/pack defects	Film, foam, hydrocolloid, hydrogel, collagen	Hydrogel, other hydrating impregnated gauzes, wound fillers with composite or film cover dressing, contact layer
Moderate to heavy	Inflammatory or proliferative	Maintain a moist environment Absorb exudate Protect periwound skin Fill/pack defects	Foam, hydrocolloid, alginate, hydrofiber, alginate with film or composite cover dressing, pouch	Alginate, foam cavity dressing, absorbent impregnated gauze, hydrofiber, superabsorbent, contact layer, wound fillers with cover dressing
Yellow				
None to minimal	Inflammatory	Debride Maintain a moist environment Hydrate or provide minimal absorption	Hydrogel, film, composite, enzyme debrider	Hydrogel, hydrating impregnated gauze
Moderate to heavy	Inflammatory	Debride Maintain moist environment Absorb exudate Fill/pack defects	Alginate, hydrofiber, superabsorbent, pouch	Alginate, foam cavity dressing, absorbent impregnated gauze, hydrofiber, superabsorbent, contact layer, wound fillers with cover dressing, pouch
Black				
None to minimal	Inflammatory	Debride Hydrate	If completely black, unable to determine; hydrogel or hydrating impregnated gauze with film or composite cover dressing, enzymatic debrider	

monly a pearly white color, may be misinterpreted as slough.

The type of dressing used to achieve debridement varies depending on the form of debridement selected. Dressing choices may include all of the dressing categories in the formulary except for dry gauze. The dressing is selected to maintain a moist wound bed and is based on volume of exudate and the architecture of the wound. Debridement is discussed in detail in Chapter 7.

Condition of Wound Edges. Tissue at the perimeter of the wound represents the wound edge. This area may be attached to the wound bed, unattached, or rolled downward into the wound. Attached wound edges are the ideal state. However, edges that are unattached or roll downward with epithelialization (referred to as a *closed wound edge*, or *epibole*) require extended healing times and often represent a nonhealing wound. Management of the unattached wound edges is similar to management of undermining; gentle packing is required. Removal of an epithelialized rolled wound edge is recommended and may be achieved by applying silver nitrate to the edge or by surgical excision.

Volume of Exudate. The volume and type of wound exudate represent a macroscopic index that is a critical point for local wound-care decisions and a key element in wound algorithms. Dressings designed for dry wounds hydrate the tissue. Conversely, exudative wounds require absorbent dressing materials (Watret, 1997). Several dressings are available that are designed to manage the full range of exudate volume (minimal to heavy amounts). Adequate containment of exudate is critical to manage increased bioburden in the wound, protect the periwound skin, control odor, and avoid overuse of wound-care products. In addition, the prolonged presence of excessive amounts of moisture in the wound may increase the patient's risk for developing hyperplasia. Methods of exudate management include moisture vapor transmission, wicking, and entrapment.

Condition of Periwound Skin. The periwound skin can be intact, dry, cracked, macerated, erythematous, or infected (e.g., candidiasis). Each assessment influences the type of wound-care products selected. For example, dry and cracked skin may require a moisturizer before applying the wound dressing. Intact skin, particularly vulnerable intact skin such as with the elderly, can be protected from adhesives and wound exudate with the use of skin protectants and sealants.

Skin integrity is also affected by the technique used to apply and remove adhesives (Chapter 6). When appropriate, less frequent dressing changes are preferred to prevent unnecessary exposure of the skin to adhesive removal. The presence of maceration indicates that wound exudate is not adequately contained or managed. Prolonged contact of wound fluid with the periwound skin also predisposes the patient to develop a fungal infection (most commonly candidiasis) or erythema at the periwound site. To correct this situation, either the type of dressing used should be modified to a more absorbent dressing, or the frequency of dressing change should be increased. Skin sealants also protect the periwound skin from damp or saturated wound dressings. Occasionally the patient will require an antifungal powder or lotion to treat the fungal infection, although milder cases may resolve spontaneously when the excessive wound exudate is managed effectively. Appropriate use of absorbent dressings or pouching to manage wound exudate reduces the incidence of periwound maceration, erythema, and candidiasis (Dealey, 1995).

Infection. The presence of a wound infection significantly influences decisions concerning topical wound management. Therefore signs and symptoms of an infection should be assessed with each dressing change. When the wound is infected, a complete systemic assessment and appropriate treatment should be instituted.

Local dressings selected for use should have an indication for infected wounds listed on the product package insert. This does not apply to other wound-care products such as cleansing agents and periwound skin-care products. Generally, occlusive dressings are not recommended for infected wounds, semiocclusive dressings should be monitored closely and changed more frequently than generally anticipated, and nonocclusive dressings are indicated as the most conservative topical wound-care approach (Browne and

Sibbald, 1999; Haimowitz and Margolis, 1997; Rolstad, Aronovitch, and Krasner, 1997). Wound cleansing is necessary at each dressing change.

Antimicrobial nonprescription dressings are also available that have demonstrated, to a limited extent, evidence of clinical benefit (Bale, 1997; Bale and Jones, 1997; Falanga, 1999; Mertz et al, 1994). For further discussion of wound infections, dressing selection, and the use of topical antibiotics, refer to Chapter 8.

Presence of Odor. The presence of odor occurs to varying degrees in numerous wound-care situations (Poteete, 1993). Odor is commonly associated with an infected wound. Highly colonized wounds, such as fungating lesions or pressure ulcers with necrotic debris, may also be malodorous. However, slight odors occur normally at dressing changes when wounds are occluded and are associated with the use of certain types of dressings (e.g., hydrocolloids). Also, odor may occur from dressing strikethrough (e.g., leakage), poor hygiene, and inappropriate dressing use (e.g., extending dressing wear time beyond that which is recommended.)

In the fungating wound, topical debridement, topical antibiotics, antimicrobial dressings, or odor-absorbent dressings are effective (Haughton and Young, 1995; Poteete, 1993). When leakage, hygiene, or inappropriate dressing use are the problem, patient and caregiver education is needed.

Extent of Wound Pain. Pain at the wound site must be adequately described and quantified objectively before the nurse can understand the origin of the pain and identify appropriate pain-control measures (Dallam et al, 1995). Chronic pain, such as with ischemia, requires maintenance pain control measures; additional analgesics may be required during wound-care procedures. Pain at the wound site may be relieved or minimized by the use of moisture-retentive dressings; analgesics given before the dressing change may also be indicated. However, pain that occurs during dressing changes should also prompt assessment of technique and wound-care product choices (Szor and Bourguignon, 1999). Skin sealants protect skin from mechanical forces during dressing removal. Nonetheless, caregiver technique in the removal of tape (i.e., proper use of adhesives and supporting the tissue during dressing removal) has a dramatic effect on the patient's pain experience.

Product Performance Parameters

Today's wound-care product armamentarium is designed to provide a physiologic microenvironment for the wound that promotes cutaneous regeneration and repair. Product performance parameters (i.e., functional characteristics) address the needs of the wound, patient, and caregiver (Bergstrom et al, 1994; Ovington, 1998b). Needs of the wound are addressed by matching the characteristics of the wound with the performance parameters of the wound-care product. General performance parameters of the ideal wound-care product include 1) healing or attainment of the highest possible function, 2) infection control, 3) pain relief or reduction, 4) safety, and 5) ease of use (Field and Kerstein, 1994; Rolstad and Harris, 1997; Thomas, 1994).

A critical performance parameter for all wound dressings is some level of occlusion to maintain tissue hydration, which reduces or relieves pain and promotes autolysis. Semiocclusive dressings provide a barrier function that protects the wound and periwound skin from microbial and physical insult. They also provide thermal insulation, odor control, compression, and delivery of antimicrobial agents.

Patient-Related Individualization

Needs of the patient are addressed in numerous ways, including product safety, esthetics, availability, and reimbursement. Safety features indicate that products are free from toxic chemicals and fibers (Collier, 1996; Flanagan, 1997) and that product biocompatibility has been tested and reported by the manufacturers. Safety should also demonstrate that the product does not increase the patient's risk of morbidity or mortality. The nurse's role in safety includes correct use of the product as recommended by the manufacturer (including FDA-approved clinical indications) and proper education of the caregiver.

The caregiver's needs are considered in product design regarding ease of use. The National Family Caregivers Association estimates that family caregivers provide approximately 75% of the home care in the United States (Turnbull, 1999). Hence patient and caregiver familiarity with the application of the wound-care product is essential. To enhance compliance with recommended wound care, products and procedures need to be easy to understand and perform. Wound-care products that require infrequent dressing changes with a limited number of steps in the application process and that use straightforward, simple procedures are most likely to be performed as instructed. Conveniently, dressings meeting these performance parameters are frequently more cost-effective as well.

Summary

A frequently stated axiom in wound care is that "all wounds are not the same." Consequently, many aspects of local wound management differ. Operationalizing this axiom yields the recognition that numerous elements affect physiologic local wound treatment decisions. Therefore one treatment protocol is not appropriate for all wounds and may require numerous modifications as wound characteristics change.

Moisture-retentive dressings (which emerged in the 1970s) are currently staples in the wound-care portfolio representing approximately 63% of the market of wound-care dressings sold in the United States in 1997 (Medical Data International, 1997). In the late 1980s and early 1990s, "bioactive" dressings were introduced. Growth factors and collagen, examples of bioactive materials, are designed to provide the benefits of interactive dressings while attempting to stimulate some aspect of the healing cascade and thereby accelerate healing (Krasner, 1997; Turner, 1997). Although bioactive products hold promise, most wound-care dressings in clinical use in the United States are interactive or passive. Advances in physiologic care also signaled the demise of outdated, traditional wound treatments such as antacids, dry dressings, iodine packing, and heat lamps.

It has been 30 years since Winter provided in vivo evidence that wounds heal faster in a moist environment, with subsequent validation from other researchers regarding the importance of a physiologic wound environment. Unfortunately, nonphysiologic approaches and inappropriate product use remain commonplace (Ballard-Krishnan, van Rijswijk, and Polansky, 1994; Bux and Malhi, 1996). A 1994 study of home health care nurses reported that dry gauze was the dressing of choice 77% of the time (Turner et al, 1994). Medical Data International (1992, 1997) predicted that gauze would represent 59% of the market share in 1997 as compared with 69% in 1992. Change in practice patterns has been slow and may be attributed to many factors. A key factor may be the failure on the part of health care clinicians to acknowledge that wounded skin is a complex pathophysiologic condition that commands a specific knowledge base, which includes assessments and interventions to achieve appropriate outcomes for the wound (Beitz, Fey, and O'Brien, 1999).

WOUND CARE PRODUCT SELECTION

Dressings are primary (placed in direct contact with the wound), secondary (placed over a primary dressing), or a contact layer (placed in direct contact with the wound and left in place while secondary dressings are changed). In some situations, a primary dressing is also the secondary dressing (e.g., hydrocolloid used over a shallow wound).

Although dressings alone do not heal wounds, the correct selection and use of dressings can facilitate wound healing (Bolton et al, 1990). Which dressing, for which wound, and at which phase are the clinical questions in decision making and are frequently deliberated topics in the wound-care literature (Barr, 1995; Cho and Lo, 1998; Krasner, 1997; Lapioli-Zufelt and Morris, 1998; Rolstad, 1997). Most of the literature suggests that there is a high degree of confusion, complexity, and cost associated with these decisions.

Standardization of Products

Currently, there are more than 60 Health Care Finance Administration Common Procedure Coding System (HCPCS) codes for surgical dressings based on type and size. Although only about a dozen generic dressing categories exist (e.g., film, collagen, gauze), substantial performance and design variations occur within each category. For example, alginates are available in rope or pad form, in gelling or high integrity form, with lateral or vertical absorption, and with high or moderate absorption capabilities.

At one time, decision-making was simple because personal preference ruled. However, this was an expensive and nonstandardized approach, which is not compatible with today's capitated health care delivery system. In an attempt to simplify decisions, the "quick-fix, cookbook" approach with a "one size fits all" approach has been observed in some settings. However, standardization of products and wound treatments yields benefits, particularly when protocols and clinical pathways are established collaboratively based on 1) recent published guidelines, 2) a review of the literature for available research, or 3) best practice.

In general, wound-care decisions concerning the type of dressings to be used (hydrogel, alginate, transparent film, etc.) should be based on wound characteristics, wound location, and the patient's situation. A 1994 survey of extended care facilities reported that product availability and reimbursement are more likely to influence dressing choice than the characteristics of the wound and patient condition (Ballard-Krishnan, van Rijswijk, and Polansky, 1994). Specific brand product choices, however, are influenced by a variety of factors. For example, product choices are frequently made based on clinician familiarity and comfort with use.

Attempts to standardize the process of product selection are increasingly common, and the desired objective is to reduce the clinician-to-clinician variability so that costs can be contained without compromising outcomes. Methods of decision analysis for wound-care product selection translate research into clinical practice: algorithms, flow charts, collaborative pathways (also known as clinical pathways), and decision trees (Greer and Siezenis, 1989). Decision-making tools are beneficial in that they can improve the accuracy of decisions making, guide treatment selection, and serve to educate the clinician concerning a particular disease entity (Letourneau and Jensen, 1998). The decision-making tools are usually accompanied by definition of terms to enhance clarity and require policies and procedures and standing orders so that they can be operationalized by the specific caregiver.

Algorithm. The algorithm presents a practical, visual guideline for the flow of care and appropriate use of resources. Numerous algorithms have been published (Bergstrom et al, 1994; Maklebust and Sieggreen, 1996; Miller, 1996). An algorithm organizes thinking by presenting simple, sequenced decisions with an automatic series of actions. The starting point is well defined (e.g., a chronic wound) with crucial decision points (e.g., volume of exudate, depth) and end points that are standard methods of management. Caveats or precautions should also be noted within the algorithm. Validation of wound care algorithms is scarce, yet it is an important process to undertake before implementing the algorithm to be assured, for example, that the terms are understandable to the user (Beitz and van Rijswijk, 1999).

The three principles of wound management and the objectives for local wound management may be incorporated into an algorithm to guide local wound management (Figure 5-1). At each patient contact, elements of the model are reviewed (such as local wound objectives) and treatment decisions are derived based on the wound diagnosis and goal. Optimal wound management will be possible only when the objectives for local wound management are used to guide the selection of topical wound care products.

Flow Chart. A flow chart may start with the type of tissue present in the wound bed; critical decision points are then linked to interventions. However, the flow chart is not usually as visual as an algorithm and may represent fewer steps to the outcome with less detailed information included. Table 5-4 demonstrates a type of flow chart that was developed based on the premise that the color of the wound indicates the type of tissue present and reflects the current phase of wound healing (Cuzzell, 1995). In this flow chart, the RYB classification system has been modified to include exudate level as an additional descriptor (Krasner, 1995; Sussman, 1998). The RYB system relies on assessment of the wound bed tissue type and exudate levels to determine local wound-care objectives and care decisions. When a wound has combined colors, the most problematic color is used in the grid.

A flow chart may also be based on the phases of wound healing. This physiologically based flow chart is useful for wound-care specialists but may prove too complex for general use. It relies on knowledge that the nurse is able to differentiate among the inflammatory, proliferative, and remodeling/maturation phases of wound healing (Barr, 1995; Thomas, 1997). However, once the phase is differentiated, clinical needs are identified (objectives) and treatment options are provided (see Table 5-3).

Collaborative Pathway. A collaborative pathway is a care delivery tool that sequences the delivery of routine care for a patient with a specific illness episode, thereby facilitating the potential to achieve desired outcomes within an ideal time frame. An interdisciplinary team typically designs these tools so that all health care activities and disciplines relevant to the management of this illness are represented in the pathway (Hill, Labik, and Vanderbilt, 1997; Lovejoy, Bussey, and Sherer, 1997; Springett and Heaney, 1999). Relevant outcomes for the illness episode are stated, and specific parameters of care pertinent to achieving that outcome are listed. Within each parameter of care, the caregiver is directed to provide selected interventions (e.g., risk, skin care) within specific timeframes.

Wound Care Product Decisions: Understanding Products

Once the patient and wound assessments are complete and the wound needs are identified, the nurse must determine which wound-care products can best meet those needs. Table 5-5 lists the various wound-care product parameters (based on the needs of the wound); these parameters are then cross-linked with categories of wound-care products. This table can serve as a quick reference guide for the care provider.

A key role of the wound-care clinician in any health care system is to standardize and organize wound-care products available within that system. Products are classified by generic categories typically used, and the resulting document is used as a product formulary (Andrychuk, 1998; Hess, 1997; Ovington, 1998a, 1998b; Rolstad and Borchert, 1995; van Rijswik and Beitz, 1998). A wound-care product formulary is set up similarly to a drug formulary: generic categories, brand-names, product description, dispensing units, indications for use, precautions, and instructions for use are included. An example of a wound-care product formulary is provided in Appendix 5.1 at the end of this chapter. Annual review of this formulary is recommended because wound-care product research and development is an ongoing and quickly paced industry (Ovington, 1999a; Salcido, 1999).

GENERAL WOUND-CARE PROCEDURES

Regardless of the type of wound or the wound dressing selected, there are fundamental procedures and techniques that apply. These include dressing removal, wound packing, dressing application, and dressing securement. Universal precautions should be used. To further minimize the risk of cross-contamination, clean nonsterile gloves should be used to remove the soiled dressing, and a new pair of gloves should be used to apply the new dressing (Stotts et al, 1993; 1997).

Dressing Removal

The goal of this procedure is to remove the dressing while protecting periwound skin and the wound base from trauma. Dressing changes are performed on a scheduled basis depending on the type of dressing in use; dressings that are oversaturated or leaking should be changed when detected. Universal precautions are indicated, and a clean technique is used. Adhesives are removed in the direction of hair growth. An edge of the dressing is gently rolled or lifted to obtain a starting edge. The tissue adjacent to the dressing is supported as the dressing is gently released from the skin. A moist gauze can be used to support the skin during removal to minimize the potential for stripping. If the dressing material is attached to the wound base, saline or a wound cleanser may be used to moisten the dressing and gently release it from the tissue. Disposal of dressing materials and contaminated gloves is performed in accordance with agency policies and procedures.

Dressing Application

After dressing removal and wound cleansing, the surrounding skin is gently cleansed and dried. A

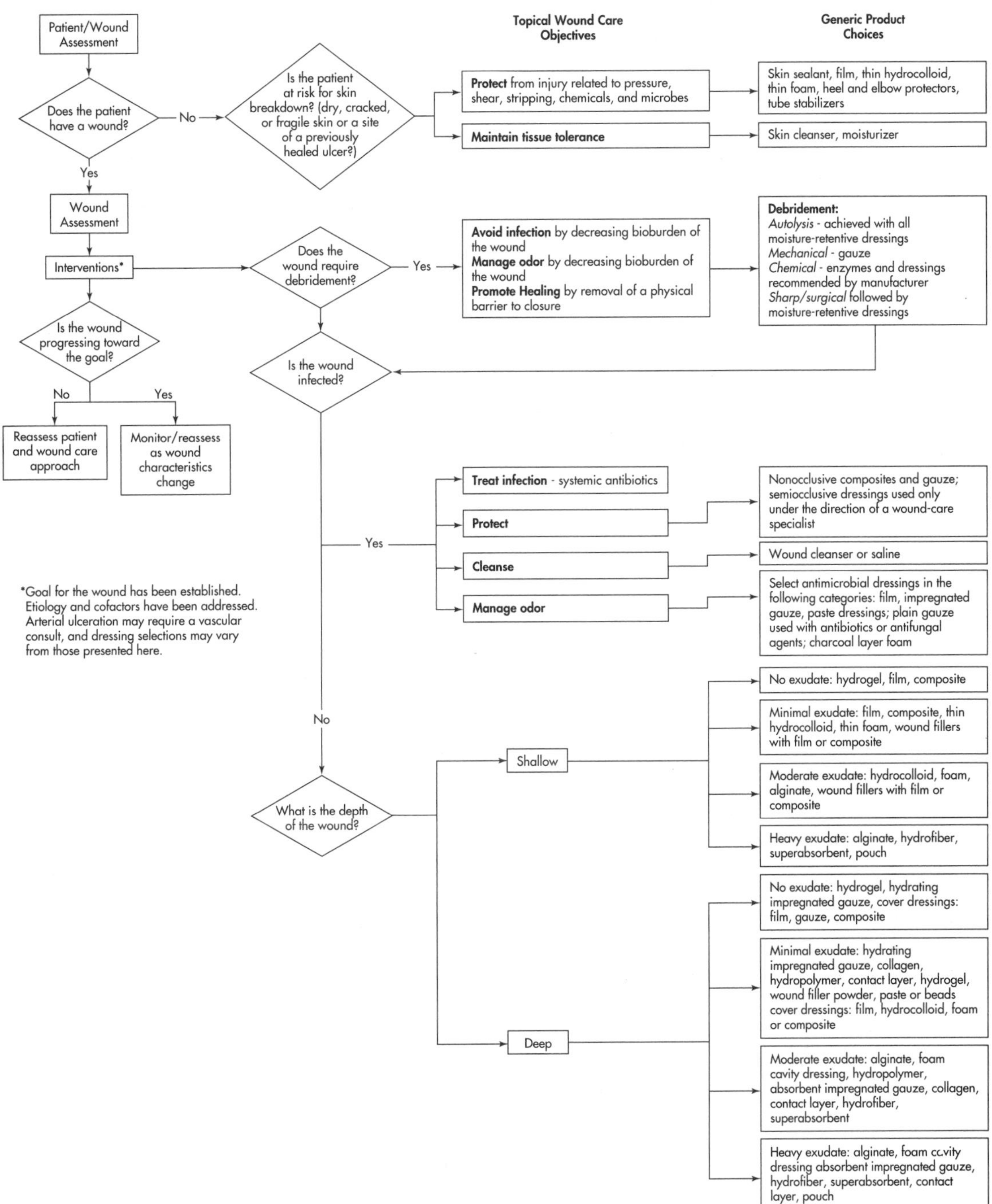

Figure 5-1 Local wound management interventions algorithm. (Courtesy Bonnie Sue Rolstad, RN, BA, CWOCN. Copyright © 2000).

TABLE 5-5 Wound Care Product Performance Parameters by Categories

	CLEANSING			DEBRIDEMENT		
CATEGORY	SKIN	WOUND	COMPRESSION	AUTOLYSIS	ENZYMATIC	MECHANICAL
Alginate				S		
Collagen				S		
Composite						
Compression: leg and wraps			P			
Contact layer						
Enzymes					P	
Foam				S		
Gauze				DD		DD
Growth factors						
Hydrocolloid				S		
Hydrofiber				S		
Hydrogel				S		
Hydropolymers				S		
Pouch						
Sealants: skin and ointments						
Skin cleanser	P					
Specialty absorptives				S		
Super-absorbents				S		
Transparent film				P		
Vaccuum-assisted closure				S		
Warming devices						
Wound cleanser		P				S
Wound filler				S		

TABLE 5-5 Wound Care Product Performance Parameters by Categories—cont'd

CATEGORY	EXUDATE MODULATION	HYDRATION MAINTENANCE*	ODOR CONTROL	PACKING	PROTECTION		WOUND HEALING†
					WOUND BED	PERIWOUND SKIN	
Alginate	P	S	DD	P			
Collagen	S	S		S			P
Composite	S	S			P	S	
Compression: leg and wraps							
Contact layer					P		
Enzymes							
Foam	P	S	DD	DD	P	S	
Gauze	P	DD	DD	P	DD		
Growth factors		DD					P
Hydrocolloid	P	S			S	S	
Hydrofiber	P	S		P			
Hydrogel	DD	P	DD	S			
Hydropolymers	P	S					
Pouch	P	S	P		P	S	
Sealants: skin and ointments						P	
Skin cleanser							
Specialty absorptives	P	S					
Super-absorbents	P	S					
Transparent film		S	DD		P	S	
Vaccuum-assisted closure	P	S	S	S	S	S	
Warming devices							P
Wound cleanser			S		S		
Wound filler	S	S	DD	P			

P, Primary performance parameter; *S*, secondary performance parameter; *DD*, dependent upon product form.
* Moisture retentive.
† Manufacturer claims.

skin sealant may be applied to the skin before dressing application to protect the skin. The selected dressing is then applied, according to manufacturer's instructions, without stretching the skin. In the gluteal fold, wafer dressings are folded in half before application to ensure that the adhesive seals into the anatomic contours. Applications of dressings at the heel or elbow may require cutting and shaping the dressing to customize the fit.

Packing Procedures

The purpose of packing the wound is to fill dead space and avoid the potential of abscess formation by premature closure of the wound. Packing materials should be conformable to the base and sides of the wound. Assessment of the depth and undermining of tunneling is completed. When tunneling is present, strip gauze packing is used to fill narrow areas while allowing for dressing retrieval. For large, deep wounds, hydrating or absorbent impregnated gauze is effective and usually requires less dressing changes than dry gauze. The packing material is fluffed and loosely placed into the wound with a cotton-tipped applicator so that the packing material is in contact with the wound edges and base. Gauze dressings may be necessary to act as an additional absorbent layer. A secondary cover dressing is then applied and secured. Overpacking of the wound should be avoided.

Dressing Securement

When dressings are nonadhesive, a method of securement is necessary to keep the dressing in place. Self-adhesive wraps, tape, Montgomery straps, gauze wraps, or tubular mesh dressings may be used. If the wound is located on the leg, a gauze wrap may be taped upon itself to avoid application of tape to the skin.

EVALUATING OUTCOMES

Routinely, the nurse must evaluate effectiveness of local wound treatments. At each patient contact, assessments are made to determine the patient's status and response to treatment. Examples of important questions include the following:

- **Is the wound progressing toward the identified goal?** If not, assess to ensure that care is being provided as recommended. Reevaluate macroscopic wound indices. If exudate has increased and autolysis is not in progress, is a more absorbent dressing required? Is the patient's condition deteriorating? Is the wound infected?
- **Is the patient and/or caregiver able to perform the procedures correctly and on schedule?** If not, review, demonstrate, and observe the caregiver doing procedures. Simplify the dressing and frequency of changes when possible.
- **Is the nonhealing wound free of infection?** If not, refer to the infection section of this text.
- **Is pain reduced?** If not, reassess to ensure that a moist wound environment is being maintained as appropriate. Reassess whether the etiology of the wound has been reduced or eliminated. Confer with other team members to consider analgesia.
- **If autolysis is in progress, is appropriate progress being achieved in a timely fashion?** If not, consider sharp and surgical methods to augment autolysis.
- **Is the topical therapy cost effective?** Cost effectiveness is not sufficiently measured by the price of the dressing (frequently, the cost per unit for an interactive dressing is higher than that for dry gauze). It must instead reflect the cost of achieving a desired outcome (Phillips, 1997). In this way, it is the cost of the outcome that is to be compared. When nursing time is factored in and healing rates are compared, moisture-retentive approaches have proven more cost-effective (Bolton, van Rijswijk, and Shaffer, 1996). Four factors should be calculated into the cost of treatment for conservatively managed chronic wounds to achieve the desired outcome: 1) cost of all dressing materials, 2) nursing time, 3) treatment costs for complications, and 4) loss of work time and other related expenses (Bolton, van Rijswijk, and Shaffer, 1996; Hermans and Bolton, 1996).

On a per-patient basis, local wound management interventions should be planned with consideration for product reimbursement for the patient. Documentation, product selection, and the care setting affect how reimbursement occurs. Some wound care items are not reimbursed (e.g., skin and wound cleansers, moisturizers) by Medicare (Turnbull, 1995). If the patient is paying out-of-pocket for these supplies, wound care may be jeopardized.

SUMMARY

The approach used to manage wounds has changed dramatically since the late 1880s but not as dramatically as in the last 20 years (since the early 1980s). Before 1980, gauze was *the* dressing available for wound care, and dressings fulfilled passive functions (e.g., to plug and conceal). Historically, passive dressing materials consisted of animal, vegetable, and mineral sources, including leaves, feathers, plant extracts, hot oil, waxes, papyrus, honey, fat, castor oil, gold, and gauze (Elliott, 1964; Leaper, 1986; Majno, 1975; Turner, 1997).

Today there are well over a dozen categories of wound care products, and each dressing contains certain performance parameters that are tailored to satisfy specific wound needs. The FDA Modernization Act of 1997 grouped products into functional categories where one dressing may be classified in more than one category (Table 5-6) (van Rijswijk, 1999). For the purposes of billing and tracking use,

TABLE 5-6 Dressing Category Definitions and Examples of Products as Presented by HIMA

CATEGORY	DEFINITION	EXAMPLES
Nonresorbable gauze/sponge for external use	• Sterile or nonsterile • Strip, piece, or pad • Woven or nonwoven mesh cotton cellulose • Simple chemical derivatives of cellulose • Intended for medical purposes	• Gauze • Sponge • Pads • Island dressings
Hydrophilic wound dressing	• Sterile or nonsterile • Nonresorbable • Material with hydrophilic properties • No added drugs or biologics • Intended to cover wound and absorb exudate	• Alginate dressings • Foam dressings • Hydropolymer dressings • Sheet gel dressings • Hydrocolloid dressings • Composite dressings • Hydrogel dressings
Occlusive wound dressing	• Sterile or nonsterile • Nonresorbable • Synthetic polymeric material with or without adhesive backing • Intended to cover wound, provide or support moist wound environment, and allow exchange of gases	• Transparent adhesive dressings • Thin film dressings • Foam dressings • Hydrocolloid dressings • Composite dressings • Hydropolymer dressings
Hydrogel wound dressing	• Sterile or nonsterile • Nonresorbable • Matrix of hydrophilic polymers or other material combined with at least 50% water • Intended to cover wound, absorb wound exudate, control bleeding or fluid loss, protect against abrasion, friction, dessication, contamination	• Alginate dressings • Hydropolymer dressings • Hydrogel dressings • Gauze dressings impregnated with hydrogel (without active ingredients)
Porcine wound dressing	• Made from pigskin • Temporary burn dressing	

From van Rijswijk L: Recommendations to change the FDA classification of various wound dressings, *Ostomy Wound Manage* 45(3):31, 1999.

the current categories and codes from the Health Care Financing Administration (HCFA) continue to be used, however. For the most current information on wound dressing categories and definitions, visit the FDA website at www.fda.gov/default.htm.

Several changes specific to the specialty of wound care have also occurred in the past decade, including the emergence of practice standardization (through practice guidelines, protocols, decision trees, algorithms, and policies and procedures), the monitoring of product selection and use (as demonstrated by the development of product formularies and interdisciplinary skin- and wound-care teams), and the monitoring or tracking of patient outcomes (Bergstrom et al, 1994; Bowman and Walton, 1996; Dwyer, 1997; Laverty 1997; Panel on Quality Determinants of Mammography, 1994; Rolstad and Borchert 1995; Strayer and Martucci, 1997; Young 1997). Understanding principles of wound management prepares a nurse to partner within interdisciplinary teams, to be capable of articulating underlying rationale, and to use a research-based approach to patient care (Bowers, 1998; Doan-Johnson, 1998; Powers, 1997).

This chapter has reviewed a holistic approach to the patient and the maintenance of a physiologic wound environment. Realistic and appropriate goals for the patient with a wound can only be set when prognostic parameters that affect the treatment plan (e.g., a large venous ulcer, lipodermatosclerosis, or long duration of disease) have been carefully considered (Tallman et al, 1997). Local wound management must be based on this holistic view of the patient. A framework and standardization for decision-making has been presented to address processes and the integration of quality care standards. Each standardized decision-making tool (e.g., wound care product formulary, decision analysis methods, and procedures) presents an opportunity to measure outcomes and conduct continuous quality-improvement activities.

SELF-ASSESSMENT EXERCISE

1. The three principles of wound management are:
   - **a.** Debridement, control of infection, and exudate management
   - **b.** Establishment of a treatment goal, wound cleansing, and physiologic local wound care
   - **c.** Assessment of the host, debridement, and physiologic local wound care
   - **d.** Addressing of etiology, support of the host, and maintenance of a physiologic local wound environment
2. Which of the following interventions indicates an attempt to control or eliminate the etiology of a venous ulcer?
   - **a.** Resizing of shoe to include orthotics
   - **b.** Applying an alginate and foam cover dressing
   - **c.** Monitoring blood glucose levels
   - **d.** Encouraging elevation of the leg three times daily
3. Two common physical factors of a physiologic wound environment are:
   - **a.** Body temperature and hydration levels
   - **b.** Body temperature and skin pH
   - **c.** Skin pH and bioburden
   - **d.** Hydration levels and bioburden
4. Three frequently used goals for wound care include:
   - **a.** Debridement, healing, and education
   - **b.** Cleansing, debridement, and physiologic local wound care
   - **c.** Healing, delayed healing, and symptom control
   - **d.** Control of infection, healing, and physiologic local wound care
5. Semiocclusive dressings are:
   - **a.** Occlusive to liquids and gases
   - **b.** Occlusive to liquids but transmit moisture vapor and gases
   - **c.** Occlusive to gases and vapors but transmit liquids
   - **d.** Inconsistent in their nonocclusive properties
6. In the patient with a new approximated surgical wound, the primary wound care objective is:
   - **a.** Absorption
   - **b.** Hydration
   - **c.** Cleansing
   - **d.** Protection

7. Dressing selection is primarily based on:
   a. Functions of the dressing
   b. Characteristics of the wound
   c. Product availability and cost
   d. Number of dressing changes required daily
8. In the patient with a highly exudative pressure ulcer, which category of dressings should be considered?
   a. Hydrocolloids
   b. Collagens
   c. Wound fillers
   d. Alginates
9. Which is the best definition of cost effectiveness?
   a. The cost of products and labor used to care for the patient
   b. The cost of achieving a desired outcome
   c. Direct and indirect costs of caring for the patient
   d. Cost of the dressing and labor for nursing procedures
10. In an integrated health care system, processes for delivering quality local wound management may best be achieved through:
    a. Guidelines and policies
    b. Collaborative, interdisciplinary teams
    c. Wound-care formularies and practice guidelines
    d. Adhering to HCFA guidelines for product use
11. Describe the relevance of a moisture vapor transmission rate to creating a physiologic wound environment.
12. State the seven objectives for local wound management, and correlate each with a type of dressing that will assist in achieving that objective.
13. Describe the purpose of and correct technique for packing wounds.

REFERENCES

Akriotis V, Biggar W: The effects of hypothermia on neutrophil function in vitro, *J Leukoc Biol* 37(1): 51, 1985.

Andrychuk M: Pressure ulcers: causes, risk factors, assessment and intervention, *Orthop Nurs* 17(4):65, 1998.

Bale S: Wound dressings. In Morison M et al: *Nursing management of chronic wounds,* ed 2, London, 1997, Mosby.

Bale S, Jones V: *Wound care nursing, a patient centered approach*, London, 1997, Baillière Tindall.

Ballard-Krishnan S, van Rijswijk L, Polansky M: Pressure ulcers in extended care facilities: report of a survey. *J Wound Ostomy Continence Nurs* 21(1):4, 1994.

Barr J: Physiology of healing: the basis for the principles of wound management, *Medsurg Nurs* 4(5):387, 1995.

Beilin B et al: Effects of mild perioperative hypothermia on cellular immune responses, *Anesthesiology* 89(5):1133, 1998.

Beitz JM, Fey J, O'Brien D: Perceived need for education vs. actual knowledge of pressure ulcer care in a hospital nursing staff, *Dermatol Nurs* 11(2):125, 1999.

Beitz J, van Rijswijk L: Using wound care algorithms: a content validation study, *J Wound Ostomy Continence Nurs* 26(5):238, 1999.

Bergstrom N et al: *Treatment of pressure ulcers: clinical practice guideline No. 15*, Rockville, Md, 1994, US Department of Health and Human Services, Public Health Service, Agency for Health Care Policy and Research. AHCPR Pub No 95-0652.

Bolton L et al: Dressing's effect on wound healing, *Wounds* (2):126, 1990.

Bolton L, van Rijswijk L, Shaffer F: Quality wound care equals cost-effective wound care: a clinical model, *Nurs Manage* 27(7):30, 1996.

Bothwell J et al: The effect of climate on repair of cutaneous wounds in humans. In Maibach H, Rovee D, editors: *Epidermal wound healing*, Chicago, 1972, Yearbook Medical Publishers.

Bowers C: Development and implementation of evidence-based guidelines: a multisite demonstration project, *J Wound Ostomy Continence Nurs* 25(4):187, 1998.

Bowman J, Walton Y: Development of specialist dermatology nurse prescribing, *Nurs Stand* 10(42):34, 1996.

Browne A, Sibbald R: The diabetic neuropathic ulcer: an overview, *Ostomy Wound Manage* 45(suppl 1A):6S, 1999.

Bux M, Malhi J: Assessing the use of dressings in practice, *J Wound Care* 5(7):305, 1996.

Chen W, Rogers A, Lydon M: Characterization of biologic properties of wound fluid collected during early stages of wound healing, *J Invest Dermatol* 99(5):559, 1992.

Cho CY, Lo JS: Dressing the part, *Dermatol Clin* 16(1):25, 1998.

Clardy CW, Edwards KM, Gay JC: Increased susceptibility to infection in hypothermic children- possible role of acquired neutrophil dysfunction, *Pediatr Infect Dis J* 4(4):379, 1985.

Collier M: The principles of optimum wound management, *Nurs Standard* 10(43):47, 1996.

Crow S: Infection control perspectives. In Krasner D, Kane D, editors: *Chronic wound care,* ed 2, Wayne, Penn, 1997, Health Management Publications.

Cuzzell J: Wound healing: translating theory into clinical practice, *Dermatol Nurs* 7(2):127, 1995.

Dallam L et al: Pressure ulcer pain: assessment and quantification, *J Wound Ostomy Continence Nurs* 22:211, 1995.
Dealey C: Common problems in wound care: caring for the skin around wounds, *Br J Nurs* 4(1):43, 1995.
Doan-Johnson S: The growing influence of wound care teams, *Adv Wound Care* 11(2):54, 1998
Doughty D: A rational approach to the use of topical antiseptics, *J Wound Ostomy Continence Nurs* 21(6):223, 1994.
Dwyer F, Keeler D: Protocols for wound management, *Nurs Manage* 28(7):45, 1997.
Elliott IMZ: *A short history of surgical dressings*, London, 1964, Pharmaceutical Press.
Falanga V: Care of venous leg ulcers, *Ostomy Wound Manage* 45(suppl 1A):33S, 1999.
Falanga V: Growth factors and wound healing, *Dermatol Clin* 11(4):667, 1993.
Faller N: *A survey exploring the ET nursing art of wound care: factors associated with clean versus sterile technique*, Amherst, 1997, University of Massachusetts. Unpublished doctoral dissertation.
Field F, Kerstein M: Overview of wound healing in a moist environment, *Am J Surg* 167(1):2S, 1994.
Flanagan M: Wound cleansing. In Morison M et al, editors: *Nursing management of chronic wounds*, ed 2, London, 1997, Mosby.
Foresman PA et al: A relative toxicity index for wound cleansers, *Wounds* 5(5):226, 1993.
Gilchrist B: Infection and culturing. In Krasner D, Kane D, editors: *Chronic wound care*, ed 2, Wayne, Penn, 1997, Health Management Publications.
Greer JM, Siezenis LMLC: Methods of decision analysis: protocols, decision trees and algorithms in medicine, *World J Surg* (13)240, 1989.
Haimowitz J, Margolis D: Moist wound healing. In Krasner D, Kane D, editors: *Chronic wound care*, ed 2, Wayne Penn, 1997, Health Management Publications.
Haughton W, Young T: Common problems in wound care: malodorous wounds, *Br J Nurs* 4(16):959, 1995.
Hellewell T et al: A cytotoxicity evaluation of antimicrobial and non-antimicrobial wound cleansers, *Wounds* 9(1):15, 1997.
Hermans M: Clinical and bacteriological advantages in the use of occlusive dressings. In Waldstrom T, editor: *Pathogenesis of wound and biomaterial-associated infections*, New York, 1990, Springer Verlag.
Hermans M, Bolton L: The influence of dressings on the costs of wound treatment, *Dermatol Nurs* 8(2):93, 1996.
Hess C: *Wound care: nurses clinical guide*, ed 2, Springhouse, Penn, 1997, Springhouse.
Hess C: Alert: wound healing halted with use of povidone iodine. In Krasner D, editor: *Chronic wound care*, Wayne, Penn, 1990, Health Management Publications.
Hess F: *Chemistry made simple*, New York, 1984, Doubleday.
Hill M, Labik M, Vanderbilt D: Managing skin care with the CareMap system, *J Wound Ostomy Continence Nurs* 24:26, 1997.
Hollinworth H: Nurse's assessment and management of pain at wound dressing changes, *J Wound Care* 4:77, 1995.
Hutchinson J: A prospective clinical trial of wound dressings to investigate the rate of infection under occlusion. In Hutchinson J: *Proceedings: advances in wound management*, London, 1993, MacMillan.
Hutchinson J: Prevalence of wound infection under occlusive dressings, a collective survey of reported research, *Wounds* 1:123, 1989.
Krasner D: Dressing decisions for the twenty-first century: on the cusp of a paradigm shift. In Krasner D, Kane D, editors: *Chronic wound care*, ed 2, Wayne Penn, 1997, Health Management Publications.
Krasner D: Wound care, how to use the Red-Yellow-Black system. *Am J Nurs* 95(5):44, 1995.
Krasner D, Kane D: Wound healing and management. In Krasner D, Kane D, editors: *Chronic wound care*, ed 2, Wayne, Penn, 1997, Health Management Publications.
Krasner D, Kennedy K: Using no-touch technique to change a dressing, *Nursing 94*, 24(8):50, 1994.
Kurz A, Sessler DI, Lenhardt R: Perioperative normothermia to reduce the incidence of surgical wound infection and shorten hospitalization, *N Engl J Med* 334(19):1209, 1996.
Lapioli-Zufelt A, Morris EJ: Skin and wound care management for a child with epidermolysis bullosa, *J Wound Ostomy Continence Nurs* 25:314, 1998.
Laverty D: Protocols and guidelines for managing wounds, *Professional Nurse* 13(2):79, 1997.
Lawrence J, Lilly H, Kidson A: Wound dressings and airborne dispersal of bacteria, *Lancet* 339(8796):807, 1992.
Lawrence J: Dressings and wound infection, *Am J Surg* 167(1A):21S, 1994.
Leaper DJ: The wound healing process. In Turner T, Schmidt R, Harding K editors: *Advances in wound management*, Chichester, 1986, Wiley.
Lehninger AL: Enzymes: kinetics and inhibition. In *Biochemistry: the molecular basis of cell structure function*, New York, 1975, Worth.
Letourneau S, Jensen L: Impact of a decision tree on chronic wound care, *J Wound Ostomy Continence Nurs* 25:240, 1998.
Lineweaver W et al: Topical antimicrobial toxicity, *Arch Surg* 120(3):267, 1985.
Lovejoy L, Bussey C, Sherer AP: The path to a clinical pathway: collaborative care for the patient with an ostomy, *J Wound Ostomy Continence Nurs* 24:200, 1997.
Majno G: *The healing hand*, Harvard, Mass, 1975, University Press.
Maklebust J, Sieggreen M: Pressure ulcers: guidelines for prevention and nursing management, ed 2, Springhouse, Penn, 1996, Springhouse Corporation.
Medical Data International: *U.S. market for wound management products*, Santa Ana, Calif, 1992, Medical Data International.
Medical Data International: *U.S. market for wound management products*, Santa Ana, Calif, 1997, Medical Data International.
Merriam-Webster's Medical Desk Dictionary, Springfield, Mass, 1993, Merriam-Webster.
Mertz P et al: Can antimicrobials be effective without impairing wound healing? the evaluation of a cadexomer iodine ointment, *Wounds* 6(6):184, 1994.

Mertz P, Ovington L: Wound healing microbiology, *Dermatol Clin* 11(4):739, 1993.

Miller M: Rationale for dressing choice, *Nursing Times* 92(suppl 37):1, 1996.

Nwomeh B, Yager D, Cohen I: Physiology of the chronic wound, *Clin Plast Surg* 25(3):341, 1998.

Ovington L: The 1998 O/WM buyers guide, *Ostomy Wound Manage* 44(7):6, 1998a.

Ovington L: The well-dressed wound: an overview of dressing types, *Wounds* 10(suppl A):1A, 1998b.

Panel on Quality Determinants of Mammography: *Clinical practice guideline number 13: quality determinants of mammography*, Rockville, Md, 1994, US Department of Health and Human Services, Agency for Health Care Policy and Research, AHCPR Publication Number 95-0632.

Phillips T: Cost effectiveness in wound care. In Krasner D, Kane D, editors: *Chronic wound care*, ed 2, Wayne, Penn, 1997, Health Management Publications.

Pieper B, DiNardo E: Reasons for nonattendance for the treatment of venous ulcers in an inner-city clinic, *J Wound Ostomy Continence Nurs* 25(4):180, 1998.

Pittet D et al: Compliance with handwashing in a teaching hospital, *Ann Intern Med*, 130(2):126, 1999.

Poteete V: Case study, eliminating odors from wounds, *Decubitus* 6(4):43, 1993.

Powers J: A multidisciplinary approach to occipital pressure ulcers related to cervical collars, *J Nurs Care Qual* 12(1):46, 1997.

Raz R et al: A 1-year trial of nasal mupirocin in the prevention of recurrent staphylococcal nasal colonization and skin infection, *Arch Intern Med* 156(10):1109, 1996.

Rodeheaver G et al: Wound cleansing by high-pressure irrigation, *Surg Gynecol Obstet* 141(3):357, 1975.

Rolstad B: Wound dressings: making the right match, *Nsg'97* 37(6):32hn 1-3, 1997.

Rolstad B, Aronovitch S, Krasner D: Appendix 2: a quick reference guide to wound care product functions and categories. In Krasner D, Kane D, editors: *Chronic wound care*, ed 2, Wayne, Penn, 1997, Health Management Publications.

Rolstad B, Borchert K: *Designing a wound care product formulary*, Poster presentation at the Clinical Symposium on Wound Management, Minneapolis, Minn, 1995.

Rolstad B, Harris A: Management of deterioration in cutaneous wounds. In Krasner D, Kane D, editors: *Chronic wound care*, ed 2, Wayne, Penn, 1997, Health Management Publications.

Rothman S: pH of sweat and skin surface. In Rothman S: *Physiology and biochemistry of the skin*, Chicago, 1954, University of Chicago Press.

Rovee D et al: Effects of local wound environment on epidermal healing. In Maibach H, Rovee D, editors: *Epidermal wound healing*, Chicago, 1972, Yearbook Medical Publishers.

Salcido R, editor: Resources in wound care: 1999 directory, *Adv Wound Care* 12(4):164, 1999.

Springett J, Heaney M: Using care pathways in pressure area management: a pilot study, *J Wound Care* 8(5):227, 1999.

Spruitt D: The water barrier and its repair. In Maebashi H, Rovee D, editors: *Epidermal wound healing*, Chicago, 1972, Yearbook Medical Publishers.

Stotts NA et al: Sterile versus clean technique in postoperative wound care of patients with open surgical wounds: a pilot study, *J Wound Ostomy Continence Nurs* 24:10, 1997.

Stotts NA et al: Wound care practices in the United States, *Ostomy Wound Manage* 39(3):53, 1993.

Strayer LS, Martucci NM: Promoting skin integrity: an interdisciplinary challenge, *Rehabil Nurs* 22(5):250, 1997.

Sussman G: Management of the wound environment. In Sussman C, Bates-Jensen B, editors: *Wound care: a collaborative practice manual for physical therapists and nurses*, Gaithersburg, Md, 1998, Aspen.

Szor JK, Bourguignon C: Description of pressure ulcer pain at rest and at dressing change, *J Wound Ostomy Continence Nurs* 26:115, 1999.

Tallman P et al: Initial rate of healing predicts complete ulcer healing of venous ulcers, *Arch Dermatol* 133:1231, 1997.

Thomas S: A guide to dressing selection, *J Wound Care* 6(10):479, 1997.

Thomas S: Functions of a wound dressing, In Thomas S: *Wound management and dressings*, London, 1990, Pharmaceutical Press.

Thomas S: *Handbook of wound dressings*, London, 1994, Macmillan.

Turnbull G: The dollars and sense of patient teaching, *Ostomy Wound Manage* 45(3):16, 1999.

Turnbull G: Weaving reimbursement of surgical dressings into the plan of treatment, *Ostomy Wound Manage* 41(7A Suppl):103S, 1995.

Turner J et al: Consistency and cost of home wound management by contract nurses, *Public Health Nurs* 11(5):337, 1994.

Turner TD: The development of wound management products. In Krasner D, Kane D, editors: *Chronic wound care*, ed 2, Wayne, Penn, 1997, Health Management Publications.

van Rijswijk L: Recommendations to change the FDA classification of various wound dressings, *Ostomy Wound Manage* 45(3):31, 1999.

van Rijswijk L: Wound assessment and documentation. In Kranser D, Kane D, editors: *Chronic wound care*, ed 2, Wayne, Penn, 1997, Health Management Publications.

van Rijswijk L, Beitz J: The traditions and terminology of wound dressings: food for thought, *J Wound Ostomy Continence Nurs* 25(3):116, 1998.

van Rijswijk L, Braden BJ: Pressure ulcer patient and wound assessment: an AHCPR clinical practice guideline update, *Ostomy Wound Manage* 45(suppl 1A):56S, 1999.

Varghese M et al: Local environment of chronic wounds under synthetic dressings, *Arch Dermatol* 122:52, 1998.

Wahl L, Wahl S: Inflammation. In Cohen IK, Diegelmann RF, Lindblad WJ, editors: *Wound healing: biochemical and clinical aspects*, Philadelphia, 1992, W.B. Saunders.

Walsh K: Decision-making in the care of cavity wounds, *Professional Nurse* 11(9):593, 1996.

Watret L: Know how . . . management of wound exudate, *Nursing Times* 93(30):38, 1997.

Wenisch C et al: Mild intraoperative hypothermia reduces production of oxygen intermediates by polymorphonuclear leukocytes, *Anesth Analg* 82(4):810, 1996.

Wiseman D, Rovee D, Alvarez O: Wound dressings: design and use. In Cohen IK, Diegelmann RF, Lindblad WJ, editors: *Wound healing: biochemical and clinical aspects*, Philadelphia, 1992, W.B. Saunders.

Wound, Ostomy, and Continence Nurses Society: *Guidelines for the management of leg ulcers: diabetic, venous and neuropathic ulcers*, Laguna Beach, Calif, 1993, Adler-Droz.

Young T: Dressing selection: use of combinations of wound dressings, *Br J Nurs* 6(17):999, 1997.

APPENDIX

5.1 WOUND CARE PRODUCT FORMULARY

Bonnie Sue Rolstad, Liza G. Ovington, & Ann Harris

The following wound-care product formulary includes major wound care product categories. ⌗ **"Precautions" denotes contraindications or special considerations that should be understood by the nurse before use.** Usage guidelines provided under "Helpful Hints For Use" are from Part B Medicare guidelines and may vary based upon wound characteristics (e.g., size, amount of exudate). However, refer to manufacturer's product insert and clinical support data before using specific products. Inclusion of a product brand name within this formulary is not intended as a product endorsement. A comprehensive listing of wound-care products is published annually.[1]

Alginate Dressings

Description

Alginates are primary dressings derived from brown seaweed. They are spun fibers available in nonwoven pads or ropes that are composed of calcium salts of alginic acid. Calcium alginate is a solid that exchanges calcium ions for sodium ions when it contacts any substance containing sodium, such as wound fluid. The resulting sodium alginate is a gel. Alginates are nonadhesive, nonocclusive, and conformable to the wound architecture. Variations exist in that some alginates become almost amorphous gels that must be irrigated from the wound, and others gel, yet they retain structural integrity and can be lifted out of the wound. Because alginates are a primary dressing, they will require a secondary cover dressing.

Indications

Alginates absorb moderate to heavy exudate and may be used to pack wounds. Therefore alginates are indicated for moderate to heavily draining wounds with or without depth. Because a moist environment is maintained with proper use of this dressing, autolysis is also promoted.

⌗ Precautions

Contraindicated for use in third-degree burns. Not recommended for use on dry or minimally draining wounds. If alginates are used on minimally draining wounds, the wound bed may become desiccated with alginate fibers imbedded in the wound. Irrigation with saline is recommended for removal. When packing deep tunnels or sinuses, strip packing gauze may be preferable since it is retrievable. Do not moisten this dressing before application.

Helpful Hints For Use

Dressings may be cut to fit the size of the wound and loosely packed. For additional absorbency, the alginate may be layered. For wounds without depth, a piece of alginate may be cut to the size of the wound and a cover dressing may be applied. Numerous cover dressings are used in combination with alginates (e.g., films, composites, hydrocolloids). As

[1]Ovington L: The 1998 O/WM Buyers Guide, *Ostomy Wound Manage* 44(7):6, 1998.

exudate decreases, evaluate for a dressing with less absorbent characteristics. Usually alginate usage is one sheet or up to 6 inches of rope at each dressing change (once per day).

Examples

Traditional Forms

Pads

KALTOSTAT Wound Dressing, ConvaTec

Restore CalciCare, Hollister, Inc.

SORBSAN, Dow Hickam Pharmaceuticals, Inc.

Rope

Manufacturers offering pads usually also offer rope forms of this dressing.

Variations

CarboFlex Odor-Control Dressing, ConvaTec (contains activated charcoal for odor control)

NutraStat Calcium Alginate Wound Dressing with Zinc, Derma Sciences (contains zinc)

PolyMem Alginate Pad, Ferris Mfg. Corp. (contains a surfactant in a foam pad)

Biosynthetic Dressings

Description

Biosynthetic dressings are composed of both man-made and biologic ingredients. The biologic components are typically animal in origin, and the man-made ingredients may be synthetic polymers or chemicals.

Indications

Depending on the specific product, these dressings may be used as temporary coverings for use before autografting or as dressings to optimize healing for burns, donor sites, or other wounds.

Precautions

Specific to individual product, may include potential allergies to ingredients.

Hints For Use

See specific products.

Examples

Biobrane, Dow Hickam Pharmaceuticals (silicone and nylon fabric coated with porcine collagen elements)

E-Z Derm Biosynthetic Dressing, Brennen Medical, Inc. (porcine dermis that has been chemically treated to crosslink the collagen)

Inerpan, Sherwood Davis & Geck (amino acids in a polymer gel)

Collagen Dressings

Description

Relatively new to the wound care market, collagen dressings are formulated with Type I bovine (cowhides or tendon) or avian collagen. Enzymatic purification renders the bovine material nonantigenic; however, most manufacturers cite sensitivity to bovine products as a contraindication for use. Collagen products are available as particles encapsulated in nonadherent pouches or in vials, gels loaded in syringes, pads, and freeze-dried sheets. Collagens require a secondary dressing. A variation in the collagen category is a formulation that also contains 10% alginate to increase product absorbency.

Indications

Collagen may accelerate wound repair. Therefore this dressing may be appropriate for recalcitrant wounds.

Precautions

Contraindicated for use in third-degree burns. Not indicated for use in wounds that are dry or eschar-covered. Contraindicated in persons sensitive to products of bovine origin.

Helpful Hints For Use

Collagen is best used when applied to a wound bed without necrotic tissue. Select the form of product that best addresses the wound size and architecture. In a dry to minimally draining wound, a gel may be applied ¼-inch thick. If the wound has depth, the gel is applied, and a saline-soaked gauze or other appropriate dressing is applied to fill the defect. In a moderate to heavily draining wound, collagen particle pouches or the collagen with alginate may be used. If the pad form is used, allow at least ¼ to ½ inch between the pad and sides of the wound to allow for expansion as exudate is absorbed. The collagen alginate form is cut to the size of the wound. Changes in exudate levels indicate the need for a less absorbent or hydrating product. Dressing-change intervals depend on formulation selected. Refer to manufacturer's instructions.

Examples

Chronicure, Medical Resources, Inc. (powder)

FIBRACOL Collagen Alginate Wound Dressing, Johnson & Johnson Medical (sheet/strips)

Medifil II Gel, BioCore Medical Technologies, Inc. (gel)

Composites

Description

Composites are dressings with distinctive structures that include at least the following: bacterial barrier; absorbent layer other than a foam, alginate, hydrocolloid, or hydrogel; either a semiadherent or nonadherent surface that contacts the wound; and an adhesive border. Composites look like Band-Aids of variable sizes. They may have semiocclusive or nonocclusive fabric covers.

Indications

May be used alone or in combination with other dressings (e.g., alginate). In wounds with depth, a primary wound filler material is required to pack the wound before securing the dressing with a composite. Some forms are useful for nonocclusive dressing procedures.

Precautions

Contraindicated for use in third-degree burns. Not appropriate for use in heavily draining wounds or as a primary dressing in full-thickness wounds.

Helpful Hints For Use

Follow package insert for specific directions. Select a dressing that extends onto intact surrounding skin at least 2.5 cm (1 inch). Do not cut the dressing because the structure of the dressing design will be compromised. Do not layer two dressings over the wound. One dressing per dressing change is usually reimbursed with dressing-change intervals up to three times per week.

Examples

Alldress Absorbent Film Dressing, Mölnlycke Health Care

Band-Aid Brand Surgical Dressing, Johnson & Johnson Medical

TELFA Plus Barrier Island Dressing, Kendall Healthcare Products Co.

Contact Layer

Description

Contact layers are composed of a single layer of woven or perforated polymer net that acts as a low-adherence material, which is placed over the wound base. The product stays in place during dressing changes, allows the passage of wound exudate through its mesh or perforations, and protects the wound bed from trauma.

Indications

These products are primary dressings for use in clean wounds without necrotic tissue.

Precautions

Contraindicated for use in third-degree burns and infected wounds. Not recommended for shallow or small wounds, dry wounds or those with viscous exudate, and wounds with tunneling and extensive undermining.

Helpful Hints For Use

Refer to manufacturer's insert for specific instructions for use. However, generally contact layer material is applied as a liner over granular wound surfaces and overlaps onto surrounding skin. The material may or may not require taping to the skin. In deep wounds, gauze packing may also be required. A secondary dressing is then applied. Contact layers are usually changed once a week.

Examples

3M Tegapore Wound Contact Material, 3M Health Care

Mepitel, SCA Mölnlycke

N-TERFACE Interpositional Surfacing Material, Winfield Laboratories, Inc.

Foam Dressings

Description

Polyurethane foams are sheets of foamed solutions of polymers that contain small open cells capable of holding fluids and pulling them away from the wound bed. The size of the cell varies. This dressing represents one of the first attempts to improve on the lack of absorbency of the early film dressings. Foams provide absorbency without compromising the moist wound environment. This category of dressings represents the most variations from one manufacturer to another. Most foams do not have an adhesive surface, but some do. Nonadhesive foams will require a secondary dressing (e.g., film) for securement. The foam may be the traditional thickness (4 to 7 mm) or newer thin formulation (<1 mm). Thin foams have adhesive surfaces and top film covers to provide a waterproof barrier. Traditional thickness foam dressings may or may not have adhesive borders. Some have a film cover for waterproofing the top surface, and one brand of foam contains a surfactant, glycerin, and a superabsorbent agent. Generally, foams are available as sheets of variable sizes or rolls. However, pads, circular, and tube-shaped foam cavity dressings are available for packing wounds. They are composed of small pieces of absorbent foam chopped up and contained in a bag of permeable material.

Indications

Foams are one of the most absorbent materials and are useful for wounds with moderate to heavy exudate. Thin foams are used to protect intact skin and for managing superficial wounds with minimal exudate. The traditional thickness foams are particularly useful for management of exudate under compression in venous ulcers. Foams without adhesive are useful for managing wounds with friable periwound skin. The dressing may be secured with a nonadhesive wrap. Thin dressings are conformable, flexible, and useful with skin tears. Foams may be used in combination with other dressings (e.g., films, absorbent pastes). Cavity dressings and some sheet formulations are used for packing wounds with depth. Foams may be used in combination with other dressing materials (e.g., pastes, films).

Precautions

Contraindicated for use in third-degree burns. Not recommended for nondraining wounds or those with sinuses and tunneling. The dressing may stick to the wound and require irrigation during removal in dry to minimally draining wounds. Cavity dressings should not be cut. Some formulations are not conformable to depth and may be difficult to use in anatomic areas that require contouring (e.g., gluteal fold).

Helpful Hints For Use

Select a dressing that extends onto intact surrounding skin at least 2.5 cm (1 inch). Foam other than cavity dressings may be cut or contoured to fit anatomic areas. Check manufacturer's instructions to determine which side of the dressing is applied to the wound surface. Dressings may require securement with tape or compression bandaging. Usual dressing change interval is up to three times a week. Dressings used as wound fillers may be changed up to once per day.

Examples

Traditional

Allevyn Adhesive Dressings, T.J. Smith and Nephew, Ltd.

Lyofoam, ConvaTec

PolyMem Non-Adhesive Dressings, Ferris Mfg. Corp.

Variations

FLEXZAN, Dow Hickam Pharmaceuticals, Inc. (extra thin)

Lyofoam C, ConvaTec (contains activated charcoal for odor control)

PolyTube "Tube Site" Dressing, Ferris Mfg. Corp. (precut foam for tubing)

Gauze

Description

This section summarizes numerous categories, including nonimpregnated gauze, gauze impregnated with water or normal saline, and gauze impregnated with substances other than water or normal saline. Gauze is available woven or nonwoven in cotton or snythetic blends. It is available sterile or nonsterile as sponges, drain sponges, pads, ribbon, strips, and rolls.

Indications

Nonimpregnated gauze may be nonwoven (particularly useful for scrubbing, prepping, wiping, absorption, and protection) or woven (preferred for wicking, debridement, and packing). Impregnated gauzes hydrate (e.g., hydrogel or saline impregnated), absorb (e.g., dry, hypertonic formulations), or act as carriers for antimicrobial agents and nutrients. New fabrics are also available for debridement.

Precautions

Avoid wet to dry gauze debridement because it is not physiologic and usually causes pain. Monitor the condition of periwound skin to avoid moisture exposure. Protection with a skin sealant or barrier may be indicated.

Helpful Hints For Use

Read manufacturer information on gauze selection to match the function to clinical indication. Particularly useful when packing deep wounds, undermining, and tunnels. Loose packing technique is always recommended. When numerous dressing changes are required daily, evaluate for a more cost-effective type of dressing.

Examples

Nonimpregnated (woven and nonwoven): All Purpose

Duform Bandage Rolls, Dumex Medical Surgical Products, Ltd.

EXCILON Dressing Sponge, Kendall Healthcare Products Co.

NU-GAUZE General-Use Sponges, Johnson & Johnson Medical

Impregnated (other than a hydrogel)

ADAPTIC Non-Adhering Dressing, Johnson & Johnson Medical

Mesalt Impregnated Absorbent Dressing, Mölnlycke Health Care

Kendall Xeroform Dressing, Kendall Healthcare Products Co.

Nonadherent

Coverlet O.R. Surgical Dressing, Beiersdorf-Jobst, Inc.

RELEASE Non-Adherent Dressing, Johnson and Johnson Medical

TELFA Dressings, Kendall Healthcare Products Co.

Elastic Support Bandages

BandNet Elastic Net Retainer, Western Medical Ltd.

ELASTINET Dressing Retainer, Brennen Medical, Inc.

Tubigrip Elastic Tubular Support Bandage, ConvaTec

Packing/Debriding

FLUFTEX Nonwoven rolls and sponges, DeRoyal Wound Care

NU-GAUZE Packing Strips Johnson and Johnson Medical

KERLIX Super Sponges

Roll/Wrapping

CONFORM Stretch Bandages, Kendall Healthcare Products Co.

KLING Conforming Gauze Bandage, Johnson & Johnson Medical

Sof-Form Conforming Gauze Bandages, Medline Industries, Inc.

Growth Factors

Description

Growth factors are short-chain proteins that are found naturally in the body. They may be autologously derived (solution of multiple growth factors isolated from the alpha granules of the platelet) or made by chemical or biochemical means outside of the body (recombinant) once identified and characterized. As proteins, they are heat sensitive (heat denatures proteins) and usually require storage at reduced temperatures. Growth factors in general affect the wound-healing process by causing certain cells to proliferate, produce a product, or migrate to a specific area. Different growth factors have different target cells that they affect, and a single growth factor may affect more than one cell. Growth factors must bind with receptors on their target cells to elicit their effects.

Indications

The indication for a particular growth factor will depend on its specific effects and on the supporting data. Currently, rh-PDGF-BB (becaplermin) is indicated for diabetic neuropathic foot ulcers.

Precautions

Growth factors are contraindicated in patients with neoplasms.

Helpful Hints For Use

Refer to manufacturer's prescribing guidelines for specific instructions. Follow dosing instructions precisely; more of a growth factor is not better.

Examples

Procuren, Curative Technologies, Inc. (autologous platelet releasate)

Regranex, Ortho-McNeil Pharmaceutical (recombinant PDGF-BB)

Hydrocolloid Dressings

Description

Hydrocolloids are formulations of elastomeric, adhesive, and gelling agents. The most common absorbent ingredient is carboxymethylcellulose, which was adapted from use in ostomy skin barriers. The surface is adhesive and may or may not have an adhesive border that extends beyond the actual hydrocolloid surface. They are covered with a transparent film that makes them impermeable to fluids. A variation to the traditional thickness of the dressing is a thin version, which is particularly conformable and flexible. Hydrocolloids may also contain alginate to increase absorption capabilities. Several shapes and sizes are available, as well as contoured dressing to address specific anatomic areas (e.g., sacrum, heels, knees, elbows). Hydrocolloids form a viscous, colloidal gel as fluid is absorbed. This is irrigated away from the wound at dressing change. Initially there were concerns that the chemicals released from the meltdown would be a deterrent to wound healing. However, reports suggest that certain hydrocolloid dressings actually interact with the endogenous growth factors to promote healing.

Indications

Hydrocolloid dressings are adhesive and absorbent. Absorbency rates vary with manufacturer. Generally, traditional-thickness wafers absorb minimal to moderate exudate levels and the thin form absorbs minimal exudate. They are able to adhere to wet and dry areas but do not stick to the moist wound bed. Hydrocolloids may be used to promote autolysis when the wound is exudative. Traditional-thickness hydrocolloids are indicated in partial- and full-thickness wounds, whereas the thin formulations are used to protect intact skin in high friction areas and for managing superficial wounds. Both forms may be used in combination with other dressing materials (e.g., absorbent powder, alginate).

Precautions

Contraindicated for use in third-degree burns. Not recommended for dry eschar management because these dressings are absorbent. Hypergranulation may occur under these dressings. When dressing are not changed at appropriate intervals, maceration of periwound skin may occur. Generally not recommended for infected wounds.

Helpful Hints For Use

Select the proper size dressing based on manufacturer instruction. The hydrocolloid material should extend onto intact surrounding skin at least 2.5 cm (1 inch). If the hydrocolloid is cut from a larger piece, the edges should be taped to avoid rolling or sticking to clothing or sheets. Avoid stretching dressing during application. Hydrocolloids are most effective when they are at body temperature. Therefore some instructions recommend holding the dressing in place with the hand for a short period of time (30 to 60 seconds) after application. Frequency of change is usually up to three times a week. Remove the dressing in the direction of hair growth, and support the skin to avoid skin stripping.

Examples

Traditional Forms

3M Tegasorb Hydrocolloid Dressing, 3M Health Care

Comfeel Ulcer Care Dressing, Coloplast Corp.

DuoDERM CGF Control Gel Formula Dressing, ConvaTec

Variations

Comfeel Plus Contour Dressing, Coloplast Corp. (flower shape)

Cutinova Thin, Beiersdorf-Jobst, Inc. (extra thin)

Restore Dressing for Psoriasis, Hollister, Inc. (same formulation as the extra thin with a psoriasis indication)

Hydrofibers

Description

Fibers of carboxymethylcellulose, which is an absorptive ingredient used in hydrocolloids, comprise this nonwoven, white, cotton-like product. The material gels quickly when in contact with wound exudate and absorbs 33% more than most alginates. It retains moisture over the wound bed and wicks vertically to avoid periwound skin maceration. Hydrofibers are available in pad and ribbon form.

Indications

Hydrofiber material is indicated in heavily draining wounds or lesser-draining wounds when extended product wear time is desired. This may be particularly useful under compression bandaging.

Precautions

Contraindicated for use in third-degree burns. Not indicated for use in dry or minimally draining wounds because dehydration of the wound may occur. Not intended for use as a surgical sponge.

Helpful Hints For Use

Requires a secondary dressing. Select the correct size dressing for the wound. Pack loosely in wounds with depth. Refer to manufacturer's package insert for specific information on use.

Examples

AQUACEL HYDROFIBER Wound Dressing, ConvaTec (currently the only product in this category)

Hydrogels

Description

Hydrogels are formulated as sheets or gels. Some are available in sterile and nonsterile versions with the nonsterile version considerably less expensive. Hydrogel sheets are three-dimensional networks of cross-linked, hydrophilic polymers. The cross-linked polymer (polyethylene oxide, polyacrylamides, and polyvinylpyrrolidone) physically entraps water to form a solid sheet. They may be up to 96% water. The sheet may feel moist but will not release water when squeezed. Hydrogels may absorb exudate by swelling but are primarily designed to hydrate the wound. Variations to the traditional hydrogel sheets are numerous. Some are adhesive; others are not. Yet another is an aloe vera hydrogel pad that is conductive and designed to disperse electrotherapy to the wound bed evenly during electrotherapy. Gel sheets are sometimes packaged so that they are protected on both sides with a polymer film, one of which should be removed before contact with the wound bed. Sheets are available with or without borders. If a border is present, it will usually be a film or foam material. Borderless foams may be attached with tape, films, stretch gauze, or tubular bandages.

Amorphous hydrogels are similar in formulation to the amorphous sheets except that the polymer has not been cross-linked to form a sheet. The absence of cross-linking means that gels do not provide the same cooling effect noticed in the sheet hydrogels. Amorphous hydrogels may be glycerin- or water-based and vary widely in viscosity. They are available in foil packages, tubes, spray bottles, and impregnated gauzes. Variations in this product group are seen with addition of ingredients such as alginate, collagen, or complex carbohydrates. However, the addition of these ingredients does not change the product category. Other variations may include aloe vera with acemannan, and one of these forms is freeze dried. All additives are designed to increase the performance parameters of the hydrogel.

Indications

Hydrogels hydrate the wound to varying degrees based on dressing formulation. They are most often indicated in full-thickness wounds. Most hydrogel formulations are indicated for use in dry to minimally draining wounds. However, some formulations may be used in moderately draining wounds (e.g., those containing alginates). A common use for hydrogels is the promotion of autolysis that occurs when these products are used to increase hydration in dry or minimally draining necrotic wounds. The design of hydrogel sheets provides a unique cooling ability and is particularly useful in painful wounds and thermal injuries. Some sheets may also be used as packing materials for wounds with depth as long as any protecting polymer films are removed first. Nonadhesive hydrogel sheets are gentle and do not disturb fragile tissue. Amorphous gels are unique in their ability to deliver hydration to eschar and thereby promote autolysis. An amorphous hydrogel covered with a film is an effective technique for promoting autolysis of slough and eschar and is also quite conformable. Amorphous hydrogels are also used in clean, granulating wounds to maintain a moist environment. A secondary dressing is required to cover and secure the amorphous hydrogel. Hydrogel impregnated gauze sponges or strip packing are indicated for wounds requiring packing and moisture.

Precautions

May be contraindicated for use in third-degree burns (check manufacturer's package insert). Hydrogels are not indicated for use in wounds with moderate to heavy exudate. Some forms of sheet hydrogels are difficult to handle and require written instructions and practice. Close monitoring of wounds for overhydration and periwound skin maceration is recommended. Amorphous gels become less viscous as they warm to body temperature. Some may liquify and lead to dressing strike-through. A skin sealant or other form of protectant may be needed to protect periwound skin. Amorphous hydrogels are not intended to fill wound spaces. This use may result in periwound skin maceration, dressing strike-through, and nonreimbursement.

Helpful Hints For Use

Select the form of product that best addresses the wound size and architecture. Sheets may be cut to the size of the wound or amorphous gels used to cover the base of shallow wounds. A film dressing may then be used as a cover. In deeper wounds, hydrogel sheets or impregnated gauzes are useful, or gel may be applied to the wound base and walls with gauze applied over to loosely fill the wound. A frequently used approach is to apply an amorphous gel directly to the gauze to impregnate it and loosely pack it into the wound. Cost will be a differentiating factor with these hydrating alternatives. During autolysis, close monitoring of the wound is important. The wound will increase in size, and sinuses, undermining, or other previously unobservable characteristics may be revealed, which may require topical therapy modifications. Usual dressing use for sheets without covers is up to once per day; for sheets with adhesive borders is up to three times a week; and for amorphous gel is approximately 3 fl oz per 30 days. Usual use for impregnated gauze is up to once per day.

Examples

Traditional Forms

Sheets

Elasto-Gel, Southwest Technologies

Nu-Gel, Johnson & Johnson Medical

Vigilon Primary Wound Dressing, Bard Medical Division, C.R.Bard, Inc.

Amorphous

IntraSite Gel, T.J. Smith and Nephew, Ltd.

Carrasyn Hydrogel Wound Dressing, Carrington Laboratories, Inc.

Restore Hydrogel Dressing, Hollister, Inc.

Impregnated Gauze

3M Tegagel Hydrogel Wound Filler with Gauze, 3M Health Care

CarraGauzeR Hydrogel Wound Dressing Pads, Carrington Laboratories, Inc.

CURASOL Hydrogel Saturated 4 × 4, HEALTHPOINT

Variations

HypergelR, Mölnlycke Health Care (hypertonic saline amorphous gel)

THINSite Border Hydrogel Dressing, B. Braun Medical, Inc. (thin sheet)

Woun'Dres Natural Collagen Hydrogel Wound Dressing, Coloplast Corp. (contains additional collagen)

HYDROPOLYMERS

Description

Another specialty absorptive dressing is a material that looks like a foam and is described as a foamed gel or hydropolymer. It is a multilayered product with a surface layer that expands into the contours of the wound as it absorbs exudate. Dynamic fluid-handling characteristics are demonstrated with this product in that exudate is wicked away into the upper layers of the dressing where it evaporates through the backing. The border adhesive is gentle yet effective and has the ability to re-adhere once it has been lifted away from the skin. Variations include a superabsorbent dressing for high exudate management and a sacral-shaped dressing.

Indications

Wounds with minimal to moderate exudate, with or without depth, are indicated for this dressing.

Precautions

Contraindicated for use in third-degree burns. Not recommended for dry wounds. If used on heavily exuding wounds, an alginate may be required to assist with fluid handling.

Helpful Hints For Use

Select the proper dressing size based on the wound. Allow adequate dressing overlap onto periwound skin. Refer to the package insert for selection and application information. Usual dressing change intervals are up to three times a week.

Examples

TIELLE Hydropolymer Dressing, Johnson & Johnson Medical (currently the only product in this category; reimbursed as a foam)

Leg Compression and Wrapping Systems

Description

A wide range of compression products is available. Generally, these products are designed to improve venous return and decrease edema in the lower extremities when venous insufficiency is present. Compression products may include the compression bandage, stocking, boot system, legging orthosis, or pneumatic pump. Compression may be elastic, short stretch, rigid, or multilayered. Compression may be low (18 to 24 mm Hg), low to moderate (25 to 35 mm Hg), moderate (30 to 40 mm Hg), or high (40 to 50 mm Hg). Compression bandages/wraps provide graduated compression when wrapped properly. Materials vary depending on the style and manufacturer. Topical dressings are frequently applied under compression bandages/wraps and stockings.

Indications

Used for venous insufficiency and other conditions resulting in chronic edema in the legs and feet.

Precautions

Consult with physician before instituting compression therapy in patients with known ischemic disease of the lower limbs. Do not use more than low compression (5 to 15 mm Hg) in patient with combined venous/ischemic wound when the ankle-brachial index (ABI) is below 0.8. Monitor closely in patients without palpable pedal or posterior tibial pulses. Use cautiously in the patient with severe congestive heart failure.

Helpful Hints For Use

Follow manufacturer's instructions for the type and level of compression and application techniques.

Examples

CIRCULON System Step 2 Venous Ulcer Kit, ConvaTec (a hydrocolloid-impregnated compression wrap and a hydrocolloid wafer are included in the kit)

Gelocast Unna Boot, Beiersdorf-Jobst, Inc. (paste bandage)

Profore Four Layer Bandage System, Smith & Nephew, Inc. (includes a wound contact layer and four separate layers; one layer pads, and the next is slightly conformable; the third provides light compression, and the outer layer provides cohesive compression)

Skin Substitutes

Description

Skin substitutes are also referred to as *skin equivalents*, *artificial skin*, or *allografts*. They are usually composed of a bioabsorbable matrix (such as collagen or suture material), which has been populated with living dermal cells (fibroblasts) and/or epidermal cells (keratinocytes) from a human source other than the patient. Neonatal foreskins have provided a source of cells that can then be cultured and expanded in vitro. If the skin substitute contains only fibroblasts, it is referred to as a *dermal substitute*; if it contains both fibroblasts and keratinocytes, it is referred to as a *full-thickness substitute.*

Indications

Currently, there is only one commercially available living skin substitute, which has an indication for venous leg ulcers.

Precautions

Living cells are fragile and sensitive to extremes of temperature. They also have a finite lifetime once shipped from the manufacturer.

Helpful Hints For Use

In some cases, meshing the allograft, or "pie-crusting" by creating slits with a scalpel, will assist in adherence by allowing the passage of any wound drainage through the graft rather than potentially lifting the graft by accumulating beneath it. Refer to manufacturer's guidelines for specific instructions.

Examples

Apligraf, Organogenesis, Inc.

Specialty Absorptive Dressings

Description

A broad range of product forms is represented by this category. Unique films, cover dressings, an antimicrobial gel, and pad and pillow are examples. The common function of this category is absorption. There is no traditional form; all members of this category are variations on other categories.

Indications

Wounds with moderate to heavy exudate and wounds requiring antimicrobial dressings.

Precautions

Precautions are unique to the dressings found in this category. Refer to the package insert.

Helpful Hints For Use

Refer to package insert.

Examples

EXU-DRY Wound Dressing, Smith & Nephew, Inc.

IODOFLEX Gel Pad Absorbent Antimicrobial Dressing, HEALTHPOINT

OsmoCyte PCA Pillow Dressing, Bard Medical Division, C.R. Bard, Inc.

Superabsorbents

Description

Dressing material formulation that has a high absorbency rate and capacity. Like materials used in the diaper industry, superabsorbent particles entrap fluid within the dressing. There is currently one dressing on the market that meets this description and one foam and one hydropolymer that claim to incorporate this technology.

Indications

Wounds with heavy exudate or situations where extended wear time is needed (e.g., under an Unna boot).

Precautions

Contraindicated for use in third-degree burns. Not recommended for dry or minimally exudative wounds. Use a packing material under this dressing as necessary.

Helpful Hints For Use

Allow the dressing to extend 1¼ inch onto the periwound skin. Do not cut the dressing.

Examples

CombiDERM ACD Absorbent Cover Dressing, ConvaTec

Tielle Plus Dressing, Johnson & Johnson Medical

Transparent Film Dressing

Description

Thin, transparent polyurethane sheets coated on one side with acrylic, hypoallergenic adhesive. The adhesive will not stick to moist surfaces, such as the wound bed or moist periwound skin, because it becomes inactivated by moisture. Film dressings are impermeable to fluids and bacteria but are semipermeable to gas, such as oxygen and water vapor. Variations on the basic form include products with perimeter adhesive and a nonadhesive center. Film moisture vapor transmission rates (MVTRs) may also differ. Traditional films have MVTRs ranging from 400 to 800 g/m^2/day. The high-permeability films have MVTRs of 3000 g/m^2/day and above. The high-permeability films are used over intravenous sites but may be used in a minimally exudative wound or as a secondary dressing over an absorbent material. Variations also exist in the delivery method and ease of use. A new antimicrobial film dressing incorporates timed-released polymers to deliver noncytotoxic quantities of ionic silver to the wound.

Indications

Films are useful for prophylaxis on high-risk intact skin. They are also indicated for superficial wounds with little or no exudate and wounds with eschar to facilitate autolysis. They are commonly used in combination with other dressing materials as a secondary (e.g., cover) dressing. Films with high MVTRs are indicated for intravenous sites. Films with antimicrobial agents are indicated in highly contaminated wounds to help protect from methicillin-resistant *staphylococcus aureus* (MRSA) and *Escherichia coli* infection.

Precautions

Contraindicated for use in third-degree burns. Films have no absorbent capacity when used alone. They may be used in combination with other dressings (e.g., alginate) with moderate to heavily exuding wounds or sinus tracts and tunneling (e.g., impregnated gauze). Remove with caution to avoid pain and skin stripping. A skin sealant may be helpful to avoid skin stripping in areas with fragile tissue.

Helpful Hints For Use

Select a dressing that allows a 2.5-cm (1-inch) overlap from wound margin to intact surrounding tissue. Avoid wrinkles and stretching of the film during application. At removal, stretch the film in a direction parallel to the wound rather than pulling upward. The stretching action gently breaks the seal. Change the dressing if exudate extends beyond the edges of the wound and onto periwound skin. Usual dressing change is up to three times a week.

Examples

Traditional Form

3M Tegaderm Transparent Film Dressing, 3M Health Care

OpSite Transparent Dressing, T.J. Smith and Nephew, Ltd.

BIOCLUSIVE Transparent Dressing, Johnson & Johnson Medical

Variations

3M Tegaderm HP Transparent Dressing, 3M Health Care (high permeability)

Arglaes Film, Medline Industries, Inc. (antimicrobial product)

DermaFilm Intelligent Film Dressing, DeRoyal Wound Care (high permeability)

Wound Fillers

Description

Pastes, powders, beads, and strands that are used as wound fillers and exudate absorbers. They are primary dressings. Composition of wound fillers varies widely depending on the specific product. Manufacturer product inserts or Material Safety Data Sheets should be consulted for specific information.

Indications

For use in shallow wounds with minimal to moderate exudate. May be used in combination with other dressings (e.g., films, hydrocolloids, composites) to increase absorption or fill shallow areas.

Precautions

Contraindicated in third-degree burns. Not recommended in dry wounds or wounds with sinuses and tunnels.

Helpful Hints For Use

Refer to manufacturer's insert because instructions vary based on dressing material used. Usual dressing change may be up to once per day.

Examples

AcryDerm Strands Absorbent Wound Dressing, AcryMed, Inc.

MULTIDEX Maltodextrin Wound Dressing, ReRoyal Wound Care

BIAFINE Wound Dressing Emulsion (WDE), KCI

WOUND POUCH

Description

Sterile or nonsterile collection system based on the design used in ostomy care. Usually has a pectin-based skin barrier, has a drainable spout, and is odor-proof. Variable adhesive sizes and capacities are available.

Indications

Collection of high-volume output wounds, tube sites, and fistulas. Minimal to moderate output wound, which requires odor containment.

Precautions

Not intended for use with dry wounds.

Helpful Hints For Use

Follow manufacturer's recommendations for application and removal. Usual change is up to three times a week.

Examples

Wound Drainage Collectors, Hollister, Inc.

Wound Manager Wound Drainage Pouch with DURAHESIVE Skin Barrier, ConvaTec

Marsupial Pouch, Derma Sciences

OTHER WOUND-CARE PRODUCTS:

- Adhesives and tapes
- Adhesive removers
- Adhesive skin closures
- Antibiotics
- Antimicrobials
- Antiseptics
- Enzyme debriding agents
- Lubricating and stimulating sprays
- Moisture-barrier ointments and creams
- Skin-protectant pastes
- Moisturizers
- Ointments
- Perineal cleansers
- Skin cleansers
- Skin sealants
- Wound cleansers

CHAPTER 6

Skin Pathology and Types of Damage

RUTH A. BRYANT

OBJECTIVES

1. State at least five categories or types of skin damage.
2. Distinguish between the following lesions: macule, papule, plaque, nodule, wheal, pustule, vesicle, and bulla.
3. Differentiate between erosion and ulcer.
4. Describe four types of mechanical trauma by the extent of tissue damage associated with each.
5. Discuss at least three interventions to prevent each type of mechanical trauma.
6. For three common causes of chemical damage, describe three preventive interventions.
7. Describe the process of an allergic contact dermatitis.
8. Identify factors that predispose a patient to candidiasis.
9. Describe the types of lesions common to candidiasis, folliculitis, impetigo, and pyoderma gangrenosum.
10. Distinguish between herpes simplex and herpes zoster according to cause, onset, clinical presentation, and treatment.
11. Describe the process of tissue damage caused by vasculitus, calciphylaxis, and TEN.

Normal skin integrity can be jeopardized or compromised by several factors: mechanical, chemical, vascular, infectious, allergic, inflammatory, systemic disease, burns, and miscellaneous assaults. Each type of injury creates a complex set of skin responses, such as erythema, macule, papule, vesicle, erosion, or ulcer. Primary lesions of the skin are the first recognizable skin lesions or a basic change in the skin. Figure 6-1 provides the definition and appearance of common primary lesions. Secondary skin lesions evolve from the primary lesion either because of the natural history of the disease or because of scratching or infection. Common secondary lesions are depicted and defined in Figure 6-2. Primary lesions such as pustules and bullae can evolve into secondary lesions like erosion and, ultimately, an ulcer. Because periwound skin can develop skin complications, the nurse who cares for wounds must be familiar with these terms.

ASSESSMENT

A systematic assessment of skin lesions is essential to obtain an accurate description of the history and evolution of the skin complication. This assessment commonly will narrow the field of differential diagnoses quickly. The components to be addressed are listed in Table 6-1.

Before a treatment plan for a chronic or acute wound is initiated, it is imperative that the underlying cause for the wound be determined. Clues to the cause can be found by assessment of the following parameters: location, characteristics, distribution, and the patient's subjective comments (Table 6-2). These clues can be used to direct the subsequent tests that may be necessary to develop a definitive diagnosis. Once the cause of the wound is identified, realistic goals for the wound can be established and a comprehensive, multidisciplinary treatment plan can be devised. This section briefly describes the pathophysiologic process of key types of skin damage and appropriate interventions.

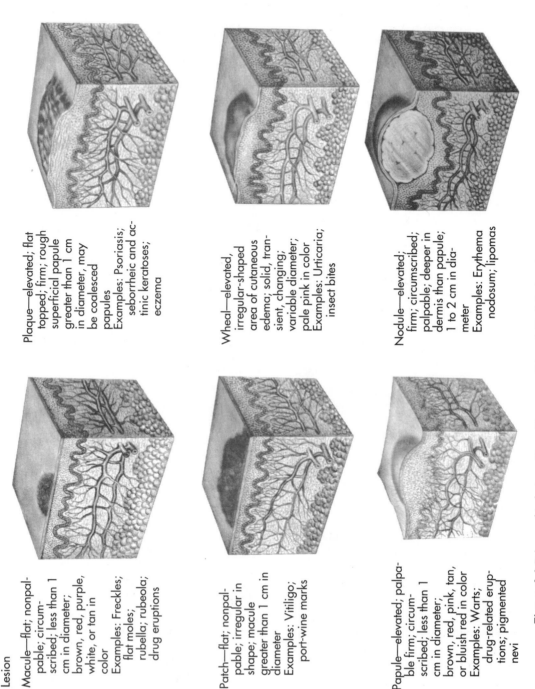

Lesion

Macule—flat; nonpalpable; circumscribed; less than 1 cm in diameter; brown, red, purple, white, or tan in color
Examples: Freckles; flat moles; rubella; rubeola; drug eruptions

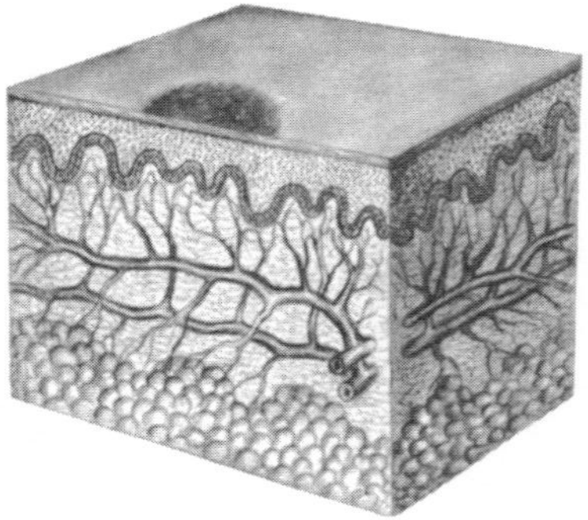

Plaque—elevated; flat topped; firm; rough superficial papule greater than 1 cm in diameter, may be coalesced papules
Examples: Psoriasis; seborrheic and actinic keratoses; eczema

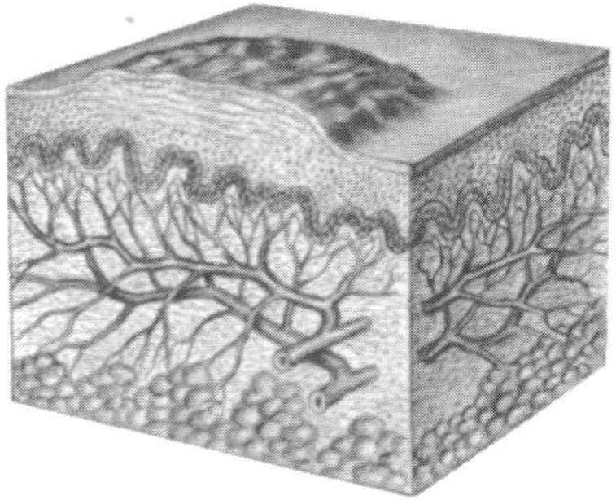

Patch—flat; nonpalpable; irregular in shape; macule greater than 1 cm in diameter
Examples: Vitiligo; port-wine marks

Wheal—elevated, irregular-shaped area of cutaneous edema; solid, transient, changing; variable diameter; pale pink in color
Examples: Urticaria; insect bites

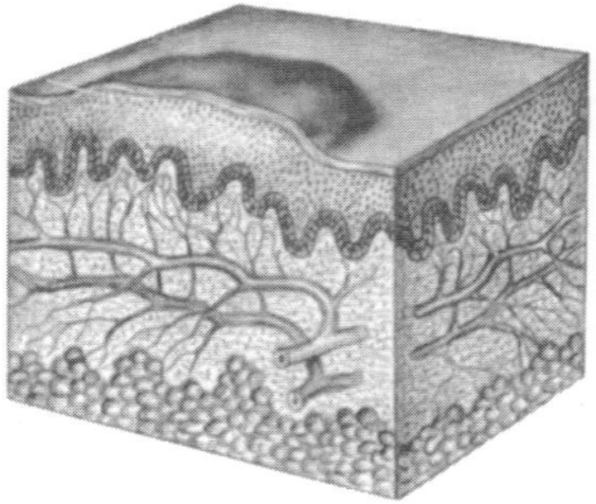

Papule—elevated; palpable firm; circumscribed; less than 1 cm in diameter; brown, red, pink, tan, or bluish red in color
Examples: Warts; drug-related eruptions; pigmented nevi

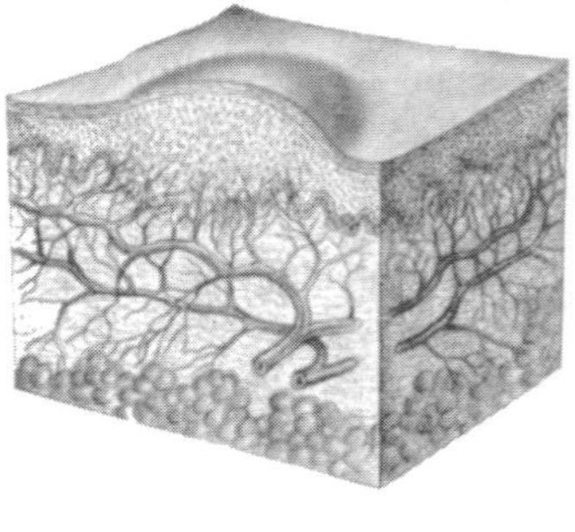

Nodule—elevated; firm; circumscribed; palpable; deeper in dermis than papule; 1 to 2 cm in diameter
Examples: Erythema nodosum; lipomas

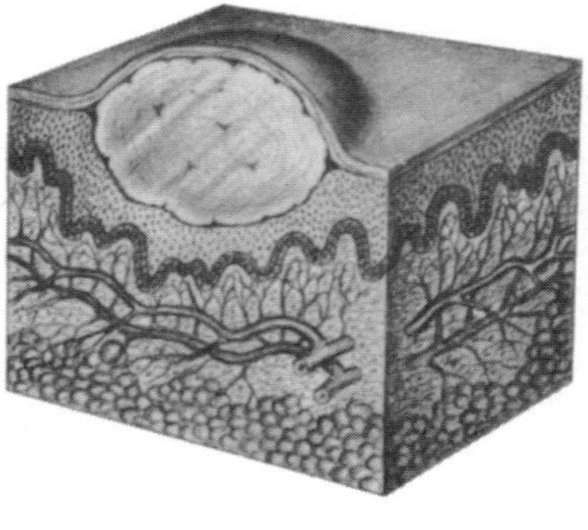

Figure 6-1 Primary skin lesions. (From Thompson JM et al: *Mosby's clinical nursing*, ed 4, St Louis, 1997, Mosby.)

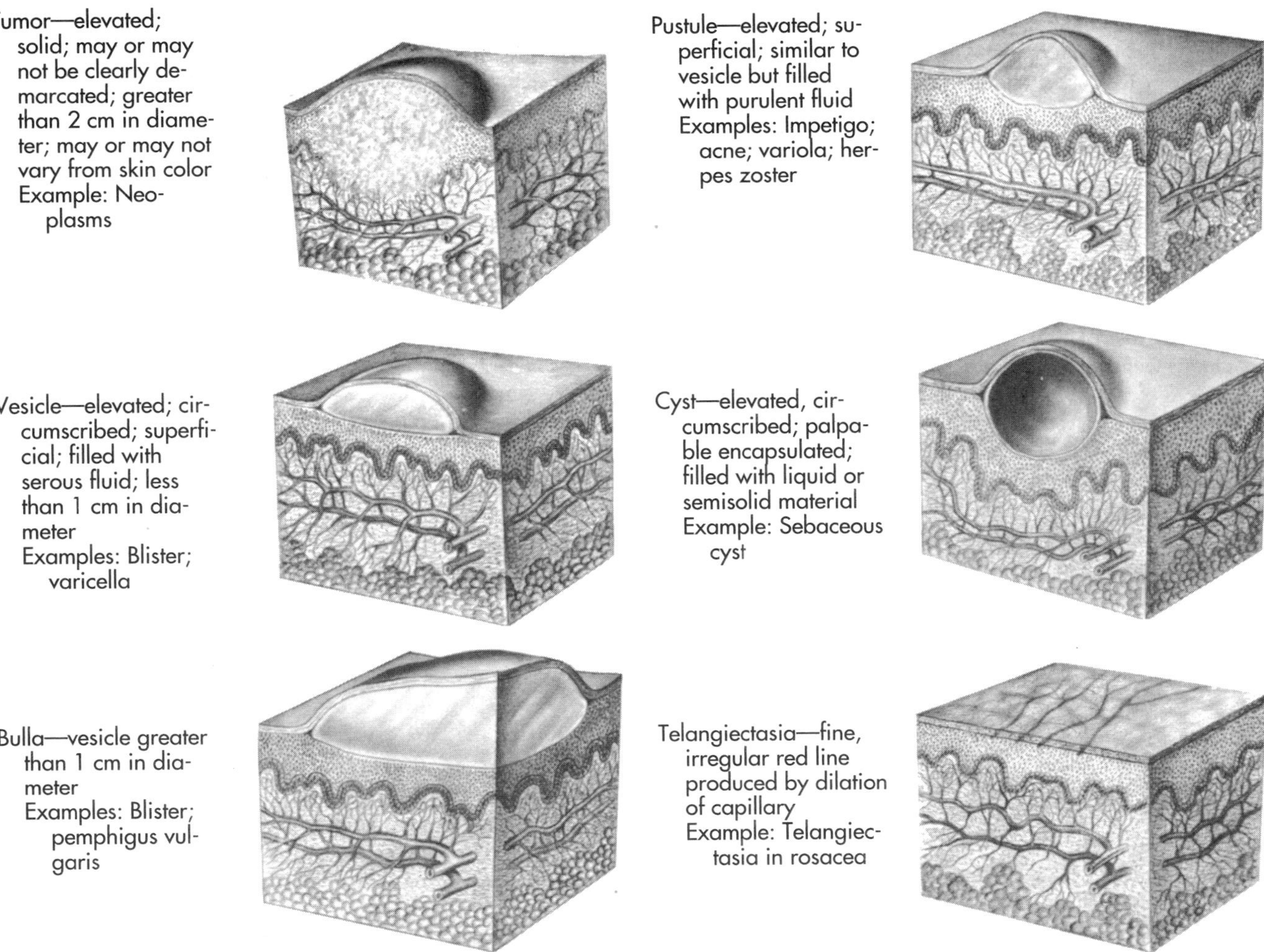

Tumor—elevated; solid; may or may not be clearly demarcated; greater than 2 cm in diameter; may or may not vary from skin color
Example: Neoplasms
Pustule—elevated; superficial; similar to vesicle but filled with purulent fluid
Examples: Impetigo; acne; variola; herpes zoster
Vesicle—elevated; circumscribed; superficial; filled with serous fluid; less than 1 cm in diameter
Examples: Blister; varicella
Cyst—elevated, circumscribed; palpable encapsulated; filled with liquid or semisolid material
Example: Sebaceous cyst
Bulla—vesicle greater than 1 cm in diameter
Examples: Blister; pemphigus vulgaris
Telangiectasia—fine, irregular red line produced by dilation of capillary
Example: Telangiectasia in rosacea

Figure 6-1, cont'd.

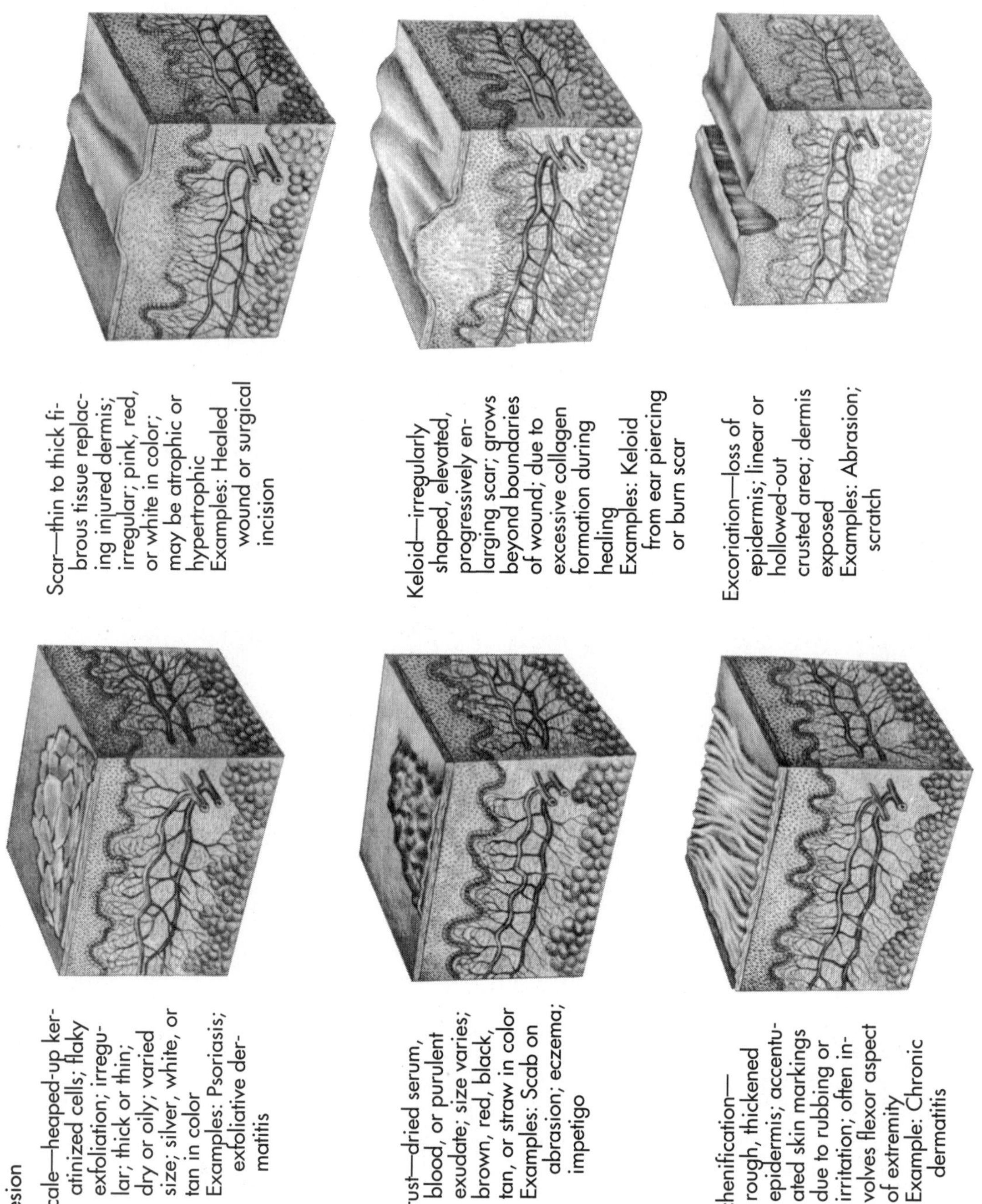

Lesion
Scale—heaped-up keratinized cells; flaky exfoliation; irregular; thick or thin; dry or oily; varied size; silver, white, or tan in color
Examples: Psoriasis; exfoliative dermatitis
Crust—dried serum, blood, or purulent exudate; size varies; brown, red, black, tan, or straw in color
Examples: Scab on abrasion; eczema; impetigo
Lichenification—rough, thickened epidermis; accentuated skin markings due to rubbing or irritation; often involves flexor aspect of extremity
Example: Chronic dermatitis
Scar—thin to thick fibrous tissue replacing injured dermis; irregular; pink, red, or white in color; may be atrophic or hypertrophic
Examples: Healed wound or surgical incision
Keloid—irregularly shaped, elevated, progressively enlarging scar; grows beyond boundaries of wound; due to excessive collagen formation during healing
Examples: Keloid from ear piercing or burn scar
Excoriation—loss of epidermis; linear or hollowed-out crusted area; dermis exposed
Examples: Abrasion; scratch

Figure 6-2 Secondary skin lesions. (From Thompson JM et al: *Mosby's clinical nursing*, ed 4, St Louis, 1997, Mosby.)

Fissure—linear crack or break from epidermis to dermis; small; deep; red
Examples: Athlete's foot; cheilosis

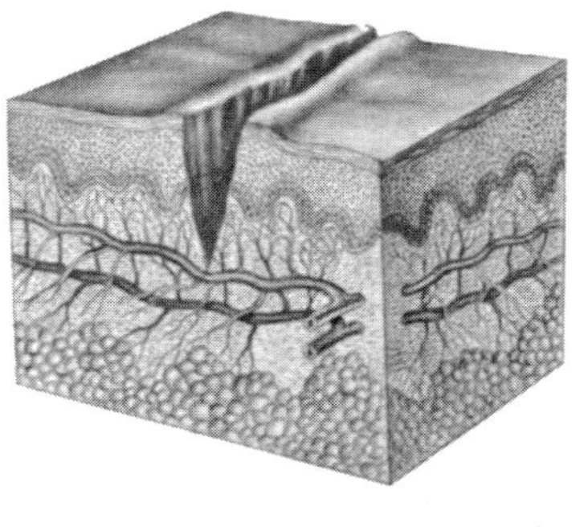

Ulcer—loss of epidermis and dermis; concave; varies in size; exudative; red or reddish blue
Example: Pressure ulcers

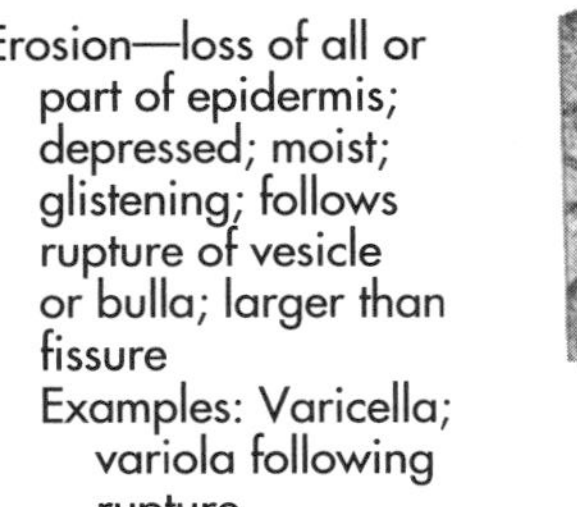

Erosion—loss of all or part of epidermis; depressed; moist; glistening; follows rupture of vesicle or bulla; larger than fissure
Examples: Varicella; variola following rupture

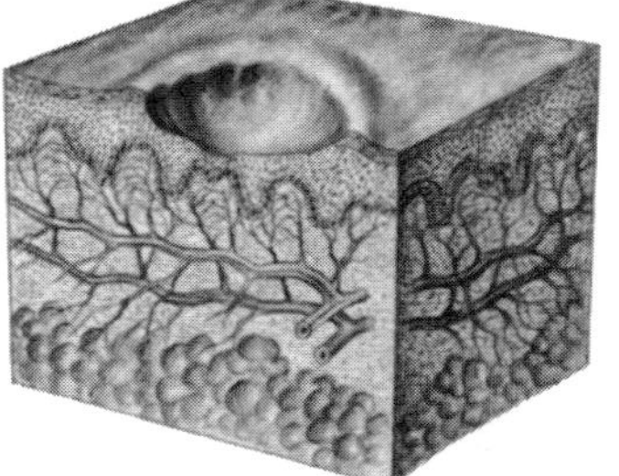

Atrophy—thinning of skin surface and loss of skin markings; skin translucent and paperlike
Examples: Striae; aged skin

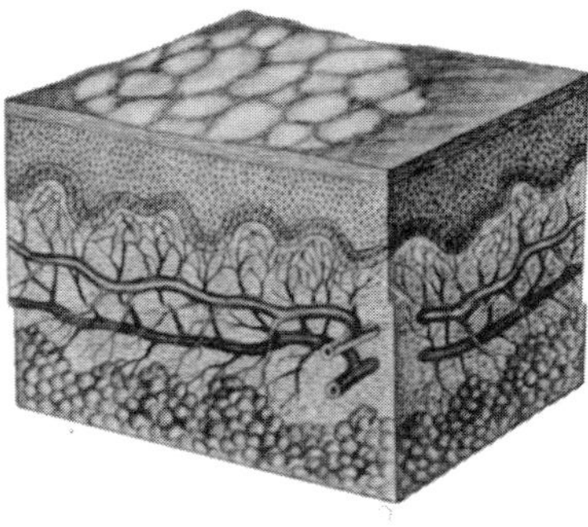

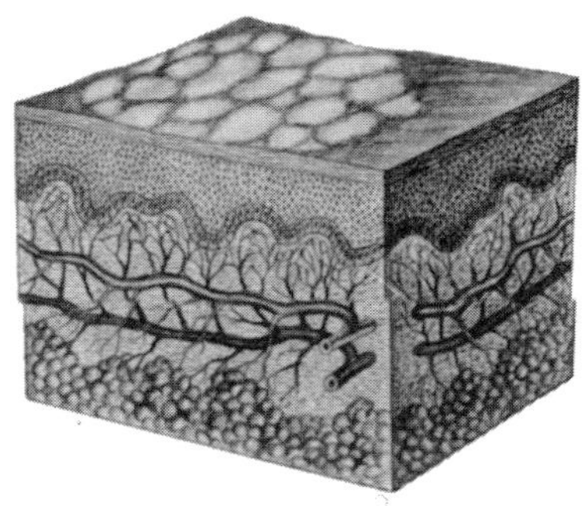

Hyperkeratosis—Abnormal skin thickening of the superficial layer of the epidermis.
Hyperpigmentation—Increased skin pigment.
Hypopigmentation—Decreased skin pigment.

Figure 6-2, cont'd.

TABLE 6-1 Systematic Assessment of Skin Lesions: Components and Descriptors

COMPONENTS OF ASSESSMENT	DESCRIPTORS
Distribution of lesions	Generalized, localized, bilateral, asymmetric, patchy
Arrangement	Discrete, confluent, grouped, well-defined
Configuration (shape or outline)	Arciform, annular (circular), polycyclic, linear, serpiginous (creeping from one place to another)
Type and evolution of primary lesion	See Figure 6-1
Characteristics of primary lesion	Dry, oozing, bleeding, color, indurated, blisters present, size, tenderness

TABLE 6-2 Common Clues to the Causes of Wounds

CAUSE	LOCATION	CHARACTERISTICS
Pressure	Bony prominence in mobility-restricted patient	Stages 1 to 4
Shear	Surfaces exposed to bed or chair surface in patient with reduced mobility or poor tissue turgor	Separation of dermal-epidermal junction (associated with pressure ulcers) May present as hematoma
Friction	Surfaces exposed to bed or chair surface	Superficial (epidermal)
Chemical (such as incontinence)	Areas exposed to urine, stool, or drainage	Superficial (epidermal, superficial dermal)
Moisture	Intertriginous areas	Maceration; superficial erosion of epidermis
Venous hypertension	Medial malleolus	Hyperpigmentation, edema, exudative wounds
Ischemia	Digits; areas of trauma	Surrounding tissue cool and pale Diminished or absent pulses Delayed capillary refill Pain
Neuropathy	Areas of sensory loss exposed to trauma or pressure (such as feet and heels)	Common in patients with diabetes Associated with abnormal gait; opening at skin level may be small, tunnels present; extensive subcutaneous tissue damage

MECHANICAL DAMAGE

Those forces that are applied externally to the skin such as pressure, shear, friction, and skin stripping (skin tears) create mechanical damage. Each may occur in isolation or in combination with other mechanical injuries. This section presents shear, friction, and skin stripping. (Pressure damage is discussed in detail in Chapter 11.)

Shear

Shear force is created by the interaction of gravity and friction (resistance) against the surface of the skin. Friction is always present when shear force is present. The classic example of shear is when a patient is in a semi-Fowler's position. While the torso slides downward to the foot of the bed, the bed surface generates enough resistance that the skin

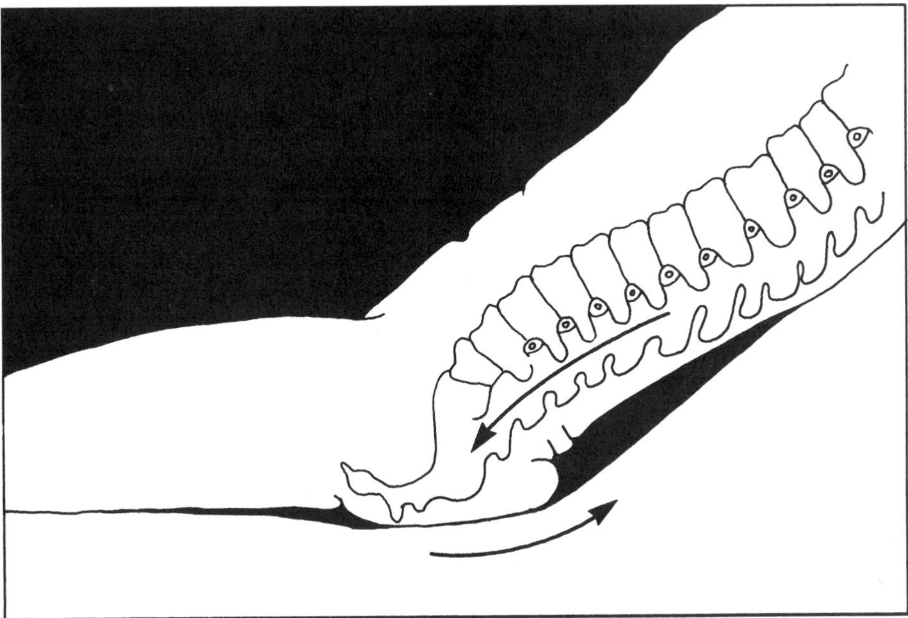

Figure 6-3 Shearing force. (From Loeper JM et al: *Therapeutic positioning and skin care*, Minneapolis, 1986, Sister Kenny Institute.)

over the sacrum remains in the same location (Figure 6-3). Ultimately, the skin is held in place while the skeletal structures pull the body (by gravity) toward the foot of the bed. Consequently, blood vessels in the area are stretched and angulated, and such changes may create small vessel thrombosis and tissue death.

Shear may cause shallow or deep ulcers and extends the tissue damage seen with pressure ulcers. This extension is manifested in the pressure ulcer by the presence of undermining (dissection or separation of tissue parallel to the skin surface).

Shear injury is predominately localized at the sacrum or coccyx and is most commonly a consequence of elevating the head of the bed or of improper transfer technique. Prevention requires an awareness of those situations in which the skin is exposed to shear force. For example, the patient with pulmonary distress requires the head of the bed to be elevated to facilitate adequate ventilation; however, the patient is at great risk for shear injury. Likewise, the patient with a cerebrovascular accident may experience shear injury when being transferred from the bed to the wheelchair.

Strategies for prevention of shear are listed in Box 6-1. However, research to substantiate these preventive measures (particularly genuine sheepskin) is lacking. Because shear is an important contributing factor to pressure ulcer development, strategies to prevent shear and pressure simultaneously are warranted. As Fontaine, Risley, and Castellino (1998) point out, "Every instance of interface pressure has a shear component and each shear force is accompanied by pressure." Many support surfaces have a slick fabric covering, which is believed to reduce shear. Unfortunately, there is no standardized method for measuring the ability of a support surface to reduce shear.

Fontaine and colleagues (1998) proposed a calculated pressure/shear factor (PSF), which would quantify support surface efficiency for the combined effect of pressure and shear reduction. PSF is calculated by adding the rounded average interface pressure (mm Hg) to the rounded average gross shear force (g) multiplied by the impact factor of 4. The equation is as follows:

$$\text{Pressure} + (4 \times \text{Shear force}) = \text{PSF} \textit{ or}$$
$$\text{mm Hg} + (4 \times \text{g}) = \text{PSF}$$

BOX 6-1 Prevention of Mechanical Skin Damage*

Pressure

1. Implement pressure reduction if the patient is able to reposition or if the wound is on only one surface. (Redistributes weight over larger surface area.)
2. Implement pressure relief if the patient is unable to reposition or if the wound is on more than one surface. (There are limited intact body surfaces that can be used to absorb and redistribute weight.)
3. Establish a turning schedule. (Compliance and continuity of care will be enhanced.)
4. Reposition patient between supine position and 30-degree lateral position. (The 30-degree lateral position does not exert pressure on any bony prominence.)
5. Keep pressure off heels by using positioning aids and pillows. (Heel interface pressures often exceed capillary closing pressure regardless of support surface.)

Shear

1. Elevate head of bed to no more than 30 degrees and for limited times. (This reduces pull of gravity and sliding of tissues.)
2. Position feet against a footboard. (This prevents sliding down in bed.)
3. Use knee gatch when head of bed is elevated. (This prevents sliding down in bed.)
4. Use lift sheet to reposition patient. (This prevents dragging of patient's skin across bed.)

Friction

1. Apply transparent dressing, thin hydrocolloid, or skin sealant to skin surface. (This provides a barrier to friction.)
2. Use sheepskin elbow or heel protectors. (This reduces exposure of skin to friction.)
3. Apply moisturizers to skin. (Adequately maintained epidermis is more resistant to stressors.)
4. Reduce shear. (Friction always occurs in combination with shear.)

Skin Stripping

1. Apply tape without tension. (This prevents blistering of skin under tape.)
2. Use porous tapes. (This allows moisture to evaporate.)
3. To remove tape, slowly peel tape away from anchored skin or pull one corner of tape at an angle parallel with skin. (This decreases trauma to the epidermis and dermoepidermal junction.)
4. Secure dressings with roll gauze, tubular stockinette, or self-adhering tape. (This avoids unnecessary tapes on skin.)
5. Use skin sealants, thin hydrocolloids, low-adhesion foam dressings, or solid-wafer skin barriers under adhesives. (This provides a protective layer over the skin for adhering tapes.)
6. Secure dressings with Montgomery straps. (This prevents repeated tape applications.)

NOTE: When protective devices are used to protect the skin from mechanical trauma, the product should be removed at regular intervals to allow inspection and assessment of the area.

*The material in parentheses represents the rationale for each intervention.

A pressure sensor and a shear sensor are required to obtain the values to put into this PSF equation. Potentially, the PSF could become a supplement to current support surface measurements, which are strictly interface pressure measurements. In this way the PSF would provide additional objective information concerning the potential for the support surface to prevent ulceration. For example, Fontaine, Risley, and Castellino (1998) studied the PSF for three support surfaces classified as group-2 devices according to the Medicare Part B policy. The PSF was calculated for a powered alternating pressure mattress overlay; a powered, zoned, air-filled mattress replacement device; and a nonpowered fluid overlay. Resulting PSFs were 939, 1043, and 331, respectively. The implication is that the nonpowered fluid overlay was more effective in reducing the pressure/shear force. However, because PSF is a newly defined variable, further research is necessary to establish validity of the variable as well as predictive value and clinical effects.

The primary intervention that nurses should employ currently to reduce shear is to use lift sheets when repositioning the patient; this method eliminates drag on the sacral skin. Elevation of the head of bed should be limited to no more than 30 degrees and for short periods of time. Sheepskin may be used; however, it should not be confused with pressure-reduction measures. Also, the knee gatch can be used to interrupt gravity's pull on the body toward the foot of the bed.

Friction

Skin injured by friction results from two surfaces rubbing together and has the appearance of an abrasion. This type of injury is frequently seen on elbows or heels because the patient easily abrades these surfaces against sheets when repositioning. Injury is characteristically very shallow and limited to the epidermis. Tissue necrosis does not occur with friction.

Interventions to prevent friction are listed in Box 6-1. These involve the use of protective sheepskin over the elbows or heels and moisturizers applied to vulnerable areas to maintain proper hydration of the epidermis. Many nurses find transparent adhesive dressings, thin hydrocolloids, low-adhesion foam dressings, and skin sealants effective at reducing friction. Adhesive dressings are contraindicated if the friction is sufficient to loosen the dressing. Braces, splints, prosthetic devices, and shoes should be assessed frequently for evidence of friction, and modifications should be implemented as needed.

Skin Stripping (Epidermal and Dermal)

Skin stripping is the inadvertent removal of the epidermis with or without the dermis by mechanical means, such as tape removal or bumping into furniture (Bryant, 1988). Payne and Martin (1990) identified these types of lesions as skin tears. The definition of *skin tear* most recently proposed by Payne and Martin (1993) is "a traumatic wound occurring principally on the extremities of older adults, as a result of friction alone or shearing and friction forces which separate the epidermis from the dermis (partial thickness wound) or which separate both the epidermis and dermis from the underlying structures (full thickness wounds)." A taxonomy for severity of skin tears is listed in Box 6-2. Distinguishing characteristics of a Category I skin tear is that the resulting skin flap or the avulsed skin can cover the exposed wound. Category II wounds are distinguished by the degree of damage to the epidermal avulsed skin. Category III lesions have no epidermal flap. Only category IA lesions are full thickness (involve the dermis).

Typically, these lesions are irregularly shaped and shallow, involving only the epidermis. The most frequent location of skin-stripping injuries is the upper extremities (73% to 80%), although they have been observed on the legs and feet (20%),

BOX 6-2 Skin Tears: Definition and Payne-Martin Classification System

Category I: Skin tear can fully approximate wound

A: *Linear skin tear.* Wound that occurs in wrinkle or furrow of skin. Both epidermis and dermis are pulled apart as if an incision has been made, exposing tissue below.

B: *Flap-type skin tear.* Partial-thickness wound in which the epidermal flap can be completely approximated or approximated so that no more than 1 millimeter of dermis is exposed.

Category II: Skin tear with partial thickness loss

A: *Scant tissue loss.* Partial thickness in which 25% or less of the epidermal flap is lost and at least 75% or more of the dermis is covered by the flap.

B: *Moderate to large tissue loss.* Partial-thickness wound in which more than 25% the epidermal flap is lost and more than 25% of the dermis is exposed.

Category III: Skin tears with complete tissue loss

A partial-thickness wound in which an epidermal flap is absent.

From Payne RL, Martin ML: Defining and classifying skin tears: need for a common language, *Ostomy Wound Manage* 39(5):16, 1993.

head (3% to 4%), and torso (3%) (Malone et al, 1991; McGough-Csarny and Kopac, 1998; Payne and Martin, 1990).

Risk factors for a skin tear include advanced age, compromised nutrition, history of previous skin tears, cognitive impairment, dependency, poor locomotion, and presence of ecchymosis (McGough-Csarny and Kopac, 1998). Daily care activities such as bathing, dressing, transfers, and toileting all require frequent handling of the patient with vulnerable skin. Therefore their potential for developing a skin tear increases. Use of equipment (e.g., mechanical lifts, wheelchairs, and geri-chairs) also increases the patient's exposure to potential trauma, which may precipitate a skin tear.

Mature and immature skin are both vulnerable to skin tears because the dermal-epidermal junction is not optimally functional. The matched groove adherence of the dermal papillae and epidermal rete pegs at the dermal-epidermal junction is critical to providing resiliency and the ability to withstand mechanical stresses. In the premature infant's skin, the dermal-epidermal junction is undeveloped and weak. As the skin ages, the epidermis thins, the dermal-epidermal junction flattens, and cohesion is diminished. In addition, the amount of collagen and elastin present in the aging skin decreases so that the skin becomes dry, wrinkled, thin, and transparent. Furthermore, vascular changes increase the fragility of capillaries in the dermal-epidermal junction. Therefore mechanical stresses can trigger a subcutaneous hemorrhage (e.g., senile purpura) between the skin layers, which results in further separation of the dermis and epidermis. Disease management regimens can also alter the skin's vitality. For example, corticosteroids reduce tissue collagen strength and elasticity and thereby increase the patient's risk to skin tears. Radiation causes epidermal atrophy, microvascular occlusions, reduced fibroblast proliferation, tissue fibrosis, and edema.

A key component to the prevention of skin tears is to recognize fragile, thin, vulnerable skin, particularly ecchymotic skin. Extreme care and a gentle touch are critical when contacting the patient or performing patient care since most skin tears occur in the course of providing routine patient care activities (e.g., bathing, dressing, transferring) (Malone et al, 1991; McGough-Csarny and Kopac, 1998; White, Karam, and Cowell, 1994).

Beyond these measures, the current focus of prevention is on the application of products to the skin to serve as a barrier between the skin and traumatic events. Skin tears resulting from adhesives can be prevented by 1) appropriate application and removal of tape; 2) use of solid-wafer skin barriers, thin hydrocolloids, low-adhesion foam dressings, or skin sealants under adhesives; 3) use of porous tapes; and 4) avoidance of unnecessary tapes (see Box 6-1). Additional protection of ecchymotic skin can be provided by applying transparent dressings, thin hydrocolloids, or low-adhesion foam dressings; keeping the arms and legs covered with roll gauze; or wearing long sleeves and pants. However, when adhesive dressings are used on intact skin to prevent skin tears, the protocol should clearly indicate that the dressing is not changed routinely. It should be left undisturbed and allowed to fall off. As the edges of the dressing loosen, the loosened edges should be clipped rather than removing the entire dressing and applying a new dressing. More research is needed to explore the prevention of skin tears, such as the role of humectants, emollients, moisturizers, and skin cleansers (Mason, 1997).

The body of evidence concerning treatment of skin tears is sparse but growing. In a recent study, Thomas, Blume, and Forman (1999) report that dressings with a high moisture vapor transmission rate (MVTR), such as with a low adhesive foam dressing, result in complete healing of 94% (16 of 17) category II and III skin tears within 21 days. This is in comparison with complete healing of only 65% (11 of 17) of skin tears using a film dressing. The researchers suggest that film dressings keep the skin tear excessively moist and exacerbate the separation of the epidermis from the dermal papillae. However, these results and recommendation remain to be further studied and replicated.

Appropriate tape application and removal techniques can also help prevent skin stripping. Proper tape application implies that the tape is applied without tension or "pinching" of the epidermis. Often tape is applied appropriately after a surgical procedure, but as edema develops at the surgical site over the ensuing 24 hours, the tape begins to pull on the underlying skin. Blisters then develop under the tape. To alleviate the tension that develops as the skin becomes normally edematous after surgical manipulation, it may be advisable to remove and reapply dressings 24 hours postoperatively.

Proper tape removal entails slowly peeling the tape away from the skin while stabilizing the skin. Solvents can be used to break the adhesive skin bond, although solvents have a drying effect on the skin. Plain tap water can often serve this purpose effectively. Some manufacturers recommend loosening the tape by pulling on one corner of the tape at an angle parallel with the skin. Solid-wafer skin barriers and thin hydrocolloids can also be applied to frame the wound; wound dressings are then secured by anchoring the tape to the surface of the barrier. One can easily apply and reapply the tape without traumatizing the epidermis. These skin barriers and hydrocolloid dressings can remain in place for several days.

Skin sealants may be applied to the skin before the tape is applied to provide protection from skin tears. Only alcohol-free skin sealants should be used when the skin is denuded or when contact with the wound edges is likely because alcohol content can cause intense stinging. It is important to allow the skin sealant to dry completely before applying tape. Many central-line dressing kits are prepackaged with a skin sealant.

Unnecessary use of adhesives and tapes should be avoided, particularly on vulnerable, fragile skin. Nurses can be creative when securing dressings without applying tape to the skin. For example, tubular stockinette, roll gauze, or self-adhering tape can be used. In general, it is best to avoid applying adhesives in an area receiving radiation. A standardized care plan for patients at high risk for skin tears is provided in Box 6-3.

CHEMICAL FACTORS

The presence of chemicals on the skin is a common source of skin damage and can result from fecal incontinence, harsh solutions such as povidone-iodine complex (Betadine), improper use of products such as skin sealants or skin cements, and drainage around percutaneous tubes or drains. The presence of these solutions or secretions on the skin destroys or erodes the epidermis. Early manifestations start with erythema or an erythematous macular rash and can quickly progress to denudement if exposure continues (Plate 11).

Chemical irritation or dermatitis is also referred to as an *irritant contact dermatitis.* Skin damage may be evident in only a few hours in the presence of a strong irritant (such as small bowel discharge). In fact, infants may develop an irritant dermatitis as soon as they pass a loose stool into the diaper. In other situations, repeat exposures over several days may be necessary when the irritant is weak. Chemical dermatitis can be distinguished from an allergic reaction by its irregular borders and always requires the presence of drainage or chemicals. Lesions are distributed in the areas that have been exposed to the offending agent. Subjectively, chemical dermatitis is very uncomfortable for the patient because of the shallow (epidermal and dermal) nature of the lesions.

Chemical irritation can be prevented by 1) identification of patients at risk for chemical irritation, 2) prevention of drainage around catheters or drains from contacting the skin, 3) avoidance of the presence of harsh substances on the skin, and 4) appropriate use of skin-care products (soaps, barriers, adhesives, or solvents).

Moisture-barrier ointments, gentle skin cleansing, and creative uses of skin barriers, thin hydrocolloids, or low-adhesion foam dressings are the cornerstone to the prevention of chemical irritation when patients are determined to be at risk. For example, it should be anticipated that the patient with a low serum albumin level who is receiving antibiotics is at risk for developing diarrhea once enteral feedings are initiated. The nurse should initiate a care plan of gentle skin cleansing (no harsh soaps or rough cloths) and ointments to prevent chemical irritation (Habif, 1996). The infant with increased stooling frequency requires more frequent diaper changes, gentle cleansing, and appropriate use of ointments. Likewise, the adult may experience diarrhea for several reasons, such as gastrointestinal bleeding or antibiotic therapy. In most situations, diligent and appropriate use of

BOX 6-3 Standardized Care Plan for Patients at High-Risk for Skin Tears

1. Provide a safe environment
   a. Free room of obstacles that obstruct pathway around bed and bathroom.
   b. Provide adequate lighting in resident's room.
   c. Leave night-light on in bathroom with the door open.
   d. Leave side rails down at night.
   e. Make hourly rounds on resident.
   f. Provide safe area for wandering.
   g. Have resident wear anklet alarm.
   h. Install bed alarm.
   i. Provide well-fitting supportive shoes with skid-free soles.
   j. Have family bring loose-fitting adaptive clothing with back closure.
   k. Ensure that resident wears protective clothing for arms and legs (e.g., fleece-lined jogging suits, knee-length athletic socks, stockinette doubled).
   l. Protect all areas of purpura.
   m. Remove name tag when determined to be the cause of skin tears.
2. Maintain nutrition and hydration
   a. Obtain dietary consult.
   b. Obtain physician's order for double portions or high protein between meals.
   c. Keep intake and output records.
   d. Offer fluids between meals two times every shift.
   e. Encourage fluids at every meal.
   f. Use lotion on arms and legs twice daily.
   g. Obtain order for absorbic acid and zinc if resident is prone to skin tears with poor healing (vitamin C, 500 mg four times a day; zinc chelate, 50 mg four times a day).
   h. Perform body checks twice daily, in AM and at bedtime.
3. Protect from self-inflicted injury or injury incurred during routine care
   a. Use wheelchair for transport only.
      1) Pad wheelchair footrests.
      2) Pad rough edges of tabletops and wheelchair trays.
      3) Position resident with pillows and folded blankets to prevent head and arms from dangling over side of chair.
      4) Use sling around chair legs to prevent resident's feet from falling off footrests.
      5) Ensure smooth vinyl on wheelchair and recliner arms.
      6) Pad wheelchair and recliner arms.
      7) Use padding or cozy comforter to provide cushioning and protect skin while resident is up in recliner.
   b. Use mechanical lift to transport resident.
   c. Protect resident's arms and legs while in bed by padding side rails.
   d. Get occupational or physical therapy consult if needed for positioning for safety.
   e. Use lift sheet for positioning and moving resident.
   f. Move resident by using palm of hands.

Reprinted with permission from White et al: Skin tears in frail elders: a practical approach to prevention, *Ger Nurs* 15(2):95-99, 1994.

moisture-barrier ointments can help prevent denudation or ulceration.

When the frequency or volume of diarrhea overwhelms moisture-barrier ointments, moisture-barrier pastes and rectal pouches may be indicated temporarily to protect the skin from diarrhea. Rectal pouches are adhesive ostomy pouches specifically designed to fit the perianal contours and contain the incontinent stool. These products can be extremely cost-effective by providing skin with pro-

BOX 6-4 Rectal Pouching Procedure

1. Assemble equipment: nonsterile gloves, pouch, skin-barrier paste, clip, cloth, bag for waste, razor.
2. Prepare pouch:
   a. Remove paper backing from skin barrier and tape.
   b. Apply a thick bead of paste around the center opening; set aside.
3. Apply nonsterile gloves.
4. Remove and apply pouch:
   a. Loosen tape and gently push skin away from adhesive.
   b. Discard used pouch and save clip (if one is used).
   c. Remove any paste residue using a dry tissue.
   d. Wash skin with soft cloth and warm water; be sure to remove any greasy residue using a gentle soap and water. Rinse and dry thoroughly.
   e. Shave perianal hair, if present.
   f. To create a smooth adhesive surface, apply a bead of paste in the gluteal fold and between the anal opening and the scrotum or vagina.
   g. Before applying pouch, fold skin barrier surface of pouch vertically (lengthwise).
   h. Align pouch between scrotum or vagina and anal opening, and apply to skin.
   i. Slowly unfold pouch and adhesive to apply to skin in smooth fashion.
   j. Encourage seal by massaging the adhesive for 1 minute.
   k. Attach clip to open end of pouch or attach spout to straight drainage.
5. Change pouch only if it leaks.
6. Reposition patient carefully to avoid undue stress on pouch seal.

NOTE: Skin-barrier powders must be used to dry denuded skin, when present, before the pouch is applied.

tection from chemicals and moisture build-up, reducing linen changes, freeing up nursing time for other types of care and activities, and preserving the patient's dignity. Step-by-step instructions to apply a rectal pouch are listed in Box 6-4.

Drainage around catheters and tubes should be managed in such a way that the drainage is either eliminated when possible or the skin is not directly exposed to the drainage. For example, when leakage occurs around a gastrostomy tube, the first step is to ascertain proper placement and stabilization of the tube. If drainage persists once this is accomplished, appropriate use of skin barriers (particularly moisture-barrier ointments, solid-wafer skin barriers, thin hydrocolloids, or foam dressings) is indicated. A solid-wafer skin barrier, hydrocolloid, or foam dressing can be trimmed to fit around a tube site, remain in place for several days, and be changed only as it loosens at the tube site. When ointment is the selected treatment, it should be reapplied periodically throughout the day to ensure adequate skin protection. However, ointments can never be used under an adhesive dressing. Regardless of the type of skin protection selected, gauze dressings are applied over the barrier to absorb drainage and are changed when damp.

Solutions such as acetic acid and Betadine, although controversial, are at times used in wounds. The constant prolonged presence of such substances against the skin can also jeopardize skin integrity and create chemical damage.

Damage can be prevented by 1) monitoring appropriate dressing technique so that gauze dressings contact only the wound bed and are not contacting surrounding intact skin and 2) bracketing the wound with skin barriers (ointments, solid wafers, skin sealants, or hydrocolloids).

Improper use of skin-care products such as skin cleansers, solvents, adhesives, and skin sealants can contribute to chemical irritation. Skin cleansers and solvents must be thoroughly rinsed from the skin to prevent build-up of harmful substances. Skin cleansers or soaps should be used sparingly to avoid disruption of the normal acid pH of the skin (Bettley, 1960; Frosch and Kligman, 1974; White, Jenkinson, and Lloyd, 1987). Adhesives, such as cements, and skin sealants must be allowed to dry adequately so that solvents evaporate before other products are applied.

VASCULAR DAMAGE

Ulcerations, particularly on the legs or feet, also occur as a result of venous hypertension, arterial insufficiency, or neuropathy, or a combination of these factors. Although these types of lesions commonly develop incidentally to benign trauma (i.e., by bumping against the leg of a chair), each ulcer has distinct distinguishing features, pathologic processes, and treatment regimen. Arterial ulcers, venous ulcers, and lymphedema wounds are discussed in detail in Chapter 12. Neuropathic ulcers, such as diabetic ulcers, are discussed in Chapter 13.

INFECTIOUS FACTORS

Many skin rashes or ulcers are indicative of an infectious process and can occur around wounds or be misinterpreted as a result of pressure, shear, friction, or chemical irritation. Infections can be categorized according to infecting organism: fungus, bacteria, virus, or arthropod. The wound-care nurse may be the first person to observe some of these infections. In many cases, the wound-care nurse will be responsible for identifying and managing the infections. A few key skin infections are summarized in this section.

Fungus

Candidiasis. Cutaneous candidiasis represents an epidermal infection with *Candida* spp., most commonly *C. albicans* (Plate 11). The primary lesion with candidiasis is a pustule. Secondary lesions are papules, which result from abraded pustules, and plaque. Erythema and maceration are common. Lesions are typically beefy red, with satellite erythematous papules and pustules. When located in the skin folds (intertriginous areas), solid plaques of moist red lesions are commonly observed. Satellite lesions (outside the advancing edge of candidiasis) are an important diagnostic feature of candidiasis (Habif, 1996). Intact pustules are not always visible because opposing skin and clothing may unroof them. Pruritus is common and may be severe.

Predisposing factors include the presence of a moist environment, a hot humid environment, tight underclothing, diabetes, and antibiotic therapy. Damp surgical dressings, the perineum, the perineal area, and intertriginous areas (beneath pendulous breasts, overhanging abdominal folds and inguinal skin folds) are typical moist areas and provide an excellent medium for yeast growth. Diabetes predisposes the patient to develop candidiasis because the associated increase in the amount of glucose in the saliva, sweat, and urine prevents bacteria from inhibiting yeast growth (Hooper and Goldman, 1999). Antibiotics predispose the patient to develop candidiasis by removing the competing organisms, which increases yeast growth. An altered skin pH also increases susceptibility to yeast infection. Immunosuppressed patients and patients with psoriasis or atopic dermatitis are also vulnerable to candidiasis.

Folliculitis and contact dermatitis can be confused with candidiasis and can be distinguished by the presence or absence of papules, pustules, or erythema. Folliculitis, the asymptomatic inflammation of a hair follicle, is characterized by isolated pustules with a hair piercing each pustule, whereas erythema and papules are atypical of folliculitis. Manifestations of contact dermatitis include erythema with papules, whereas pustules are observed only with candidiasis. Distribution can also help distinguish between contact dermatitis and candidiasis because a contact dermatitis is limited to the area in contact with the irritant.

Candidiasis is most often determined clinically by the signs, symptoms, and predisposing factors. Pruritus and burning at the site are common. The most relevant laboratory test to confirm candidiasis is a potassium hydroxide (KOH) preparation scraping. Scrapings from an intact pustule and the contents are needed to yield the best results. Budding spores and elongated pseudohyphae are observed. Because the skin can be colonized with *C. albicans* but not infected, swab cultures for *Candida* are not informative because such cultures cannot distinguish between infection and colonization (Habif, 1996).

Nonpharmacologic treatment includes reduction of predisposing factors, such as humidity, moisture, antibiotics, hyperglycemia, and tight-fitting clothes. Body powders (e.g., Zeasorb-AF) or wide-mesh gauze can be placed in intertriginous areas to absorb moisture. Prevention of moisture build-up is the most important intervention to prevent candidiasis. Box 6-5 lists strategies to prevent moisture build-up.

Burrow's solution soaks followed by air-drying are soothing when maceration or severe pruritus are present. Topical antifungal creams may be ap-

BOX 6-5 Strategies to Prevent Moisture Build-Up

- Dust intertriginous skin folds with absorbent powders.
- Separate intertriginous skin folds with skin sealants (spray or wipes) and/or soft gauze.
- Use skin sealants, thin hydrocolloids, low-adhesion foam dressings, or solid-wafer skin barriers beneath dressings and around wounds.
- Change dressings before they become saturated.
- Use a support surface (if needed) with air-vent capabilities.

plied twice daily for limited involvement, and antifungal powders may be used in less severe cases. When creams are used, they should be applied sparingly to reduce moisture entrapment. Because ointments can further trap moisture and therefore exacerbate the candidiasis, they may not be preferred. Recalcitrant or severe fungal infections require oral therapy.

Bacterial

Folliculitis, impetigo, erysipelas and staphylococcal scalded skin syndrome (SSSS), toxic shock syndrome, and necrotizing fasciitis are not necessarily frequently encountered in the typical practice of a wound-care nurse. However, they pose significant complications and should be familiar to the wound-care nurse. Many of the bacterial skin infections are caused by *Staphylococcus aureus*. Although *S. aureus* is frequently recovered from normal intact skin, it is rarely a true member of resident bacterial flora (Leyden and Gately, 1995).

Folliculitis. Folliculitis is a bacterial infection that involves the hair follicle. *S. aureus* is the most common organism. The primary lesion is a pustule that is pierced by a hair, and secondary lesions are crusts and erythema. Folliculitis may be limited to the superficial area of the hair follicle or progress deeper into the follicle. Although most common on the scalp or extremities, folliculitis may develop on any hairy body location, particularly under adhesive wound dressings.

Risk factors for developing folliculitis are diabetes mellitus, obesity, malnutrition, immunodeficiency, and chronic staphylococcal infections. Folliculitis may also develop as a secondary infection in the presence of excoriated skin (e.g., scabies, insect bites, and eczema).

Nonpharmacologic treatment includes the use of warm compresses three to four times daily for mild cases. Adhesives in the affected area should be avoided, and hair should be clipped rather than shaved. Oral antibiotics are required for deep folliculitis.

Impetigo. Impetigo is most commonly seen in children and is caused by gram-positive bacteria (usually *S. aureus*). The initial onset is a pustule with little or no surrounding erythema. Lesions quickly form a yellow-tan crust when disrupted. Beneath the crust is a superficial glistening base; ulcerations are not present because the infection is superficial and barely extends below the stratum corneum. Impetigo can occur anywhere but is most common on the face.

It is important to distinguish impetigo from a streptococcal infection and from herpes simplex. Culture and appearance are used to determine streptococcal infections. Clinically, streptococcal skin infections are deeper, extending through the epidermis so that an ulcer is seen when the crust is removed. Furthermore, streptococcal skin infections are commonly surrounded by erythema. Herpes simplex can be distinguished from impetigo by culture and by early manifestations; herpes simplex begins with grouped, clear vesicles that are uniform in size, and it recurs at the same site.

Treatment involves topical or systemic antibiotics. Small limited lesions may be effectively managed with topical 2% mupirocin; deeper infections require 7 to 10 days of erythromycin or penicillin-resistant penicillins (such as dicloxacillin).

Bullous Impetigo. Bullous impetigo is an infection that results from certain strains of *S. aureus* that produce a specific toxin. These toxins induce superficial, fragile, clear bullae that become pustular. When these bullae rupture, a thin crust develops and a rim of the bulla roof often remains, encircling the crust. Satellite lesions may develop by autoinoculation. Extensive toxin production can precipitate a scarlatina-type rash or a generalized erythematous eruption with splitting in the outer epidermal layers (i.e., SSSS) (Leyden and Gately, 1995). Common locations include the face, neck, and extremities and may be typified by pruritus. Predisposing factors include poor hygiene and inadequate attention to skin injury.

As with deeper impetigo infections, systematic antibiotics with penicillinase-resistant penicillins (e.g., dicloxacillin) or erythromycin are usually preferred because lesions develop rapidly over multiple body sites. Spontaneous healing occurs without antibiotics over 3 to 6 weeks.

Erysipelas. Erysipelas is a form of cellulitis that occurs as a complication of a break in skin integrity. It is a skin infection that develops from the invasion of group A β-hemolytic streptococcus into the dermis and subcutaneous tissues. This disease has a very high morbidity rate if left undiagnosed (up to 80% in infants and 75% in the elderly) (Hooper and Goldman, 1999).

Erysipelas most commonly occurs in infants, young children, and older adults. Additional risk factors include patients with malnutrition, alcoholism, recent infections, stasis dermatitis, lymphedema, nephrotic syndrome, and diabetes mellitus. Small, seemingly insignificant breaks in the skin can serve as a portal of entry for the infection. The extremities and face are the most common sites.

Erysipelas means "red skin," and the involved body part is characterized by well-demarcated erythema. (In contrast, cellulitis is less well-marginated.) The classic primary lesion is a plaque, and the surrounding skin is erythematous, edematous, and painful. Secondary lesions are vesicles, bullae, and cutaneous hemorrhage. Lymphatic involvement as demonstrated by the presence of "streaking" may be prominent.

Erysipelas is usually diagnosed by clinical findings: sharply marginated erythema, edema, and/or streaking. Accompanying systemic complaints of fever, chills, malaise, and localized pain are also suspicious for the disease. A culture (via needle aspiration) of any drainage from the advancing edge and skin biopsies are appropriate although often uninformative. When septicemia is suspected, a white blood cell count and blood cultures are warranted.

Nonpharmacologic interventions include bed rest, elevation of the affected extremity, and hot packs. Burrow's solution can be applied topically to lessen pain. Uncomplicated cases of erysipelas can be treated with oral antibiotics, whereas toxic, debilitated, and elderly patients or children with extensive facial involvement often require intravenous antibiotics. Pain control measures are essential.

Staphylococcal Scalded Skin Syndrome. SSSS is a superficial blistering disease that results in superficial necrosis. SSSS is a cutaneous response to a circulating toxin released from a staphylococcal infection that may be distant from the affected area. The primary lesion is superficial bullae that may occur on the face, neck, axillae, and groin. Secondarily, lesions become scales. Desquamation develops subsequent to the significant erythema. The skin also has a sandpaper feel.

Although it has been reported in adults, SSSS most commonly occurs in healthy children younger than 6 years of age (Beers and Wilson, 1990). Mortality approaches 3% in adults with renal failure and in those who are immunocompromised.

Staphylococcal cultures from suspicious sites (nose, eyes, ears, throat, vagina) are needed to confirm the diagnosis, and bullae are usually negative. A frozen section of sloughing skin is needed to differentiate SSSS from a drug-induced skin reaction (toxic epidermal necrolysis). Full-thickness necrosis is consistent with the drug-induced process (Leydon and Gately, 1995).

Debridement and antibiotics are essential to manage the infection. Topical management of the resulting desquamated skin should address exudate management, pain control, and maintaining a moist environment. Foam dressings, superabsorbent dressings, sheet hydrogels, and alginates are preferred dressing options, and adhesives should be avoided. When massive tissue loss is apparent, the wound should be managed according to the principles for burn therapy as outlined in Chapter 10.

Toxic Shock Syndrome. Toxic shock syndrome is a bacterial infection with acute onset and widespread macular erythematous eruptions. The most common pathogen for this serious infection is *S. aureus*. Desquamation of the skin is highly characteristic of toxic shock syndrome and occurs 10 days to 3 weeks after onset. The primary body sites are the fingertips and plantar surface of the palms (Leyden and Gately, 1995). Treatment requires aggressive antibiotic therapy, and the mortality rate is approximately 7%. Local wound management is based on wound needs (e.g., exudate absorption), and topical dressings should be nonocclusive and nonadhesive.

Necrotizing Fasciitis. Necrotizing fasciitis is an uncommon subcutaneous tissue infection that spreads rapidly along the superficial fascial plane. The overall mortality rate from this infection is 47%; early diagnosis (within 4 days of onset) reduces the rate to 12% (Leyden and Gately, 1995). Necrotizing fasciitis is characterized by widespread necrosis of the fascia and deep subcutaneous tissue with thrombosis of nutrient vessels and sloughing of overlying tissue. It usually occurs in the extremities after a minor operation or injury.

Initial signs of necrotizing fasciitis are pain, swelling at the site of the wound, chills, fever, toxemia, and rapidly spreading painful cellulitis. The skin appears normal over the cellulitis, but as the infectious process compromises blood supply the skin becomes erythematous, edematous, and reddish-purple to patchy blue gray. Bullae form within 3 to 5 days from onset, which progress to necrosis of the skin, sloughing, and frank cutaneous gangrene.

Necrotizing fasciitis can be detected by its dramatic clinical presentation and by probing the wound. When the affected area is probed with a hemostat through a limited incision, the instrument passes easily along a plane of superficial to deep fascia. This examination also helps to distinguish necrotizing fasciitis from cellulitis. This infection may be a monomicrobial infection caused by *Clostridium* spp., *S. pyogenes*, *S. aureus*, or group B streptococcus. Polymicrobial infections that include anaerobic bacteria are also causative for necrotizing fasciitis (Leyden and Gately, 1995).

Treatment is surgical intervention to debride all nonviable fascia and tissue. Surgical debridement must be prompt, extensive, and aggressive. Local wound care consists of close monitoring for further dissection, which indicates progression of the infection. Topical dressing recommendations are largely expert opinion based or preference based. Dressings should be used that meet the needs of the wound (e.g., fill dead space, absorb exudate), allow for frequent monitoring of the wound, and are nonadhesive and nonocclusive.

Virus

Viral infections, particularly herpes simplex virus (HSV) and varicella-zoster virus (VZV), are commonly triggered by stress and illness. It is important to recognize these highly contagious infections to facilitate prompt appropriate treatment and prevent spread to others.

Herpes Simplex. HSV infections of the epidermis are highly contagious and can be spread when a susceptible noninfected person comes into direct contact (mucous membrane or broken skin) with a person shedding the virus. Viral shedding occurs even in the absence of symptoms. Most transmission of HSV occurs during periods of asymptomatic shedding (Whitley, Kimberlin, and Roizman, 1998). Consequently, HSV infection should be considered a chronic process rather than an intermittent process, and all HSV-infected people should be treated as potentially contagious. Furthermore, because the primary infection is often subclinical, a negative history of vesicles or blisters does not rule out previous HSV infection (Chandrasekar, 1999).

HSV is typically classified as either HSV-1 (oral herpes) or HSV-2 (genital herpes). HSV-1 is associated with cold sores (fever blisters); genital and perianal herpes is caused by HSV-2. However, genital lesions from HSV-1 and oral lesions from HSV-2 are becoming more common, a trend that may be a consequence of sexual freedom and ease of transmission. Ultimately, HSV lesions are not limited to the lips and genital area and may occur anywhere on the skin.

HSV infections have two phases: primary infection and secondary phase. During the primary infection, the virus becomes established in a nerve ganglion; HSV-1 most often occurs during childhood, whereas HSV-2 commonly occurs after sexual contact in sexually active individuals. Symptoms of the primary infection range from being undetectable to localized pain, headache, generalized aching, malaise, and tender regional adenopathy. Uniform, grouped vesicles develop on an erythematous base; the vesicles contain large numbers of infective viral particles. Vesicles soon become pustules that erode, drain, and crust (Plate 12). Primary lesions last for 2 to 6 weeks and heal without scarring. As the lesion heals, the virus enters the skin nerve endings and ascends through peripheral nerves to the dorsal root ganglia where it remains in a latent stage.

Reactivation of the virus can occur in response to local trauma (abrasion, ultraviolet light) or systemic changes (such as stress, illness, fatigue, fever, and compromised immune system). The virus then travels back down the peripheral nerve to the site of, or in the vicinity of, the initial infection to trigger a recurrence. Prodromal symptoms of burning at the site may precede the recurrence. The reactivated virus presents as vesicles on an erythematous base, or ulcers. Crusts cover the eruptions within 2 to 4 days and are shed in approximately 8 days, exposing a reepithelialized surface.

Clinical presentation of grouped vesicles on an erythematous base is a key indicator of HSV and can be confirmed with a Tzanck smear. However, the reliability of the Tzanck smear is best when the lesion sampled is a vesicle and becomes less reliable with pustules, crusts, or ulcers.

Primary HSV-1 infections are generally asymptomatic. When symptoms are present, the lesions include painful vesicles or shallow ulcers on the lips or lower face or in the oral cavity, and they last for 2 to 3 weeks. Recurrent HSV-1 infections are forewarned with pain and tingling or a burning sensation 2 to 24 hours before the eruption of vesicles (Chandrasekar, 1999). Recurrent HSV-1 lasts about 2 days as vesicles, and they then progress to pustules, ulcers, and eventually crusts. Complete healing occurs in 8 to 10 days.

Primary genital herpes (typically HSV-2 infection) are initially macules and papules followed by vesicles, pustules, and ulcerations. Lesions may occur on the genitalia, perineum, and buttocks; are extremely painful; and persist for about 2 weeks. Spontaneous resolution of the primary infection is common. Recurrent genital herpes is less pronounced and lasts for 8 to 10 days. Ulcers are shallow and may or may not be painful.

Perianal ulcers are commonly misinterpreted as the result of pressure, chemical damage, or scabies (Plate 13). Therefore the differential diagnosis for ulcers located in the perianal area or on the buttocks must include HSV (Chandrasekar, 1999). Genital herpes can be distinguished from pressure sores in that the lesions are not limited to a bony prominence and are more typical over the fleshy part of the buttocks. Genital herpes in the perianal area can also be distinguished from chemical irritation (such as with diarrhea) by the presence of several isolated ulcers rather than the confluence of superficial denudement or erythema that impinges on the anal opening.

Clinical presentation (grouped vesicles on an erythematous base) are highly suspicious for HSV regardless of body site. The most definitive method of confirming the infection is to culture the vesicular fluid from intact vesicles that have been unroofed. Rapid testing (within a few hours) can also be done with direct fluorescent antibody (DFA) examination. Commercially available kits also distinguish HSV-1, HSV-2, and VZV.

Antiviral medications are effective in treating HSV infection and are available in topical, oral, and intravenous administration. Early initiation of oral acyclovir for genital herpes decreases healing time, viral shedding, and duration of pain.

Nursing care should be directed at keeping lesions dry, avoiding trauma, and providing comfort. Burrow's solution (aluminum acetate) soaks and refrigerated hydrogel dressings can relieve the topical pain commonly associated with genital herpes lesions. When shedding HSV lesions are present, skin cleansing should be done cautiously so that spreading of the virus is avoided, particularly when the lesions are present on the buttocks.

Varicella-Zoster Virus. VZV causes varicella (chicken pox) and herpes zoster (shingles). VZV is highly contagious and is transmitted by direct contact with either vesicular fluid or airborne droplets from the infected host's respiratory tract. Airborne transmission is a very serious mode for spreading VZV. Spread of varicella with no direct contact has been reported; the sole exposure was to air that flowed from the room of the infected individual to

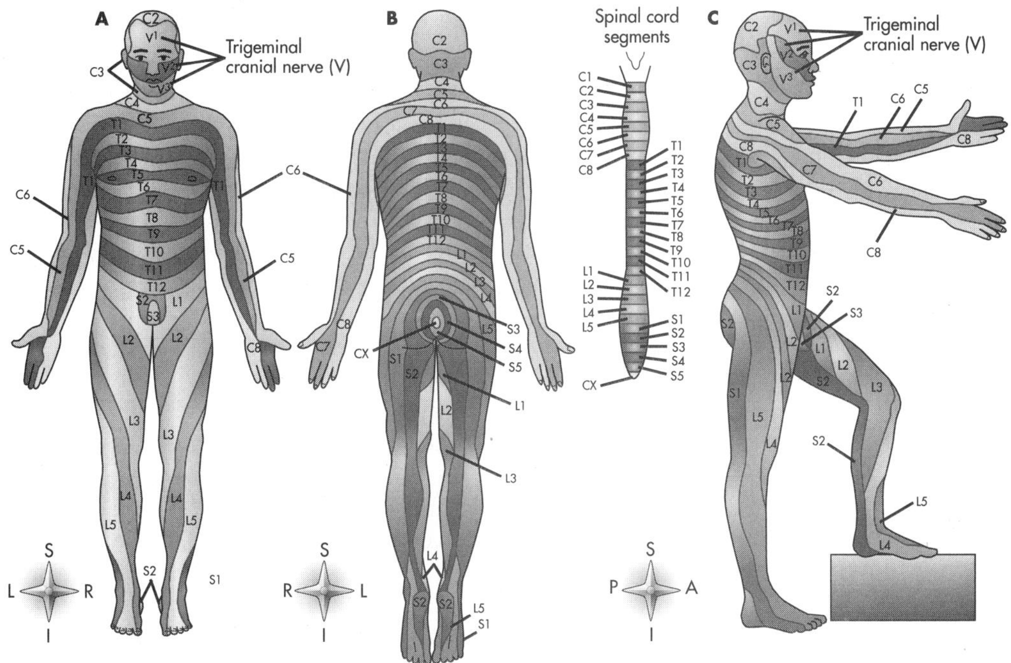

Figure 6-4 Segmental dermatome distribution of spinal nerves to the front, back, and side of the body. Dermatomes are specific skin surface areas innervated by a single spinal nerve or group of spinal nerves. *C*, Cervical segments; *T*, thoracic segments; *L*, lumbar segments; *S*, sacral segments; *CX*, coccygeal segment. (From Thibodeau GA, Patton KT: *Anatomy and physiology*, ed 4, St Louis 1999, Mosby.)

another room. Patients with herpes zoster are less contagious than patients with varicella (Cohen et al, 1999).

Herpes zoster is an infection within the epidermis that occurs along one or two adjacent dermatome distributions (Figure 6-4). Eruptions result from the reactivation of the VZV that entered the cutaneous nerves and has remained dormant in the dorsal root ganglia after a bout with chicken pox. Reactivation can occur as a result of immunosuppression, fatigue, and emotional trauma and occurs in 15% of people (Cohen et al, 1999). The elderly may be predisposed to herpes zoster as a consequence of a potential decline in immunologic function. Individuals who are immunocompromised are at risk of developing VZV and experience more severe infections. These patients are more likely to develop disseminated disease with extensive skin lesions, pneumonia, hepatitis, or encephalitis (Cohen et al, 1999). Diagnosis is most often based on clinical appearance.

Herpes zoster has characteristic manifestations, including a unilateral vesicular rash along one or two dermatomes (Plate 14). Vesicles may develop in clusters and vary in size. Over the next few days, vesicles become filled with purulent fluid (pustules) followed by rupturing and crusting. In some debilitated patients, the eruption may become more extensive and inflammatory, with necrosis or secondary infections developing. Pain that persists beyond 1 month is called *post-herpetic neuralgia*.

Treatment of herpes zoster is similar to HSV with antiviral medications and Burrow's solution to act as an astringent on the lesions. Lesions should not be occluded because this delays their healing (Chandrasekar, 1999). Analgesics may be necessary to control the pain associated with herpes zoster.

Arthropod

The brown recluse spider bite initially presents with swelling and erythema. Because of the release of a necrolytic toxin, purpura and subsequent extensive necrosis follows. The most common body location for the brown recluse spider bite is on the extremities but can also be found on the buttocks or genitalia.

Treatment is controversial, but the following measures are indicated (Smith, Ickstadt, and Kucera, 1997):

1. Ice pack on the affected area (no heat)
2. Antibiotics to treat the secondary infection
3. Pain control
4. Tetanus toxoid
5. Nonocclusive dressings to facilitate debridement and fill tissue loss

Patients should be observed for systemic reactions, which can occur 2 to 3 days after the bite. Systemic reactions may include renal failure or coagulation disorders such as disseminated intravascular coagulopathy (DIC) (Goldstein and Goldstein, 1997).

ALLERGIC FACTORS

Numerous allergic responses, local and systemic, can be manifested on the skin. Because the wound care nurse is in a likely position to observe such a reaction, it is important to be able to describe the manifestations accurately and to report the assessment to the physician in a timely fashion. This section focuses on those allergic responses that are localized reactions to such things as adhesives, wound-care products, or a solution. These types of skin damage are commonly referred to as *allergic contact dermatitis.*

Allergic contact dermatitis is an immunologic response to an allergen. Contact dermatitis occurs more readily in the presence of preexisting skin changes such as atopic dermatitis and is therefore more common in adults than in children.

A true allergic dermatitis requires exposure to an allergen and has two phases:

1. The *sensitization phase* (exposure to a substance or chemical to the skin of a nonsensitized individual) requires 5 to 21 days to transpire. Small molecules from the allergen pass through the epidermis and attach to an epidermal protein found on the surface of the Langerhans' cell. From here these cells migrate through the dermis to the lymph nodes where the allergen is exposed to T lymphocytes (the site of effector, memory, and suppressor T lymphocyte production). Here the body develops the ability to recognize the antigen when it reappears on the skin.
2. When reexposed to the allergen, the *elicitation phase* occurs within 1 to 2 days. Once the Langerhans' T cell delivers the antigen to memory T cells in the skin, effector T cells begin to produce lymphokines. Inflammatory cells are summoned by the lymphokines, and allergic manifestations can be observed. Suppressor T cells are believed to end the inflammatory reaction.

An acute inflammatory response occurs within 48 hours of exposure to an allergen. Clinical manifestations begin with erythema followed by pruritus. Primary lesions are vesicles, bullae, papules, plaques, and wheals. Secondary lesions include moist desquamation, edema, fissure, excoriation, and crust (Plate 15). An acute reaction usually resolves in days to weeks after the allergen has been removed.

The cause or source of the allergen may be obvious or obscured by other concurrent processes. A careful detailed assessment and interview are imperative to identify the skin reaction as an allergic response. Common allergic sensitizers include poison ivy, nickel (used in jewelry), rosins, rubber compounds (used in elastic, gloves), benzocaine (used in antipruritic creams), paraphenylenediamine (a dye used to color hair), and preservatives (such as ethylenediamine, which is a preservative found in Mycolog cream, aminophylline, some insecticides, or synthetic waxes). Topical preparations with one of the following ingredients are also common allergic offenders: vitamin E, aloe vera, fragrances, parabens, quarternium 15, diphenhydramine (Benedryl spray or Caladryl lotion), neomycin (Neosporin), and para-aminobenzoic acid (PABA) (Young, Newcomer, and Kligman,

1993). Overuse of soaps, cleansers, moisturizers, and cosmetics can produce reactions. Many chemicals of similar structure cross-react; therefore a person who is sensitive to one product may be sensitive to several other products.

The location of the skin damage is an important clue in identification of the causative agent. Allergic contact dermatitis is localized to the skin where the product is applied, and involved areas typically have sharp margins. Therefore an allergic reaction to an adhesive, for example, will be the shape of the adhesive and will have well-defined borders. Allergic contact dermatitis can spread from the original site of application through inadvertent transfer of the allergen by the hands or, as the disease progresses, by the circulating T lymphocytes. However, the skin reaction begins and remains most severe in the area in which contact with the antigen occurred (Burgdorf, 1994).

Patch tests can be conducted to confirm the suspected agent that is causing the allergic reaction; however, these tests must be properly conducted and interpreted. Suspected allergens are applied to the skin and secured with tape. The patient's back is usually the preferred site for patch testing. After 48 hours, the patches are removed and the test site is assessed for skin damage, which is graded using a standard scale as described in Box 6-6. Although the patch test seems simple to apply and read, it is a complicated procedure that requires training and experience to obtain valid results (Rietschel and Fowler, 1995).

BOX 6-6 Scale for Interpretation of Patch Test Results

+	=	Weak (nonvesicular) positive reaction: erythema, infiltration, possibly papules
++	=	Strong (edematous or vesicular) positive reaction
+++	=	Extreme (spreading, bullous, ulcerative) positive reaction
−	=	Negative reaction
IR	=	Irritant reactions of different types
NT	=	Not tested
Doubtful reaction (macular erythema only)		

Adapted from Habif T: *Clinical dermatology: a color guide to diagnosis and therapy,* ed 3, St Louis, 1996, Mosby.

Allergic contact dermatitis can be prevented by simply avoiding contact with allergens. However, recognizing or identifying the potential allergen is the key to prevention and may not be an easy task. When a patient reports having "sensitive skin," patch testing of adhesives is valuable to prevent a potential skin reaction, which would complicate recovery.

When an allergic response is suspected, the offending product or chemical should be discontinued. Often a substitute can be used. Use of antiinflammatory agents may be warranted topically or systemically and is usually determined based on the severity of the allergic reaction.

INFLAMMATORY

Inflammatory ulcers include the various manifestations of pyoderma granulosum and vasculitides and must be carefully assessed to avoid being misinterpreted as a venous or arterial ulcer.

Pyoderma Granulosum

Pyoderma granulosum (PG) is a chronic neutrophilic inflammatory disease that can cause painful ulcerative lesions. Although associated with immune reaction and underlying systemic disorders (Box 6-7), 40% to 50% of cases are idiopathic (Goldstein and Goldstein, 1997; Margolis, 1993). When PG accompanies a systemic disease, it does not necessarily parallel the underlying disease. The pathophysiologic mechanism of PG is unknown. Histologically, the presence of numerous polymorphonuclear leukocytes creates a dense

BOX 6-7 Systemic Diseases Associated with Pyoderma Granulosum

Ankylosing spondylitis
Rheumatoid arthritis
Sarcoidosis
Chronic active hepatitis
Inflammatory bowel disease
Monoclonal gammopathies
Myeloma

infiltrate of the dermis that can extend from the superficial dermis to the subcutaneous tissue (Kerdel, 1993).

PG has several different manifestations (Powell, Su, and Perry, 1996). The most common presentation is the classical (ulcerative) form. This particular manifestation is commonly associated with inflammatory bowel disease or arthritis. These extremely painful PG lesions begin with pustules or bullae that develop significant induration and erythema and progress to ulcers. Another variant of PG is a bullous form. Lesions begin as gray vesicles and bullae that ulcerate into superficial ulcers. This manifestation of PG is associated with myeloproliferative disease.

Common characteristics of all PG lesions is that the wound margins are ragged, elevated, and violaceous (Plate 16). Ulcers are exudative and extremely tender, and wound edges are undermined. A band of erythema may extend from the wound edge, which defines the direction in which the ulcer will extend (Hoffman, 1999). Healing may be present along one edge of the ulcer while enlargment occurs along another edge. Ulcers heal slowly and leave an atrophic, irregular scar. The most common sites are the lower extremities (particularly the lower legs), although PG may also occur on the buttocks, abdomen, face, and hands. A diagnostic characteristic of PG is a phenomenon known as *pathergy*, the abnormal and exaggerated inflammatory response to noxious stimuli. Patients often report the lesion developing after minor trauma, such as a bump against a piece of furniture.

PG is difficult to diagnose and is basically a disease of exclusion. It can be misdiagnosed as venous, arterial, neuropathic, vasculitic, or neoplastic wounds (Lorentzen and Gottrup, 1998). Diagnosis is based on clinical manifestations and a thorough examination in which other ulcerative skin disorders (e.g., vasculitis and infections) and psychosomatic illnesses have been excluded. A history and physical examination, skin biopsy for histology and microbiology, and an investigation for an associated illness constitute a thorough workup. The histopathologic findings are not specific for PG; however, they are supportive of the disease. Furthermore, the ulcer biopsy needs to be obtained from the erythematous margin of the wound to best demonstrate these histopathologic findings (Hoffman, 1999). This biopsy may result in enlargement of the ulcer as a result of the pathergy response; however, biopsy is important to rule out vasculitic, vasoocclusive, and infectious causes (Hoffman, 1999). Laboratory tests for antineutrophilic cytoplasmic antibodies (ANCA), antiphospholipid antibodies (anticardiolipin antibodies, lupus anticoagulant, RPR) are important to obtain, again for the purpose of excluding other diseases that could account for these lesions. The diagnosis of pyoderma granulosum is reached only after this workup is complete.

Several treatments have been used to manage PG with no one treatment emerging as clearly effective. However, PG is not an infectious disease process, nor is it a disease to be managed by debridement (Hoffman, 1999). Systemic corticosteroids are generally required and reliably lead to improvement. Unfortunately, their use is limited by their significant side effects. With minimal disease, intralesional injections of corticosteroids may be effective with intermittent doses of oral steroids. Patients with severe disease may require immunosuppressants (e.g., Imuran, cyclosporine, tacrolimus, and chlorambucil), antimicrobials (dapsone, clofazimine, minocycline, sulfasalzine), and cytotoxic agents (azathioprine) (Cooley et al, 1996; Goldstein and Goldstein, 1997; Hoffman, 1999; Margolis, 1993).

Topical wound management should address wound needs, which include exudate management, protection from trauma, and a moist wound environment. Because of the extreme pain that typifies PG, nonadhesive dressings are preferred. Debridement is achieved only through autolysis and regression of the disease process itself. Local care should be delivered with great caution because of the tendency for pathergy.

Vasculitis

Vasculitis comprises a group of disorders that have in common the pathologic feature of vascular inflammation and necrosis (Kerstein, 1996). Vessels of any type can be affected, so any organ or system may be involved, resulting in a wide array of symptoms and clinical presentations (Jennette and Falk, 1997). Vasculitic ulcers that result in skin lesions are usually the sign of a complex process and may indicate a systemic disorder (Roenigk and Young, 1996). The size of the vessels involved (large, medium, or small) usually categorizes vasculitis; however, there is significant overlap among the different categories. Immunologic features are believed to be a part of the pathogenesis of most vasculitic syndromes. Although the pathology involved in vasculitis is not yet clearly known, when immune complexes are deposited on the vessel walls, the ensuing leukocyte infiltration and release of enzymes can cause necrosis of the vessel wall (Erlich, 1993; Jennette and Falk, 1997; Kerstein, 1996).

Vasculitides is a broad term that refers to systemic disorders that result in vasculitis. The vasculitides that cause skin ulcers involve small- and medium-sized vessels (Roenigk and Young, 1996). Specific diseases include rheumatoid arthritis, systemic lupus erythematosus, polyarteritis nodosa, hypersensitivity vasculitis, Wegener's granulomatosis, Sjögren's syndrome, cryoglobulinemic vasculitis, and dermatomyositis (Roenigk and Young, 1996; Rubano and Kerstein, 1998).

The general signs and symptoms of vasculitis are fever, myalgias, arthralgias, and malaise. Patients sometimes describe a vague, flulike illness. Peripheral neuropathy may also be present. Other symptoms depend on the organ involved, which is determined by the specific disease. For example, cryoglobulinemic vasculitis is likely to involve renal and skin problems, Wegener's granulomatosis may lead to respiratory involvement, and Sjögren's syndrome produces severe oral and ocular dryness (Erlich, 1993; Jennette and Falk, 1997).

The cutaneous features of vasculitis can vary depending on the disease, but there are certain common characteristics. The lesions can range from erythematous macules and/or nodules to hemorrhagic vesicles and palpable purpura to necrotic lesions and ulceration (Erlich, 1993; Roenigk and Young, 1996). Skin biopsy is critical and is best taken from the early purpuric lesions. Two or three sites might be needed to obtain the correct diagnosis (Roenigk and Young, 1996). Skin ulcers associated with vasculitis are frequently located on the lower extremities, particularly near the malleoli, making it difficult to distinguish these lesions from venous ulcers (Plate 17).

Treatment of vasculitic ulcers is aimed at control of the underlying disease process. Steroids and immunosuppressive agents are often prescribed. In severe cases, plasmapheresis might be necessary to remove the circulating immune complexes. Topical therapy includes debridement of necrotic tissue, prompt identification and treatment of infection, maintenance of a moist wound base, absorption of excess exudate, packing of any dead space, insulation, and protection from further trauma. The application of topical vitamin A may be of benefit to counteract the antiinflammatory effects of steroid therapy.

There are many similarities among the various vasculitic syndromes; however, there are some specific differences unique to some of the diseases. The unique features of rheumatoid arthritis, systemic lupus erythematosus, and polyarteritis nodosa are presented in Table 6-3.

Drug reaction

In approximately 10% of patients with vasculitis, the cause is a drug reaction rather than a disease process. Drug-induced vasculitis is usually confined to the skin and will appear about 1 week after administration of the drug. The drugs bind to serum proteins, causing an immune-complex vasculitis (Jennette and Falk, 1997). The typical presentation is purpura and ulceration involving the lower extremities. Once systemic disease has been ruled out, treatment involves removal of the precipitating drug and symptomatic treatment. Antihistamines and nonsteroidal antiinflammatory drugs (NSAIDs) are most often prescribed. Steroids may be added for more severe symptoms. Wound care is based on wound needs, and ulcers resolve spontaneously once the drug is removed.

DISEASE

Skin wounds may also develop as a manifestation of a disease process or as a complication associated with the treatment of a disease. In this section, four rare diseases that can trigger massive skin loss or skin necrosis and two blood dyscrasias are discussed.

TABLE 6-3 Characteristics of Skin Lesions with Vasculitic Disorders

VASCULITIC DISORDER	DESCRIPTION	ULCER CHARACTERISTICS
Rheumatoid arthritis	• Not well understood • Associated with high levels of rheumatoid factor (RF) (Ikeda et al, 1998; Yamamoto, Ohkubo, and Nishioka, 1995) • Evidence of venous insufficiency (McRorie, Ruckley, and Nuki, 1998) • Limited ankle movement contributes to poor calf-muscle pump function and may place patient at risk for venous ulcer development	• Begin as palpable purpura and ecchymosis • May progress to ulceration • Shallow, well demarcated, painful, and slow to heal (Erlich, 1993) • May require addition of compression therapy (McRorie, Ruckley, and Nuki, 1998)
Systemic lupus erythematosus (SLE)	• Chronic immune disorder • Characterized by exacerbation and remission • Affects multiple organs (skin, serosal surfaces, CNS, kidneys) and red blood cells. • Circulating immune complexes and autoantibodies cause tissue damage and organ dysfunction • No single cause; influenced by environment, host immune responses and hormones • Common symptoms include fatigue, weight loss, fever, malaise • Butterfly rash (facial edema over cheeks and nose) is typical • Potential manifestations include seizures, hemiparesis, pericarditis, pleuritis, renal failure, nausea, vomiting, abdominal pain, and arthralgias	• Present as palpable purpura • Progress to ulceration • Occur on the malleolar area • Present as round lesions with erythematous borders • Wound may also have atrophy and loss of pigmentation (Rubano and Kerstein, 1998)
Polyarteritis nodosa (PAN)	• Medium and small vessel vasculitis • Necrotizing arteritis affecting small and medium-sized arteries of most organs • Involved organs commonly include kidney, liver, intestine, peripheral nerves, skin, and muscle • Characterized by fresh and healing lesions • Clinical manifestations include anorexia, weight loss, fever, and fatigue • Organ-specific manifestations include abdominal pain, myalgia, arthralgia, or paresthesia • Subcutaneous painful nodules of lower extremities may develop	• Skin involvement occurs in approximately 40% of patients • Lesions have a "punched out" appearance • Painful • Lesions may begin as purpura with urticaria before progressing to ulceration • May be a "starburst" pattern extending from the ulcer • Painful subcutaneous nodules present (Roenigk and Young, 1996; Rubano and Kerstein, 1998)

Epidermolysis Bullosa

Epidermolysis bullosa (EB) is the name given to several genetically determined diseases that have a tendency to develop blisters and erosions in the skin, and sometimes in mucous membranes, after mild trauma (Eady, 1992). EB mainly affects keratinizing stratified squamous epithelium of the skin; however, virtually any mucosal surface can be involved. It is known to affect every epithelial structure in the body, including the eyelids, conjunctivae, corneas, bowels, skin, and gums. A lack of significant autoimmunity characterizes the disease.

EB is divided into three broad categories: simple (SEB), junctional (JEB), and dystrophic (DEB). At least 23 distinctive phenotypes of EB have been identified. Differences between the three categories are based on ultrastructural levels of the skin within which blisters develop after minor mechanical trauma (Fine, 1992). The electron microscope is most reliable in establishing the diagnosis. Distinctive characteristics of EB are provided in Box 6-8. DEB (both recessive and dominant) is the most life-threatening variant.

Extracutaneous manifestations are common and may be gastointestinal, opthalmologic, or hematologic. The severity of these manifestations varies with the category of EB as well as the subtype within that category. Gastrointestinal complications are a major source of symptoms and morbidity for all EB patients. The most severe problems are related to the oropharynx, esophagus, and proximal gut. The simple process of using eating utensils and the passage of foods results in bullae formation that rupture, erode, and heal with scar formation. Strictures are inevitable, and nutritional problems develop.

Anemia is another major problem with EB and is multifactorial in origin. Poor nutrition resulting from painful oral blisters and esophageal strictures precipitates a deficiency in iron, trace metals, and protein, which contributes to anemia. Protein and blood are also lost through the chronic skin lesions typical of JEB and DEB.

The patient with EB is deprived of an epidermal barrier to bacterial invasion. *S. aureus* and other pathogens often colonize the chronic nonhealing wound. Sepsis is a serious complication, especially in the infant. Judicious use of topical antibiotics is warranted to decrease bacterial flora and minimize the risk of soft tissue infection. Silver sulfadiazine cream is contraindicated in newborns under 8 weeks of age because of the increased risk of kernicterus

BOX 6-8 Characteristics of Epidermolysis Bullosa (EB) by Category

EB Simplex (EBS)

- Intraepidermal blisters
- Heals without scar formation
- Nails and teeth normal
- Occasional cutaneous blistering
- Autosomal dominant trait

Junctional EB (JEB)

- Autosomal recessive trait
- Blisters form at lamina lucida (between basal cell plasma membrane and lamina densa)
- Several subtypes with distinct clinical manifestations

Recessive Dystrophic EB (RDEB)

- Also known as dermolytic EB
- Dystrophic scarring is distinctive feature that serves as clinical marker
- Separation at basement membrane zone deep to the lamina densa (dermal side of the lamina densa)
- Recessive inheritance
- Blister formation results from even minimal mechanical trauma
- Blisters may be hemorrhagic
- Blisters eventually rupture to form slow-to-heal superficial ulcers that continue to be exposed to minimal mechanical trauma
- Healing always involves scarring so skin has atrophic and wrinkled appearance
- Elbows, knees, hands, and feet are sites of repeated trauma
- Predisposes patient to squamous cell cancer

Dominant Dystrophic EB (DDEB)

- Formation of blisters below lamina densa
- Autosomal dominant inheritance
- Trauma-induced blisters form at birth or shortly thereafter
- Blisters heal without scar formation
- Predispose patient to squamous cell cancer

(Caldwell-Brown et al, 1992). Topical antibiotics should not be used as a lubricating ointment because they are for open lesions only. In the presence of cellulitis, systemic antibiotics are necessary (Lin and Carter, 1992). Close monitoring of lesions and bacteriologic studies are imperative.

Phenytoin may be administered to decrease blistering. A long-observed side affect of phenytoin is that it inhibits collagenase activity and consequently stimulates fibroplasia. Collagenase activity is unusually increased in EB, specifically patients with recessive DEB (RDEB), so phenytoin appears to be beneficial. Systemic corticosteroids are used in all three types of EB with mixed results on cutaneous blistering. Skin grafts are proving to be a promising treatment option. The role of vitamin E and zinc in the treatment of EB is inconclusive.

The primary objective in the care of EB patients is to minimize and protect the patient from mechanical trauma (Caldwell-Brown et al, 1992). Special precautions to minimize cutaneous trauma during select clinical procedures can be found in Table 6-4. Interventions such as convoluted foam to pad rails, sheepskin, an air-fluidized support surface, and joint protectors are important to use routinely. Low-adherence foam dressings or thin hydrocolloids may also be appropriate to protect the hands or feet. However, if these are used, the dressing should be left in place and allowed to fall off rather than removed and reapplied on a regular basis.

No single approach to wound care has been demonstrated to be effective for managing EB lesions (Caldwell-Brown et al, 1992). Nonadherent dressings are most appropriate and should be secured with roll gauze, tubular gauze, or a stockinette. Creative dressing techniques are often necessary for difficult locations such as the digits or face. Temporary skin substitutes hold a great deal of promise for this dangerous disease. For further information about this disease, the Dystrophic Epidermolysis Bullosa Association of America (DEBRA) can be contacted at 141 Fifth Ave, New York, New York, 10010 (212-995-2220).

Calciphylaxis

Calciphylaxis, a rare and lethal complication associated with end-stage renal disease, is characterized by indurated, painful necrotic lesions with a violaceous discoloration. An estimated 1% of dialysis patients develop this disease annually (Levin, Mehta, and, Goldstein, 1993). Initially, patients develop painful, mottled skin lesions that progress to subcutaneous nodules and ulcerations that eventually become gangrenous. Subsequent infection and gangrene contribute to the high mortality rate associated with this disease (60%) (Budisavljevic, Cheek, and Ploth, 1996; Burkhart, Burkhart, and Mian, 1999). A distinctive finding with calciphylaxis is that peripheral pulses are intact because blood flow distal to the necrosis or deeper than the necrosis remains intact. This clinical assessment is critical in distinguishing the disease from other forms of peripheral vascular disease.

Histologically, microvascular calcification of the intima layer of the arteriole (and occasionally the media layer) is found. These calcifications precipitate a narrowing of the lumen, and arterial thrombosis is also occasionally observed. However, complete occlusion of the arteriole seldom develops. The primary cause for the accompanying ischemia is hyperplasia, another histologic change that occurs within the intima lining of the arteriole. The combination of microvascular calcification of the media layer and hyperplasia within the intima of arterioles with a diameter of approximately 0.04 to 0.1 mm is considered a histologic marker for calciphylaxis. These findings assist in differentiating this disease from peripheral arterial occlusion. Arteriole hyperplasia and microvascular calcification have also been reported in patients with normal renal function who have diabetes, multiple myeloma, breast cancer with hypercalcemia, or primary parathyroidism (Hafner et al, 1995; Khafif et al, 1990).

The etiology of calciphylaxis is as yet unknown. Hypercalcemia, hyperphosphatemia, and hyperparathyroidism are associated with the syndrome, although it also occurs in the absence of these abnormalities (Budisavljevic, Cheek, and Ploth, 1996; Ruggian, Maesaka, and Fishbane, 1996). Protein C functional deficiencies that precipitate thrombosis in small blood vessels has been studied as a risk factor for calciphylaxis, although this deficiency is not consistently found with calciphylaxis (Hafner et al, 1995).

TABLE 6-4 Special Precautions to Minimize Cutaneous Trauma During Select Clinical Procedures

PROCEDURE	SUGGESTIONS
Blood pressure (BP) monitoring	Apply dressing under BP cuff.
Electrocardiogram monitoring	Use a nonadhesive plastic film such as Omiderm (which does not interfere with electrical conduction) as a barrier between the patient's skin and the adhesive of the electrode pads.
Urine collections (young children)	Wring out cloth diaper; do not apply urine bags containing adhesives.
Blood drawing	To cleanse skin, allow alcohol or Betadine swab to remain in place for 5 min without rubbing; place tourniquet over padding to protect skin; or apply direct pressure on vein using thumb in a parallel position to skin.
Parenteral therapy	Cut a piece of hydrocolloid dressing (Extra Thin Duoderm or Resolve) into a horseshoe shape and put dressing with adhesive backing side in contact with skin. Start the IV between the legs of the horseshoe bandage and tape the tubing onto the dressing. Secure IV with roller gauze, or place a snug-fitting piece of tube gauze such as Bandnet on extremity adjacent to IV and secure with tape to tube gauze.
Preoperative preparations: operating room, table, surgical drapes, and surgical scrub	Operating room table should be well padded. Sheepskin covered by a table-sized burn pad such as Exudry, which has a double layer of meshed material to minimize friction, is advised. If positioning with pillows is necessary for patients with joint contractures, place Exudry pad between pillow and patient's skin. Sterile sheets of nonadherent mesh (Exudry Mesh or N-terface) are placed under sterile drapes to protect exposed skin from friction. Fold mesh over edge of drape and secure with clamps as usual. Adhesive drapes are contraindicated. Apply antimicrobial solution to surgical site. Allow to remain on skin for 5 min, then irrigate to rinse. Repeat this process three times.
Mask-delivered anesthesia	Protect skin on face from possible shearing with a nonadhesive polyurethane film, such as Omiderm, which adheres to any damp surface and is easily removed by rewetting; or apply copious amount of petrolatum to face before applying mask.

Reprinted with permission from Caldwell-Brown D et al: Nursing aspects of EB: a comprehensive approach. In Lin AN, Carter DM, editors: *Epidermolysis bullosa: basic and clinical aspects,* New York, 1992, Springer-Verlag.

Treatment of calciphylaxis is neither universally standardized nor necessarily effective. Prompt recognition and treatment yield the best results. Systemically, normalization of abnormal calcium and phosphorus levels is warranted. Severe hyperparathyroidism may be managed pharmacologically or surgically. Antibiotics should be implemented to treat wound infection and to prevent sepsis. Most individuals who develop calciphylaxis require limb amputation and reconstructive surgery (Burkhart, Burkhart, and Mian, 1999).

Topical wound management should address specific wound needs: fill dead space, provide physiologic environment, and absorb exudate. Aggressive debridement is indicated to reduce the potential for wound infection. Severity of wound-related pain should be assessed regularly, and control measures for the pain should be implemented routinely and during wound procedures.

Toxic Epidermal Necrolysis

Toxic epidermal necrolysis (TEN) is a rare condition in which there is widespread loss of sheets of epidermis involving more than 10% of the body surface. TEN is seen in adults or children usually as a drug reaction. Three main drug categories have been associated with TEN: antibiotics (sulfonamides, allopurinol, and ampicillin), anticonvulsants (phenytoin, carbamazepine, and phenobarbitol) and analgesics (acetaminophen) (Burgdorf, 1994; Habif, 1996). The mortality rate is high with TEN (20% to 30%), and death is usually the result of sepsis (Goldstein and Goldstein, 1997).

Clinically, a generalized maculopapular rash develops suddenly followed by widespread erythema. Within hours the skin becomes painful. With slight thumb pressure, the skin wrinkles, slides laterally, and separates from the dermis, a sign known as *Nikolsky's sign* (Habif, 1996). Large sheets of skin are sloughed. The entire epidermis is usually involved as well as mucous membranes (oral ulcers), the eyes (purulent conjunctivitis), and the respiratory tract (bronchopneumonia).

Diagnosis of TEN is by skin biopsy, and full-thickness epidermal damage is revealed. The differential diagnosis for TEN must include SSSS, which is distinguished by skin biopsy, and graft-versus-host disease (GVHD) of the skin, which is distinguished by history.

The patient with TEN should be managed as a burn patient because temperature regulation problems, electrolyte disturbances, and propensity for wound or skin infections (Burgdorf, 1994; Habif, 1996). See Box 6-9 for a recommended treatment protocol. Temporary skin coverage is warranted, and systemic corticosteroids are not recommended.

BOX 6-9 Treatment Protocol for Toxic Epidermal Necrolysis

1. Patient is taken to the operating room on an urgent basis.
2. All loose skin and blisters are wiped vigorously with a rough washcloth moistened with normal saline solution. No detergents are used.
3. Porcine xenografts are applied to all raw surfaces and stapled in place.
4. The patient is transferred to a warmed air-fluidized bed in the burn unit.
5. Initial fluid resuscitation is not required, but careful fluid and electrolyte monitoring is important.
6. The administration of oral steroids is stopped unless medically necessary; they are tapered if possible.
7. Internal alimentation is established through a nasogastric feeding tube.
8. Systemic antibiotics are used only for specific infections.
9. Intense pulmonary toilet is established.
10. Physical therapy is begun on the day after operation.
11. Dislodged xenografts are replaced.
12. Pain is managed with a pain cocktail of methadone, hydroxyzine, and acetaminophen in cherry syrup. Intravenous narcotics are given as necessary. With the dermis covered, the wound becomes essentially pain free.
13. Meticulous eye care is provided hourly. Each day the ophthalmologist removes conjunctival synechiae with a glass rod.
14. Central venous and bladder catheters are avoided.
15. The xenograft becomes brittle and desiccates as the wounds heal beneath it. These areas are trimmed each day.

Reprinted with permission from Habif TP: *Clinical dermatology: a color guide to diagnosis and therapy,* ed 3, St Louis, 1996, Mosby.

Graft-Versus-Host Disease

After allogeneic bone marrow transplantation (bone marrow from another individual), the transferred immune competent cells have the potential to produce a severe reaction in the transplant patient. Clinically, acute GVHD can develop within 30 days after bone marrow transplantation. Risk factors that predispose the bone marrow transplantation patient to GVHD include recipient age (over 40 years), recipient history of blood transfusions, the conditioning regimen, the prophylaxis protocol, and the number of T cells infused (Alcoser and Burchett, 1999; Sullivan, 1999).

GVHD affects the skin, gut and liver. In the skin, cutaneous manifestations include a maculopapular rash that usually begins in the axillae, then spreads to the palms, soles, chest, shoulders and ears (Plate 18). These may be pruritic or painful. In severe cases, generalized erythema, bullae and desquama-

TABLE 6-5 Characteristics of Skin Lesions with Blood Dyscrasias

BLOOD DYSCRASIA	PATHOLOGY	ULCER CHARACTERISTICS	TREATMENT
Sickle cell anemia	• Sickled blood cells are rigid • May clump together occluding the microcirculation • Damage to endothelium leads to thrombus formation (Eckman, 1996) • Altered vasomotor response, which can lead to a rise in capillary pressure and edema formation (Mohan et al, 1997)	• Exact etiology of the ulceration remains unclear • Lower leg near the malleolus • May be single or multiple • Can range significantly in size • Ulcers are well defined, vary in depth, and have raised borders (Eckman, 1996; Kerstein, 1996; Roenigk and Young, 1996) • Tend to be slow to heal • High rate of recurrence (Eckman, 1996)	• Control of edema (compression therapy and/or bed rest) • Systemic management of the underlying disease process (address anemia either pharmacologically or by transfusion) • Debridement • Prevention of infection • Protection from trauma • Pain management • Moist wound healing (such as with hydrocolloids [Cackovic, 1998; Chung , Cackovic, and Kerstein, 1996; Eckman, 1996])
Thalassemia	A microcytic anemia common in people of Mediterranean descent	Etiology related to a decreased hemoglobin and increased iron loading, making patients more susceptible to trauma	• Blood transfusions and iron-chelation therapy (Kerstein, 1996) • Topical care based on wound needs and moist wound-healing principles • Emphasis on insulating wound to prevent hypothermia • Protect wound from further trauma

tion may be present. GVHD may have the appearance of SSSS as well as a drug reaction. A skin biopsy is beneficial to differentiate among these three possibilities (Sullivan, 1999).

Treatment of GVHD requires a combination of immunosuppressants and antiviral medications. To stimulate adequate neutrophil levels with these treatment regimens, growth-colony–stimulating factor is also given. Topical wound care requires attention to infection control, maintaining a physiologic wound environment, and pain management. Adhesive occlusive dressings are seldom desirable. Topical wound management should be determined collaboratively with input and discussion from the marrow transplantation team involved. For more detailed information concerning this disease, additional resources can be accessed (Chao and Schlegel, 1995; Thomas, 1999; Whedon, 1991)

Blood Dyscrasias

Two types of blood dyscrasias may lead to chronic leg ulceration. Sickle cell anemia and thalassemia; etiology, ulcer characteristics, and treatment are summarized in Table 6-5.

SUMMARY

The intact skin provides the first line of defense against microbial invasion and trauma. Different factors can jeopardize the skin's integrity. It is important to be able to recognize the skin-related signs of these factors so that the factor can be eliminated or the intensity of the factor can be reduced substantially. Most of the time, the type of skin damage that the wound-care nurse encounters is mechanical or vascular. Only with an in-depth skin assessment and history of the skin eruption can the etiology of the skin damage be identified and the negative sequelae arrested through appropriate prevention and treatment interventions.

Because the more rare inflammatory, infectious, or disease-related skin lesions often require prompt treatment to be effective, they should also be familiar to the wound-care nurse. Although the underlying disease is the critical determinant for wound healing in these situations, the wound-care nurse is an important partner and interdisciplinary team member because they can provide valuable recommendations for wound management that will best address the needs of the wound and the patient.

SELF-ASSESSMENT EXERCISE

1. List seven categories of factors known to damage the skin.
2. A lesion that is raised, solid, and less than 0.5 cm in diameter is a:
   - **a.** Macule
   - **b.** Papule
   - **c.** Pustule
   - **d.** Nodule
3. A blister that measures 1.5 cm in diameter may also be called a:
   - **a.** Bulla
   - **b.** Pustule
   - **c.** Vesicle
   - **d.** Wheal
4. Distinguish between erosion and ulcer according to depth of tissue damage.
5. List at least four interventions to prevent skin stripping.
6. List three treatment options to prevent chemical skin irritation in a patient with diarrhea.
7. Which of the following accurately characterizes chemical skin irritation?
   - **a.** Erythema with satellite lesions
   - **b.** Erythema and erosion of skin
   - **c.** Ulcerations with necrotic tissue in wound bed
   - **d.** Ulcerations with pustules
8. VZV is characterized as a disease that:
   - **a.** Requires prior exposure to genital herpes
   - **b.** Is reactivated by mechanical trauma
   - **c.** Consists of a bilateral vesicular rash
   - **d.** Develops along one or two dermatomes
9. State the two phases of an allergic contact dermatitis.
10. Candidiasis can be described as a:
    - **a.** Macular rash with ulcerations
    - **b.** Papular rash within the hair follicle
    - **c.** Pustular erythematous rash
    - **d.** Vesicular rash with plaque formation
11. Which of the following statements is true of herpes simplex virus?
    - **a.** Initially develops as papules
    - **b.** Secondary lesions consist of necrotic plaques
    - **c.** Erythema signifies a secondary infection
    - **d.** Vesicles are uniformly shaped and grouped
12. List three disease processes that can result in massive loss of epidermis.

REFERENCES

Alcoser PW, Burchett S: Bone marrow transplantation, *Am J Nurs* 99(6):26, 1999.

Beers B, Wilson B: Adult staphylococcal scalded skin syndrome, *Int J Dermatol* 29:428, 1990.

Bettley FR: Some effects of soap on the skin, *Br Med J* 1:1675, 1960.

Bryant RA: Saving the skin from tape injuries, *Am J Nurs* 88(2):189, 1988.

Budisavljevic MN, Cheek D, Ploth DW: Calciphylaxis in chronic renal failure, *J Am Soc Nephrol* 7:978, 1996.

Burgdorf WHS: *Atlas of dermatology*, ed 3, Philadelphia, 1994, Lea & Febiger.

Burkhart CG, Burkhart CN, Mian A: Claciphylaxis: a case report and review of literature, *Wounds* 11(2):58, 1999.

Cackovic M et al: Leg ulceration in the sickle cell patient, *J Am Coll Surg* 187(3):30, 1998.

Caldwell-Brown D et al: Nursing aspects of EB: a comprehensive approach. In Lin AN, Carter DM, editors: *Epidermolysis bullosa: basic and clinical aspects*, New York, 1992, Springer-Verlag.

Chandrasekar PH: Identification and treatment of herpes lesions, *Adv Wound Care* 12(5):254, 1999.

Chao NJ, Schlegel PG: Prevention and treatment of graft-versus-host disease, *Ann NY Acad Sci* 770:130, 1995.

Chung C, Cackovic M, Kerstein M: Leg ulcers in patients with sickle cell disease, *Adv Wound Care* 9(5):46, 1996.

Cohen JI et al: Recent advances in varicella-zoster virus infection, *Ann Intern Med* 130:922, 1999.

Cooley HM et al: Resolution of pyoderma gangrenosum using tacrolimun (FK-506), *Aust NZ J Med* 26:238, 1996.

Eady RAJ: Current perspectives and differential diagnosis in epidermolysis bullosa. In Lin AN, Carter DM, editors: *Epidermolysis bullosa: basic and clinical aspects*, New York, 1992, Springer Verlag.

Eckman J: Leg ulcers in sickle cell disease, *Hematol Oncol Clin North Am* 10(6):1333, 1996.

Erlich M: Vasculitic ulcers: a complication of collagen-vascular disorders, *Ostomy Wound Manage* 39(1):12, 1993.

Fine JD: Pathology and pathogenesis of epidermolysis bullosa. In Lin AN, Carter DM, editors: *Epidermolysis bullosa: basic and clinical aspects*, New York, 1992, Springer Verlag..

Fontaine R, Risley S, Castellino R: A quantitative analysis of pressure and shear in the effectiveness of support surfaces, *J Wound Ostomy Continence Nurs* 25:233, 1998.

Frosch PJ, Kligman AM: The soap chamber test: the irritancy method for assessing the irritancy of soaps, *J Am Acad Derm* 1:35, 1974.

Goldstein BG, Goldstein AD: *Practical dermatology*, ed 2, St Louis, 1997, Mosby.

Habif TP: *Clinical dermatology: a color guide to diagnosis and therapy*, ed 3, St Louis, 1996, Mosby.

Hafner J et al: Uremic small-artery disease with medial calcification and intimal hyperplasia (so-called calciphylaxis): a complication of chronic renal failure and benefit from parathyroidectomy, *J Am Acad Dermatol* 33:954, 1995.

Hoffman MD: Pyoderma gangrenosum, *Wounds* 11(suppl B):2B, 1999.

Hooper BJ, Goldman MP: *Primary dermatologic care*, St Louis, 1999, Mosby.

Ikeda E et al: Rheumatoid vasculitis in a patient with seronegative rheumatoid arthritis, *Eur J Dermatol* 8(4):268, 1998.

Jennette J, Falk R: Small-vessel vasculitis, *N Engl JMed* 337(21):1512, 1997.

Kerdel FA: Inflammatory ulcers, *J Dermatol Surg Oncol* 19:772, 1993.

Kerstein M: The non-healing leg ulcer: peripheral vascular disease, chronic venous insufficiency, and ischemic vasculitis, *Ostomy Wound Manage* 42(suppl 10A):19S, 1996.

Khafif RA et al: Calciphylaxis and systemic calcinosis: collective review, *Arch Intern Med* 150:956, 1990.

Levin A, Mehta RL, Goldstein MB: Mathematical formulation to help identify the patient at risk of ischemic tissue necrosis: a potentially lethal complication of chronic renal failure, *Am J Nephrol* 13(6):448, 1993.

Leyden JJ, Gately LE III: Staphylococcal and streptococcal infections. In Sanders CV, Nesbitt LT: *The skin and infection*, Baltimore, 1995, Williams and Wilkins.

Lin AN, Carter DM: Epidermolysis bullosa simplex: a clinical overview. In Lin AN, Carter DM, editors: *Epidermolysis bullosa: basic and clinical aspects*, New York, 1992, Springer Verlag.

Loeper JM et al: *Therapeutic positioning and skin care*, Minneapolis, 1986, Sister Kenny Institute.

Lorentzen H, Gottrup F: Misclassification errors of ulcerative pyoderma gangrenosum, *Wound RepReg* 6:A475, 1998.

Malone ML et al: The epidemiology of skin tears in the institutionalized elderly, *J Am Geriatr Soc* 39(6):591, 1991.

Margolis DJ: Dermatology of the lower extremity, *Ostomy Wound Manage* 39(5):36, 1993.

Mason SR: Type of soap and the incidence of skin tears among residents of a long-term care facility, *Ostomy Wound Manage* 43(8):26, 1997.

McGough-Csarny J, Kopac CA: Skin tears in institutionalized elderly: an epidemiological study, *Ostomy Wound Manage* 44(suppl 3A):14S, 1998.

McRorie E, Ruckley C, Nuki G: The relevance of large-vessel vascular disease and restricted ankle movement to the aetiology of leg ulceration in rheumatoid arthritis, *Br J Rheumatol* 37(12):1295, 1998.

Mohan J et al: Postural vasoconstriction and leg ulceration in homozygous sickle cell disease, *Clin Science* 92:153, 1997.

Payne RL, Martin ML: Defining and classifying skin tears: need for a common language, *Ostomy Wound Manage* 39(5):16, 1993

Payne RL, Martin ML: The epidemiology and management of skin tears in older adults, *Ostomy Wound Manage* 26:26, 1990

Powell FC, Su WPD, Perry HO: Pyoderma gangrenosum: classification and management, *J Am Acad Dermatol* 34:395, 1996.

Rietschel RL, Fowler JF Jr: *Fisher's contact dermatitis*, ed 4, Baltimore, 1995, Williams & Wilkins.

Roenigk H, Young J: Leg ulcers. In Young J, Olin J, Bartholomew J, editors: *Peripheral vascular diseases*, ed 2, St Louis, 1996, Mosby.

Rubano J, Kerstein M: Arterial insufficiency and vasculitides, *J Wound Ostomy Continence Nurs* 25(3):147, 1998.

Ruggian JC, Maesaka JK, Fishbane S: Proximal calciphylaxis in four insulin-requiring diabetic hemodialysis patients, *Am J Kidney Dis* 28:409, 1996.

Smith DB, Ickstadt J, Kucera J: Brown recluse spider bite, *J Wound Ostomy Continence Nurs* 24(3):137, 1997.

Sullivan KM: Graft-versus-host disease. In Thomas ED, Blume KG, Forman SJ, editors: *Hematopoietic cell transplantation*, ed 2, Malden, Mass, 1999, Blackwell Science.

Thibodeau GA, Patton KT: *Anatomy and physiology*, ed 4, St Louis 1999, Mosby.

Thomas ED, Blume KG, Forman SJ, editors: *Hematopoietic cell transplantation*, ed 2, Malden, Mass, 1999, Blackwell Science.

Thompson JM et al: *Mosby's clinical nursing*, ed 4, St Louis, 1997, Mosby.

Whedon MB editor: *Bone marrow transplantation: principles, practice and nursing insights*, Boston, 1991, Jones & Bartlett.

White MI, Jenkinson DM, Lloyd DH: The effect of washing on the thickness of the stratum corneum in normal and atopic individuals, *Br J Dermatol* 116:525, 1987.

White MW, Karam S, Cowell B: Skin tears in frail elders: a practical approach to prevention, *Geriatr Nurs* 15(2):95, 1994.

Whitley RJ, Kimberlin DW, Roizman B: Herpes simplex virus, *Clin Infect Dis* 26:541, 1998.

Yamamoto T, Ohkubo H, Nishioka K: Skin manifestations associated with rheumatoid arthritis, *J Dermatol* 22(5):324, 1995.

Young EM, Newcomer VD, Kligman AM, editors: *Geriatric dermatology: color atlas and practitioner's guide*, Philadelphia, 1993, Lea & Febiger.

CHAPTER 7

Wound Debridement

JANET RAMUNDO & JUDY WELLS

OBJECTIVES

1. Describe the importance of debridement in the wound-healing process.
2. Distinguish between selective and nonselective debridement.
3. Compare and contrast how debridement is achieved with autolysis, enzymes, maggots, wet-to-dry dressings, and wound irrigation.
4. Describe the appropriate technique for wet-to-dry dressings, conservative sharp debridement, and high-pressure wound irrigations.
5. List debridement options for an infected wound.
6. Describe at least five factors to consider when selecting a debridement approach.
7. For each method of debridement, list two advantages, disadvantages, and relevant precautions.

Debridement is the removal of nonviable tissue and foreign matter from a wound and is a naturally occurring event in the wound-repair process. During the inflammatory phase, neutrophils and macrophages digest and remove "used" platelets, cellular debris, and avascular injured tissue from the wound area. However, with the accumulation of significant amounts of damaged tissue, this natural process becomes overwhelmed and insufficient. Build-up of necrotic tissue then places considerable phagocytic demand on the wound and retards wound healing. Consequently, debridement of necrotic tissue is an essential objective of topical therapy and a critical component of optimal wound management (AHCPR, 1994; Goode and Thomas, 1997; Robson, 1997; Stotts and Hunt, 1997).

Although it has not been adequately researched, debridement is believed to achieve several objectives:

1. Debridement reduces the bioburden of the wound. Because devitalized tissue supports the growth of bacteria, the presence of necrotic tissue places the patient at risk for wound infection and sepsis. Using external measures to remove the necrotic tissue and foreign matter reduces the volume of pathogenic microbes present in the wound.
2. Debridement controls and potentially prevents wound infections, particularly in the deteriorating wound.
3. Debridement facilitates visualization of the wound wall and base. In the presence of necrotic tissue, accurate and thorough assessment of the viable tissue is hampered (Rolstad and Harris, 1997).
4. At a molecular level, debridement interrupts the cycle of the chronic wound so that protease and cytokine levels more closely approximate those of the acute wound (Schultz, 1999).

Necrotic tissue can appear in various forms. Eschar has the firm, dry, leathery appearance of desiccated and compressed tissue layers (Plate 19). When the tissue is kept moist, the devitalized tissue remains soft and may be brown, yellow, or gray in appearance, which is called *slough* (Plate 20). Slough may be adherent to the wound bed and edges or loosely adherent and stringy (Plate 21). Components of slough include fibrin, bacteria, intact leukocytes, cell debris, serous exudate, and significant quantities of deoxyribonucleic acid (DNA) (Thomas, 1990b). Once the eschar is removed, slough is often visible covering the wound bed. Maintaining a moist wound environment is essential because continued exposure to air dehydrates slough, returning to a hard, leathery state (Bale, 1997a).

Debridement is indicated for any wound, acute or chronic, when necrotic tissue (which may be slough or eschar) or foreign bodies are present. It is also indicated when the wound is infected. Once the wound bed is clean and viable tissue is present, debridement is no longer indicated. Two contraindications to debridement exist. Pressure ulcers located on the heel, in which a dry eschar covers the ulcer should not be debrided (AHCPR, 1994). Also, dry, stable (i.e., noninfected; nonfluctuant) ischemic wounds or those with dry gangrene should not be debrided until perfusion to the extremity has been improved (Bale, 1997b; Bates-Jensen, 1998). Measurement of vascular status, including an ankle-brachial index (ABI), is an important component of the assessment process when considering debridement in a patient with a lower leg ulceration.

METHODS OF DEBRIDEMENT

Several methods of debridement are available for removal of devitalized tissue from necrotic wounds. Debridement methods are classified as either selective (only necrotic tissue is removed) or nonselective (viable tissue is removed along with the nonviable tissue). More specifically, debridement is classified by the actual mechanism of action: autolysis, chemical, mechanical, or sharp (conservative or surgical). Although one method of debridement may the primary approach selected to rid the wound of necrotic tissue, debridement typically occurs by using a combination of debridement methods.

AUTOLYSIS

Description

Autolysis is the lysis of necrotic tissue by the body's white blood cells and enzymes, which enter the wound site during the normal inflammatory process. Proteolytic, fibrinolytic, and collagenolytic enzymes are released to digest the devitalized tissue present in the wound (Rodeheaver et al, 1994). Autolysis is a selective method of debridement that leaves healthy tissue intact.

Autolysis, a naturally occurring physiologic process, occurs in the presence of a moist, vascular environment. The primary requirements for debridement via autolysis include a moist wound environment, adequate leukocyte function, and an adequate neutrophil count. Autolysis is enhanced or supported by applying a moisture-retentive dressing to the necrotic wound and allowing it to remain undisturbed for a reasonable length of time. By maintaining a moist wound environment, the cellular structures that are essential for phagocytosis (neutrophils and macrophages) remain intact and are not prematurely destroyed through desiccation. Since an important role of macrophages is to produce growth factors, the presence of healthy macrophages in the wound fluid supports the continued production of growth factors.

Directions for Use

Dressings support autolysis if they add or maintain moisture at the wound surface. Dressing selection is based on the condition of the wound base, depth of the wound, volume of wound exudate, and the patient's condition. When the wound base is dry, a dressing that will add moisture, such as a hydrogel, should be used. If absorption is needed, a dressing should be selected that will absorb excess exudate without dehydrating the wound surface, such as an alginate dressing for a highly exudative wound or a hydrocolloid for a moderately exudative wound. Transparent adhesive dressings trap enzyme-rich wound exudate at the wound site and are very effective at loosening eschar from the surrounding skin and wound base. However, transparent adhesive dressings become dislodged with moderately to highly exudative wounds and are most effective with nonexudative or low-exudative wounds.

Autolysis can be used alone or in combination with other debridement techniques. Autolysis is automatically employed any time a moisture-retentive dressing is used. However autolysis as a sole method of debridement is only recommended for noninfected wounds with a limited volume of necrotic tissue. The moisture-retentive dressing selected to achieve autolysis is dependent upon the wound needs as described in Chapter 5. Many times it becomes necessary to combine dressings to meet the wound needs and achieve debridement. For example, an alginate dressing and composite dressing may be best for an exudative wound that has tissue depth (Bryant and Rolstad, 1998). Promotion of autolysis is an important adjuvant to all debridement modalities so that cellular desiccation through air exposure and the resulting build-up of necrotic tissue are avoided. For example, after surgical sharp debridement of a pressure ulcer, the application of a hydrogel-impregnated gauze maintains a moist wound environment, thus preventing tissue desiccation and promoting continued softening and loosening of residual necrotic tissue.

Autolysis is generally considered a slower process than other debridement methods (Mosher et al, 1999). The time frame for autolysis to occur varies depending on the size of the wound and the amount and type of necrotic tissue. Generally, progress should be observed within 72 to 96 hours (Alvarez, 1988). Initially, the black eschar will loosen from the edges, become soft, change to brown or gray in color, and eventually transform into stringy yellow slough. It is critical to monitor the wound closely during the autolysis process because as the wound debrides, the full wound bed and walls are exposed and the true extent of the wound is revealed.

Consequently, the wound will increase in length, width and depth necessitating a change in the therapy. Reassessment of the wound needs based on the changing wound dimensions is essential so that the most appropriate and effective dressing is used.

Precautions

It is important to use the most appropriate dressing for the wound when the objective is to debride by autolysis. Autolysis can be achieved with occlusive dressings and with moisture-retentive nonocclusive and semiocclusive dressings such as hydrogels. The type of dressing used for autolysis must be selected based on the wound needs and the patient's status. Considerations for each dressing as discussed in Chapter 5 must also be followed. For example, a transparent dressing is inappropriate for debridement of a wound that has depth and is exudative. Instead, a dressing such as an alginate is warranted because it will fill the wound depth and absorb the exudate. Likewise, a patient who is severely neutropenic (absolute neutrophil count of less than 500 mm^3) is at risk for severe infection or sepsis (Bodey et al, 1966). In these patients, it may be prudent to avoid occlusive dressings for debridement because the number of viable neutrophils available in the wound fluid may be diminished and could be overwhelmed by even the slightest increase in the number of bacteria present at the wound site. Whether debridement is pursued with the use of a nonocclusive moisture-retentive dressing or delayed until the absolute neutrophil count increases is a decision that should be made in consultation with the patient's physician.

Autolysis should not be the primary method of debridement in a wound with advancing cellulitis because of the length of time it takes to debride. The goal is to debride the wound as quickly as possible. In addition, if the infection is due to anaerobic bacteria, any dressing that maintains a layer of fluid between the wound bed and dressing will provide some degree of occlusion, which may promote further growth of the anaerobic bacteria. However, if the infection is addressed, and local symptoms have subsided (e.g., decreased erythema, induration, and odorous exudate), autolysis may be used safely. The type of dressing may be nonocclusive (such as gauze) or semiocclusive (transparent film).

Debridement by autolysis compares favorably with other methods of debridement in terms of effectiveness (Colins, Kurning, and Yuon, 1996; Mulder et al, 1993). However, there are some precautions for the nurse to note. Periwound maceration can develop when wound exudate has continued contact with intact skin. Logically, the potential for maceration is increased in the more exudative wound, such as the infected wound or a venous ulcer. Liquid barrier film or skin barriers should be applied to the surrounding skin as prophylaxis. In addition, dressings should be selected and changed at appropriate intervals so as to manage exudate levels and reduce the likelihood of maceration of the periwound skin.

Fear and lack of familiarity with the process can also present problems. Clinicians, patients, and family members unfamiliar with the process of autolysis can misinterpret the collection of wound exudate and the accompanying odor as indicative of an infection. Consequently, they may want to change the dressing as soon as fluid appears, so reassurance and education is necessary. It is important to emphasize that the wound exudate contains phagocytic cells and growth factors that are essential to wound repair. The fear that occlusive dressings promote an infection must be corrected. In fact, wounds treated with semiocclusive dressings are less likely to become infected than wounds treated with conventional dressings (Hutchinson, 1989). The proposed mechanisms for this effect include the impermeability of dressings to exogenous bacteria, the increased number of viable neutrophils in the wound fluid, the accumulation of natural substances in wound fluid that inhibit bacterial growth, and the reduction of necrotic tissue (Eaglstein, 1993; Hutchinson, 1989; Lawrence, 1994).

CHEMICAL

Wounds can be debrided chemically with the use of enzymes, sodium hypochlorite (Dakin's solution), and maggots. These methods remove the necrotic tissue through a chemical process.

Enzymes

Description. Topical application of exogenous enzymes is a selective method of debridement. Enzymes are derived from various sources (e.g., krill, crab, papaya, bovine extract, and bacteria) and are applied topically to the necrotic tissue. They are capable of inducing changes in the substrate against which they are effective and result in the breakdown of necrotic tissue. Commercially available enzymes include collagenase, papain/urea, and a fibrinolysin and deoxyribonuclease combination. Table 7-1 provides a description of commonly used enzymes for wound debridement.

Enzymes work in one of two ways: 1) by directly digesting the components of slough (e.g., fibrin, bacteria, leukocytes, cell debris, serous exudate, and DNA) or 2) by dissolving the collagen "anchors" that secure the avascular tissue to the underlying wound bed (Boxer et al, 1969). Ideally the type of enzyme selected should correlate with the type of tissue found on the wound surface. Unfortunately, there is little information available to guide the identification of the predominant substrate in the wound bed and therefore the most appropriate enzyme.

Directions for Use. Enzymes require specific conditions, which vary from product to product, to be effective. Manufacturer's guidelines must be followed carefully to optimize the enzyme's effectiveness. The presence of heavy metals, which can be found in many wound cleansers and other commonly used topical wound products, inactivates enzymes. Examples of heavy metals include silver and zinc. These products should be rinsed thoroughly from the wound before applying an enzyme. The amount and frequency of enzyme application is type-specific and ranges from three times daily to once daily.

Enzymes require a specific pH range, which necessitates testing the pH of the wound surface with litmus paper, but this is not a common practice. Because enzymes are not effective in dry environment, eschar must be crosshatched to allow penetration of the enzyme and the wound surface must be kept moist. Crosshatching the eschar is achieved by using a scalpel to make several slits the length and width of the eschar. To avoid damaging the viable wound base beneath the necrotic tissue and causing pain, these slits are shallow and do not penetrate the depth of the necrotic tissue. Once the eschar begins to separate or demarcate from the surrounding skin, the enzyme can be applied to the wound edges along the line of demarcation to hasten separation. At this point, conservative sharp debridement can be used to remove softened necrotic tissue. Enzymes can then be continued, or another debridement technique such as autolysis can be instituted. Enzymes must be discontinued once viable tissue is revealed and necrotic tissue is removed.

Dressing changes daily to three times daily are required depending on the type of enzyme used. The most appropriate type of cover dressing to use is not well researched. According to manufacturer's guidelines, moist gauze dressings are used to cover the enzymes. However, these recommendations are based on safety and efficacy studies conducted before the advent of modern moisture-retentive dressings (Boxer et al, 1969; Lee and Ambrus, 1975; Rao, Sane, and Georgier, 1975).

Most dressings can be used safely with enzymes, including gauze, hydrogels, and transparent film dressings. The cover dressing that is selected should require the same frequency of application as the enzyme. Because enzymes are typically applied daily or twice daily, dressings that are intended to remain in place for several days are not cost-effective in combination with enzyme preparations. Enzymatic debridement can be augmented by using a moisture-retentive dressing so that autolysis can be supported. However, although this appears to facilitate more rapid debridement, the wound should be observed frequently and assessed carefully for infection.

Because these enzymes are selective in nature, damage to viable tissue in the wound bed should not occur if the dressing is continued once debridement is completed and viable tissue is exposed, although this practice is not advocated. More appropriate dressings are available at a fraction of the cost and should be implemented once the wound is debrided. Transient erythema and irritation, particularly when preparations containing papain come into contact with intact skin, have been reported (Berger, 1993). Ointments may be used to protect the periwound intact skin

Precautions. Enzymatic debridement has several disadvantages. Enzymes are a prescription item, so there are cost and reimbursement implications with their use. The frequent dressing changes dictate considerable commitment on the part of the caregiver (the patient, family, or staff) that may not always be reasonable or acceptable. Enzymatic debridement is slow; the length of time required to achieve debridement may range from several days to weeks.

The major frustration about enzymatic debridement is the lack of research to guide clinical use and decision making. As previously mentioned, there is little research to guide the selection of the type of enzyme to use. Although the enzyme active ingredient is effective against specific types of necrotic tissue (e.g., denatured protein, denatured collagen, fibrin), it is unclear how this affects the enzyme's clinical effectiveness. It is very difficult to identify the specific type or predominant type of tissue present in the necrotic material. Currently, decisions about which product to use are based on availability, cost, ease and frequency of application, and familiarity with the product.

Few clinical trials comparing the effectiveness of enzymatic debridement with other enzymes and other debridement methods are available. In a recent animal study, researchers compared a collagenase enzyme with a fibrinolysin and deoxyribonuclease combination enzyme; both enzymes are active against denatured protein (Mekkes, Zeegelaar, and Westerhof, 1998). They reported the fibrinolysin and deoxyribonulcease combination enzyme to be no more effective than placebo when compared with collagenase. In another in vitro study, greater debriding action was reported in a 24-hour period with papain/urea versus collagenase or the fibrinolysin and deoxyribonuclease combination (Hobson et al, 1998). In a nonexperimental design using a complicated statistical technique employing decision analysis and computer modeling, Mosher and colleagues (1999) reported collagenase to have a greater likelihood of achieving a complete debridement of a full-thickness noninfected pressure ulcer at 2 weeks than fibrinolysin, autolysis, or wet-to-dry dressings. This report, however, is difficult to apply clinically and needs clinical validation. Existing research uses several research designs and reports various endpoints, so consistency or consensus concerning effectiveness outcomes such as time to debride is lacking (Glyantsev and Adamyan, 1997; Hobson et al, 1998; Mekkes, Zeegelaar, and Westerhof, 1998; Mosher et al, 1999).

Dakin's Solution

Dakin's solution (diluted sodium hypochlorite solution) has a long history of being used to cleanse and debride wounds and was originally used as a topical disinfectant for wounds sustained in war. The primary action of Dakin's solution is to exert antimicrobial effects and odor control. As a debriding agent, Dakin's solution is nonselective because of its cytotoxic properties.

TABLE 7-1 Enzyme Comparison

ENZYME	DESCRIPTION	SOURCE	MECHANISM OF ACTION	DOSAGE	APPLICATION GUIDELINES
Collagenase	Sterile enzyme debriding agent containing collagenase in white petrolatum (e.g., Stantyl ointment)	Derived from *Clostridium* bacteria	• Digests native and denatured collagen, therefore effective on the "holding strands" and denatured collagen in the slough • Does not attack collagen in healthy tissue and newly forming granulation tissue	Administer once daily	• Optimal pH range: 6 to 8 • Activity adversely affected by detergents; hexachlorophene, and heavy metal ions such as mercury and silver will inactivate the enzyme; flush wound with saline before applying enzyme • Avoid soaks containing metal ions or acidic solutions such as Burrows solution; metal ion and low pH will inactivate enzyme • Hydrogen peroxide and Dakin's solution compatible with enzyme • In wounds with depth, apply with tongue depressor; if wound is shallow can apply enzyme directly to gauze dressing • Cross hatch eschar with #10 blade to allow penetration

Papain/urea combination	• Combined papain and urea in a hydrophilic ointment base (e.g., Accuzyme, Panafil White) • Also available in combination with chlorophyllin copper complex sodium (e.g., Panafil ointment)	Derived from papaya	• Papain is a proteolytic enzyme that digests nonviable protein and is harmless to viable tissue • Papain is ineffective alone and requires activators to stimulate digestive potency • Urea is a denaturant of proteins and works as an activator to render the protein more susceptible to enzymatic attack by papain • Chlorophyllin copper complex sodium controls inflammation and reduces wound odor	Daily or twice daily application	• Hydrogen peroxide may inactivate • Salts of heavy metals such as lead, silver, and mercury may inactivate • Active at pH range from 3 to 12
Fibrinolysin and deoxyribonuclease combined	• An enzyme combination of two lytic enzymes (fibrinolysin and deoxyribonuclease) in ointment base of liquid petrolatum and polyethylene (e.g., Elase ointment) • Also available in combination with chloramphenicol ointment (e.g., Elase-Chloromycetin ointment)	• Fibrinolysin derived from bovine plasma • Deoxyribonuclease is isolated in a purified form from bovine pancreas	• Directed against denatured protein, fibrin, and deoxyribonucleic acid found in slough • Chloromycetin provides a broad-spectrum antibiotic activity against gram positive and gram negative organisms	Requires application one to three times daily because of rapid reduction in enzyme activity once applied	Monitor for patient sensitivity

Description. Dakin's solution denatures protein, therefore rendering it more easily removed from the wound. Loosening of the slough also facilitates debridement by other methods.

Directions for Use. Dakin's solution is applied by saturating gauze with the solution, lightly packing it into the wound, and applying a gauze cover dressing. It is changed twice daily if the goal is debridement. Periwound skin protection should be provided with ointments, liquid skin barrier film dressings, or solid skin barrier wafers.

Dakin's solution is probably most appropriately used when there is a large amount of slough on the wound bed and the wound is infected or malodorous. Dakin's solution should be considered a short-term treatment (less than 10 days). Once infection and odor are under control, another debridement method should be selected to complete the process. Alternative dressing and debridement techniques should be implemented as the amount of slough decreases, exposing viable tissue.

The use Dakin's solution for debridement is controversial (Monroe, 1992). Thomas (1990a, 1991) considers hypochlorites to be ineffective for the purpose of debridement based on his report that approximately 100 ml of 0.25% chlorine solution was needed to liquefy 1 g of slough and that necrotic tissue remained unchanged after 24 hours of immersion in a chlorine solution.

Precautions. There is conflicting evidence linking the use of Dakin's solution and cytotoxicity, but some studies indicate that at a dilution of 0.025%, sodium hypochlorite can be an effective antimicrobial and still remain noncytotoxic (Heggers et al, 1991). Concentrations greater than 0.025% should be avoided bacause higher concentrations may be toxic and pose a risk of damage to fibroblasts, resulting in an impaired wound-healing process (Rodeheaver, 1990).

Maggots

Another method of chemical debridement includes the use of maggots, which was originally used on battlefields. Physicians noted anecdotal reports from medics who observed the rapid removal of necrotic tissue when maggots were present on the wound bed. This technique has also been referred to as *biologic debridement*, or *biosurgery*. Because its mechanism of action is chemical in nature, the maggot therapy is discussed as a means of chemical debridement in this text.

Description. Therapeutic maggot therapy involves sterilizing the fly eggs. Once they hatch (again, under sterile conditions) the sterile larvae are introduced into the wound bed. It is theorized that larvae secrete proteolytic enzymes, including collagenase, that break down the necrotic tissue. It is also believed that the larvae ingest microorganisms, which are then destroyed. Because of this reported action and the emergence of resistant organisms, there is renewed interest in maggot therapy in some centers, particularly in Europe (Thomas et al, 1996).

Directions for Use. Generally maggot therapy is considered for use in wounds that have not responded to conventional methods of debridement. The main benefit is the rapid debridement of necrotic tissue along with odor control. There may be some antimicrobial effects as well, but again this is based on anecdotal reports.

Precautions. Although there are no reported side effects, care should be taken to avoid having the larvae come in contact with healthy skin, since this could result in damage caused by the proteolytic enzymes. The main disadvantage to maggot therapy is the sensation of crawling that some patients experience, but confinement of the larvae to the wound bed decreases this sensation. One dressing that has been devised for use with maggot therapy is comprised of hydrocolloid to protect the periwound skin, a mesh net over the wound to contain the larvae, and an absorbent pad to contain exudate (Sherman, 1997).

MECHANICAL

Mechanical modes of debridement include wet-to-dry gauze dressings, irrigation, and whirlpool. These techniques represent selective and nonselective modes of debridement.

Wet-to-Dry Debridement

Description. Wet-to-dry dressings have been the conventional treatment for debridement for decades (Mulder 1995; Turner, 1997). This method removes necrotic tissue and absorbs small amounts of exudate, but as a nonselective method of debridement, exposed healthy tissue in the wound may be damaged.

Directions for Use. Wet-to-dry mechanical debridement is most commonly used with heavily necrotic wounds. It is also used with infected wounds, thus allowing frequent visualization of the affected area. However, once the infection has resolved, a more selective method of debridement should be initiated.

Wet-to-dry debridement consists of applying saline-moistened gauze to the wound bed and allowing it to dry on the wound, trapping debris. Once dry, usually 4 to 6 hours after application, the dressing is pulled off of the wound along with the trapped debris, the wound is cleansed, and the saline-moistened gauze reapplied. This process is continued until viable tissue is apparent, which takes several days to weeks.

Appropriate technique and dressing materials are critical for effective wet-to-dry debridement. Gauze should be moistened (not dripping wet) when applied to the wound, and while the gauze should contact the entire wound surface, it should not be packed tightly into the wound. Wet-to-dry gauze dressings must be allowed to dry out before removal, hence the need to avoid oversaturation of the gauze.

The most effective type of dressing material for wet-to-dry gauze dressings is an open weave cotton fabric because it provides a combination of mildly abrasive qualities and adherent properties (Hall and Ponder, 1992; Mulder, 1995; Ponder and Krasner, 1993). Nonwoven gauze is generally ineffective because the fiber composition does not allow tissue adherence. One type of nonwoven gauze is specific for selective debridement (Nu-Brede, Johnson and Johnson Medical, Inc.) because it combines elements of a woven gauze with larger openings in the weave and is characterized by increased absorbency and decreased linting and shredding.

Precautions. Several disadvantages are associated with wet-to-dry debridement. To be effective, the procedure for preparing, applying, and removing the wet-to-dry dressing must be strictly followed. Unfortunately, the dressing change is rarely performed correctly. Gauze that is moistened immediately before removal minimizes the removal of debris (Goode and Thomas, 1997). The removal of the dressing can trigger acute noncyclic wound pain (see Chapter 17) for the patient and necessitate analgesia. Wet-to-dry dressings are a nonselective mode of debridement so that granulation tissue and epithelial tissue are also removed along with the necrotic tissue. When moistening the gauze before application, excess saline is often used, which prevents the dressing from drying out as it should and macerates of the periwound tissue (Rodeheaver et al, 1994). Additionally, when the wound is exudative, wet-to-dry gauze dressings provide insufficient absorption, again macerating periwound skin. Wet-to-dry dressings are labor intensive because they must be changed more than once per day. This technique is also complicated in that there are many steps involved that require a judgement call to be performed correctly. Finally, the steps involved in moistening the gauze provide ample opportunity to contaminate the gauze and break sterile technique or even clean technique, thus posing a risk of infection.

The use of wet-to-dry dressings is a controversial debridement method. Some wound care experts even consider gauze to be contraindicated as a wound contact dressing (Turner, 1997). However, wet-to-dry dressings remain a prevalent technique. This may be due to the ready availability of gauze, the perception that it is inexpensive, training, or simply force of habit. For most clinicians, until randomized clinical trials comparing wet-to-dry debridement with other methods of debridement are conducted, the appropriateness and effectiveness of wet-to-dry dressings will continue to be debated. Nonetheless, most experts in wound care agree that the use of wet-to-dry dressings should be restricted to heavily necrotic wounds and discontinued when viable tissue is present.

Irrigation

Another method of removing debris mechanically is through wound irrigation with pressurized fluids. There are two common methods of wound irrigation: high pressure irrigation and pulsatile high-pressure lavage.

High-Pressure Irrigation

Description. Irrigation of the necrotic wound with fluid delivered at 8 to 12 pounds per square inch (psi), such as with a 35 ml syringe and a 19-gauge angiocatheter, is referred to as *high-pressure irrigation*. This procedure provides adequate force to remove debris without damaging healthy tissue or inoculating the underlying tissue with bacteria (Wheeler et al, 1976). Pressures below 4 psi, such as that provided by a bulb syringe, are not sufficient to remove eschar and slough from the wound base. These recommendations are also outlined in the *AHCPR Pressure Ulcer Treatment Guideline* (1994) (see Appendix C).

Directions for use. High-pressure irrigation is particularly well-suited for sloughy wound beds as compared with eschar, and it should be discontinued when the wound base is clean. Normal saline is the most commonly recommended irrigant. Occasionally, antimicrobial solutions such as Dakin's solution may be used for a short-time period when the wound is infected. Although these solutions precipitate cytotoxic effects on healthy wound cells, Rodeheaver (1990) also suggests that unless an antiseptic is particularly toxic, brief contact with tissue will not impair wound healing. However, Lawrence, a Senior Research Fellow at the Wound Healing Research Unit at the University of Wales College of Medicine in Cardiff, states that "there is little evidence to suggest that irrigating with antiseptics significantly alters the bacteriological content of wounds" (1997). In a study conducted by Stringer, Lawrence, and Lilly (1983), no bacteriologic benefit was noted among "dirty wounds" irrigated with one of three popular antiseptics or physiologic saline.

High-pressure irrigation can be achieved with commercially available products that attach to saline bags so that a continuous flow of irrigation solution can be delivered to the wound at consistent, acceptable pressures (Irrijet, Ackrad Labs). Prepackaged cannisters of pressurized saline are also available and deliver the wound irrigant at an appropriate range of pressure.

Precautions. Delivering fluid under pressure to the wound bed can cause dissemination of wound bacteria over a wide area, exposing the patient and care provider to potential contamination. Consequently, personal protective equipment (e.g., mask, gloves, gown, and goggles) should be worn by the care provider during this procedure.

Pulsatile High-Pressure Lavage

Description. An alternative to high-pressure irrigation is pulsatile high-pressure lavage (e.g., Pulsavac, Zimmer, Inc.; Simpulse, Davol, Inc.). These machines provide intermittent high-pressure irrigation combined with suction to remove the irrigant and debris. The apparatus allows adjustment of pressure to higher levels to remove debris.

Directions for use. Pulsatile high-pressure lavage loosens necrotic tissue, facilitating removal by other methods of debridement and may be used as an alternative to whirlpool. The amount of solution needed depends on the size of the wound. Moist gauze is the most commonly used dressing; the frequency of treatment should be considered when selecting a dressing. Pulsatile high-pressure lavage is an effective tool for removing larger amounts of debris, but efficacy studies are needed to determine its place in debridement and effects on wound healing. Pulsatile high-pressure lavage is best discontinued once the wound is clean.

Precautions. The main disadvantage to pulsatile high-pressure lavage is the cost. The hose and tip are designed for one-time use and necrotic wounds may require twice-daily treatments. Pressure settings should be maintained at 8 to 15 psi for debridement. Higher pressures are not appropriate because there may be inoculation of surrounding tissue and damage to any granulation tissue (AHCPR, 1994). Caution should be used when irrigating with pulsatile high-pressure lavage to avoid blood vessels, graft sites, and exposed muscle, tendon, and bone. Patients on anticoagulant therapy should be observed carefully for any bleeding, and treatment is immediately discontinued if bleeding occurs. As with high-pressure irrigation, personal protective equipment is necessary. However with pulsatile high-pressure lavage, treatment should be delivered in an enclosed area separate from any other patients to avoid contamination with mist (Loehne, 1998).

Whirlpool

Description. Whirlpool is commonly used to remove bacteria and debris from the surface of large wounds. Additional benefits include softening and loosening of adherent necrotic tissue and cleansing and removal of wound exudate. The vigorous action and hydration may contribute to the debridement effects, however research to support this is minimal (Frantz, 1997).

Directions for use. Whirlpool is indicated for trunk or extremity wounds located on a body area that can be immersed into the tank. Wounds appropriate for whirlpool are usually large with a significant amount of necrotic material covering the wound surface. Water is the most common type of solution used with an optimal temperature of 37° C (Sussman, 1998).

Questions about the efficacy of whirlpool alone in removing bacteria and debris from the wound surface have been raised (Frantz, 1997; Sussman, 1998). Although there is some reduction in bacterial load, this is actually thought to be the result of forceful rinsing after immersion rather than the action of the whirlpool alone (Neiderhuber, Stribley, and Koepke, 1975). Therefore it is probably the irrigation action rather than the whirlpool that decreases the surface bacteria.

Precautions. Vasodilatation, which leads to increased circulation to the affected area, naturally occurs with whirlpool. However, vasodilatation is not always desirable. McCulloch and Boyd (1992) demonstrated an increase in lower leg edema in patients with venous ulcers after whirlpool therapy. This effect was attributed to a combination of the whirlpool itself and the dependent position of the leg during the therapy. Consequently, the pathophysiology of the wound must be considered before selecting whirlpool therapy. Increasing circulation in the extremity of patients with venous insufficiency contributes to venous congestion. In the presence of advanced arterial disease, the vessels in the leg are likely to be maximally dilated, so there is questionable benefit, and the added stress locally may increase metabolic demands. Also, whirlpool therapy needs to be used cautiously in the patient with diabetes who may not be able to detect temperature changes because of sensory or autonomic neuropathy.

Concerns about cross contamination between patients who use the whirlpool also exist. According to Lawrence (1997), "wound bacteria readily contaminate bath water . . ." Although it is common practice to add antiseptic solution to the water, these additives may exhibit deleterious effects on the wound.

SHARP

Sharp debridement is also referred to as *instrumental debridement* and requires the use of surgical instruments. Sharp debridement can be done sequentially in a conservative fashion (conservative sharp wound debridement), or it can be done surgically (surgical sharp debridement).

Conservative Sharp Wound Debridement

Description. Conservative sharp wound debridement, also known as *conservative instrumental debridement*, is a selective debridement method for removal of loosely adherent, nonviable tissue using sterile instruments (e.g., forceps, or "pick-ups," scissors, and scalpel with #10 and #15 blades). Conservative sharp debridement is probably the most aggressive type of debridement performed by nonphysician health care providers such as wound care nurses. When done correctly, the procedure is not aggressive enough to expose viable tissue and there is little likelihood of blood loss. Therefore the risks to the patient are minimal.

Professional and educational qualifications required to perform conservative sharp debridement have been proposed by numerous experts (Fowler, 1992; Gordon, 1996; Razor and Martin, 1991; Thomaselli, 1995). A position statement by the Wound Ostomy Continence Nurses Society is provided at the end of this chapter (Appendix 7.1). Most states consider conservative sharp debridement to be within the scope of practice for registered nurses. A variety of other requirements may also need to be satisfied depending on the specific state nurse practice act and the employer's requirements.

Directions for Use. The basic principles of conservative sharp debridement include the following:

1. Decrease the likelihood of infection by using sterile instruments, using sterile technique, and preparing the site for debridement with an antiseptic (e.g., Betadine or a chlorhexidine solution such as Hibiclens).
2. Establish a plane of dissection by holding the necrotic tissue taught to clearly visualize the plane of dissection.
3. Avoid all vascular tissues and tissues that are not clearly identified.
4. Irrigate the wound following the procedure.

Conservative sharp debridement has several advantages. It removes the necrotic tissue more quickly than the previously discussed methods and can be accomplished in a serial manner. This method of debridement can be combined with other debridement techniques (autolysis or enzymatic) to shorten this phase of wound care. Theoretically, a more rapid approach to debridement decreases the body's expenditure of energy during a time of high resource use. Additionally, because of the low risk involved, conservative sharp debridement can be performed in a variety of settings by nonphysician clinicians who are skilled and credentialed in this technique. Therefore conservative sharp debridement of necrotic wounds is a viable option for patients residing in nonacute care settings and does not require transfer to a hospital.

It is impossible to make a "blanket statement" about the exact requirements that must be met for a nurse to be authorized to perform this procedure. Wound care nurses and physical therapists interested in seeking approval to perform conservative sharp debridement should consult their applicable state practice acts and individual facility requirements. In addition, answers to the following questions should be pursued:

1. Is conservative sharp debridement covered under the clinician's state practice act?
2. Are specialty education, training, and credentials in conservative sharp debridement required by the state or employer?
3. Are formal knowledge and skill updates required on a periodic basis?
4. Has the individual's professional organization or employer delineated specific guidelines related to conservative sharp debridement?
5. Are policies, procedures, and protocols in place for conservative sharp debridement?
6. Is conservative sharp debridement considered part of the clinician's clinical privileges or is a physician's order required for each incident of conservative sharp debridement?
7. What level of physician supervision, if any, is required for conservative sharp debridement?
8. Does the employer provide malpractice insurance coverage for conservative sharp debridement?
9. Does the clinician carry malpractice insurance to cover conservative sharp debridement?

A sample policy and procedure on conservative sharp debridement is provided in Box 7-1. Before implementing these policies and procedures, they should be evaluated and approved by the organization in which the wound care specialist contracts or is employed.

Precautions. A disadvantage of conservative sharp debridement is that, depending on the size of the ulcer and amount of necrotic tissue involved, it could conceivably take weeks to remove all of the nonviable tissue. It may also be an uncomfortable procedure for the patient, so the need for analgesia either topically or systemially should be considered.

Although blood loss is not expected during conservative sharp debridement, it remains a possibility. As a result, the patient should be assessed for factors that place him or her at risk for clotting problems if a vessel is accidentally severed. Factors to consider include medications (e.g., heparin, warfarin, high-dose NSAIDS, and antibiotics) and pathologic conditions (e.g., thrombocytopenia; impaired liver function; vitamin K deficiency; and malnutrition). When any of these factors is present, the wound care specialist should confer with the physician before proceeding with conservative sharp debridement.

Infected wounds present unique considerations for conservative sharp debridement. In general, there is the potential for transient bacteremia after debridement of wounds, particulary when the wound is infected. Transient bacteremia in a patient who is nutritionally compromised, leukopenic, or otherwise immunocompromised can be devastating. Unfortunately, there is a lack of research concerning the relationship between sharp debridement and transient bacteremia. Therefore the nurse should exercise caution and employ a conservative approach.

Theoretically, surgical sharp debridement is the preferred method of debriding most infected wounds. Realistically, this is not always an option because of either the patient's condition or the setting. In these situations, serial conservative sharp debridements can be conducted by the nonphysician wound care provider but only in conjunction with appropriate antibiotic coverage. Although systemic antibiotics may not penetrate the necrotic tissue to reduce the bacterial load in the wound, they should reduce the potential for dissemination of the pathogens systemically. Topical antiseptic solutions may also be instrumental in reducing the bioburden of the wound. The nurse should be in compliance with any policies contained within the facility or agency that concern the management of infected wounds and with the state nurse practice act.

Surgical Sharp Wound Debridement

Description. Surgical sharp wound debridement, also known as *surgical debridement*, is usually reserved for those cases requiring the removal of massive amounts of tissue or involving a life-threatening infectious process that dictates immediate removal of necrotic tissue to effectively treat the patient (Haury et al, 1978). Surgical debridement inherently implies aggressive removal of necrotic tissue. In most cases, it is a one-time procedure carried out by a surgeon in the operating room, although there are necrotic processes (e.g., necrotizing fasciitis) that require serial debridement. If the patient is unstable or unable to withstand the anesthesia required for such procedures, surgical debridement may be performed under a local or spinal anesthetic. When indicated, the surgeon may choose to perform a less-aggressive sharp debridement at the bedside using a local anesthetic.

Directions for Use. Surgical debridement is the fastest method for removing large amounts of necrotic tissue. It has also been demonstrated to stimulate wound repair in diabetic ulcers, which is theorized to be due to correcting the imbalance of cytokines and proteases in chronic wound fluids, thus converting the detrimental molecular environment of a chronic wound into a pseudoacute wound molecular environment (Schultz, 1999; Steed et al, 1996).

Surgical debridement is beyond the scope of practice of most wound care nurses and physical therapists. In fact, few nonsurgeon physicians perform surgical debridement. There may be some instances when advanced practice nurses (e.g., nurse practitioners, clinical nurse specialists) or physician assistants have the education and training required to perform such aggressive interventions.

Precautions. Disadvantages of surgical debridement include increased direct risks to the patient in terms of anesthesia risks, bleeding, and sepsis. As stated previously, it is common to see transient bacteremia after a wound is debrided. Most healthy subjects can withstand such events. Unfortunately, many infected wounds occur in people who are not in optimal health; therefore the transient bacteremia could progress to systemic infection and patient death. Nurses should be aware of the possibility of transient bacteremia and incorporate measures to prevent or control it, such as using sterile technique and instruments and perioperative antibiotics. Because of its obvious aggressive nature, some viable tissue may be sacrificed during surgical debridement (Linder and Morris, 1990).

Another disadvantage of surgical debridement is that it may add tremendously to the overall costs of treating the patient. The condition of the patient, the aggressive nature of this procedure, and the higher level of care required after debridement often require hospitalization

Laser Debridement

Description. Laser debridement, a form of surgical sharp debridement, uses focused beams of light to cauterize, vaporize, or slice through tissue. Several light sources for lasers are available: argon, CO_2, neodyminum yttrium aluminum garnet (Nd:YAG), and tunable (Habif, 1996) Each type of laser emits light at a specific wavelength, and different body tissues absorb different wavelengths. The

Box 7-1 Policy and Procedure: Conservative Sharp Wound Debridement

I. Purpose

The purpose of this policy and procedure is to outline the process by which an RN with certification in wound care may remove devitalized tissue by conservative sharp wound debridement.

II. Policy

- Any RN performing conservative sharp wound debridement will have additional didactic education in the skill.
- Any RN performing conservative sharp wound debridement will have additional laboratory education to develop the skill.
- Any RN performing conservative sharp wound debridement will participate in a clinical practicum involving patients with wounds.
- Documentation of the above will be filed with the individual's other credentialling information. (This is determined by practice setting.)

III. Authority and Responsibility

- The individual performing conservative sharp wound debridement will provide documentation of education and competency.
- An order from the attending physician will be obtained before the procedure, or physician practice protocols will be in effect permitting the procedure.
- Obtain consent from the patient or appropriate representative. (This is determined by practice setting.)

IV. Definitions

Conservative sharp wound debridement is the removal of loose, avascular tissue using surgical instruments (e.g., scissors, scalpel, forceps) without inflicting pain or precipitating bleeding.

V. References

- State nurse practice act
- Thomaselli N: WOCN position statement: conservative sharp wound debridement for registered nurses, *J Wound Ostomy Continence Nurs* 22(1):32A, 1995.

part of the tissue that absorbs the light is called the chromophore (e.g., water is the chromophore for the CO_2, laser, and hemoglobin is the chromophore for the argon laser). When the chromophore absorbs the light, it is quickly heated and vaporized. When the beam of light is tightly focused, it is capable of cutting through human tissue like a knife (Raz, 1995).

Directions for Use. The choice of which laser to use is often dictated by the type of problem at hand (e.g., the extent of the necrosis, location of the wound). Historically, the continuous wave CO_2 lasers were often used to debride necrotic tissue. Advantages of laser debridement are that the wound bed is sterilized and that most severed vessels are cauterized (Flemming, Frame, and Dhillion, 1986; Slutzki, Sharif, and Bornstein, 1977).

Precautions. Disadvantages of laser debridement include injury to adjacent healthy tissue and delayed healing process. More current work with pulsed laser beams rather than the continuous laser beams has decreased these negative effects (Glatter et al, 1998; Smith et al, 1997). Unfortunately, this method is not available in all settings.

SELECTION OF DEBRIDEMENT METHOD

The method of debridement selected is affected by individual patient situations and by clinician skill. Three general principles guide the selection of the

Box 7-1 Policy and Procedure: Conservative Sharp Wound Debridement—cont'd

VI. Procedure

1. Explain procedure to patient
2. Obtain consent (this is determined by practice setting)
3. Assemble equipment
   a. Forceps with teeth
   b. Scalpel handle with #10 and #15 blades
   c. Silver nitrate sticks
   d. Curved iris scissors
   e. Surgical gel foam
   f. Gauze sponges
   g. Normal saline
   h. Clean gloves
   i. Sterile gloves
4. Wash hands
5. Prepare work surface
6. Position patient for procedure
7. Ensure adequate lighting
8. Apply clean gloves
9. Remove old dressing and discard
10. Wash hands
11. Don sterile gloves
12. Prep site with antiseptic (betadine or Hibiclens if iodine allergy)
13. Grasp loosely adherent tissue with forceps; pull tautly, exposing a clear line of dissection
14. Cut or snip loose tissue
15. Irrigate wound with normal saline
16. For minor bleeding, apply silver nitrate, gel foam, or pressure for any bleeding
17. Re-dress wound
18. Document procedure and patient's response to procedure
19. Advise staff of any relevant issues

most appropriate debridement process: 1) urgency of need for debridement, 2) the skill level of the care provider, and 3) availability of products and supplies. Clinicians must assess the wound characteristics, wound-treatment goals, patient status or comorbidities, and the clinician's own clinical experience and competence.

Wound Characteristics

The type of necrotic tissue in the wound guides the debridement method selected. Eschar responds to autolysis, enzymes (with cross-hatching), wet-to dry dressings, and either conservative or surgical sharp debridement. Slough is most commonly managed with autolysis and conservative sharp debridement, although wet-to-dry dressings can also be used. When slough is unresponsive to these techniques, enzymes can be considered. High-pressure wound irrigation or lavage are adjunctive and should always accompany dressing changes in the necrotic wound.

The presence of wound infection is another critical determinant in method selection. Infection dictates that debridement is imperative, but certain methods are more appropriate for the infected wound and are selected after considering the patient's condition. Autolysis is generally not rapid enough in the infected wound, and the infection can be exacerbated by the presence of anaerobes. When the wound is infected, conservative sharp debridement may be performed by the surgeon; it is not, however, in the scope of practice of nonphysician wound care specialists until the infection is resolved or at least treated for 2 to 3 days. Wet-to-dry dressings, enzymes, Dakin's solution, and irrigation may be used with concomitant antibiotic therapy.

Wound-Treatment Goals

The overall goals for the wound should also be considered. First it must be decided whether debridement is appropriate and, if appropriate, whether it should be pursued immediately or delayed. This depends on the wound treatment goal (whether the goal is to heal the wound or to prevent deterioration of the wound).

Occasionally, it may be necessary to forego debridement in light of other more urgent needs of the patient. Such a decision must include input from the patient, the patient's significant others, and the primary care provider. Even if the goal is not to heal the wound, debridement of necrotic tissue will also control malordorous wounds, making the environment more comfortable for the patient, family, and caregivers.

Wound debridement may be delayed in some circumstances. For example, when a necrotic but noninfected ulcer is found on a patient who is critically ill, unstable, or severely neutropenic, it may be prudent to delay the debridement until the patient's condition improves. Because necrotic tissue harbors microbes, transient bacteremia can still occur after debridement of noninfected wounds and overwhelm the patient's immune system. Postponement of debridement can help to reduce this likelihood.

When eschar covers a stable, noninfected wound on an ischemic extremity and when dry eschar covers a pressure ulcer located on the heel, debridement is contraindicated (AHCPR, 1994). The subsequent finding of a wound infection dictates reevaluation of the plan of care.

Patient Status and Comorbidities

The patient's history and coexisting morbidities, such as neutropenia and clotting disorders, also affect the method of debridement selected. Autolysis should not be expected in the presence of severe neutropenia (absolute neutrophil count of less than 500 mm_3) because there is an insufficient number of neutrophils available to respond to the wound demands. Generally, the wound will appear stagnant during this time. Debridement should be postponed until the neutrophil count climbs over 1000 mm^3. Knowledge of clotting disorders or anticoagulant medication use is also critical when considering conservative sharp debridement.

Wound pain is another critical determinant of debridement method selection. Patients experiencing wound pain may benefit from the less painful debridement modalities such as autolysis or enzymatic debridement. Other types of debridement such as wet-to-dry, conservative sharp and surgical sharp may trigger or exacerbate pain. The patient's pain status during dressing changes and while resting should be assessed; analgesia should be administered topically or systemically prophylatically.

Clinician Experience and Competence

Although debridement methods such as autolysis, wound irrigations, wet-to-dry dressings, and enzymes are ideally initiated under the direction of the physician or wound care specialist, they are procedures that can be performed by nurses, physical therapists, the patient, and caregivers. However, the more aggressive methods of debridement, specifically sharp debridement, require a level of skill and competence. Conservative sharp debridement should be performed only by a wound care nurse who has demonstrated and documented competence with this technique and is in compliance with their scope of practice, state nurse practice act, and institutional policies. In addition, they should maintain their clinical skill level and be comfortable with the procedure. Surgical sharp debridement and laser debridement are only performed by physicians.

ASSESSMENT OF THE DEBRIDEMENT PROCESS

The methods of wound debridement typically employed by the nonphysician wound care specialist do not immediately yield a completely clean wound; therefore the wound must be closely monitored for indicators of progression of the debridement process. Deterioration of the wound requires reevaluation of the treatment selected. Assessment parameters include wound dimensions, volume of exudate, odor, type of tissue present, and condition of the periwound skin. Wound dimensions typically increase as the necrotic tissue is removed from the wound. Early in the debridement process, the wound is commonly exudative; this should decrease as the necrotic tissue is removed. As the underlying tissue is exposed, healthy viable tissue in the wound base should be present. When using autolysis, enzymes or wet-to-dry dressings, a gradual transition in the type of necrotic tissue present in the wound base should be observed and documented. Hydrated eschar becomes gray and soft; firmly adherent slough becomes loose and stringy. When the wound is infected, a decrease in the periwound erythema and induration should be observed. If the patient was febrile or had leukocytosis before initiating debridement, a decrease should be observed as the necrotic tissue is removed and the bacterial load is reduced. However, these clinical changes may also be attributed to antibiotic therapy.

SUMMARY

Debridement is a critical component of topical therapy for necrotic wounds. The nurse should be knowledgeable about the various methods available for debridement and discuss their options with the patient's physician and the patient so that the most appropriate wound-management choice can be made. Debridement methods are not used in isolation; rather, they are used in combination and modified as the wound conditions change. For example, an eschar-covered noninfected wound may be crosshatched and covered with a hydrogel sheet. As the eschar softens, it may then be possible to use conservative sharp debridement to facilitate removal of the bulk of the residual eschar and to continue use of the hydrogel or select another moisture-retentive dressing, depending on the wound needs. Close supervision of the patient and accurate wound assessments during the debridement phase are essential to ensure an outcome consistent with the stated wound goals.

SELF-ASSESSMENT EXERCISE

1. Which of the following methods of debridement is nonselective?
   a. Autolysis
   b. High-pressure irrigation
   c. Enzymes
   d. Sharp
2. High-pressure wound irrigation requires:
   a. A bulb syringe
   b. Daily dressing changes
   c. Personal protective gear
   d. Expensive equipment
3. List three precautions in the use of enzymatic debridement.
4. Selection of debridement approach is guided by all of the following EXCEPT:
   a. Patient's age
   b. Presence of wound infection
   c. Extent and type of necrotic tissue
   d. Clinician experience
5. The risk of transient bacteremia is associated with which of the following debridement techniques?
   a. Autolysis
   b. Conservative sharp
   c. Enzymes
   d. Wet-to-dry dressings

REFERENCES

Agency for Health Care Policy and Research: *AHCPR pressure ulcer treatment guideline: clinical practice guideline, no 15*, Rockville, Md, 1994, US Department of Health and Human Services, Public Health Service,. AHCPR Pub No 95-0652.

Alvarez O: Moist environment for healing: matching the dressing to the wound, *Ostomy Wound Manage* 21:64, 1988.

Bale S: A guide to wound debridement, *J Wound Care* 6(4):179, 1997a.

Bale S: Principles of wound intervention. In Bale S, Jones V, editors:*Wound care nursing: a patient-centred approach*, London, 1997b, Baillière Tindall.

Bates-Jensen B: Management of necrotic tissue. In Sussman C, Bates-Jensen B, editors: *Wound care*, Gaithersberg, Md, 1998, Aspen.

Berger M: Enzymatic debriding preparations, *Ostomy Wound Manage* 39(5):61, 1993.

Bodey GP et al: Quantitive relationship between circulating leukocytes and infection in patients with acute leukemia, *Ann Intern Med* 64(2):328, 1966.

Boxer A et al: Debridement of dermal ulcers and decubiti with Collagenase, *Geriatrics* 24:75, 1969.

Bryant R, Rolstad BS: *Autolysis white paper*, St Paul, Minn, 1998, 3M Health Care.

Colins D, Kurning P, Yuon C: Managing sloughy pressure sores, *J Wound Care* 5(10):44, 1996.

Eaglstein WH: Occlusive dressings, *J Dermatol Surg Oncol* 19:715, 1993.

Flemming A, Frame J, Dhillion R: Skin edge necrosis in irradiated tissue after carbon dioxide laser excision of tumor, *Lasers Med Sci* 1:263, 1986.

Fowler E: Instrumental/sharp debridement of non-viable tissue in wounds, *Ostomy Wound Manage* 38(8):26, 1992.

Frantz R: Adjunctive therapy for ulcer care, *Clin Geriatr Med* 13(3):553, 1997.

Glatter D et al: Carbon dioxide laser ablation with immediate auto-grafting in a full-thickness porcine burn model, *Ann Surg* 228(2):257, 1998.

Glyantsev SP, Adamyan AA: Crab collagenase in wound debridement, *J Wound Care* 6(1):13, 1997.

Goode P, Thomas D: Pressure ulcers: local wound care, *Clin Geriatr Med* 13(3):543, 1997.

Gordon B: Conservative sharp wound debridement, *J Wound Ostomy Continence Nurs* 23(3):137, 1996.

Habif TP, editor: *Clinical dermatology: a color guide to diagnosis and therapy*, ed 3, St Louis, 1996, Mosby.

Hall S, Ponder R: Non-woven wound care products, *Ostomy Wound Manage* 38(6):24, 1992.

Haury B et al:. Debridement: an essential component of traumatic wound care, *Am J Surg* 135(2):126, 1978.

Heggers JP et al: Bacteriocidal and wound healing properties of sodium hypochlorite solutions: the 1991 Lindberg Award, *J Burn Care Rehabil* 12:420, 1991.

Hobson D et al: Development and use of a quantitative method to evaluate the action of enzymatic wound debriding agents in vitro, *Wounds* 10(4):105, 1998.

Hutchinson JJ: Prevalence of wound infection under occlusive dressings: a collected survey of reported research, *Wounds* 1(2):123, 1989

Lawrence JC: Dressings and wound infection, *Am J Surg* 167(1A):215, 1994.

Lawrence JC: Wound irrigation: an update on irrigating fluids and their effect on wounds, *J Wound Care* 6(1):23, 1997.

Lee L, Ambrus J: Collagenase therapy for decubitus ulcers, *Geriatrics* 30:91, 1975.

Linder M, Morris D: The surgical management of pressure ulcers: a systematic approach based on staging, *Decubitus* 3(2):32, 1990.

Loehne HL: Pulsatile lavage with concurrent suction. In Sussman C, Bates-Jensen B, editors: *Wound care*, Gaithersburg, Md, 1998, Aspen.

McCulloch J, Boyd V: The effects of whirlpool and the dependent position on lower extremity, *J Orthop Sports Phys Ther* 16(4):169, 1992.

Mekkes J, Zeegelaar J, Westerhof W: Quantitative and objective evaluation of wound debriding properties of collagenase and fibrinolysin/deoxyribonuclease in a necrotic ulcer animal model, *Arch Dermatol Res* 290:152, 1998.

Monroe D: Hypochlorites: a review of the evidence, *J Wound Care* 1(4):44, 1992.

Mosher BA et al: Outcomes of 4 methods of debridement using a decision analysis methodology, *Adv Wound Care* 12(2), 1999.

Mulder G: Evaluation of three non-woven sponges in the debridement of chronic wounds, *Ostomy Wound Manage* 41(3):62, 1995.

Mulder G et al: Controlled randomized study of a hypertonic gel for the debridement of a dry eschar in chronic wounds, *Wounds* 5(3):112, 1993.

Neiderhuber S, Stribley R, Koepke G: Reduction of skin bacterial load with use of the therapeutic whirlpool, *Phys Ther* 55(5):482, 1975.

Ponder R, Krasner D: Gauzes and related dressings, *Ostomy Wound Manage* 39(5):48, 1993.

Rao D, Sane P, Georgier E: Collagenase in the treatment of dermal and decubitus ulcers, *J Am Geriatr Soc* 23(1):22, 1975.

Raz K: Laser physics, *Clin Dermatol* 13:11, 1995.

Razor B, Martin L: Validating sharp wound debridement, *J ET Nurs* 18(3):105, 1991.

Robson M: Wound infection: a failure of wound healing caused by an imbalance of bacteria, *Surg Clin North Am* 77(3):637, 1997.

Rodeheaver GT: Influence of antiseptics on wound healing. In Wesley AJ, Thomson PD, Hutchinson JJ, editors: *International forum on wound microbiology*, Princeton, 1990, Excerpta Medica.

Rodeheaver GT et al: Wound healing and wound management: focus on debridement, *Adv Wound Care* 7(1):22, 1994.

Rolstad BS, Harris A: Management of deterioration in cutaneous wounds. In Krasner D, Kane D, editors: *Chronic wound care*, ed 2, Wayne, Penn, 1997, Health Management Publications.

Schultz G: Molecular regulation of the wound environment. In Bryant RA, editor: *Acute and chronic wounds: nursing managment*, ed 2, St Louis, 1999, Mosby.

Sherman R: A new dressing design for use with maggot therapy, *Plast Reconstr Surg* 100(2):451, 1997.

Slutzki S, Sharif R, Bornstein L: Use of the carbon dioxide laser for large excisions with minimal blood loss, *Plast Reconstr Surg* 60:250, 1977.

Smith K et al: Depth of morphologic skin damage and viability after one, two, and three passes of a high-energy, short pulse CO_2 laser (Tru-Pulse) in pig skin, *J Am Acad Dermatol* 37(2):204, 1997.

Steed DL et al: Effect of extensive debridement and treatment on the healing of diabetic foot ulcer, *J Am Coll Surg* 183:61, 1996.

Stotts N, Hunt T: Managing bacterial colonization and infection, *Clin Geriatr Med* 13(3):65, 1997.

Stringer MD, Lawrence JC, Lilly HA: Antiseptics and the casualty wound, *J Hosp Infect* 4:410, 1983.

Sussman C: Whirlpool. In Sussman C, Bates-Jensen B, editors: *Wound care*, Gaithersberg, Md, 1998, Aspen.

Thomas S: Eusol revisited, *Dressing Times* 3:1, 1990a.

Thomas S: Evidence fails to justify use of hypochlorite, *J Tissue Viabil* 1:9, 1991.

Thomas S: *Wound management and dressings*, London, 1990b, The Pharmaceutical Press.

Thomas S et al: Using larvae in modern wound management, J *Wound Care* 5(2):60, 1996.

Thomaselli N: WOCN position statement: conservative sharp wound debridement for registered nurses, *J Wound Ostomy Continence Nurs* 22(1):32A, 1995.

Turner TD: The development of wound management products. In Krasner D, Kane D, editors: *Chronic wound care*, ed 2, Wayne, Penn, 1997, Health Management Publications.

Wheeler C et al: Side effects of high pressure irrigation, *Surg Gynecol Obstet* 143(5):775, 1976.

APPENDIX

7.1 WOCN POSITION STATEMENT: CONSERVATIVE SHARP WOUND DEBRIDEMENT

The initial treatment goal for full-thickness wounds with necrotic tissue is debridement. There are several methods to achieve debridement, including surgical debridement, conservative sharp debridement, enzymatic debridement, autolysis, and mechanical debridement.

Conservative sharp wound debridement is a technique used by many professionals. As the professional organization for nurses specializing in wound care, the Wound, Ostomy, and Continence Nurses Society (WOCN) recognizes the need to clarify the role of the wound care nurse in regard to performance of conservative sharp wound debridement. *Conservative sharp wound debridement* is defined as removal of loose avascular tissue without pain or bleeding. This procedure does not require the administration of general anesthesia. Many states permit the nurse to use topical anesthesia.

The wound, ostomy, and continence (WOC) nurse and nurse specializing in wound care are prepared to perform conservative sharp wound debridement once they have satisfactorily completed didactic and clinical instruction in the sharp debridement procedure from an accredited Wound Ostomy Continence Nursing Education Program (WOCNEP), wound-management specialty course, or a continuing education (CE)-approved course in debridement. The WOC nurse and nurse specializing in wound care may perform conservative sharp wound debridement when the following criteria are met:

- The WOC nurse and wound care nurse confirm that their state nurse practice act recognizes debridement to be within the domain of nursing. It may be the nurses' preference to obtain a letter from the state board of nursing to be kept on file with the employer.
- A policy and procedure is in place with the employing institution or contracting agency, which addresses educational preparation, certification, and a validation process for conservative sharp wound debridement.
- Conservative sharp wound debridement is conducted with the awareness the patient's primary health care provider. In some health care settings and states, an order for conservative sharp wound debridement may be necessary from the physician.
- To further refine the technical skill of conservative sharp wound debridement, it is recommended that the WOC nurse and wound care nurse collaborate with physicians such as plastic surgeons, dermatologists, or surgeons.

The indication for conservative sharp wound debridement is the presence of loose necrotic tissue in a dermal ulcer. The etiology of the ulcer includes, but is not limited to, pressure, neuropathy, and arterial and venous insufficiency. Contraindications to conservative sharp wound debridement include the following situations:

- Densely adherent necrotic tissue in which the interface between viable and nonviable tissue cannot be clearly identified.
- The patient who is at an increased risk of bleeding, such as the individual with an impaired clotting mechanism.
- The noninfected ischemic ulcer that is covered with dry eschar. In this setting, tissue oxygenation is insufficient to support infection control and wound healing, therefore placing the patient at risk for a serious infectious complication. Examples include, but are not limited to, arterial ulcers or diabetic ulcers with dry gangrene.

CHAPTER 8

Wound Infection: Diagnosis and Management

NANCY A. STOTTS

OBJECTIVES

1. Define *wound infection.*
2. Compare and contrast contamination, colonization, and wound infection.
3. Compare and contrast signs and symptoms of infection in acute and chronic wounds.
4. Identify risk factors for wound infection.
5. Describe how to identify a wound infection.
6. Describe how to obtain a wound culture by biopsy, aspiration, and swab.
7. Interpret laboratory data indicative of a wound infection.
8. Understand the therapies that can be used to treat wound infection.

INFECTION AS A SIGNIFICANT PROBLEM

Infection is a serious wound-healing problem. It results in delayed healing, disruption of wound tensile strength, pain, increased length of hospital stay, and additional cost of care. Infection increases the patient's risk of bacteremia, sepsis, multisystem organ failure, and death (Bryan, Dew, and Reynolds, 1983; Garibaldi, Brodine, and Matsumiya, 1981; Thomas et al, 1996).

Acute and chronic wounds are both at risk of infection. Acute wounds are those that have a rapid onset and normally heal as predicted (Lazarus et al, 1994). Surgical wounds are the predominant acute wound. More than 27 million surgeries are performed in the United States annually. Infection is the most frequent postsurgical complication, and 38% of those diagnosed with infection have a wound infection. Most deaths caused by wound infection involve infection of organs or body cavities (Mangram et al, 1999).

Chronic wounds are those that do not heal in a timely manner to full functional and structural integrity (Lazarus et al, 1994), and they consist primarily of pressure ulcers, vascular ulcers, and diabetic ulcers. In the chronic wound population, pressure ulcers and vascular ulcers are the most frequent wounds. In one study of persons with pressure ulcers in seven skilled nursing facilities, local infection is reported in about 6% of patients (Garibaldi, Brodine, and Matsumiya, 1981). Osteomeyelitis is seen in 17% to 26% of patients with nonhealing ulcers (Darouiche et al, 1994). Bacteremia, sepsis, and death are seen as a part of the pressure ulcer continuum (Thomas et al, 1996). In one study when the pressure ulcer was the most likely site of sepsis, 56.9% of patients died as a result of the infection (Bryan, Dew, and Reynolds, 1983).

Vascular disease results in alterations in blood flow, often to the lower extremities. About 70% to 80% of vascular ulcers are venous, 10% to 15% are arterial, and the rest are mixed. Trauma to ischemic lower extremities results in an ulcer. The underlying vascular pathology produces a relative hypoxia that contributes to delayed healing and infection (Stadelmann, Digenis, and Tobin, 1998).

Diabetic patients are at risk for foot ulcer infection because of high glucose level, neuropathy, and small vessel disease. The ulcer often occurs because of repeated trauma to an insensate foot. Necrosis occurs deep in the foot architecture, and when the wound necrosis extends through to the skin, the wound becomes contaminated. The wound often is deep, warm, and full of necrotic material, an ideal environment to support organisms. Cultures often show multiple organisms, including gram-positive and gram-negative organisms, aerobes, and anaerobes (Steed, 1998). Amputation often is needed because of uncontrolled infection in the lower extremities of persons with diabetes.

Contamination, Colonization, and Infection

Contamination is the presence of microorganisms on the wound surface. It is often found in surface debris such as feces and soil. The contaminants themselves are not visible to care providers and do not elicit a response from the body. At times, surface contaminants multiply on the tissue surface and then the wound is considered colonized. The microorganisms that colonize wounds do not contribute to the chronicity of the wound, and only occasionally is the same organism that colonizes the wound shown to be the one causing the infection (Mertz and Ovington, 1993). When microorganisms invade the tissues, infection is present. Usually signs of local inflammation and pus or exudate are present. If the organisms are gram negative, unusual odor often occurs. Fever and leukocytosis may be present. Occasionally with infection, hypothermia is seen, indicating a poor central nervous system response and poor potential for a positive outcome. Generally it is agreed that culture results for wound infection show $>10^5$ organisms/gram of tissue (or as few as 10^3 organisms/gram of tissue if a virulent organism such as β-hemolytic streptococcus is present) (Robson, 1997).

Host-Microorganism Defenses

Infection occurs when the homeostatic balance among the host, organism, and environment is disrupted (Robson, 1997). The host's first line of defense is the skin, which is not intact in those who have a wound. Microorganisms are present on all wounds, yet the presence of organisms on the surface of the wound does not necessarily mean an infection will result.

The relationship between microorganisms and the host is kept in balance by the host defense mechanisms. When organisms invade tissues, the body's immune system is stimulated. The inflammatory response occurs and brings white blood cells (WBCs) and enzymes into the affected tissues. Neutrophils are mobilized, and the host's neutrophils phagocytose invading organisms. Lymphocytes are stimulated and release lymphokines that recruit neutrophils and monocytes to the area of injury. Exudate increases because of the capillary permeability and the increased number of cells recruited to the area. If the individual was previously exposed to the same organism, antibodies are activated to fight the organism. The interleukins mediate the acute phase response that is characterized by redness, warmth, swelling, pain, and impaired function.

The host's response leads to resolution of the problem, a localization of the infection, or chronic inflammation. When the chronic inflammatory response occurs, monocytes and lymphocytes are brought to the area. The monocytes are converted to tissue macrophages and become the long-term clean-up cells in the wound. Fibroblast proliferation is supported during this phase, leading to increased fibrotic tissue in the area of chronic inflammation.

Microorganisms have several weapons to fight the body's defenses. The organisms' ability to cause infection is related to several factors, including toxins, adherence factors, evasive factors, and invasive factors.

Toxins. Toxins destroy or alter the normal function of the host's cells and are described as exotoxins and endotoxins. Exotoxins are proteins released form the bacteria that enzymatically inactivate or modify cells, causing their death or dysfunction. Endotoxins are lipids and polysaccharides that are located in the cell wall of gram-negative organisms. When released, they activate the regulatory systems of the body (e.g., clotting, inflammation). Excessive activity in these systems may result in shock.

Adherence Factors. Infection depends on the adherence of the organism to the host's body. Attachment requires that the organisms bond with a receptor using a ligand (the substance that binds to the receptor). Some are site specific (e.g., mucous membrane), others are cell specific (e.g., T lymphocytes), and others are nonspecific (e.g., moist surface). Colonization and ultimately invasion of the

TABLE 8-1 Criteria for Incisional and Organ/Space Surgical Site Infection

SUPERFICIAL SSI	DEEP INCISIONAL SSI	ORGAN/SPACE SSI
• Purulent drainage • Positive wound culture • At least one of the following signs or symptoms of infection: pain or tenderness, local swelling, redness, or heat; superficial incision is deliberately opened by a surgeon unless incision is culture negative • Diagnosis by surgeon or attending physician	• Purulent drainage • Incision dehisces or is opened by physician when the patient had one of the following: fever, local pain, tenderness (unless the site is culture negative) • An abscess or other evidence of infection found on examination, x-ray, or histopathology • Diagnosis by surgeon or attending physician	• Purulent drainage • Positive wound culture • Abscess or other evidence of infection found on examination, x-ray, or histopathology • Diagnosis by surgeon or attending physician

tissue by microorganisms cannot occur without attachment.

Evasive Factors. Some organisms can alter the environment in which they live so that the host's immune system cannot locate them and/or has difficulty destroying them. These evasive factors include capsules, slime, and mucous layers. Others such as *Staphylococcus aureus* have the capacity to produce a surface protein that immobilizes the host's immunoglobulin, making it difficult for the host's antigens to reach the organism.

Invasive Factors. Invasive factors are the fourth type of microorganism defense. They allow the microorganism to penetrate the host tissue. Most of these invasive factors are enzymes (e.g., proteases) that break down cells and allow the microorganism to invade the tissue (Porth, 1998). The host defenses and the microorganism's mechanisms compete. If the microorganism overwhelms the host's defenses, infection occurs (Robson, 1997).

Effects of Infection

Microorganisms in wound tissue use nutrients and oxygen that were intended for repair. In this way they rob the tissues of nutrient flow. In addition, microorganisms release enzymes that break down the protein. The enzymes degrade fibrin that is essential for fibroblast migration and maintenance of macrophage activity.

The presence of necrotic material and slough increases the deleterious effects of the organisms. Dead tissue provides a medium for the growth of microorganisms. They stimulate the inflammatory mediators and cytokines. Thus the inflammatory response is augmented and prolonged. Enzymes are released that result in the breakdown of the fibrin matrix needed for fibroblast migration, and they also inactivate growth factors. Exotoxins also are released from the organisms and inhibit migration of keratinocytes and fibroblasts (Stadelmann, Digenis, and Tobin, 1998). Debridement of necrotic material is critical to reverse infection because debridement reduces the bacterial burden and decreases the factors that inhibit growth factors and migration of cells.

Infection in Surgical Wounds

Surgical wound infection has been termed *surgical site infection* (SSI) and occurs within 30 days of surgery or within 1 year if an implant has been inserted and the infection involves the site of the surgery. SSI is an incisional infection or organ/space infection (Mangram et al, 1999). Incisional infection involves only skin or subcutaneous tissue at the incision. Deep incision infection involves the deep tissues, including the muscles and fascia. Infection of the organ/spaces involves organs or body cavities that were manipulated during surgery. Criteria for diagnosing various types of SSI are listed in Table 8-1. A stitch abscess, infection of an episiotomy or newborn circumcision site, and an infected burn are not classified as SSIs (Mangram et al, 1999).

BOX 8-1 Signs and Symptoms of Infection in Chronic Wounds

Drainage excess, change in color/consistency
Redness
Warmth around the wound
Poor granulation tissue
Pain or tenderness
Unusual odor
Sudden high glucose in patient with diabetes

Infection in Chronic Wounds

Chronic wounds often are more highly contaminated than surgical wounds. This may be because they are open to the environment, often have necrotic material present, and have irregular surfaces that house microorganisms. Usually they are manipulated for dressing changes and thus are exposed to the potential for cross-contamination (Kerstein, 1996). Although not well studied in the literature, these wounds may occur in persons who are debilitated and their ability to respond to the organism may be impaired.

The signs of infection in chronic wounds are listed in Box 8-1 (Kerstein, 1996; Mertz and Ovington, 1993). The erythema, edema and pain are secondary to the inflammatory response. The elevated neutrophil count and local wound pus reflect the WBC response to invasion by microorganisms. Change in the color of the exudate usually reflects a change in the organism present. Uncharacteristic odor usually is secondary to the presence of gram-negative organisms and anaerobes (Ademiluyi et al, 1988). Elevated glucose levels may be due to the insulin resistance that accompanies stress (Stotts and Whitney, 1999).

There is controversy about the meaning of the number and types of organisms in chronic wounds, but most authors agree that $>10^5$ organisms/gram of tissue is diagnostic of infection (Kerstein, 1996; Stadelmann, Digenis, and Tobin, 1998; Steed, 1998). Clinically this becomes a moot point because wound cultures are not routinely performed in most settings. Usually a culture is taken when signs of infection are present or when a clean wound does not show any progress in healing in 2 weeks (Panel on the Treatment of Pressure Ulcers, 1994). On the other hand, some providers do not obtain a culture but treat the patient empirically.

DIAGNOSIS OF INFECTION

The diagnosis of wound infection is made using a combination of history, physical examination, and laboratory work. This triad gives the provider a holistic view of the patient.

History

The history is critical in the diagnostic process because the findings from it focus the physical examination and the laboratory work. The history is obtained from the patient and/or caregiver and available records. The initial focus is on when the wound occurred, how it occurred, the environment in which it occurred, the presence of a systemic infection, and the effects of prior treatments on healing and infection. The provider needs to understand whether the wound is chronic or acute because this information will help direct the plan of treatment. Important data to elicit in the history pertain to the patient and systemic characteristics. Factors to include are age, cognitive ability, functional ability, level of mobility, caregiver ability, medications, nutritional status, and concurrent conditions, such as diabetes, venous and arterial disease, and liver and kidney function (Stotts and Whitney, 1999). Risk factors for wound infection are listed in Box 8-2.

Physical Examination

The physical examination is pivotal in the diagnosis of infection. Along with the classic signs of inflammation, the nurse should also pay close attention to the characteristics of the drainage from the wound. The inflammation process is natural and expected; however, if inflammation persists for 5 days, infection should be suspected. Immunosuppressed patients, such as those who are malnourished, diabetic, or receiving steroids or chemotherapy, may have a slower or less pronounced inflammatory response.

Data from the physical examination for surgical patients needs to be categorized according to the Criteria for Diagnosis of Incisional and Organ/

BOX 8-2 Risk Factors for Wound Infection

Deficiencies of vitamins and minerals: vitamins A, B, C, D, or K; minerals zinc, copper, or magnesium
Diseases: liver, kidney, or heart failure; diabetes
Drugs: steroids, nonsteroidal antiinflammatory, chemotherapeutic agents
Foreign debris: sutures
Immunodeficiency
Ischemia
Hypoxia
Hypothermia
Necrotic material
Remote infection
Smoking/tobacco use

Plus the following for surgical patients:
Prolonged preoperative stay
Preoperative nares colonization with *Staphylococcus aureus*
Perioperative transfusion

BOX 8-3 Clinical Indications for a Wound Culture

Local signs of infection: pus, change in odor or character of exudate, redness, induration, change in wound odor
Systemic signs of infection: fever, leukocytosis
Suddenly high glucose
Pain in neuropathic extremity
Lack of healing after 2 weeks in a clean wound

Space SSI that were created by the Centers for Disease Control and Prevention (CDC) (see Table 8-1). Chronic wounds may present with more subtle symptoms. The nurse should be alert to a change in the amount or character of exudate, redness, and warmth around the wound; poor quality granulation tissue; pain and tenderness that did not previously exist; and change in wound odor. A sudden high glucose level also is a heralding sign of infection. Table 8-1 and Box 8-1 list the signs of acute and chronic wound infection.

Laboratory Tests

Laboratory tests also play an important role in the diagnosis of infection. The categories of tests that are important in the diagnosis of wound infection are blood work and wound culture. A complete blood count (CBC) should be obtained when infection is suspected. It is a quick and relatively noninvasive test that with infection shows an increase in the number of WBCs. The differential may show an increase in bands or immature neutrophils. This is called a "shift to the left" and denotes an impending infection.

A wound culture is performed to identify the number of organisms present, to diagnose infection, to identify the organism causing the infection, and to identify the antibiotic that will kill the organism. Clinical indications for culture are listed in Box 8-3. Wound culture is used to examine tissue for aerobic and anaerobic organisms. It also can be used to obtain a specimen for a Gram's stain, a method recognized as a rapid diagnostic technique to identify infection (Duke, Robson, and Krizek, 1972; Levine et al, 1976). For a Gram's stain, the tissue fluid is placed on a slide, treated with various stains, and viewed under a microscope. In wounds where swabs yielded $<10^5$ organisms, a Gram's stain shows no bacteria and the culture is negative. Results from a Gram's stain can be expected in 20 minutes, a preliminary culture report in 24 hours, and a final culture and sensitivity within 48 hours.

The wound culture needs to be taken from clean, healthy-appearing tissue (Stotts, 1995). Because infection involves the tissue, it is important to culture the tissue rather than pus, slough, eschar, or necrotic material. Although a laboratory report will be produced if pus, eschar, or necrotic tissue is cultured, the results will reflect the microflora of that site and will not provide an accurate profile of the microflora in the tissue. In fact, the results will be a false report—the only question is the type of error. It could be false positive (organisms present in the area that is cultured but not present in the tissue), false negative (organisms not present in the area that is cultured but present in the tissue), or a chance agreement (area that is cultured and tissue have the same result). A false negative is problematic in that the patient has an infection and needs to have it treated. The patient's condition may deteriorate if not treated. A false positive is problematic in that the patient is treated when there is not a need, increasing the risk of side effects of the antibiotic and the development of organism resistance. The probability that the number and type of organism in the area that is cultured is the same as that in the tissue is small because data indicate that even within the same wound tissue, the number and type of organisms vary (Levine et al, 1976).

The three major types of wound cultures are tissue culture, aspiration culture, and swab culture. Tissue biopsy for culture is removal of a piece of tissue with a scalpel or punch biopsy. The wound may be anesthetized topically or by injection. Topical anesthetic is preferred because it does not affect the fluid balance in the tissue and so will not affect the culture results. The open wound is cleansed with a nonantiseptic sterile solution. A biopsy specimen is taken from the tissue, and bleeding is controlled. Once in the laboratory, the specimen is processed and plated (Robson and Heggers, 1969).

Needle aspiration involves insertion of a needle into the tissue adjacent to the wound to aspirate tissue fluid. If organisms are present in the tissue, they can be detected in the tissue fluid (Lee, Turnidge, and McDonald, 1985). Intact skin next to the wound is disinfected and allowed to dry. Fanning the area to speed drying is not recommended because it allows the organisms in the environment to settle on the biopsy tissue. Equipment needed is a 10 ml disposable syringe and a 22-gauge needle. About 0.5 ml of air is drawn into the syringe, and the needle is inserted through intact skin adjacent to the wound. Suction is applied by withdrawing the plunger to the 10 ml mark. The needle is moved backward and forward at different angles for 2 to 4 explorations. After the needle is withdrawn from the tissue, the plunger is gently returned to the 0.5 ml mark and the syringe is capped. The aspirated fluid is plated in the laboratory. If tissue is extracted using this technique, it is processed as described for tissue biopsy.

The swab technique often has been criticized as a method that provides data about the organisms on the ulcer surface rather than in the tissue. In part this may be an accurate appraisal because the swab technique has been performed inconsistently. Frequently, the eschar, pus, or exudate has been cultured before wound cleansing (Morison, 1992; Pagana and Pagana, 1992) or the culture is obtained using a "Z technique" (side to side across the wound from one edge to the other) after the wound was cleansed (Alvarez, Rozint, and Meehan, 1990; Cuzzell, 1993). Others irrigate the wound with sterile water or saline and press the swab against the wound margin or ulcer base to elicit fresh exudate (Association for Professionals in Infection Control and Epidemiology, 1996).

BOX 8-4 Tips on Wound Culturing

- Obtain the culture before administering antibiotics.
- Obtain the culture from clean tissue.
- Collect the specimen using sterile technique.
- Do not contaminate the specimen when placing it in the container.
- Collect sufficient specimen for examination.
- If a Gram's stain will be done, obtain enough specimen.
- Place the specimen in an appropriate container.
- Complete the laboratory slip to provide clinical data for the microbiologist.
- Transport quickly to the laboratory to keep the organisms viable.

The method of Levine and colleagues (1976) is recommended for swab culture. The wound is cleansed with a sterile nonantiseptic solution. The swab or applicator is moistened with normal saline (without preservative) because the moistened swab provides more precise data than a dry swab (Georgiade et al, 1970). The end of a sterile alginate applicator is rotated in 1 cm^2 of clean tissue in the open wound. Pressure is applied to the swab to elicit tissue fluid. When the tip of the swab is saturated, it is inserted into the appropriate sterile container and transported to the laboratory. If a Gram's stain is to be performed, a second swab is obtained from the same clean tissue site.

Of these three techniques, the tissue biopsy for culture is the gold standard. Obtaining a piece of the tissue and identifying the organisms present is the most optimal approach to wound culture. A physician or nurse with special training must perform a biopsy.* One of the limitations of the technique is that many facilities do not process tissue for culture and therefore the method cannot be used. In addition, obtaining a tissue culture requires disruption of the wound, so healing may be delayed and it may cause the patient pain because it requires cutting living tissue.

Aspiration and swab are alternative approaches to wound culture. Aspiration technique underestimates the bioburden, whereas swab technique overestimates the tissue burden. With aspiration technique, the operator needs to understand the structures being penetrated by the needle. The risk is that the needle will inadvertently cause damage to a nerve or other structure and result in iatrogenic damage. Box 8-4 lists tips for successful and accurate wound culture.

PRINCIPLES OF TREATMENT OF WOUND INFECTION

Wounds do not heal until infection is eradicated. Thus the goal of treatment in wound infection is to kill the microorganisms without damaging healthy tissue while precipitating the fewest possible side effects.

Treatment can be local and systemic. Local treatment of the wound focuses on reduction of bioburden. Debridement is the most important local treatment because it removes dead tissue and foreign materials. Debridement can be performed surgically, chemically, or autolytically. In addition to removing dead tissue, sharp debridement also changes a chronic wound into an acute wound, stimulating the inflammatory process and healing.

Surgical debridement is a method of rapidly removing necrotic material. A physician or nurse with special training must perform it.* The advantage of surgical debridement is that it rapidly and efficiently removes dead tissue from the wound. The major limitation of the technique is that viable tissue may unintentionally be resected. It also may be accompanied by pain when viable tissue is removed.

Enzymatic debridement is the breakdown of necrotic material using exogenous enzymes that are applied topically. It is a slower process than surgical debridement but is not accompanied by the potential loss of viable tissue nor the pain and discomfort that are seen with sharp debridement.

Autolysis is the use of body's own immune system to debride, holding the body fluids in place with dressings. This is a very slow process but is appropriate when small areas need debridement. The strength of the technique is that a moist environment is provided, and debridement with this technique takes part of the normal local care of the wound.

Topical agents can be used to treat wound infection. The agent should be carefully selected, based on the specific organism that has been identified. Sensitivity testing can be performed for topical antimicrobials such as silvadine and bacitracin and should be used in the selection of the agent (Stadelmann, Digenis, and Tobin, 1998). The formulation of the agent is important in its effectiveness. For example, elemental iodine kills a number of cells important to healing, but when formulated as cadexomer iodine gel, it contains microspheres that absorb bacteria while slowly releasing iodine (Stadelmann, Digenis, and Tobin, 1998).

The goal of care during this phase of the healing trajectory is reduction of bioburden. Once the bioburden falls to $<10^5$ organisms/gram of tissue, the patient's immune system usually is able to complete the cleanup. At that point, healing becomes the goal of care. However, although reduction of bioburden is the goal of care, it may make sense in some situations to cleanse the wound with antiseptics to reduce those organisms on the surface of the wound so that they do not become adherent, colonize the wound, and then cause infection. There are no studies, however, that support this perspective.

The dressing selected should keep the wound moist but not allow exudate to accumulate on the wound surface or on the periwound tissue. Exudate on the wound becomes a media for the microorganisms to proliferate, and exudate that extends

* The state nurse practice act must stipulate that nurses with special training are allowed to perform this procedure. Also, the institution or agency needs to address who can perform this procedure in its policies and procedures.

beyond the wound will lead to maceration of surrounding tissue, making that intact tissue more susceptible to invasion by microorganisms.

The wound should be cleansed routinely. This is a treatment not aimed specifically at curing the infection but rather at reducing the surface contaminants. As with routine cleansing of the wound, the pressure should be between 4 and 15 psi. Normal saline is the recommended agent to use when cleansing a wound. If the slough is thick, commercial wound cleansers may be used because they contain surfactants that enhance their effectiveness. Whirlpool should be considered if the slough is thick and adherent or when necrotic tissue is not readily removed by other means (Panel on the Treatment of Pressure Ulcers, 1994).

Antibiotics are appropriate when there is a systemic response to infection, such as cellulitis, leukocytosis, or fever (Stadelmann, Digenis, and Tobin, 1998). When antibiotics are used, it is critical that the blood level be maintained so the therapeutic effect can be achieved. This means that the timing of administration of antibiotics is critical.

Other systemic therapies are important to control infection, and these focus on therapies to support nutrient blood flow to the wound (Hunt and Hopf, 1997). Adequate perfusion needs to be provided so that blood flow can get to the wound and the local environment will contain the macrophages and lymphocytes to clean up the area. This means that intravascular volume needs to be maintained through oral or intravenous fluids. Nutrients are provided to support cellular activities. Pain management is critical to the perfusion because pain control overcomes vasoconstriction and supports nutrient blood flow. Keeping the area warm but not hot also optimizes blood flow (Hunt and Hopf, 1997).

There are limited data about patients' psychologic response to having a wound infection, the sociologic adaptations that take place, and the effect of the wound infection and its treatment on the family unit. Addressing psychosocial issues and inclusion of the family and/or involvement of social services in the plan of care may prove to be pivotal to patient outcomes. Effective recovery may require comprehensive assessment and mobilization of the needed resources to address the patient and the wound infection.

CASE STUDY

Mr. G is a 75-year-old Hispanic man who has been admitted to your service with a right trochanteric pressure ulcer that cannot be staged. He became dizzy and fell at home. He could not arise and was trapped in the bathtub for 30 hours. The ulcer is 4 cm in diameter and is filled with malodorous yellow-gray slough. By history, Mr. G has type I diabetes mellitus and glaucoma. The etiology of his dizziness is unknown.

The immediate goal of care for the pressure ulcer is to control bacterial burden in the ulcer. The necrotic tissue must be removed, and you consider the time and resources required for each type of debridement (surgical, enzymatic, and autolytic). Surgical debridement is indicated because the depth and extent of the ulcer cannot be known until the base of the wound is visible and the patient is at risk for bacteremia and sepsis should this area become infected. After debridement, the wound is 5 cm deep with 2.5 cm undermining running from the 3 o'clock to 9 o'clock positions and extending to 3 cm from the 9 o'clock to 12 o'clock positions. There are no signs of infection, so culture is not indicated. Local care after debridement includes the use of Silvadene in course mesh gauze. Because of the large amount of tissue insult, close monitoring and management of his diabetes are paramount for subsequent healing.

SELF-ASSESSMENT EXERCISE

1. Infection is when microorganisms:
   - **a.** Reside on the surface of the wound
   - **b.** Invade the tissue
   - **c.** Multiply on the wound
   - **d.** Reside on the surface and multiply there
2. Which of the following statements accurately characterizes colonization of a wound?
   - **a.** Colonization is associated with a fever
   - **b.** Colonization is manifested by local inflammation of the wound

   c. Colonization is diagnosed with a culture result of $>10^5$ organisms/gram of tissue
   d. Colonization is often present without clinical signs of an infection
3. Mr. H is a 35-year-old man with an open wound of his foot after he was dragged by a tractor in a farm accident 3 days ago. He does not have insurance and so did not seek medical assistance at the time of the injury. He comes today because he has shaking chills. By history he is a healthy active adult. On physical examination you find that he has abrasions over his legs, but x-ray examination shows no fracture. The wound involves the plantar surface of his foot where a triangular flap is visible, but the wound is filled with eschar and its depth cannot be evaluated. The entire foot is reddened, swollen, and hot. He is alert, oriented, and concerned. The major risk factor for infection in this man is:
   a. Local wound environment because of the contamination
   b. Malnutrition because he has not eaten well as a result of his fever
   c. Ischemia resulting from trauma to the foot and leg
   d. Immunosuppression resulting from the stress of the injury
4. All of the following define *surgical site infection except:*
   a. $>10^5$ organisms/gram of tissue
   b. Redness, induration, and local warmth surrounding a wound
   c. Purulent drainage
   d. Increased WBCs
5. Infection in a neuropathic ulcer located on the left plantar surface of a 63-year-old man with diabetes could be diagnosed with:
   a. Pain at the ulcer site
   b. Sudden low glucose level
   c. $<10^3$ organisms/gram of tissue
   d. Redness and induration
6. You inadvertently contaminated a culture when you were obtaining it. How should the findings be interpreted?
   a. False positive. The laboratory work shows infection when it really is not present
   b. False negative. The laboratory work shows no infection when in fact it is present
   c. False. You cannot know if the patient had infection because of the contamination
   d. Accurate. A little contamination is expected because the skin is always contaminated
7. In a culture obtained by aspiration, you would expect the number of organisms to be:
   a. More than by swab culture
   b. More than by tissue biopsy
   c. The same as by swab culture
   d. Fewer than on tissue biopsy
   e. Accurate because comparisons do not matter
8. To get the most accurate culture, it is important that the specimen be taken from:
   a. Pus
   b. Necrotic tissue or slough
   c. Exudate
   d. Healthy-looking tissue
9. Comprehensive wound treatment of a 47-year-old patient with an open wound of the abdomen secondary to retroperitonneal abscess includes:
   a. Pain control
   b. Regular dressing changes
   c. Nutritional support
   d. Adequate oral/IV intake
   e. All of the above

REFERENCES

Ademiluyi SA et al: The anaerobic and aerobic bacterial flora of leg ulcers in patients with sickle-cell disease. *J Infect* 7(2):115, 1988.

Alvarez O, Rozint J, Meehan M: Principles of moist wound healing: indications for chronic wounds. In Krasner D editor: *Chronic wound care,* King of Prussia, Penn, 1990, Health Management Publications.

Association for Professionals in Infection Control and Epidemiology: *Infection control and applied epidemiology: principles and practice,* St Louis, 1996, Mosby.

Bryan CS, Dew CE, Reynolds KL: Bacteremia associated with decubitus ulcers, *Arch Intern Med* 143(11):2093, 1983.

Cuzzell JZ: The right way to culture a wound. *Am J Nurs* 93(5):48, 1993

Darouiche RO et al: Osteomyelitis associated with pressure sores, *Arch Intern Med* 154(7):753, 1994.

Duke WF, Robson MC, Krizek TJ: Civilian wounds, their bacterial flora and rate of infection, *Surg Forum* 23(0):518, 1972.

Garibaldi RA, Brodine S, Matsumiya S: Infections among patients in nursing homes: policies, prevalence, problems, *N Engl J Med* 305(13):731, 1981.

Georgiade NG et al: A comparison of methods for the quantification of bacteria in burn wounds, *Am J Clin Pathol* 53(1):35, 1970.

Hunt TK, Hopf HW: Wound healing and wound infection: what surgeons and anesthesiologists can do, *Surg Clin North Am* 77(3):587, 1997.

Kerstein M: Wound infection: assessment and management, *Wounds* 8(4):141, 1996.

Lazarus GS et al: Definition and guidelines for assessment if wounds and evaluation of healing, *Arch Dermatol* 130: 489, 1994.

Lee P, Turnidge J, McDonald PJ: Fine-needle aspiration biopsy in diagnosis of soft tissue infections, *J Clin Microbiol* 22(1):80, 1985.

Levine NS et al: The quantitative swab culture and smear: a quick simple method for determining the number of viable aerobic bacteria on open wounds, *J Trauma* 16(2):89, 1976.

Mangram AJ et al: Guideline for prevention of surgical site infection, *Am J Infect Control* 27(2):97, 1999.

Mertz PM, Ovington LG: Wound healing microbiology, *Dermatol Clin* 11(4):739, 1993.

Morison MJ: *A colour guide to the nursing management of wounds,* Oxford, 1992, Blackwell Scientific.

Pagana KD, Pagana TJ: *Mosby's diagnostic and laboratory test reference,* St Louis, 1992, Mosby.

Panel on the Treatment of Pressure Ulcers: *Clinical practice guideline: treatment of pressure ulcers,* Number 15, Rockville, Md, 1994, U.S. Department of Health and Human Services, AHCPR Pub No 95-0652.

Porth CM: *Pathophysiology,* ed 5, Philadelphia, 1998, J.B. Lippincott.

Robson MC: Wound infection: a failure of wound healing caused by an imbalance of bacteria, *Surg Clin North Am* 77(3):637, 1997.

Robson MC, Heggers JP: Bacterial quantification of open wounds, *Mil Med* 134:19, 1969.

Stadelmann WJ, Digenis AG, Tobin GR: Impediments to wound healing, *Am J Surg* 176(suppl 2A):39S, 1998.

Steed DL: Foundations of good ulcer care, *Am J Surg* 1998(suppl 2A):20S, 1998.

Stotts NA: Determination of bacterial burden in wounds, *Adv Wound Care* 8(4):28, 1995.

Stotts NA, Whitney JD: Identifying and evaluating wound infection. *Home Healthcare Nurse* 17(3):159, 1999.

Thomas DR et al: Hospital acquired pressure ulcers and risk of death, *J Am Geriatr Soc* 44(12):1435, 1996.

CHAPTER 9

Acute Surgical And Traumatic Wound Healing

JUDITH M. WEST & MICHAEL L. GIMBEL

OBJECTIVES

1. State two factors from current research known to impair acute wound-repair processes.
2. Describe the microcirculation of an acute surgical or traumatic wound environment.
3. Discuss the effects of an activated sympathetic nervous system on acute wound-repair processes.
4. Differentiate among the roles of wound tissue oxygen and arterial oxygen in wound repair.
5. Describe five interventions to increase tissue oxygen in acute surgical and traumatic wounds.

BACKGROUND

The phenomenon of healing is an inescapable component of the human experience. The challenge of repairing bodily injury is complex. Tissue injury, whether accidental or planned, initiates a series of biochemical events directed toward reestablishing vascular and cellular integrity. During tissue repair, wound healing is vulnerable to a number of factors. Failure at any step of the sequence may impair wound healing and confer significant morbidity and cost.

A great deal has been learned about tissue repair over the last decade, although much of the information that has been acquired has not become standard in everyday clinical practice. The literature is a guide to a new understanding of the importance of adequate blood flow to peripheral tissues to supply oxygen for optimal wound healing and resistance to infection. This chapter addresses the autonomic nervous system, fluids and hydration, hypothermia, warming, and effective methods for achieving better wound-tissue perfusion.

OXYGEN

Availability of oxygen (Po_2) is essential for wound-healing processes, including oxidative bacterial killing and resistance to infection (Babior, 1978; Hohn et al, 1976; Knighton, Halliday, and Hunt, 1984), collagen synthesis and fibroplasia (Niinikoski, 1969), angiogenesis (Knighton, Silver, and Hunt, 1981), and epithelization (Pai and Hunt, 1972). Decreased local wound oxygen (tissue hypoxia) is a major contributor to wound complications (Goodson et al, 1987; Jonsson, Hunt, and Mathes, 1988; Knighton, Halliday, and Hunt, 1984).

Peripheral tissues may become hypoxic from direct traumatic or surgical injury to vessels or from blood volume loss and vasoconstriction of regional vasculature. Wound-tissue oxygen delivery may be impaired unless conditions of diminished peripheral perfusion are anticipated and corrected. Correction of adrenergic vasoconstrictive stimuli, particularly cold, pain, and volume loss, elevates Po_2 (Hopf et al, 1997; West, 1994) and leads to fewer postoperative infections (Kurz et al, 1996). The degree of regional tissue perfusion regulates the supply of oxygen and is therefore the prime determinant of the competency of wound healing. Strategies to optimize perfusion by addressing specific sympathetic nervous system activators are described in Table 9-1.

Arterial oxygen levels are not necessarily reflective of tissue oxygen delivery. Although the Pao_2 of 90 mm Hg in a healthy volunteer breathing room air maintains a wound Po_2 of 50 mm Hg or greater, the postoperative patient experiencing pain, cold, fear, or periodic desaturation will exhibit predictably low oxygen levels within the wound. This

TABLE 9-1 Optimizing Perfusion: Correcting Sympathetic Nervous System (SNS) Activation

SYMPATHETIC NERVOUS SYSTEM ACTIVATORS	INTERVENTIONS TO OPTIMIZE PERFUSION
Cold	Increase warmth by covering feet with socks or slippers, applying blankets or sweaters, and facilitating postoperative warming with warm blankets. Prevent heat loss, and prevent shivering.
Pain	Medicate for comfort (adequate pain control). Seek additional measures for pain control such as repositioning, relaxation, etc.
Fear	Provide patient teaching to reduce fear related to procedures or knowledge deficits. Administer medications as needed to reduce anxiety and fear.
Pharmacologic	Discontinue beta blockers.
Smoking	Refer patient to a tobacco cessation program. Encourage successful completion of entire program.

observation led to an approach to adrenergic activation as an etiology for wound hypoxia (West, 1990).

SURGICAL STRESS

Stress may be defined as the body's primitive protective response to injury or anticipated injury. Cannon (1970) revealed the mechanisms that activate the autonomic nervous system to respond to stress. He directly observed the constriction of blood vessels in peripheral tissues during stress in animals. The mediators of the sympathetic and adrenal response to stress, epinephrine and norepinephrine, induce profound vasoconstriction in subcutaneous and skin blood vessels supplying peripheral tissues (Rowell, 1986). Sympathetic activation in the postoperative period is a function of severing of afferent nerves, hypovolemia, fear, pain, and cold rather than anesthesia (Halter, Pflug, and Porte, 1977). Catecholamines may remain elevated for days after surgery (Derbyshire and Smith, 1984; Halter, Pflug, and Porte, 1977), and concentrations vary with length and severity of surgery (Chernow et al, 1987). Norepinephrine is increased three-fold in the early postoperative hours (Derbyshire and Smith, 1984), peaking with the patient's first expression of pain (Niinikoski, Heughan, and Hunt, 1972).

Infusion of exogenous epinephrine in healthy subjects, designed to mimic the body's response to stress, decreased subcutaneous tissue oxygen 45%, whereas heart rate and arterial PO_2 did not markedly change (Jensen et al, 1985). The relationship of tissue oxygen and perfusion of various tissues is well established in animal models (Gosain et al, 1991; Gottrup et al, 1987) and in humans (Jonsson et al, 1991).

Cutaneous capillary blood flow is determined chiefly by the direct effects of temperature on the amount of vasomotor tone. Local cooling increases norepinephrine affinity to alpha-adrenergic receptors on vascular smooth muscle, augmenting the response of cutaneous vessels to autonomic activation, increasing constrictive vessel tensions up to five-fold (Vanhoutte, Verbeuren, and Webb, 1981).

Hypothermia-induced vasoconstriction decreases subcutaneous oxygen tension in anesthetized volunteers (FIO_2 of 0.6 mm Hg) to a mean of 50 mm Hg (Sheffield et al, 1992). Furthermore, a lower blood temperature also shifts the oxyhemoglobin curve to the left, thereby increasing the amount of oxygen carried in the blood but decreasing the amount of oxygen released (Severinghaus, 1958). This effect may exacerbate tissue hypoxia induced by peripheral vasoconstriction.

A rapid initial decrease in core temperature (1° C to 2° C) during the first hour after the induction of anesthesia is characteristic of both general and regional anesthesia (Sessler, 1993) because virtually all anesthetic agents are vasodilators. Internal redistribution of body heat from core to periphery is exacerbated by conductive and evaporative losses as a result of visceral exposure in a cold environment (Roe, 1971). The rapid initial body heat loss may be limited by heating the operating room and aggressive preoperative warming (Morris, 1971) and may be nearly prevented by preinduction warming (Hynson and Sessler, 1992).

Adverse consequences of perioperative body heat loss include prolonged hypothermia and postoperative warming time in elderly patients and shivering. Shivering in the elderly, although rare, is dangerous because oxygen demand may increase by 400% to 500% (Bay, Nunn, and Prys-Roberts, 1968), thereby increasing cardiac workload. Increased oxygen consumption has been shown to coincide with core decrements of 0.3° C to 1.2° C (Roe et al, 1966). Prolonged postoperative hypothermia is associated with increased mortality (Slotman, Jed, and Burchard, 1985) and myocardial ischemia (Frank et al, 1993). Animal studies demonstrate that the harmful effects of cooling are proportional to the duration of the cooling period. In a series of canine studies comparing incised wounds of cooled limbs with contralateral uncooled limbs similarly wounded, there was a higher incidence of infection after delayed primary closure of the cooled limbs (Large and Heinbecker, 1944). The cooled limb wounds had less tensile strength, and sections taken immediately after cooling showed no histologic evidence of response to injury (inflammation).

Aggressive intraoperative warming and rapid postoperative warming are effective modalities for minimizing the risks of prolonged hypothermia (Hynson and Sessler, 1992). Sympathetic vasoconstriction can be overcome by warmth to provide uncomplicated healing. In a large study combining intraoperative and postoperative warming, wound infection rates were reduced by 60% (Kurz et al, 1996). Local radiant heating also increases subcutaneous blood flow in human wounds (Ikeda et al, 1998; Rabkin and Hunt, 1987; West, 1996).

Clinicians must demonstrate awareness and understanding of the ways in which the injured may be at risk for wound complications given his or her constellation of preinjury vulnerabilities. Wound-tissue hypoxia occurs to some extent at the time of injury in everyone, regardless of age or state of health (Silver, 1980). Early recognition and treatment of perfusion deficits translate to improved clinical outcome.

ACUTE WOUND

Human wounds can be characterized by the type and extent of tissue loss. Whether the surgeon's scalpel or other trauma causes a wound, viability of tissue will determine the course and quality of healing. Primarily closed incisional wounds resulting from elective surgery with the best of aseptic conditions and wound edge approximation appear to have the least reparative obstacles to healing. However, any tissue injury disrupts vascular supply. All wounds are relatively hypoxic at the center, in the range of 0 to 5 mm Hg (Silver, 1969). After oxygen leaves the red blood cells (RBCs) in the capillaries, it diffuses into the wound space. The driving force of diffusion is partial pressure. In wounds, damage to the microvasculature, vasoconstriction, and intravascular fluid overload markedly increase intercapillary distances (Goodson et al, 1979; Heughan, Ninikoski, and Hunt, 1972; Hunt and Hopf, 1997). In animal studies done in ear chamber wounds, the mean oxygen tensions were 0 to 3 mm Hg in the wound center dead space, 5 to 15 mm Hg in the growing edge, and 20 to 30 mm Hg in the newly vascularized area with early fibroblast proliferation. The steepest fall in oxygen occurred in the tissue within the first 25 microns of the wound edge (Niinikoski, Heughan, and Hunt, 1972; Silver, 1969).

Clinicians may assume that tissue hypoxia is present in all wounds. In most perioperative circumstances, healing can be enhanced (Chang et al, 1983; Hopf et al, 1997; Kurz et al, 1996; West, 1990). All surgical and traumatic wounds warrant concern and effort. The acute surgical wound is often cited as an example of a healthy, potentially "uncomplicated" wound that will heal "uneventfully" if left unperturbed. However, the most of the clinically relevant literature on healing addresses chronic or problematic wounds. At what points is the repair process stressed, compromised, or aborted? When and why does an acute wound, expected to have an uncomplicated and fairly predictable course, make the transition to a chronic and problematic wound? Hunt and Silver (Silver, 1969; Silver, 1980) focused attention on the study of events in the cellular microenvironment to discover how living tissue repairs itself when damaged. Explanation of the nature of the healing vs. nonhealing wound environments continues to be the major thrust of current wound-healing research (Gimbel and Hunt, 1999).

Comorbidities

Another important factor contributing to the potential for infection and failed healing is diabetes mellitus, which affects a large portion of the increasingly aging population undergoing surgical procedures. Elevated blood glucose levels are associated with significant reduction in the phagocytic ability of neutrophils and diminished wound strength (Goodson, 1979). Perhaps the single most advantageous action nurses can take to minimize risk is maintaining blood glucose levels at less than 200 mg/dl. Careful monitoring and control of diabetes should extend well into the postoperative period to optimize the healing environment during the months of collagen remodeling.

Presurgical morbidity is another critical variable, which may dramatically tip the balance against a favorable healing outcome. Poor nutrition before surgery correlates with decreased quality and quantity of collagen deposition (Goodson et al, 1987). Rapid preoperative replenishing of nutrients is effective in reducing postoperative wound complications (Hopf et al, 1997).

Fluid Status

A growing number of researchers have suggested that inspiration of increased oxygen concentration (FiO_2) be routinely prescribed for postoperative patients during the first few days after surgery to increase oxygen delivery to the reparative site. This practice is especially emphasized in patients undergoing lengthy abdominal or pelvic procedures. Correcting tissue hypoxia requires more than simply providing increased FiO_2 to increase the arterial saturation (SaO_2). Wound PO_2 may remain unchanged even while breathing additional oxygen. In one study of patients who underwent general surgery, approximately 30% had reduced tissue oxygen tension levels despite adequate urine output and arterial oxygen levels (Chang et al, 1983). This finding results from the early postoperative compartmental fluid shifts, in which kidney perfusion is restored at the expense of peripheral vasculature vasoconstriction. In addition, Jonsson and colleagues (1987) demonstrated that tissue oxygen levels could be corrected with infusion of fluids, and that a fluid bolus of 250 ml of normal saline was sufficient in most cases. In well-perfused patients, tissue oxygen pressure continues to rise as PaO_2 rises.

In a prospective randomized trial, aggressive postoperative warming and pain control increased the wound PO_2 to 70 mm Hg within 4 to 6 hours, a level nearly equal to that of normal volunteers (West, 1994). In addition, the actively rewarmed patients having undergone lengthy abdominal surgeries were given a 1-liter fluid bolus to replace fluids lost as urine during the diuresis, which commonly accompanies hypothermia and vasoconstriction. Trauma patients have demonstrated improved regional perfusion after warming and adequate fluid resuscitation (Knudson et al, 1997). Patients who are well perfused and oxygenated rarely get wound infections (Hopf et al, 1997).

Hypovolemia is a powerful physiologic vasoconstrictor. Therefore volume replacement must coincide with postoperative warming to benefit peripheral perfusion. Core temperature is not a clinically useful indicator in this equation. Skin surface temperatures do correlate with fingertip blood flow; a forearm-minus-fingertip difference of $>4°$ C defines a state of peripheral vasoconstriction. However, this method is not yet commonly used in practice (Rubinstein and Sessler, 1990).

Primary Dressing

Regardless of origin, wounds progress through the same phases of the reparative process: inflammation, angiogenesis, fibroplasia and matrix deposition, and epithelization. Knowledgeable assessments of the patient's surgical incision site include evaluation of the primary dressing, epithelial resurfacing, wound closure, healing ridge, and local changes at the wound site that may signal infection.

Theoretically, incisional dressings become unnecessary eventually. Despite this fact, many patients prefer that the wound remain covered. As healing evolves, some incisions begin to itch as a result of wound contraction or simply dry skin. Desire to view the surgical scar is personal. The presence of a dressing allows these patients to gradually incorporate changes in body image. Although an incisional dressing may no longer be necessary once epithelial cells have resurfaced the wound, a soft dressing placed over the suture line often limits local irritation and provides additional comfort and support, particularly as the patient begins to wear street clothes.

Because of the presence of intact epithelial appendages, such as hair follicles, and the relatively short distance that cells in the interrupted epithelial tissue must traverse, resurfacing of the wound closed by primary intention occurs relatively soon after wounding. Most incisions closed by primary intention are resurfaced within 2 to 3 days after surgery. Although the incisional wound does not have the structural integrity (tensile strength) to withstand force at this time, it is resurfaced and impenetrable to bacteria.

Healing Ridge

Deposition of collagen in the wound begins immediately in the inflammatory phase and peaks during the proliferative phase approximately 4 to 21 days after wounding. When healing progresses normally the clinician can detect the accumulation of new tissue synthesis by palpating what is referred to as the *healing ridge* (induration beneath the skin extending to about 1 cm on each side of the wound between 5 and 9 days after wounding). This is an expected positive sign. Lack of a ridge is cause for concern, and interventions to reduce mechanical strain on the wound need to be instituted promptly.

Hunt and Dunphy (1979) point out that "almost all dehiscences occur by the fifth to eighth postoperative day in patients who have not yet developed a cutaneous healing ridge and about half are associated with infection." Furthermore, they state that when a healing ridge is present, even retention sutures can be removed because the risk of separation has passed.

PATIENT EDUCATION

The knowledgeable nurse employs a theory-based assessment and coordinated therapeutic plan to optimize wound care within the context of a larger plan, including patient teaching and necessary follow-up. Patients in acute care settings require instruction in wound care, fluid replacement, avoidance of dehydration, and practical ways to conserve body heat. Unfortunately, this instruction occurs frequently at a time when the patient is fatigued and somewhat overwhelmed by the entire surgical experience. Teaching, in this case, is best done succinctly and should be reinforced by providing the patient or family member with written guidelines.

WOUND AS AN ORGAN

One problem in making clinically useful decisions about wounds is that the wrong things may be measured at the wrong times. In the wound microenvironment, what is happening *in* the wound may be discovered by sampling the wound itself (wound fluid, tissue, or oxygen tension). Infection, for example, is a function of bacteria *in* the tissue, not *on* the tissue. Just as myocardial dysfunction is confirmed by enzymes in the blood and thyroid alterations may be detectable by blood analysis, wound oxygen has become a useful measure of perfusion. Wound oxygen is a clinically valid and reliable index that responds more rapidly to intravascular fluid shifts than do blood pressure and pulse. When adequate oxygen is available for wound fibroblasts, collagen formation and wound tensile strength can be achieved. Collagen maturation then continues for months after wounding.

Although low initial periwound oxygen is a feature of most wounds, continued, unexplained hypoxia is of particular importance. Wound healing is proportional to local oxygen tension. Transcutaneous oxygen tension ($TcPo_2$) is a useful, noninvasive way to assess the adequacy of tissue oxygenation near a wound or suture line in relationship to Fio_2 (Plate 22).

Defining the contribution of hypoxia in the context of the recent history of the patient and time from wounding enables the nurse to explain why wound Po_2 is low. Tests can be conducted to reveal the wound's responsiveness to factors such as local

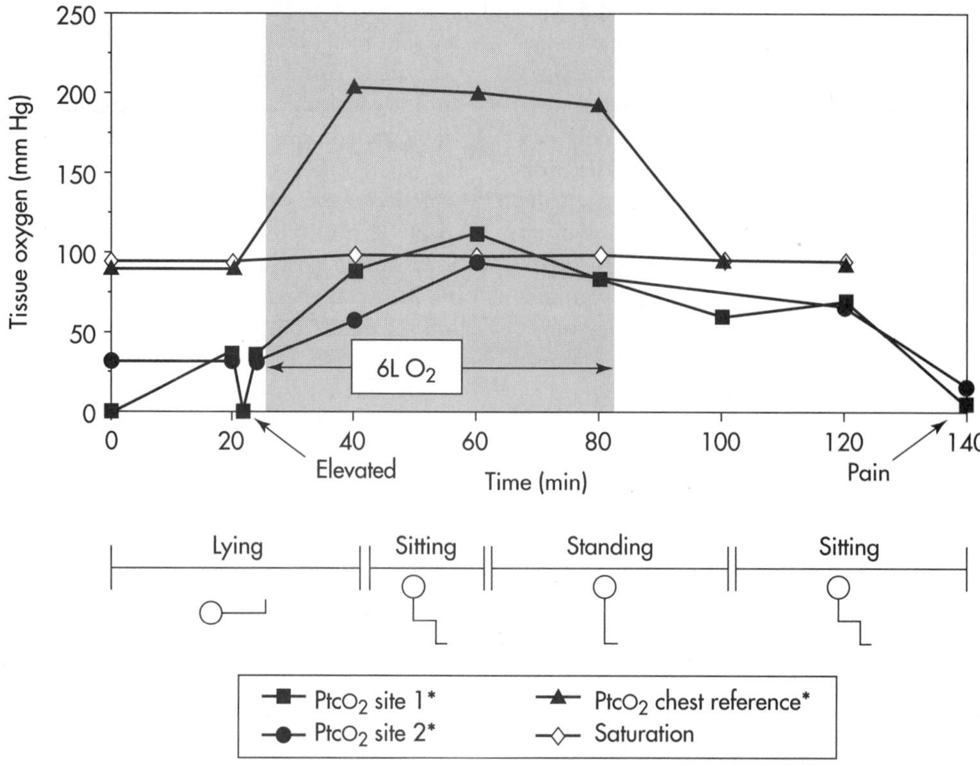

Figure 9-1 Graph demonstrating wound responsiveness to position changes and oxygen challenge. Wound Po_2 measurement with the patient breathing Fio_2 0.21 (room air), and then with a supplemental challenge at Fio_2 0.50 or greater, allows one to see how the periwound microvasculature is able to respond. Notice that only the oxygen challenge, not the chest reference, is affected by position changes. The $Ptco_2$ for site 1 is lower than for site 2 and for the chest reference in both the lying and sitting positions. However, it does demonstrate a response to 6 liters of oxygen.

warming, vasodilating drugs, oxygen therapies, sympathetic blockade, positioning, pain, and anxiety management (Figure 9-1). For example, during an oxygen challenge in the absence of vasoconstriction, there will be significant oxygen diffusion into the capillary-perfused wound edge. Simple, effective, and conservative corrective therapy can then be initiated. Since improved wound Po_2 is a real measure of wound healing progress, serial measurements of damaged tissue can be obtained during the course of healing.

SUMMARY

All components of repair must be enhanced, step by step, to keep the wound "healing." From the onset of injury, any interference with oxygen delivery to any degree will proportionately compromise reparative processes and increase susceptibility to infection (Hunt and Dunphy, 1979).

SELF-ASSESSMENT EXERCISE

1. State two wound-healing outcomes that require molecular oxygen.
2. Define three observable characteristics of a healing acute surgical wound.
3. True or false. Urine output >50 ml/hr correlates well with adequate wound Po_2.
4. True or false. Pao_2 is a measure of tissue oxygen (Po_2).

5. State four nursing interventions to optimize wound-tissue perfusion.
6. Describe the significance of the healing ridge in an acute surgical wound.
7. State five contributors to sympathetic nervous system activation.
8. To optimize the phagocytic ability of neutrophils, blood glucose levels should be maintained:
   - a. Between 40 and 80 mg/dl
   - b. Between 80 and 130 mg/dl
   - c. Less than 150 mg/dl
   - d. Less than 200 mg/dl

REFERENCES

Babior BM. Oxygen-dependent microbial killing by phagocytes, *N Engl J Med* 198:659, 1978.

Bay J, Nunn JF, Prys-Roberts C: Factors influencing arterial Po_2 during recovery from anaesthesia, *British Journal of Anaesthesia* 40:398, 1968.

Cannon WB: *Bodily changes in pain, hunger, fear and rage: an account of recent researches into the function of emotional excitement*, College Park, Md, 1970, McGrath.

Chang N et al: Direct measurement of wound and tissue oxygen tension in postoperative patients, *Ann Surg* 197:470, 1983.

Chernow B et al: Hormonal responses to graded surgical stress, *Arch Intern Med* 147(7):1273, 1987.

Derbyshire D, Smith G: Sympathoadrenal responses to anaesthesia and surgery, *Br J Anaesth* 56:725, 1984.

Frank SM et al: Unintentional hypothermia is associated with postoperative myocardial ischemia: the Perioperative Ischemia Randomized Anesthesia Trial Study Group, *Anesthesiology* 78:468, 1993.

Gimbel M, Hunt T: Wound healing and hyperbaric oxygen. In Kindwall E, Whelan H, editors: *Hyperbaric medicine practice*, Flagstaff, Az, 1999, Best Publishing.

Goodson W: Wound healing and the diabetic patient, *Surg Gynecol Obstet* 149:600, 1979.

Goodson W et al: The influence of a brief preoperative illness on postoperative healing, *Ann Surg* 205:250, 1987.

Goodson W et al: Wound oxygen tension of large vs small wounds in man, *Surg Forum* 30:92, 1979.

Gosain A et al: Tissue oxygen tension and other indicators of blood loss or organ perfusion during graded hemorrhage, *Surgery* 109:523, 1991.

Gottrup F et al: Directly measured tissue oxygen tension and arterial oxygen tension assess tissue perfusion, *Crit Care Med* 15:1030, 1987.

Halter JB, Pflug AE, Porte D Jr: Mechanism of plasma catecholamine increases during surgical stress in man, *J Clin Endocrinol Metab* 45(5):936, 1977.

Heughan C, Ninikoski J, Hunt TK: Effect of excessive infusion of saline solution on tissue oxygen transport, *Surg Gynecol Obstet* 135:257, 1972.

Hohn DC et al: Effect of O_2 tension on microbicidal function of leukocytes in wounds and in vitro, *Surg Forum* 27:18, 1976.

Hopf HW et al: Wound tissue oxygen tension predicts the risk of wound infection in surgical patients, *Arch Surg* 132:997, 1997.

Hunt TK, Dunphy JE: *Fundamentals of wound management.* New York, 1979, Appleton Century Crofts.

Hunt TK, Hopf H: Wound healing and wound infection: what surgeons and anesthesiologists can do, *Surg Clin North Am* 77:587, 1997.

Hynson JM, Sessler DI: Intraoperative warming therapies: a comparison of three devices, *J Clin Anesth* 4:194, 1992.

Ikeda T et al: Local radiant heating increases subcutaneous oxygen tension, *Am J Surg* 175:33, 1998.

Jensen JA et al: Epinephrine lowers subcutaneous wound oxygen tension, *Curr Surg* 42(6):472, 1985.

Jonsson K et al: Assessment of perfusion in postoperative patients using tissue oxygen measurements, *Br J Surg* 74:263, 1987.

Jonsson K et al: Tissue oxygenation, anemia, and perfusion in relation to wound healing in surgical patients, *Ann Surg* 214:605, 1991.

Jonsson K, Hunt TK, Mathes SJ: Oxygen as an isolated variable influences resistance to infection, *Ann Surg* 208:783, 1988.

Knighton DR, Halliday B, Hunt TK: Oxygen as an antibiotic: the effect of inspired oxygen on infection, *Arch Surg* 119:199, 1984.

Knighton DR, Silver IA, Hunt TK: Regulation of wound-healing angiogenesis-effect of oxygen gradients and inspired oxygen concentration, *Surgery* 90:262, 1981.

Knudson MM et al: Use of tissue oxygen tension measurements during resuscitation from hemorrhagic shock, *J Trauma* 42:608, 1997.

Kurz A et al: Perioperative normothermia to reduce the incidence of surgical-wound infection and shorten hospitalization, *N Engl J Med* 334:1209, 1996.

Large A, Heinbecker P: The effect of cooling on wound healing, *Ann Surg* 120:727, 1944.

Morris RH: Influence of ambient temperature on patient temperature during intraabdominal surgery, *Ann Surg* 173:230, 1971.

Niinikoski J: Effect of oxygen supply on wound healing and formation of experimental granulation tissue, *Acta Physiol Scand* 1969:1, 1969.

Niinikoski J, Heughan C, Hunt TK: Oxygen tensions in human wounds, *J Surg Res* 12:77, 1972.

Pai MP, Hunt TK: Effect of varying oxygen tensions on healing of open wounds, *Surg Gynecol Obstet* 135:756, 1972.

Rabkin JM, Hunt TK: Local heat increases blood flow and oxygen tension in wounds, *Arch Surg* 122:221, 1987.

Roe CF: Effect of bowel exposure on body temperature during surgical operations, *Am J Surg* 122:13, 1971.

Roe CF et al: The influence of body temperature on early postoperative oxygen consumption, *Surgery* 60:85, 1966.

Rowell LB: *Human circulation: regulation during physical stress*, New York, 1986, Oxford University Press.

Rubinstein EH, Sessler DI: Skin-surface temperature gradients correlate with fingertip blood flow in humans, *Anesthesiology* 73:541, 1990.

Sessler DI: Perianesthetic thermoregulation and heat balance in humans, *FASEB J* 7:638, 1993.

Severinghaus J: Oxyhaemoglobin dissociation curve correction for temperature and pH variation in human blood, *J Appl Physiol* 12:485, 1958.

Sheffield CW et al: Thermoregulatory vasoconstriction decreases subcutaneous oxygen tension in anesthetized volunteers, *Anesthesiology* 77:A96, 1992.

Silver IA: The measurement of oxygen tension in healing tissue, *Prog Resp Res* 3:124, 1969.

Silver IA: The physiology of wound healing. In Hunt T, editor: *Wound healing and wound infection: theory and surgical practice*, New York, 1980, Appleton-Century-Crofts.

Slotman GJ, Jed EH, Burchard KW: Adverse effects of hypothermia in postoperative patients, *Am J Surg* 49:495, 1985.

Vanhoutte PM, Verbeuren TJ, Webb RC: Local modulation of adrenergic neuroeffector interaction in the blood vessel well, *Physiol Rev* 61:151, 1981.

West JM: *The effect of postoperative forced-air rewarming on subcutaneous tissue oxygen tension and wound healing in hypothermic abdominal surgery patients*, San Francisco, 1994, University of California, San Francisco.

West JM: Wound healing in the surgical patient: influence of the perioperative stress response on perfusion, *AACN Clin Issues Crit Care Nurs* 1(3):595, 1990.

West JM, Hopf H, Hunt T: A radiant-heat bandage increases abdominal subcutaneous oxygen tension and temperature, *Wound Repair Regen* 4:A134, 1996.

CHAPTER 10

Massive Tissue Loss: Burns

RUTH WILSON

OBJECTIVES

1. Discuss the three periods of burn care, including the actions for each and the fluid shifts that can be anticipated.
2. Differentiate among thermal, chemical, and electrical burns.
3. Identify the three zones of tissue damage.
4. Differentiate between first-, second-, and third-degree burns and superficial, partial-, and, full-thickness burns.
5. Describe the common methods to calculate the total body surface area of a burn.
6. Describe the advantages and disadvantages of at least four topical burn care products and dressings, including skin replacements.
7. Distinguish among the following surgical procedures for burn wounds by identifying the indication and technique for each procedure: escharotomy, fasciotomy, surgical excisions, and grafts.
8. Describe one intervention for at least three complications specific to the burn wound.
9. Identify the types of burns that can be treated in an outpatient setting.

Care of the burn patient requires a multidisciplinary team consisting of physicians, a nurse, dieticians, a physical therapist, case managers, an occupational therapist, a pharmacist, and social workers that manage the needs of a patient with a burn injury. A burn injury creates a significant alteration in the functioning and structural integrity of the skin. All team members must be knowledgeable of the concepts of wound management, the biology of wound healing, and pathophysiology. Team members also need to be aware of the psychologic stages that a person undergoes when recovering from an acute illness and the rehabilitation that follows.

EPIDEMIOLOGY

At least 1.4 million people are burned every year and require medical attention because of burn- and fire-related incidents (Carrougher, 1997). These injuries result in approximately 53,000 hospitalizations annually. About 75% of these people have burns of less than 10% of the total body surface area (TBSA). There are rarely hemodynamic problems except in the elderly or in those suffering from smoke inhalation (Monafo, 1996). In-hospital fatality rates have declined; now only about 4% are associated with burns. The cost of the daily medical care, economic loss, and damage to the psychologic and social well-being of the victim are tremendous. These negative effects are significant considering that 50% of burn injuries occur during the formative and productive years (in children from 1 to 5 years of age and in males from 17 to 30 years of age) (Kottke and Lehmann, 1990).

PATHOLOGY

Major burns affect all body systems, and understanding the systemic response is essential for treatment. The assessment of the burn victim includes the cause of the burn, amount of area involved, depth, and severity. The calculation of the area burned is expressed as a percentage of the TBSA.

Burn care is divided into three overlapping periods: emergent, acute, and rehabilitation. The *emergent period* refers to the first 2 to 4 days after injury.

Care during this period centers on fluid replacement, maintaining pulmonary function, and wound management. The *acute period* begins with the patient diuresing the large amounts of fluid received during the emergent period. The acute period lasts until the full-thickness wounds are grafted. Partial-thickness wounds heal by epithelialization, resurfacing by epidermal cell migration in about 10 to 20 days (Doughty, 1992). Wound management during the acute phase consists of debridement and closure. Complications that can occur during this period include wound infection, sepsis, pulmonary insufficiency, and multiorgan failure. The *rehabilitation period* is concerned with returning to society and may last several years. The cosmetic and functional problems caused by contractures and scar tissue formation are dealt with during this period.

Although there are multiple causes of burns (chemical, electrical or thermal), the pathophysiology and treatment are similar. Public education that stresses prevention is very important and needs to be supported.

TYPES OF BURN INJURY

Thermal Burns

Thermal burns are the most frequent type of burn. Thermal injury results from exposure or contact with a flame, hot liquids, or radiation, and the severity of injury is related to the temperature and duration of contact. Temperatures up to 45° C (113° F) may be tolerated for relatively long periods of time without injury, but higher temperatures cause damage more quickly. As little as 10 seconds of exposure to water at 70° C (158° F) can result in a full-thickness injury (Carrougher, 1997; Jordan and Harrington, 1997).

Burns to the upper body can be caused during cooking, while burning trash or leaves, and often with the misuse of gasoline. The mishandling of firecrackers can cause burns to the hands and face. House fires may be due to faulty electrical systems, use of space heaters, and unsafe fireplaces. Kitchen accidents are common, including scald injuries. The elderly are vulnerable because of decreased reaction time, limited mobility and strength, and decreased vision, especially during cooking, bathing, or smoking. Unsupervised children are at risk for accidental burns. In addition, physical abuse can take place in the form of a burn injury.

Chemical Burns

Chemical burns account for only 2.1% to 6.5% of burn unit admissions. Chemical burns are usually smaller than thermal burns but are more likely to be full-thickness in depth. The depth of the burn takes several days to develop. The severity of the burn depends on the manner and duration of skin contact, how much skin is involved and the area of the body involved, the concentration of the chemical, and how the incident occurred. The deeper depth results from the continuation of tissue damage after the initial exposure until the chemical can be inactivated with irrigation. The most common treatment for most chemical burns is copious irrigation with water. An exception to this is in a burn involving phenols (carbolic acid), in which dilution with water causes more rapid absorption. Phenols are found in chemical disinfectants. Burns caused by a phenol need to be irrigated with 50% polyethylene glycol. Vegetable oil or glycerol may be substituted but is less effective (Woods et al, 1989). Inactivation or neutralization of the burn with another chemical is dangerous and not recommended unless the exact agent is known. Neutralizing chemicals may generate more heat and result in further tissue loss.

Contact with acids, alkalis, or organic substances such as petroleum distillates also causes burns. The amount of tissue damage depends on the strength of the chemical. Acid burns result in coagulation necrosis and protein precipitation, limiting the extent of tissue injury (Kottke and Lehmann, 1990).

Acids are found in rust removers, drain cleansers, and swimming pool chemicals. Muriatic acid (hydrochloric acid) is found in masonry cleaners. Hydrofluoric acid is a weak inorganic acid used in industry and household products for cleaning or rust removal. This substance is extremely hazardous. Contact with the skin releases fluoride ions, which can quickly penetrate to the muscle or bone. Calcium and magnesium from the tissue bind with the fluoride ions and produces cardiac arrhythmia from hypocalcemia or hypomagnesemia (Lim et al, 1998). Areas involving as little as 2.5% of the body can result in cardiac death (Woods et al, 1989).

Alkaloid burns undergo liquefaction necrosis, denaturation of protein, and loosening of tissue planes, allowing for deeper spread than acid burns. Alkalis are present in industrial cleansers such as drain and oven cleansers, swimming pool chemicals, cement, some fertilizers, and paint removers. Organic compounds (e.g., petroleum products, such as gasoline, diesel fuel, and creosote) can be absorbed into the skin becaue of their fat-solvent actions, causing cutaneous damage or systemic toxicity, which can lead to renal or hepatic failure.

Electrical Injury

Patients with injuries caused by contact with electricity comprise 4% to 6% of admissions to burn units. Electrical injuries are most commonly caused by alternating current, the type of current found in homes and industries. The alternating or cyclic current flow can produce cardiac arrhythmias, respiratory arrest, loss of consciousness, seizures, or tetany of the skeletal muscles, which makes it difficult for the victim to let go of the live wire. The severity of electrical injury is due to the voltage (force) and amperage (strength) of the current. Tissue injury occurs when the electrical energy is converted to heat (Lim et al, 1998). Moist or sweating skin is less resistant to current flow than dry skin. Approximately two thirds of electrical injuries are low voltage (less than 1000 volts); these occur in the home and can range from minor to life threatening. High-voltage injuries occur through contact with power lines or industrial or commercial circuitry. These injuries result in massive tissue damage, leading to multiple-extremity amputation or death.

Damage from electrical contact is normally more severe in the extremities than in the trunk because of the smaller surface area and relates to the combined effects of current passage, heat generation, and compression of vital structures (Lim et al, 1998). Thermal burns can occur when electricity passes through moist skin (Woods et al, 1989). Because of the electrolyte-rich solutions in blood vessels and nerves, these structures readily conduct current. Small blood vessels may undergo coagulation necrosis, but larger vessels can usually dissipate heat because of higher blood flow and not be injured. Edema can develop in fascia compartments, and the pressure results in further circulatory compromise.

Bone and muscle resist the passage of current but continue to radiate heat, and thermal damage takes place in nearby muscle and adjacent structures. Dead muscle may be found near undamaged bone while the superficial muscle is still viable. Heat dissipates through the skin and prevents skin damage. Nonviable tissue may be present under intact skin and lead to amputation. Electrical injuries have a point of entrance and exit that can be identified by edematous areas surrounded by shriveled, depressed skin with low-voltage shocks. High-voltage shocks are characterized as dry, shriveled, and charred.

Renal failure can be attributed to muscle damage, which releases potassium and results in hyperkalemia. Damaged erythrocytes or myocytes release myoglobin or hemoglobin into the bloodstream; these large proteins lead to acute tubular necrosis. Fluid resuscitation must be adjusted to reduce the damage. Other organ dysfunction can occur within or near the path of current.

Long-term effects of electrical injury, such as late peripheral mononeuropathy or polyneuropathy, may result from ischemia and degeneration, leading to fibrosis of the involved nerves. Reflex sympathetic dystrophy has been reported after minor electrical injury. Neurologic injury after the initial insult can manifest as severe headaches, posttraumatic stress disorders, and impairment of attention, concentration, memory, or learning abilities. Ocular diseases, such as cataracts, glaucoma, recurrent iritis, macular holes, and central retinal artery occlusion, have been reported when the path of current traverses the head (Woods et al, 1989). An eye examination at the time of injury can document the absence of preinjury cataracts and will assist with compensation in a work-related injury.

EVALUATION OF THE BURN INJURY

Zone of Tissue Damage

The zone of tissue damage describes the extent of the injury from the superficial or outermost area to the deepest or most severely damaged area (Carrougher, 1997; Jordan and Harrington, 1997). The three zones of tissue damage are zone of coagulation, zone of stasis, and zone of hyperemia.

TABLE 10-1 Comparison of Severity of Burn with Stage of Wound Repair

DEGREE OF BURN	CLASSIFICATION OF BURN DEPTH	STAGE OF WOUND HEALING
First	Superficial	Defensive, proliferative
Second (superficial)	Superficial partial-thickness	Defensive, proliferative
Second (deep)	Deep partial-thickness	Defensive, proliferative, maturation
Third	Full-thickness	Defensive, proliferative, maturation
Fourth	Full-thickness	Defensive, proliferative, maturation

The *zone of coagulation* is the area of greatest damage, is closest to the heat source, and is characterized by coagulation of the cells. Damage to the cells from heat results in protein denaturation. This area indicates a full-thickness injury. If the zone of coagulation is above the level of the dermal appendages, healing by reepithelialization will occur and wound grafting will not be necessary.

The *zone of stasis* surrounds the zone of coagulation and involves the vascular system in the area. Thrombosis and vasoconstriction cause transient dermal ischemia. Adequate perfusion and prevention of infection aid in preserving this zone. If the area is protected from further damage, such as infection, drying from exposure to air, rough handling during turning or moving, or pressure, circulation will return and tissue health will be restored.

The *zone of hyperemia* is the outermost area, and usually no cellular death occurs because this area is only minimally damaged. Cells in this zone recover in 7 to 10 days. The area is reddened because of vasodilatation and inflammation. The zone of hyperemia is similar to a first-degree burn and/or superficial partial-thickness burn.

Severity of the Burn Wound

The treatment of the burn wound is based on the amount, depth, and severity of the injury. The depth of the injury is based on the number of cells injured or destroyed and on the functional capacity of the level of the skin. The traditional classification of burns as first, second, or third degree has been replaced by the designations of superficial, superficial partial-, partial-, deep partial-, and full-thickness injury (Jordan and Harrington, 1997; Mertens et al, 1997).

Superficial burns heal without scar formation, pigmentation changes, or contractures. The classic signs of inflammation, pain, swelling, heat and redness are present. The area blanches with pressure. This type of burn occurs from overexposure to sunlight or a brief scalding with hot liquids (Staley and Richard, 1997). After a few days, the outer layer of injured cells peels away from totally healed new skin (Table 10-1).

With a *superficial partial-thickness burn*, there is a great deal of pain because of sensitivity to air and temperatures. It is characterized by blister formation and weeping. The basal layer of the dermis is intact, and after opening of any blisters present or allowing the fluid to reabsorb, healing occurs rapidly by epidermal regeneration.

Partial-thickness burns involve the epidermis with portions of the burn extending into the dermis. This type of burn will heal in about 2 weeks with little scar formation. Dermal structures such as nails, hair follicles, nerves, and oil and sweat glands are intact and functional. There is pain, weeping, and blanching.

A *deep partial-thickness* burn requires a longer time to heal, and there maybe scarring and disruption of the appearance and function of nails, glands, and hair. It is difficult to distinguish a deep partial-thickness burn from a full-thickness burn. The wound appears red with cheesy white patches, large blisters, and pain. The injury to the dermis is partial, so healing by primary intention without grafting can occur. The tissue that forms may not be able to withstand strong insult since the tensile strength of the scar is reduced and hypertrophic scarring can form. Ischemia in the area can convert a deep partial-thickness burn to a full-thickness burn during the emergent phase (Kottke and Lehmann, 1990). Itching and hypersensation in the scar are common complaints of the patient.

A *full-thickness burn* results in the destruction of the entire dermis. Healing will only occur at the wound margins and by grafting. The heat-coagulated blood vessels leave the tissue avascular so the appearance of the burned tissue is a waxy white to gray color (Thompson et al, 1997). If the burn extends into the fat or has been exposed to a prolonged flame source, the color is brown or black with a leathery charred appearance. A full-thickness burn lacks pain sensation because of death of the nerves; this sign is often used to distinguish a full-thickness burn from a partial-thickness burn. As stated previously, the zones of stasis and hyperemia surround the actual burn area. The area can be converted from partial to a full thickness by hypoxia, decrease in blood flow, or infection. Pain can be felt in the outer zones and varies with each burn and with each individual.

The fourth-degree burn is a full-thickness burn that results from an incineration-type exposure and electrical burns in which the heat is sufficient to destroy tissues below the skin. The damage includes fascia, muscle, or bone. This type of burn requires not only skin grafts, but also local or regional flaps to cover the area definitively (Jurkeiwicz et al, 1990; Winfree and Barillo, 1997).

Calculation of Area

There are two methods of determining the extent of a burn injury: the Lund and Bower chart (Figure 10-1) and the Rule of Nines (Figure 10-2). The Lund and Bower chart is the preferred method because it is more exact. Areas of the body that are burned are identified as first, second, or third degree. This is done on admission to determine fluid requirements and repeated after 72 hours to recalculate any areas that have extended. The Rule of Nines is used in the prehospital setting because it is simple and quick. The Rule of Nines is based on each anatomic region (of which there are 11) representing 9% of the TBSA. By adding the areas of partial and full-thickness burn, the entire area is calculated. The TBSA is expressed as a percentage and helps estimate the extent of the injury for diagnosis and treatment and for prognosis and statistical analysis. Superficial burns are not included in the calculation of the TBSA. This method can serve as a reference for transportation and fluid resuscitation.

The Rule of Nines is modified in children because of the differences in head and chest size as compared with the extremities. The head is approximately 18% TBSA in a small child, as compared with 9% in an adult.

The American Burn Association has categorized burns as minor, moderate, and major (Table 10-2). Major burns, or specific indicators such as those listed in Box 10-1, require treatment in a specialized center. A burn center is a facility with a burn physician as director and a highly trained, multidisciplinary staff.

Patients with burns located on the face, hands, feet, and perineum, even if minor, should be referred to a burn center. Airway difficulties and delayed respiratory distress can occur with burns near the eyes, ears, nose, or mouth. Hand burns require close attention to splinting, elevation, physiotherapy, and wound care to restore full function. Injuries to the feet or lower legs can interfere with mobility, and edema may delay healing. The age of the victim and associated injuries are the most substantial variables in determining survival. Critical ages are younger than 3 years of age and older than 60 years of age.

One last method may be used as a crude approximation of the size of the burn: to use the palm of the patient's hand with fingers closed as 1% of the body surface area. Erythema is not included (Fowler, 1998; Mertens et al, 1997).

PATHOPHYSIOLOGY

As with other wounds, the burn area goes through the three phases of wound healing: 1) defensive, or inflammatory, phase; 2) proliferative, or fibroblastic, phase, 3) and remodeling, or maturation. The inflammatory response occurs immediately, with the injured cells releasing various vasoactive and chemotactic agents that affect the vascular system, fluid balance, hemodynamics, and metabolism. The helper T cells form mediators, or cytokines that act on other cells of the immune system (Carrougher, 1997). Important cytokines such as interleukin-1 (IL-1), IL-2, IL-6, and tumor necrosis factor are

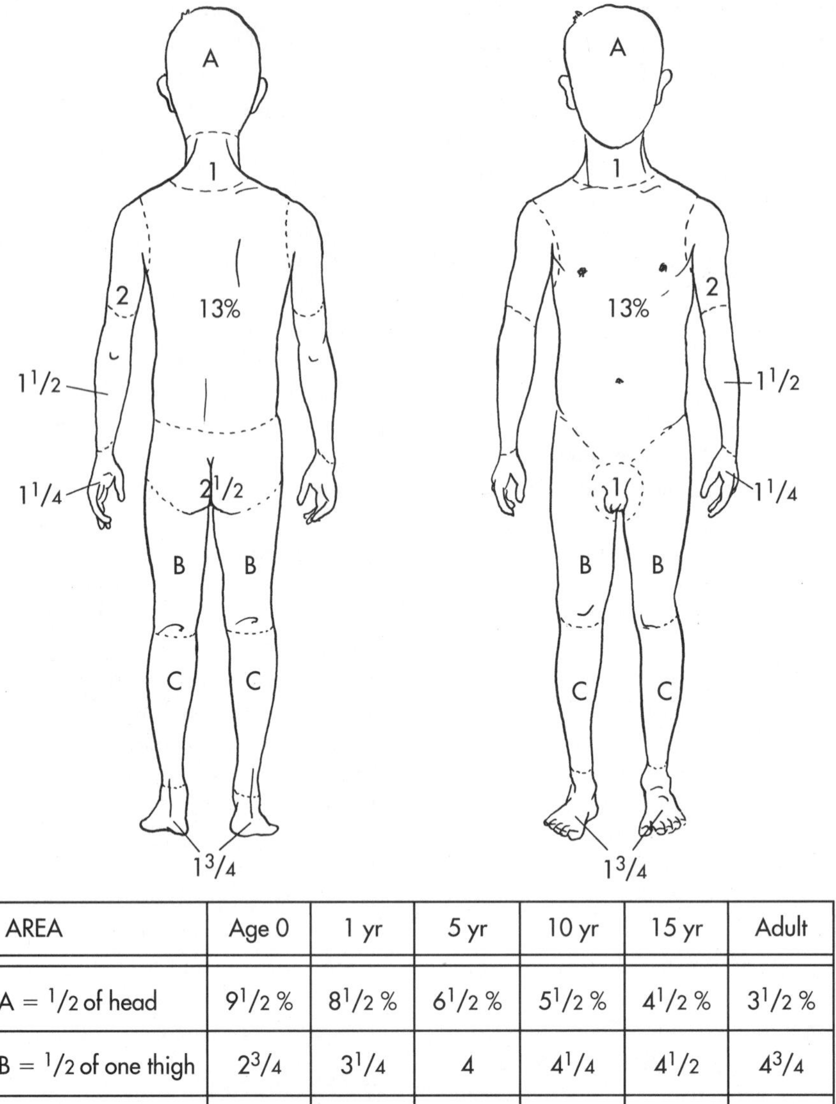

AREA	Age 0	1 yr	5 yr	10 yr	15 yr	Adult
A = $\frac{1}{2}$ of head	$9\frac{1}{2}$ %	$8\frac{1}{2}$ %	$6\frac{1}{2}$ %	$5\frac{1}{2}$ %	$4\frac{1}{2}$ %	$3\frac{1}{2}$ %
B = $\frac{1}{2}$ of one thigh	$2\frac{3}{4}$	$3\frac{1}{4}$	4	$4\frac{1}{4}$	$4\frac{1}{2}$	$4\frac{3}{4}$
C = $\frac{1}{2}$ of one leg	$2\frac{1}{2}$	$2\frac{1}{2}$	$2\frac{3}{4}$	3	$3\frac{1}{4}$	$3\frac{1}{2}$

Figure 10-1 Estimation of burn size; relative area changes significantly with age. (Modified from Trott AT: *Wounds and lacerations*, ed 2, St Louis, 1991, Mosby.)

released, initiate the inflammatory response, and exacerbate a hypermetabolic state. Interleukin levels often reflect the body's response to injury. IL-1 and IL-6 are highest during the first postburn week and decline over time. IL-1 levels increase in relation to the extent of the burn. Elevated IL-6 levels have been shown to correlate to mortality, with nonsurvivors having significantly higher levels (Jordan and Harrington, 1997).

The proliferative phase occurs 4 to 20 days after the burn, which is during the acute phase. Collagen is secreted to provide strength and structure to the

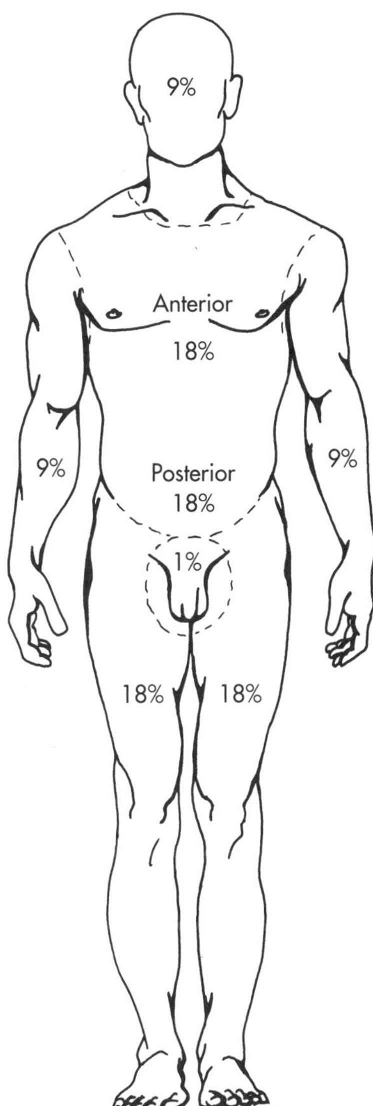

Figure 10-2 Rapid estimation of extent of burn can be determined by the "rule of nines." Only partial-thickness (second-degree) and full-thickness (third-degree) burns are considered. (From Trott AT: *Wounds and lacerations,* ed 2, St Louis, 1991, Mosby.)

wound. Macrophages stimulate angiogenesis and epithelialization. As with other wounds, epithelial cells migrate across the wound from the wound margins or undamaged dermal appendages in partial-thickness burns. With meshed grafted wounds, epidermal cells migrate into the open spaces. Maturation of the scar tissue and grafted areas continues throughout the rehabilitation period.

Tissue edema is usually limited to the burn wound if the total size is less than 25% of the TBSA. When larger areas are affected, a generalized body edema occurs (Carrougher, 1997). Although direct thermal damage to vessels increases permeability within the injured tissue, hypoproteinemia is probably the cause of generalized body edema. Capillary permeability returns to normal roughly 18 to 24 hours after injury.

Hypovolemic shock develops in patients with a burn wound of at least 15% to 20% TBSA unless interventions are started (Lim et al, 1998). Before knowledge of fluid replacement principles, burns of 30% or greater were fatal. Fluid losses of burns with smaller areas can be managed orally. Evaporative fluid loss caused by loss of the integrity of the skin is 4 to 20 times the normal rate, which leads to hypovolemia; this fluid loss continues until all the wounds are closed. In the first 6 to 8 hours after injury, edema is most rapid but continues for 18 to 24 hours. The inflammatory response of the platelets, macrophages, and leukocytes contributes to local and systemic hyperpermeability of the microcirculation. Blood flow increases in the area, causing an increase in capillary pressure. Osmotic and hydrostatic gradients are created, resulting in further wound edema. Red blood cells escape into the area, but blood loss requiring transfusion is rare. Treatment is directed toward restoration and maintenance of intravascular volume with fluid similar to that which is lost in the tissues.

MANAGEMENT

Early Interventions

During the emergent period, the first 24 hours is devoted to fluid resuscitation and ventilatory and hemodynamic stability of the patient. The rare exception is in the case of a chemical burn, which requires removal of the substance to prevent further injury. The usual burn care given during this period is to cleanse the areas with a nonirritating detergent and rinse with warm water in a warmed treatment room. Hypothermia is prevented so that the patient's metabolic rate is not further increased. Loose

TABLE 10-2 American Burn Association (ABA) Categories of Burn Injury*

MINOR BURNS	MODERATE BURNS	MAJOR BURNS
• Adults: ≤15% TBSA • Children and elderly: ≤10% TBSA • <2% TBSA full-thickness burns not involving cosmetic or functional risk or impairment of the face, ears, eyes, feet, hands, or perineum	• Adults: 15% to 25% TBSA, mixed partial/full-thickness • Children <10 years of age or adults >40 years of age: 10% to 20 % TBSA • <10% TBSA full-thickness burns not involving cosmetic or functional risk or impairment of the face, ears, eyes, feet, hands, or perineum	• All patients: >25% TBSA • Children or adults >40 years of age: 20% TBSA • >10% TBSA full-thickness • All burns of face, eyes, ears, hands, or perineum, especially if functional or cosmetic impairment exists • All high-voltage electrical burns • All burns with inhalation injury or major trauma • Poor-risk patients

*Also adopted by the American College of Surgeons.

BOX 10-1 American Burn Association (ABA) Criteria for Burn Center Referral

>10% TBSA when <10 years of age
>10% TBSA when >50 years of age
>20% TBSA for all other ages
>5% full-thickness burns
Any involvement of hands, feet, face, perineum
Circumferential burns of chest or extremities
Electric or chemical injury
Significant associated injuries
Any inhalation injury
Major preexisting diseases

necrotic or devitalized tissue is lightly debrided, and intact bullae of more than 2 cm are opened. Debridement is only conducted to the point of minimal pain or bleeding. Body hair in the area is shaved out to 3 to 4 inches from the wound. The burned area is examined, and the percentage of TBSA is calculated along with extent and depth. Body weight is obtained and the amount of fluid for resuscitation is calculated. Intravenous analgesic agents are provided for pain control and are tolerated safely provided that fluid resuscitation is on target. Wounds are usually dressed with a topical antimicrobial agent; systemic prophylactic antibiotics are not routinely used without identification of specific organisms at this time.

Fluid Resuscitation

The need for fluid replacement is due to vascular changes and tissue loss that precipitate fluid shifts. Generalized increased capillary permeability occurs in burns greater than 15% to 25% TBSA. The loss of plasma is greatest during the first 12 hours (Kottke and Lehman, 1990).

The hypovolemic stage occurs during the first 24 to 48 hours, or the emergent period. Fluid and serum protein from the vascular compartment shift into the interstitial spaces causing edema, blisters, and weeping of fluid and a decrease of the circulating blood volume. Sodium moves into the tissues along with water resulting in hyponatremia and hyperkalemia. To prevent hypovolemic shock and maintain adequate cardiac output and renal and tissue perfusion, the fluid must be replaced. The amount of fluid for replacement depends on the extent and depth of the burn, the patient's age, and the patient's medical history. If the burn area involves less than 20% TBSA, intravenous fluid therapy may not be needed. Standard formulas are used to estimate fluid replacement needs (Table 10-3). As an alternative, Gordon and Goodwin (1997) use the following formula to calculate fluid needs:

$$4 \text{ ml} \times \text{body weight (kg)} \times \text{TBSA}$$

TABLE 10-3 Common Formulas for Estimating Resuscitation

	ELECTROLYTE	COLLOID	GLUCOSE IN WATER
First 24 Hours			
Evans	Normal saline 1.0 ml/kg/% TBSA	1.0 ml/kg/% TBSA	2000 ml
Brooke	Lactated Ringer's solution	0.5 ml/kg/% TBSA	2000 ml
Modified Brooke	Lactated Ringer's solution 2 ml/kg/% TBSA	0.3-0.5 ml/kg/% TBSA	D_5W to maintain urine output
Modified Brooke (pediatric)	Lactate Ringer's solution 3 ml/kg/% TBSA plus maintenance fluid	0.3-0.5 ml/kg/% TBSA	$D_5$1/2 NS titrated to maintain urine output
Parkland	Lactated Ringer's solution 4 ml/kg/% TBSA	None given	2000 ml
Second 24 Hours			
Evans	½ first 24-hr amount	½ first 24-hr amount	2000 ml
Brooke	½ to ¾ first 24-hr amount	½ to ¾ first 24-hr amount	2000 ml
Parkland	None given	20% to 60% of calculated plasma volume	To maintain urine output

Fluid requirements may be greater in pediatric patients with extensive injuries, comorbidities, or smoke inhalation.

The type of fluid for replacement must be similar to plasma (Monafo, 1996). This is commonly a balanced salt solution; a serum albumin is added to replace protein. The correct amount of fluid is achieved when blood pressure and urinary output are normal without overloading of the vascular system. Solutions containing glucose are not given to adults in the first 24 hours to avoid osmotic diuresis (Peck and Ward, 1997).

After the first 24 hours the crystalloid fluid is changed to a hypotonic solution, usually 5% glucose for adults and 5% glucose/0.45% saline for children younger than 6 years of age. Sodium may need to be added to maintain intravascular volume and reduce cellular edema (Peck and Ward, 1997).

Beginning the second day, plasma colloid or protein is repleted. Replacement with albumin is calculated at 0.5 ml/kg/% TBSA if the burn is larger than 30% TBSA. Not all institutions give colloids; some controlled trials have shown no clear advantage and may increase the rate of pulmonary complications because of pulmonary edema (Monafo, 1996). Significant protein loss (up to 1.2 mg/BSA/% TBSA per day) can occur through the wound; replacement can range from 1.5 to 4 g/day and can be delivered either parentally or enterally (Jordan and Harrington, 1997).

The emergent period ends when the patient begins diuresing, usually around 4 or 5 days after injury. Maintenance fluids are then initiated and should be based on 1500 ml/m^2/day to replace insensible losses through the burn wounds.

Assessing Resuscitation Adequacy. Adequacy of resuscitation is determined by routine and frequent surveillance of urinary output, heart rate, pulse oximetry, and blood pressure via intraarterial cannulas (Box 10-2). Invasive hemodynamic monitoring (central venous pressure or pulmonary arterial pressure) is usually only required when the patient fails to respond to fluid resuscitation (Pessina and Ellis, 1997) as calculated by burn formulas (Gordon and Goodwin, 1997).

Neuroendocrine Response

The body responds to a thermal injury with a classical hemodynamic response. There is almost an immediate fall in cardiac output, metabolic rate,

BOX 10-2 Clinical Indicators for Assessing Fluid Resuscitation (Adult)

Clear cognitive function: Orientated × 3
Heart rate: <120 beats/min
Urine output: 30 to 50 ml/hr
Peripheral pulses: Palpable (or detected by Doppler flow meter)
Blood pressure: Normal for age and comorbid condition
Capillary refill: <2 seconds

oxygen consumption, fluid imbalance, cellular shock, and blood pressure for 3 to 7 days. This is followed by a slow increase to a hypermetabolic state with elevated catecholamine, glucocorticoid, and glucagon levels and a decrease in insulin. The increase in metabolic rate causes an increase in protein catabolism, gluconeogenesis, and lipolysis. This response is characterized by increased heat loss, negative nitrogen balance, and weight loss (Carrougher, 1997). Aggressive nutritional support is essential, and requirements decrease as the wound heals. The severity and duration of the hypermetabolic activity is directly proportional to the extent of injury. The peak occurs in the first 2 weeks and slowly returns to normal with closure of the wound.

Cardiovascular Response

As stated previously, the cardiovascular system responds to a major thermal injury with tachycardia and an increase in peripheral vascular resistance. Cardiac output may fall to as low as 50% of normal. It increases with resuscitation but does not return to normal for 18 to 24 hours after injury. When the patient enters the hypermetabolic phase, cardiac output increases to two to three times normal and hypertension may develop, requiring treatment (Carrougher, 1997). In the early postburn period, blood is shunted away from the skin to the viscera. Measures to prevent pressure ulcer development should be implemented. Most patients with extensive burns are placed on pressure relief/reduction mattresses or surfaces.

Pulmonary Response

Pulmonary response to burn injury involves damage to the upper and lower airways. Pulmonary dysfunction is a major cause of morbidity and mortality in the burn patient. Inhalation injury and the associated complications can account for 20% to 84% of burn mortality (Carrougher, 1997). Respiratory problems are common when burns are located on the upper body and also result from smoke inhalation. Bronchospasm from inhaled noxious gases; pulmonary congestion; distended pulmonary vessels; and damage to nasal mucosa, oral mucous, and the pharynx all contribute to inefficient gas exchange, upper airway obstruction, upper airway edema, and ventilation-perfusion imbalance.

Mechanical ventilation is often necessary to provide adequate oxygenation until the edema resolves. Acute respiratory distress can be the result of a deep burn with eschar to the anterior and lateral chest, which restricts movement of the chest during breathing. A chest escharotomy, which involves splitting the eschar vertically, can release the restricted rib motion and increase expansion.

Pulmonary symptoms that develop 24 to 48 hours after injury are the most serious because of the inhalation of noxious gases and incomplete products of combustion (Carrougher, 1997). Unless laryngeal edema presents on admission, clinical development can require 12 to 24 hours or more as mucosa sloughs, secretions accumulate, the airway obstructs, and atelectasis progresses. If signs of laryngeal edema appear, such as hoarseness, brassy cough, or stridor, immediate endotracheal intubation is required (Monafo, 1996).

Renal Response

Oliguria is the early response of the kidney to decreases in blood flow as a result of loss of intravascular volume. If fluid resuscitation is inadequate, hypovolemia will progress and acute renal failure will occur. Occasionally early acute renal failure is due to damage of the renal tubules. With adequate resuscitation, renal blood flow and cardiac output increase and extravascular fluid is reabsorbed.

Early fluid replacement within 2 hours will moderate kidney damage, prevent the severe manifestations of renal hypoperfusion, and offset the vasoconstrictive response of the inflammatory system (Chrysopoulo et al, 1999). If acute renal dysfunction is identified later than the first week after the burn injury, the cause is usually secondary to sepsis and is commensurate with multiorgan failure or with disseminated intravascular coagulopathy.

Gastrointestinal Response

Function of the gastrointestinal tract can be altered in a burn victim because of severe splanchnic vasoconstriction, causing an ileus. After thermal injuries of 20% to 25% TBSA or greater, blood flow to the mesenteric bed is diminished as a result of bowel edema and hypoperfusion. This edema can lead to increased transfer of bacteria into the lymphatic or portal venous system, which triggers the release of cytokines and exacerbates the systemic inflammatory response. The presence of food in the gut is thought to prevent the translocation of bacteria (Peck and Ward, 1997). With adequate resuscitation, gastrointestinal function and motility return to normal in 24 to 28 hours. Gastroduodenal ulceration caused by stress is less frequent because of improved resuscitation, early enteral feedings, and the use of antacids to decrease acidity and protect the gastric mucosa (Molnar et al, 1983).

Nutrition

Burns are associated with an increase in metabolic rate of 50 to 100 times normal. By 5 or 6 days after the burn injury, caloric needs double. Aggressive nutritional support is essential to minimize the weight loss of thermal injury, facilitate wound healing, support optimum functioning of the immune system, and reduce mortality rates.

The preferred route for nutritional support is the gastrointestinal tract. Feedings are usually started after the fluid resuscitation is achieved. Transpyloric tube feedings can be started earlier than gastric feedings, decreasing the need for parental nutrition, and do not need to be withheld before surgery, which helps sustain caloric intake (Mertens, 1997; Peck and Ward, 1997). In the presence of an ileus, the parenteral route is used until the ileus resolves.

A nutritionist is invaluable in estimating nutritional requirements, determining the formula, and adjusting the exact daily protein and calorie needs of the patient. Nutritional requirements can also be estimated as 1) 24 kcal/kg, 2) 40 kcal/% TBSA, 3) 20 g nitrogen/m^2 body surface/day, and 4) 2% to 4% daily calories as linoleic acid (Jurkiewicz et al, 1990). Supplemental enteral feedings are commonly required to satisfy nutritional requirements. The goal is to maintain the patient's preburn weight. Serial transferrin and prealbumin blood values are necessary to monitor the patient's nutritional status.

Pain and Anxiety Management

Pain management is part of the entire burn experience and particularly critical during admission. If the pain and anxiety are adequately managed before the first wound debridement, then subsequent procedures will be better tolerated. Pain scales are used to determine the level of pain, the intolerable level of pain, and the amount of pain relief that is expected, possible, and achieved. Emotional support and education for the patient and family decrease fear and anxiety, which contribute to pain.

Initially, during the hypermetabolic phase, opiods such as morphine sulfate are best administered in small, repetitive boluses. Patient-controlled analgesia (PCA) devices are effective in the delivery of opioids and allow the patient a sense of control. Anxiolytic agents are commonly given to augment pain medication in addition to diversionary activities, imagery, and relaxation, particularly during dressing changes (Davis and Sheely-Adolphson, 1997).

Supplemental pain-control measures are necessary to control background or procedural pain. Morphine, the neuromuscular blocking agent remifentanil, benzodiazepines, acetaminophen with codeine, and nonnarcotic medications such as nonsteroidal antiinflammatory drugs (NSAIDs) are used (Davis and Sheely-Adolphson, 1997). Aspirin and NSAIDs are not routinely given during the acute phase because of the adverse effect on the coagulation system and propensity for gastric ulceration.

Topical Wound Management

The goals of wound care are to control the growth of microorganisms, reduce the potential for invasive wound infection, prevent the wound from being a source of sepsis, and prepare the area for closure. Injured and nonviable tissue provide a medium for microorganisms; gram-positive organisms can become colonized by the fifth day of injury. Topical agents delay the colonization and keep wound flora to a minimum. Ideally the topical agent will penetrate the eschar, have wide activity against colonizing organisms, not interfere with healing, and have minimal systemic absorption and toxicity (Kinney, 1998) (Table 10-4).

Silvadene (silver sulfadiazine), a 1% suspension of silver sulfadiazine in a water-miscible cream, is the most widely used agent because of its relatively low toxicity and painless, easy application. The ac-

TABLE 10-4 Comparison of Topical Agents

AGENT	APPLICATION	ACTIVITY	ADVANTAGES	DISADVANTAGES
Silvadene (1% silver sulfadiazine)	• qd or bid • Cleanse and remove between applications • Apply to depth of 1/16 inch	• Gram-positive and gram-negative • Bacterial cell wall synthesis	• Painless • Convenient for outpatient • Applied with or without dressings • Wide spectrum	• Only partial penetration through eschar • 5% to 7% hypersensitivity • Transient leukopenia • Potential cross sensitivity with other sulfonamides
Sulfamylon (mafenide acetate)	• qd or bid • No dressing • Cleanse and remove between applications • Apply to depth of 1/16 inch	• Gram-positive and gram-negative • Interferes with bacterial cell wall synthesis	• Penetrates full-thickness eschar • Easy (no dressing) • Wound visible • Full ROM possible • Persistent activity against pseudomonas • Wide-spectrum, resistance does not develop	• Unable to use dressings • Painful upon application for 15-20 min • Metabolic acidosis may develop • Irritation of new skin
Silver nitrate (0.5%) (dilute with distilled water)	• Wet-moist dressings • Dampen q2h • Change dressing bid/tid	• Wide range of pathogens • Fungus	• No hypersensitivity • Painless on application • No resistant organism reported • Evaporative water and heat loss minimized with use of required dressings	• Does not penetrate eschar • Labor intensive • Limited joint movement • Discoloration of wound • Complicates wound assessment • Environmental staining is permanent • Potential fluid and electrolyte imbalance

Modified from Jordan BS, Harrington DT: Management of the burn wound, *Nurs Clin North Am* 32(2):251, 1997.

tive ingredient, sulfadiazine complex, and silver ion provide a wide spectrum of antimicrobial activity but must be applied twice a day since it is inactivated after approximately 12 hours. Silvadene can cause a transient leukopenia and has a reported hypersensitivity incidence of 5% to 7%. Even with continued use, the leukopenia will resolve after the first week. However, prolonged or exclusive use of Silvadene may allow for the development of resistant strains of *Enterobacter cloacae* and *Pseudomonas aeruginosa*, necessitating discontinuation of the agent.

Sulfamylon (mafenide) is an 11.1% suspension of the acetate salt of mafenide and is water miscible. Because it readily penetrates eschar, Sulfamylon is ideal for full-thickness areas with poor vascular supply, such as the cartilaginous structures of the ears (Jordan and Harrington, 1997). Sulfamylon has broad-spectrum activity and is effective against *P. aeruginosa*. The complications associated with the use of Sulfamylon include pain when applied to partial-thickness areas, a maculopapular rash in 5% of the patients (it resolves when Sulfamylon is discontinued), and a mild metabolic acidosis. Limiting its use to 25% TBSA prevents metabolic acidosis. It is frequently applied before escharotomy to minimize bacteremia. Mafenide is used less frequently now since invasive burn wound infections are rare.

A solution of 0.5% silver nitrate is an effective antimicrobial agent that is bacteriostatic and provides a broad spectrum of coverage against pathogens and fungal agents. It is painless upon application, has no hypersensitivity or resistance, but has little eschar-penetrating capacity. Silver nitrate is a hypotonic solution and pulls electrolytes from the tissue through the open wound, stains, and requires extensive dressings. Irrigation is required every 2 hours and requires a vast amount of nursing time to apply (Jordan and Harrington, 1997). For these reasons it is rarely used except when allergic responses are experienced with the other topical agents.

Surgical Procedures

Escharotomy. Burns that encircle an extremity or the torso may require an escharotomy to relieve pressure. Edema forms under the fixed eschar in the tissues, which can retard blood flow. The pressure from the fluid leaking into the tissues can exceed capillary closing pressure and result in ischemia. In addition, neurologic and vascular deficits may develop if the tight muscle compartments are not relieved. Hourly monitoring for cyanosis, delayed capillary refill (more than 5 seconds), and progressive unrelenting paresthesia is essential.

The ultrasonic flowmeter may be used to assess arterial blood flow, monitor vascular compromise before and after escharotomy, and avoid unnecessary escharotomies. Direct measurement of compartment pressures can be performed by placing a needle or specially designed wick catheter into each compartment (Jordan and Harrington, 1997). Normal compartment pressures are 9 mm Hg; pressures more than 30 mm Hg require a surgical escharotomy. Elevation and active exercise of the extremity for about 5 minutes each hour decrease edema and usually prevent compartment syndrome.

The escharotomy is a linear incision through the full-thickness wound dividing the eschar. The incision is only as deep as necessary to split the eschar and should not result in excessive bleeding or exposure of additional subcutaneous tissue to bacterial invasion. Full-thickness eschar lacks nerve endings, so pain is minimal, although small doses of narcotics are given intravenously to control anxiety and background pain. This procedure can be done at the bedside with a sterile field and scalpel. The small amount of bleeding present can be controlled with pressure or electrocautery. Major vessels, tendons, and nerves should be avoided, but involved joints need to be included to prevent vascular obstruction in these areas. More than one incision, usually a contralateral incision, may be necessary (Jordan and Harrington, 1997). The incisional wounds are dressed with a topical agent and packed.

Fasciotomy. When the burn injury extends to the muscle, such as with a high-voltage electrical injury or skeletal trauma, edema develops beneath the fascia and muscle compartment, which precipitates tissue ischemia and nerve damage. A fasciotomy, or surgical incision of the fascia, is then necessary. This procedure is conducted in the operating room under general anesthesia.

Burn Excision. Early excision of the burn wound has been associated with the most significant increase in survival of seriously burned patients. The goal is to remove the burned nonviable skin as soon as possible to reduce the risk of bacterial colonization and decrease the metabolic response to the burn injury. Excisions of burns that involve more than 40% TBSA may be staged.

Tangential or sequential excision involves removing thin layers of nonviable tissue until a bleeding wound bed is reached with a knife or guarded dermatome. This "shaving" away of the eschar preserves as much as possible the surrounding healthy tissue. It is often used for excision of deep partial-thickness wounds that may reach into the superficial portions of the subcutaneous fat.

Fascial excision consists of the surgical removal of the burned tissue down to the level of the muscle fascia rather than adipose tissue. The excised fat will not regenerate, and edema formation may become problematic as a result of the disruption of the lymphatic system in the area. Fascial excision provides a better wound bed for graft adherence but a poorer cosmetic appearance; distinct imperfection between the burned and nonburned area will be apparent. Fascial excision is indicated in the presence of an invasive life-threatening infection, such as with the *Aspergillus* or *Candida* fungi.

Wound Closure Techniques

To reduce the risk of complications such as infection, reduce fluid loss, and expedite the patient's recovery, prompt closure of the extensive wounds is imperative. In general, dressings used for massive tissue loss may be categorized as permanent, such as an autograft or skin graft from the patient, or temporary (Box 10-3). Temporary dressings are further categorized as follows (Hansbrough and Rennekampff, 1997):

1. *Homografts, or allografts.* Transfer of skin from human cadavers
2. *Xenografts, or heterografts.* Transfer of skin from other species, such as a pig
3. *Biosynthetic dressings.* Synthetic dressings integrated with cells such as fibroblasts and keratinocytes
4. *Biologic skin replacements.* Composite epidermal-dermal skin grafts

BOX 10-3 Types of Skin Substitutes Used as Wound Coverings

Permanent Wound Coverings

Sheet autograft. Thin, intact layer of skin (epidermis and dermis) used for small or cosmetic areas, including portion of dermis.

Meshed autograft. Thin layer of skin with small holes that allow for expansion in order to cover more area, including portion of dermis.

Cultured epithelial autograft. Patient's own keratinocytes laboratory grown into sheets of cells. Used when patient's own skin is limited; lacks dermis (fragile).

Temporary Wound Coverings

Allograft/homograft. Human cadaver skin donated and harvested after death; becomes vascularized but rejected.

Heterograft/xenograft. Porcine skin harvested after slaughter; cryopreserved or lyophilized for storage; develops collagen bond; not vascularized.

Biologicals

Integra. Permanent dermal replacement; bovine hide collagen and chondroitin 6-sulfate obtained from shark collagen; neodermis; degrades and grafted with epidermal cells.

DermaGraft. Permanent dermal replacement made from fibroblasts of neonatal foreskin.

Apligraf. Cultured skin equivalent containing keratinocytes and fibroblasts (derived from neonatal foreskin).

Before graft application, adequate hemostasis must be obtained. Hemostasis can be accomplished by pressure, topical vasoconstrictors, ligation or electrocautery, topical thrombin, or nonadherent sponges soaked with epinephrine (Laing, 1997). After application of a permanent or temporary cover and/or dressing, the area needs to be assessed continually for sites of bleeding. Hematomas beneath grafts can prevent graft adherence.

Autologous Skin Graft. An autograft, or a graft of the patient's own skin, is the most desirable burn cover because it is permanent and will not be rejected. Sheets of the epidermis with a thin layer of the dermis are removed from an area of unburned skin (the donor site) with a dermatome. The graft is laid down flat onto the wound bed without overlapping onto the intact skin so that adherence of the wound margins is not jeopardized (Gallico et al, 1984). A donor site is essentially a superficial partial-thickness wound and may be harvested several times, usually 7 to 10 days after injury. If the area is repeatedly harvested, healing will take longer and there is a risk of hypertrophic scarring.

Autografts are prepared as either a sheet or meshed. Sheet grafts provide a more durable covering and are more cosmetically pleasing. They are used on the face, hands, feet, neck, and joints, although it is also difficult to apply a sheet graft on an irregular area. Care of a sheet graft requires meticulous care to remove any fluid accumulation under the graft (Sulton, 1997). A triple antibiotic ointment is applied to keep the graft moist, especially around staples or sutures. Sheet autografts are not covered with a dressing.

For large burn areas, the skin graft is meshed to allow more coverage with fewer donor sites. A solid strip of skin is placed through a device that creates a mesh pattern, or small holes, to expand the size of the strip to a 5:1, 4:1, 3:1 or 2:1 size; the larger the size the longer the healing time. Epidermal cells migrate in between and leave a typical pattern after healing; the wider the mesh the more noticeable the pattern. The mesh graft is secured with staples or sutures, kept moist for cell growth and adherence (usually with a triple antibiotic ointment), and covered with a nonadherent dressing. Prevention of shear is essential. The postoperative dressing is typically left in place for 5 to 7 days and then carefully removed, and the graft is inspected and redressed. The dressing is then changed daily.

Skin grafts are stable 10 to 14 days after grafting. Once stable, splints are worn continuously until the wound is mature enough to decrease wound contraction. Extremities are padded and splinted to prevent movement. After passive range of motion (ROM) exercises are started, the splints may be worn only at night.

A pressure garment allows the graft to heal flatter and with a more uniform appearance. Pressure aids the graft junction and prevents immature collagen from producing hypertrophic scarring.

The donor site is a partial-thickness wound. These donor sites bleed easily and can be a source of blood loss. An absorptive dressing, such as a calcium alginate with a transparent film as the secondary dressing or a hydrocolloid, may be used.

When skin donor sites are limited because of the extensive nature of the burns, the excised area is not acceptable to immediate grafting, or the overall patient condition does not permit immediate grafting with autologous skin, alternative biologic and synthetic grafts and/or dressings must be considered.

Allograft. The allograft is cadaver-procured tissue and may be purchased as fresh or cryopreserved. As the "gold standard" for temporary coverage of excised burn wounds, the allograft is durable, fosters vascularization, and prepares the wound for definitive autografting. Cadaver skin allografts have been necessary for survival of patients with burns over 80% TBSA. Unfortunately, rejection of the foreign keratinocytes in the allograft is inevitable. In most patients, rejection can occur within several weeks of placement unless the patient is immunosuppressed; in some studies rejection is reported as soon as 5 to 9 days after placement (Hansbrough et al, 1997; Purdue et al, 1997). In addition to rejection, allografts are associated with limited supply, variable quality, and the potential for disease transmission (Hansbrough and Rennekampff, 1997; Kealey et al, 1996; Kearney, 1998). Cadaver skin can be easily obtained from almost any body that has been kept cold in a morgue for a few days (May and DeClement, 1981). Unfortunately cadaver skin has a limited market in part because skin banking or transplantation has not been as well publicized as that of other solid organs (Heck, 1997; Kealey, 1997).

Xenograft. A xenograft (e.g., pigskin) is useful on partial-thickness burns that will eventually heal on their own. The xenograft is not as effective as the cadaver allograft but augments reepithialization and, because it is occlusive, reduces pain. This graft must be removed and reapplied every 3 to 7 days. If left in place too long, the xenograft can become incorporated into the wound, making removal difficult. Xenografts do not establish vessel-to-vessel connections and thus undergo necrosis and slough, which leads to an increased number of bacteria under the graft (Pruitt, 1997). It can also become dry and adhere to the wound, restricting ROM (Helm and Fisher, 1998). Plates 23 and 24 demonstrate the temporary application of a porcine xenograft followed by a split-thickness skin graft at a later date.

Biologic, Synthetic, and Biosynthetic Skin Replacements. Biosynthetic dressings are used with superficial partial-thickness burns rather than heterografts or homografts. Their particular advantages are that they are readily available, nonallergenic, relatively inexpensive, easily removed, have a permeable membrane, and are packaged in large conformable sheets. Biobrane (Dow Hickam Pharmaceutical, Sugarland, Texas) is a very thin, meshlike, synthetic dressing consisting of a silastic membrane bonded to one surface of a nylon mesh and coated with porcine collagen. This dressing is applied directly to the wound, covered with a compression dressing to ensure adherence, and left in place until epithelialization occurs (Jurkiewicz et al, 1990). After the dressing is adherent, usually in 1 to 2 days, the compression dressing is removed. To test for adherence, a small section is uncovered and the dressing is palpated with a sterile gloved finger. If considerable exudate is present or after 24 to 48 hours the dressing is not adherent, the presence of infection is suspected or the wound is deeper than assessed. As epithelialization occurs, the edges of the dressing loosen and are trimmed away. Unfortunately, reliable closure of large areas of full-thickness excised burn wounds is difficult because of lack of adherence and subgraft supparation (Purdue et al, 1997).

When an infection is present, fine mesh gauze with an absorbing pad, such as the specialty absorptive nonadherent dressing Exu-Dry, is used. A topical agent, such as silver sulfadiazine, is used with parenteral antibiotics to control and treat infection. Applying the cream directly to the dressing rather than to the wound is less painful. This cream can be gently removed during hydrotherapy.

Cultured keratinocyte grafts. Also known as cultured epithelial sheets or cultured epidermis, keratinocyte grafts can be harvested from the unburned skin of the victim (cultured epidermal autograft [CEA]) or from donor skin such as neonatal foreskin (cultured epidermal allograft) and then expanded. Cell expansion, whereby a 2 cm by 2 cm biopsy specimen can increase by a factor of 10,000, takes 3 to 4 weeks. While waiting for the cultured skin, the wounds are excised and covered with available frozen human cadaver skin, allografts, or other temporary coverings.

Keratinocyte grafts are clipped in place, covered with petrolatum, and left in place for 7 to 10 days. Cultured epidermal allografts act as occlusive dressings and release growth factors into the wound bed to induce epithelialization from the wound edges. After application of a CEA, physical therapy and rehabilitation are postponed because of the 7 to 10 days of immobilization required. Even after this period of delay, blister formation and graft loss can occur with resumption and progression of physical therapy.

Closure of excised burn wounds with cultured keratinocytes has met with varied success. The cultured sheets are fragile, difficult to handle, and difficult to affix to the wound (Hansbrough and Rennekampff, 1997; Monafo, 1996). Transportation from the laboratory to the transplantation site is complex. Subsequent wound care is meticulous and the cultured grafts are highly susceptible to infection. "Take rates" are also low. Tompkins and colleagues (1989) reported an initial take of 51%, but then 60% of that group subsequently experienced a loss (Georgia Medical Care Foundation, 1997). In 1993, Rue and colleagues evaluated cultured derived epidermal autografts with 19 patients involving 31 wounds. The average area covered was 10.8% TBSA. Between days 21 and 28, only 30.6% of the grafts were adherent and the average area closed was 2.08%. They also found that as the size of the burn increased, the percentage of rejection also increased. Cultured epithelium is also prone to shearing and contractions once healed.

Several factors may account for poor performance of cultured keratinocytes. When cultured epidermal sheets are placed on full-thickness wounds, a delay in basement membrane formation is observed. In addition, development of ultrastructural elements that attach the dermis to the epidermis (e.g., anchoring fibrils) is delayed. The interdigitation of the epidermis and dermis (which increases the surface area of the dermal-epidermal junction) and the anchoring fibrils are important because they furnish the skin with strength and durability.

Composite (epidermal-dermal) skin grafts. To achieve optimal results for covering full-thickness wounds, replacement of the dermal layer of skin and the epidermis is necessary. Several techniques have been developed and are in various stages of clinical testing.

Synthetic bilaminates, such as BioBrane (Dow Hickam Pharmaceutical) and Integra Artifical Skin (Integra LifeSciences Corporation, Plainsboro, NJ), have an outer epithelial-type membrane that prevents desiccation and an inner layer fabricated of collagen and other dermal matrix proteins.

Dermagraft-TC (Dermagraft-Transitional Covering; Advanced Tissue Sciences, Inc.) is a temporary skin replacement consisting of human neonatal fibroblast grown on Biobrane (Dow Hickam Pharmaceutical). These fibroblasts are grown for 17 days and produce a dermal matrix. The resulting dressing is then frozen for storage (Purdue, 1997). Dermagraft-TC is easy to handle and can be sutured or stapled to the wound. Early formation of basement membrane structures, including laminin and type IV collagen, has been observed as well as resistance to tearing.

Advantages of Dermagraft-TC over cadaver allografts include less bleeding upon removal, ability to observe fluid accumulation under the transparent covering, and because the dermis is relatively nonantigenic, an absence of epidermal loss or rejection. Therefore Dermagraft-TC could be used to cover the wound for an extended period of time while planning permanent closure (Hansbrough et al, 1997). Decreased costs have been reported with Dermagraft-TC because operating room time is reduced by 30% (as a result of the ease of removal as compared with removing cadaver allograft) and since it does not slough, reapplication is eliminated (Parente, 1997).

Integra Artificial Skin is a bilayered product with a dermis composed of a cross-linked bovine collagen-glycosaminoglycan matrix, which allows for the penetration of the patient's own fibroblasts, macrophages, lymphocytes, and capillaries (Helvig, 1997). The top layer of this skin covering is a removable "epidermal" silicone layer. A neodermis is regenerated over a 2- to 3-week period as the patient's cells grow into the matrix. The silicon layer can then be removed, and a thin epidermal autograft can be conducted to complete the treatment.

Integra Artificial Skin is applied in the operating room after early surgical excision of the wound and hemostasis has been achieved. The artificial skin is not meshed and applied as an autograft and secured by staples or sutures. A silicone sheet is fastened to the outside of the product, which safeguards the graft from infection and desiccation. Care needs to be taken to protect the area from pressure and shear. The wound must be assessed for local or systemic infection and hematomas, which can form under the graft. When the dermal matrix has been replaced by the patient's neodermis, the wound appears yellow-orange. The silicone layer may be easily removed, and thin epidermal grafts are meshed, applied, and secured. Postoperative care is the same for any meshed autograft.

Apligraf (Organogenesis) is a third type of skin substitute and is also called a bilayered, allogeneic, cultured skin equivalent. This skin equivalent consists of four important elements of natural skin: a tough protective stratum corneum, an epidermis made up of multiple layers of live differentiating keratinocytes, and a dermal matrix composed of human dermal fibroblasts in a bovine collagen lattice (Choucair, Faria, and Fivenson, 1998). Both the living fibroblasts and the keratinocytes are derived from infant foreskin tissue. This dressing was designed with the hope of eliminating the need for autografting. In a study of patients with chronic venous leg ulcers, no evidence of clinical graft rejection has been observed (Choucair, Faria, and Fivenson, 1998).

Summary. Numerous types of skin coverings and grafts exist. Although autologous skin grafts are preferred, they are not always feasible because of the extensive nature of the burns or the patient's overall condition. Prompt temporary coverage of the excised burn wound is critical to reduce the risk of infection, provide pain relief, and control fluid loss through the burned skin surface. Because of their inevitable rejection, potential for transmission of disease, and disparity in quality, alternatives to cadaver allografts are sought. Tissue-engineering technology has introduced cultured epithelial sheets and biosynthetic epidermal-dermal replacements (Brown, Smith, and McGrouther, 1997; Langer and Vacanti, 1993).

COMPLICATIONS

Numerous complications can affect the burn patient, including infection, excessive scarring, contractures, skin changes, and altered body image.

Infection

In spite of major improvements in care of the burn victim, infection is still the greatest adverse outcome for this patient population. With a burn injury, the avascular eschar is moist and rich in denatured proteins, which creates the ideal environment for the unrestrained growth of microorganisms. In the emergent period, there is an increase in the total white blood cell count and a decrease in peripheral blood lymphocyte count in all burn patients. The immune system's response is hampered by the loss of plasma volume and decrease in IgG levels and in B lymphocytes; these gradually return to normal over 2 to 4 weeks. The diagnosis of infection is difficult because the normal T-helper cell to T-suppressor cell ratio is reversed.

In the burn patient, the wound and its care are primary sources for transmission of microorganisms. The most common organism responsible for burn wound infections is gram-positive bacteria; the predominant cause of burn bacteria is the gram-positive bacteria *Staphylococcus aureus*. Group A β-hemolytic streptococcus and enterococcus are gram-positive organisms that pose a specific hazard to engraftment, especially in pediatric patients who have a high incidence of nasopharyngeal colonization (Greenfield and MacManus, 1997). With the routine use of early excision and grafting, *Pseudomonas aeruginosa* (gram-negative) infection has decreased. Fungal infections have become rare, although they are the most common nonbacterial wound colonizers (Greenfield and MacManus, 1997). *Candida* infections most commonly occur in patients with large burns who required treatment with broad-spectrum antibiotics for other infections. Systemic amphotericin B may be required to treat candidemia.

Filamentous fungi (i.e. *Aspergillus* sp.), can colonize in wounds and have exceeded gram-negative pathogens as a cause of burn wound invasion. Fungi can be found throughout the environment and can be cultured from room air, nonsterile wound supplies, and laundry items. Fungal wound infections have not decreased as bacterial infections have. Fungal infections are treated with topical antifungal agents such as clotrimazole solution or ciclopiroxolamine cream twice a day, systemic amphotericin B, and surgical excision of the infected tissue (Greenfield and MacManus, 1997).

A burn wound biopsy of viable tissue in the wound (not eschar) remains the gold standard to determine the invading microorganism. This is usually done when healing is not progressing (graft or epidermal regeneration), when pain is increased upon touch, when a change in color of the wound or drainage is noted, or in the presence of fever in a previously afrebrile patient. Usual systemic signs are not reliable in burn patients because of the hypermetabolic activity present (Table 10-5).

Prevention of infection, as with other wounds, includes the use of topical antimicrobial agents, adherence to strict aseptic technique when providing wound care, debridement of necrotic tissue, and constant assessment. Universal precautions should be augmented with protective gowns, and sterile gloves, hats, shoe covers, and masks should be worn when caring for patients with open burn wounds. Hand washing is still the best preventive procedure available. Single-room patient isolation has been proven to decrease infection, with continued isolation until 20% of the burn has been closed. Patients who become antibiotic-resistant require more stringent procedures, including single-staff caregivers with days off before caring for nonisolated patients; nonresistant patients are treated in other departments before isolated patients.

Excessive Scarring

Excessive scarring can take the form of a hypertrophic scar or a keloid. Hypertrophic scarring results from an imbalance between collagen synthesis and collagen lysis. A hypertrophic scar is red, thick, hard, and raised above the level of the surrounding normal skin but within the boundaries of the

TABLE 10-5 Signs and Symptoms of Infection in the Burn Patient

	LOCAL CHANGES	SYSTEMIC CHANGES	LABORATORY FINDINGS
Noninvasive	• Change in color • Graft loss • Localized erythema or cellulitis at wound margins • Purulent or odorous exudate • Epithelial breakdown of healed areas	Temperature >101° F	Elevated WBCs (>10,000)
Invasive	• Conversion of partial- to full-thickness area • Breakdown of previously healed areas • Accelerated eschar separation • Tenderness, edema, erythema at wound margin • New necrotic areas	• Tachycardia, hypotension • Oliguria • Paralytic ileus • Changes in LOC	• Leukopenia <5000 • Leukocytosis >10,000 • Elevated blood sugar level • Positive blood cultures • Positive wound biopsy • Thrombocytopenia

Adapted from Greenfield E, MacManus AT: Infectious complications: prevention and strategies for their control, *Nurs Clin North Am* 32(2):297, 1997.

wound, burn, or incision. The collagen is disorganized and hypervascular. Hypertropic scar development is related to the patient's age, pigmentation, family history, and location of the scar (Pessina and Ellis, 1997). In contrast, keloids, which occur more frequently in African-Americans, extend above and over the margins of the burn, wound, or incision.

Pressure therapy is used to prevent excessive scarring until the scar is mature, as evidenced by being avascular, flat, and soft. Patients and their families need to be educated in the care, use, and need for compliance to achieve the benefit of the pressure therapy. They also need to understand that pressure therapy minimizes the appearance of scars but does not necessarily prevent all scar formation. To be effective, garments must be worn 23 hours a day for 1 to 2 years until the scar is fully mature. This can be difficult for many people because the garments can be hot, are confining, and once the crisis is over, many people find it difficult to continue with therapy, including pressure garments. When the patient receives follow-up care in a rehabilitation center or a clinical setting, continued exercising and use of compression garments can be reinforced.

Contractures

Contractures result from the proliferation of scar tissue in deep burns, and normal tissue is pulled into the scar area. Collagen fibers develop in circular patterns. Parallel fibers are less likely to develop contractures. Early splinting, ROM exercises, positioning, and use of pressure garments aid in the development of parallel fibers and maintaining soft-tissue length. To prevent contractures, positions are based on the anatomic tendency to contract in predicted patterns, which are shortened and flexed positions. As stated previously, splints to prevent contractures are to be worn continuously. Splints to protect and immobilize newly placed grafts are applied in the same anticontracture positions and worn at all times (Helm and Fisher, 1998). Both need to be checked for pressure areas and neurologic complications such as numbness and tingling. In less extensive burns there may be more flexibility, with splints being worn for several hours at different times during the day.

Splints in the later rehabilitation phase may differ from those in the early phase since more emphasis is placed on strength and function. Dynamic splints exert a constant stretch or pull on the joint, and their purpose may be to obtain a joint's final degree of range or allow active movement that resumes a lengthened position at rest (Helm and Fisher, 1998). This type of splint requires monitoring by the therapist and nursing staff to maintain proper position and is usually worn for no more than 4 hours at a time.

Skin Changes

Biologic changes in scar tissue affect thermal regulation, sweating, and oil secretions. Split-thickness grafting involves the epidermis and superficial dermis. Therefore the epidermal appendages, hair follicles, and sweat and oil glands are often not included in the grafted skin. Skin pigmentation will eventually return in scar tissue but not completely (DiMola et al, 1988).

Shivering and sweat production are not possible in full-thickness scar tissue. The patient with extensive grafting requires a controlled environment to avoid the extremes of hot or cold. Protection from the sun with clothing and sunscreens is essential; lanolin-based skin lotion is encouraged to provide moisture and decrease pruritus.

Body Image and Family Support

Body image disturbance can result in the patient having strong negative feelings concerning appearance. Psychosocial changes, even problems with family members or significant others, may result in feelings of doubt over appearance, body, and helplessness. A change in occupation can result in a change in lifestyle. Interventions of the team should be directed toward maintaining a positive, accepting, and realistic body image by exploring feelings about the changes and functions of the skin (Watkins et al, 1989). The patient needs to realize positive aspects of the personality rather than just the physical component. Emotional support, empathy, and a nonjudgmental attitude assist in the development of a positive, accepting, realistic body image (Fratianne and Brandt, 1997).

OUTPATIENT BURN MANAGEMENT

The American Burn Association Injury Severity Grading System classifies burns as minor, moderate, or severe, with approximately 80% to 95% of all burns being classified as minor (Box 10-4) (DiMola et al, 1988; Mertens et al, 1997). These minor burns can be managed in an outpatient setting. Minor burns, however, can be significant and can emerge into a major wound or problem. The moderate or severe burn that is treated on an inpatient basis could also be managed in a lower level of care once the wound and patient are stabilized.

BOX 10-4 Definition of Minor Burn Injury

15% TBSA. Superficial partial-thickness/deep partial-thickness in an adult (first or second degree)
10% TBSA. Superficial partial-thickness/deep partial-thickness in a child (first or second degree)
2% TBSA. Full-thickness in a child or adult not involving the eyes, ears, face, or genitalia (third degree)

Adapted from Edlich RF et al: Modification of the American Burn Association injury severity grading system, *JACEP* 7(6):226, 1978.

Patients in acute or possible respiratory distress, inhalation injury, shock, alteration in level of consciousness, or with traumatic injuries would not be appropriate for outpatient care until their condition has stabilized. The severity of the burn, the age of the patient, and any comorbidity are major factors in deciding if the wound could be treated on an outpatient basis. There are sources available to assist the nurse in determining criteria for admission versus outpatient care.

The Georgia Medical Care Foundation (1997) uses *InterQual* as a reference for providers for Medicare program review. Criteria for admission and continued admission and discharge indicators are listed in Box 10-5.

Wound Care

As with any open wound, tetanus vaccination status should be checked and updated as needed. If the wound is free of necrotic tissue or can be easily debrided, this should be performed for proper wound assessment after thorough irrigation and cleansing. A partial-thickness burn is similar to an abrasion or stage 2 pressure ulcer; any topical dressing suitable for the area may be used, keeping in mind the

BOX 10-5 Criteria for Determining Appropriate Setting for Burn Patient

A. Clinical findings* for hospital admission of burn patients
   1. Loss or damage to the skin of 15% TBSA or more
   2. High-voltage burn with devitalized skin, fat, or muscle
   3. Second- or third-degree burns of one of the following: face, hands, perineal region, encircling neck or extremities, anterior or posterior neck or limbs

B. Criteria for continued admission
   1. Presence of any one of the following:
      a. Postsurgery or procedure care 3 days or less
      b. Graft or wound care
      c. Oxygen at more than 4 liters
      d. Hyperbaric therapy
      e. Total parental nutrition (TPN)
      f. Intravenous or intramuscular therapy
      g. Fluids at 100 ml/hr or more
      h. Analgesics
      i. Antiemetics
      j. Electrolytes
      k. Plasma expanders.
   2. Or receiving at least three of the following:
      a. Blood or blood products
      b. Complex burn, graft, or wound care
      c. IV fluids at 100 ml/hr or more
      d. Restorative physical or occupational therapy more than twice a day
      e. Intravenous or intramuscular therapy such as TPN, anticoagulants, corticosteroids, or antiinfectives three times a day or more
      f. Analgesics or antiemetics more than four times a day
      g. Diuretics twice a day or more

C. Discharge indicators
   1. Vital signs stable past 8 hours
   2. Limb swelling decreasing
   3. Burns, grafts, or wounds healing or manageable
   4. Chemistry within normal limits
   5. Infection improving
   6. Pain controlled or manageable
   7. TPN tolerated
   8. Urine output greater than 350 ml in past 12 hours

D. Criteria for discharge after surgery or procedure (all of the following must be met)
   1. Vital signs stable past 8 hours
   2. Fluids tolerated
   3. Vomiting controlled
   4. Grafts or wounds healing or manageable
   5. Passing flatus or stool
   6. Voiding

**InterQual* is a reference for providers for Medicare program review.

principles of moist wound healing. The wound should also be protected from further trauma and dressed to promote optimal activity and function of the patient. The risk of infection is no greater for the burn then other chronic wounds, so systemic antibiotics are not needed. Options for burn coverage include the various wound dressings, topical agents, and ointments such as bacitracin, zinc, or polysporin and nonadherent gauze. Any hair, especially if the area is on the scalp, should be shaved to facilitate wound care and assessment. Blisters, depending on the size and location, can be left intact or removed. If it is extremely large or in an area of friction that will likely rupture, it may be best to unroof the blister and treat the wound while the patient is receiving care. Blisters that are drained have a tendency to refill.

Follow-up is based on 1- to 2-week intervals depending on the extent, depth, and ability or need for reinforcement of the patient or caregiver (Mertens et al, 1997). This is continued until wound epithelization occurs. Once healed, the interval is extended to every 6 weeks to evaluate scar maturation. The scar tissue requires frequent application of a nonperfumed moisturizing cream to prevent dryness. A factor 15 to 30 sun block is recommended to prevent hyperpigmentation.

If the wound does not heal in 3 weeks, surgical excision and grafting should be considered. If more than 2 to 3 weeks are needed to heal, there could be an increase in hypertropic scarring, blistering, and friability of the area. During this period, active use of the area is encouraged for positioning, exercise, and prevention of edema. In the lower extremities, elastic bandages and ambulation are used to promote venous return. For burns on the fingers and hands and in any involved joint, active ROM exercises are essential to maintain flexibility and function. Pressure garments are considered only if grafting is needed or if the healing time extends beyond 2 weeks. Children or older adults who may not be able to exercise may need splints for protection.

Pain should be slight once the wound is dressed. The patient may also require acetaminophen for discomfort and a lanolin-based cream for itching. Severe pruritus can be treated with diphenhydramine or hydroxyzine hydrochloride.

OUTCOME MANAGEMENT

The length of stay based on the Medicare diagnosis-related group (DRG) for nonextensive burns with wound debridement is 10.3 days, for extensive burns with an operating room procedure is 30.2 days, and for extensive burns without an operating room procedure is 8.4 days. Extensive burns are defined as involving 20% to 29% TBSA with third-degree burns or more than 50% TBSA with any degree. Some variations will apply based on individuals.

Outcome management should be based on this and on several other factors (e.g., what the patient and/or family needs or considers important, what the nurse feels is the best practice pattern for the problem, and what the third-party payers believe is of value and quality).

Outcomes for the burn victim should consider the patient's quality of life, satisfaction with the care received, relief of suffering, and restoration of function and safety while in the health care environment. Goals should be designed as steps to reach these outcomes. Clinical pathways can be used to collect these goals or clinical indicators (Box 10-6), and the outcomes can be compiled in a database. This information can then be examined for results and trends, and the process can be reevaluated for performance improvement.

SUMMARY

The wound care nurse has many opportunities to be involved in the care of a patient with massive tissue loss. Whether involved in the care of a patient with extensive major burns requiring hospitalization or with minor burns that can be managed on an outpatient basis, the wound care nurse must be familiar

BOX 10-6 Examples of Clinical Outcomes

- At time of discharge, the patient and/or significant other will be able to perform exercises as instructed.
- The patient will have acceptable pain control evaluated by use of the 1 to 10 pain scale.
- Full-thickness burns will be excised and closed with a permanent or temporary covering by day 3 of admission.

with assessment of burn severity, management options, prevention, and management of potential complications and psychosocial support needs.

SELF-ASSESSMENT EXERCISE

1. Which phases of wound healing occur in burns?
2. Which type of burn occurs in the home?
3. Which zone of tissue damage experiences the most damage?
4. What actions will prevent further damage to the zone of stasis?
   a. Prevention of infection
   b. Protection from drying and exposure
   c. Turning or moving to relieve pressure
   d. All the above
5. The treatment of a burn wound is based on the ________ , ________ , and ________ .
6. Which is the most accurate method to calculate TBSA?
   a. Lund and Bower chart
   b. Rule of Nines
   c. Palm method
   d. Harris-Benedict formula
7. The inflammatory response releases agents that affect:
   a. Urine output, blood pressure, respirations
   b. Vasoconstriction, fluid balance, metabolism
   c. Sodium retention, metabolism, temperature control
   d. Urine output, vasoconstriction, temperature control
8. The most accurate method to assess resuscitation adequacy is:
   a. Preburn body weight
   b. Blood pressure
   c. Cardiac output
   d. Urine output
9. Early excision should occur between which days after the incident?
   a. 1 and 2
   b. 3 and 5
   c. 5 and 8
   d. 9 and 12
10. Facial burns are best grafted with:
    a. 2-to-1 meshed graft
    b. Sheet graft
    c. Allograft
    d. Xenograft
11. Positioning and splinting are done to:
    a. Prevent contractures
    b. Provide comfort
    c. Reduce pain
    d. Enhance graft take
12. Which is the most common type of organism responsible for wound infections?
    a. Gram-positive bacteria
    b. Gram-negative bacteria
    c. Fungus
    d. Virus
13. Minor burns are identified as:
    a. 10% to 15% TBSA deep partial-thickness in an adult
    b. 5% to 10 % TBSA partial-thickness in a child
    c. 2% TBSA full-thickness in an adult not involving the eyes, ears, face, or genitalia
    d. All the above

REFERENCES

Brown RA, Smith KD, McGrouther DA: Strategies for cell engineering in tissue repair, *Wound Rep Reg* 5:212, 1997.

Carrougher G: Management of fluid and electrolyte balance in thermal injuries: implications for perioperative nursing practice, *Semin Perioper Nurs* 6(4):201, 1997.

Choucair M, Faria D, Fivenson D: Use of human skin equivalent in the successful treatment of chronic venous leg ulcers, *Wounds* 10(3):97, 1998.

Chrysopoulo M et al: Acute renal dysfunction in severely burned adults, *J Trauma* 46(1):141, 1999.

Davis ST, Sheely-Adolphson P: Burn management: psychosocial interventions: pharmacologic and psychologic modalities, *Nurs Clin North Am* 32(2):331, 1997.

DiMola M et al: Burns. In Kinney M, Pack D, editors: *AACN's clinical reference for critical care nursing,* New York, 1988, McGraw-Hill.

Doughty D: Principles of wound healing and wound management. In Bryant R, editor: *Acute and chronic wounds: nursing management*, St Louis, 1992, Mosby.

Fowler A: Nursing management of minor burn injures, *Nurs Standard* 12(49):47, 1998.

Fratianne R, Brandt C: Improved survival adults with extensive burns, *J Burn Care Rehabil* 18(4):347, 1997.

Gallico G et al: Permanent coverage of large burn wounds with autologous cultured human epithelium, *N Engl J Med* 311(7):448, 1984.

Georgia Medical Care Foundation: *InterQual*, Atlanta, 1997, GMCF.

Gordon M, Goodwin CW: Burn management: initial assessment, management, and stabilization, *Nurs Clin North Am* 32(2):237, 1997.

Greenfield E, MacManus AT: Infectious complications: prevention and strategies for their control, *Nurs Clin North Am* 32(2):297, 1997.

Hansbrough JF et al: Clinical trials of a biosynthetic temporary skin replacement, dermagraft-transitional covering, compared with cryopreserved human cadaver skin for temporary coverage of excised burn wounds, *J Burn Care Rehabil* 18:43, 1997.

Hansbrough JF, Rennekampff HO: Cultured skin cells for wound closure and for promoting wound healing. In Ziegler TR et al, editors: *Growth factors and wound healing: basic science and potential clinical applications*, New York, 1997, Springer-Verlag.

Heck E: Operational standards and regulations for tissue banks, *J Burn Care Rehabil* 18(1 Pt 2):S11, 1997.

Helm R, Fisher S: Rehabilitation of the patient with burns. In DeLisa H, editor: *Rehabilitation medicine: principles and practice*, ed 3, Philadelphia, 1998, J.B. Lippincott.

Helvig E: Dermal replacement: an update, *Semin Perioper Nurs* 6(4):233, 1997.

Jordan B, Harrington D: Management of the burn wound, *Nurs Clin North Am* 32(2):251, 1997.

Jurkiewicz MJ et al: *Plastic surgery: principles and practice*, St Louis, 1990, Mosby.

Kealey GP: Disease transmission by means of allograft, *J Burn Care Rehabil* 18(1 Pt 2):S10, 1997

Kealey GP et al: Cadaver skin allografts and transmission of human cytomegalovirus to burn patients, *J Am Coll Surg* 182:201, 1996

Kearney J: Quality issues in skin banking: a review, *Burns* 24:299, 1998

Kinney M: *Burns: AACN's clinical reference for critical care nursing*, St Louis, 1998, Mosby.

Kottke F, Lehmann J: *Krusen's handbook of physical medicine and rehabilitation*, Philadelphia, 1990, W.B. Saunders.

Laing H: Perioperative burn nursing, *Semin Perioper Nurs* 6(4):210, 1997.

Langer R, Vacanti JP: Tissue engineering, *Science* 260:920, 1993.

Lim J et al: Rapid response: Care of burn victims, *AAHON Journal* 46(4):169, 1998.

May SR, DeClement FA: Skin banking. Part I. Procurement of transplantable cadaveric allograft skin for burn wound coverage, *J Burn Care Rehabil* 2:7, 1981.

Mertens D et al: Outpatient burn management, *Nurs Clin North Am* 32(2):343, 1997.

Molnar J et al: Burns: metabolism and nutritional therapy in thermal injury. In Schneider H, editor: *Nutritional support of medical practice*, Philadelphia, 1983, Harper & Row.

Monafo W: Initial management of burns, *N Engl J Med* 235(21):1581, 1996.

Parente ST: Estimating the economic cost offsets of using Dermagraft-TC as an alternative to cadaver allograft in the treatment of graftable burns, *J Burn Care Rehabil* 18:18, 1997.

Peck M, Ward G: Burn injury. In Civetta J, Taylor R, Kirby R: *Critical care*, ed 3, Philadelphia, 1997, Lippincott-Raven.

Pessina M, Ellis S: Rehabilitation, *Nurs Clin North Am* 32(2):365, 1997.

Pruitt BA Jr: The evolutionary development of biologic dressings and skin substitutes, *J Burn Care Rehabil* 18(1Pt2):S2, 1997.

Purdue GF et al: A multicenter clinical trial of a biosynthetic skin replacement, dermagraft-TC, compared with cryopreserved human cadaver skin for temporary coverage of excised burn wounds, *J Burn Care Rehabil* 18:52, 1997.

Rue LW et al: Wound closure and outcome in extensively burned patients treated with cultured autologous keratinocytes, *J Trauma* 34(5):662, 1993.

Staley M, Richard R: Use of pressure to treat hypertrophic burn scars, *Adv Wound Care* 10(3):44, 1997.

Sulton L: Postoperative nursing care of the burn patient, *Sem Perioper Nurs* 6(4):236, 1997.

Tompkins R et al: Increased survival after massive thermal injuries in adults: preliminary report using artificial skin, *N Engl J Med* 17(8):743, 1989.

Thompson J et al: *Mosby's manual of clinical nursing*, St Louis, 1997, Mosby.

Trott AT: *Wounds and lacerations*, ed 2, St Louis, 1991, Mosby.

Watkins P et al: Psychological stages in adaptation following burn injury: a method for facilitating psychological recovery of burn victims, *J Burn Care Rehabil* 2(4):376, 1989.

Winfree J, Barillo D: Nonthermal injuries, *Nurs Clin North Am* 32(2):275, 1997.

Woods N et al: Supporting families during chronic illness, *Image* 21(1):46, 1989.

CHAPTER 11

Mechanical Forces: Pressure, Shear, and Friction

BARBARA PIEPER

OBJECTIVES

1. Distinguish between cumulative incidence and prevalence.
2. Describe the data reporting the prevalence of pressure ulcers in hospitals and nursing homes, in the elderly, and in patients with spinal cord injury.
3. Define *pressure ulcer.*
4. Identify the three most common locations for pressure ulcers to develop.
5. Describe the role of subcutaneous tissue and muscle in preventing pressure ulcers.
6. Identify four factors that cause pressure ulcer formation.
7. Differentiate between capillary pressure, capillary closing pressure, and interface pressure.
8. Describe the role of tissue tolerance, intensity of pressure, and duration of pressure in the development of pressure ulcers.
9. Describe the effects of the following factors on pressure ulcer development: blood pressure, temperature, smoking, psychosocial status, and age.
10. Describe the phenomena of reactive hyperemia, blanching erythema, and nonblanching erythema.
11. Describe the pathophysiologic consequences of pressure damage, including the changes that occur at the cellular level and the cone-shaped pressure gradient.
12. Discuss five variables that influence the extent of tissue damage as a consequence of pressure.
13. Differentiate between reliability, validity, specificity, and sensitivity.
14. Describe three pressure-sore risk-assessment scales, including the parameters that each scale measures.
15. Identify therapeutic features that can be provided by support surfaces.
16. Explain the relevance of capillary closing pressure in selection of support surfaces.
17. Distinguish between the three categories of support surfaces: overlay, replacement mattress, and specialty bed.
18. Identify four criteria for the use of therapeutic foam.
19. Compare and contrast the following in terms of advantages and disadvantages:
    a. Foam overlays
    b. Water overlays
    c. Gel overlays
    d. Static air overlays
    e. Low air-loss overlay
    f. Alternating air overlay
    g. Replacement mattresses
    h. Low air-loss bed
    i. Air fluidized bed
    j. Kinetic therapy bed
20. Establish two criteria for use of each of the following:
    a. Pressure-reduction device
    b. Pressure-relief device
    c. Kinetic therapy device
21. Describe the effect of repositioning on interface pressure.
22. Describe ways to support the patient during pressure ulcer treatment.
23. Identify methods to measure pressure ulcer healing.

24. Identify the potential of pain with a pressure ulcer.
25. Relate quality improvement and legal aspects of pressure ulcers.
26. Knows resources available for pressure ulcer information.
27. Identify the need to educate the patient, caregiver, and health professional about pressure ulcers.

Pressure ulcers present a significant health care threat to patients with restricted mobility or chronic disease and to older patients. The National Pressure Ulcer Advisory Panel (NPUAP, 1989) estimated that well over 1 million people in hospitals and nursing homes suffer from pressure ulcers. In 1992, 194,000 persons admitted to hospitals were diagnosed with a pressure ulcer at the time of discharge; 77% (n = 150,000) were persons 65 years of age or older (Margolis, 1995).

Facility-acquired pressure ulcers add to the patient's length of stay, delay the patient's recuperation, and increase the patient's risk for developing complications. Additionally, pressure ulcers often necessitate hospitalization (in certain patient populations such as the elderly and patients with a spinal cord injury) because of sepsis or the need for debridement or surgical repair. At a time of increasingly scarce health care dollars, pressure ulcers consume intense resources in the form of dressing changes, nursing care, physical therapy, medications, nutritional support, and physician services. Pressure ulcers have been examined in terms of their effects on mortality rates. Residents with a pressure ulcer in long-term care had a relative risk of dying of 2.37, but after adjusting for 16 other measures, the risk declined to 1.45 (Berlowitz et al, 1997). Pressure ulcers are not an independent predictor of mortality but a marker for underlying disease severity and other comorbidities (Allman, 1998; Berlowitz et al, 1997).

ECONOMIC EFFECTS

The financial cost of pressure ulcers to the U.S. health economy is a matter of conjecture. The literature reports a range of costs for pressure ulcer management. For patients in long-term care, Xakellis and Frantz (1996) calculated the cost of treating a pressure ulcer as $2731; the cost of treatment per patient was $4647. The cost of treating one occipital pressure ulcer has been calculated to be $4323 (Powers, 1997). Allman (1998) and Allman and colleagues (1999) calculated the mean cost per admission for patients who develop a pressure ulcer as $37,288 versus $13,924 for patients who did not. After adjusting for admission characteristics, the mean cost for each patient who developed a pressure ulcer was $14,260 versus $12,382 for those who did not (Allman, 1998; Allman et al, 1999). Patients who developed pressure ulcers versus patients without them were more likely to develop nosocomial infections and other hospital complications (Allman et al, 1999). Postdischarge expenses for Medicare patients were $13 higher per day for patients with pressure ulcers; this increased effect did not remain when an adjustment was done for activity (Allman, Damiano, and Strauss, 1996).

Unfortunately, the costs that are reported to be incurred while a pressure ulcer is being managed must be viewed cautiously; the studies are not all comparable. Some studies account for all costs: room, nursing care, supplies, medications, physician fees, and so forth. Other studies examine only direct costs, such as the supplies or medications specifically indicated for that particular problem. Costs of programs for prevention (training, changes in reporting, policies and procedures) may initially be $60,000 with subsequent annual costs of $10,000 (Moore and Wise, 1997). There are many opinions in the literature about costs. In summary, about 1.6 million patients each year in acute care settings develop pressure ulcers, representing a cost of $2.2 to $3.6 billion to the U.S. health care system (Beckrich and Aronovitch, 1998).

SCOPE OF THE PROBLEM

The scope of the pressure ulcer problem in the United States is as unknown as the true costs of managing the pressure ulcer. This may be attributed to two factors: 1) a pressure ulcer is not a reportable condition, and 2) institutions believe that the presence of pressure ulcers is a negative reflection on the quality of care. The quality assurance

BOX 11-1 Characteristics of Incidence and Prevalence

Cumulative Incidence

- The number of new cases that develop during a specific period of time in a population of individuals at risk for the condition.
- Used as a measure of risk; the probability that an individual will develop the condition within a given time frame.
- Requires repeated obvservations over time; considered a prospective or longitudinal measure.
- Observation is one for specific population *who are at risk* for developing the disease of interest (such as all residents of a state, all male, all patients over 60 years of age).
- Calculated as the number of patients who are initially pressure ulcer free and then develop a pressure ulcer during a specified time frame (e.g., 1 month) divided by the total number of patients who are at risk for developing a pressure ulcer; this number is then multiplied by 100 to obtain a percentage.
- Cumulative incidence is dimensionless; ranges from 0 to 1 or 0% to 100%.
- Should not be confused with incidence rate, which has units of time. For example, 10 patients out of 100 at-risk patients who are pressure ulcer free develop a pressure ulcer over a 3-month period for an incidence of 10 new cases per 3 months or a 3 month incidence rate of 10%.

Prevalence

- The number of cases (old and new) at a particular point in time.
- Used to measure burden of disease or condition.
- Requires only one observation; considered a cross-sectional measure.
- Observation is of one specific population.
- Calculated as the number of patients with a pressure ulcer on the day of data collection divided by the total number of patients in the population; this may then be multiplied by 100 to obtain a percentage.
- Prevalence is dimensionless; ranges from 0 to 1 or 0% to 100%.
- Considered to be relatively stable over time unless the frequency of the disease is changing.

Example

A survey is conducted of all the nursing homes in one city. There are 1000 nursing home residents. On May 1, 100 patients are found to have pressure ulcers. The prevalence on May 1 is 100/1000, or 10%. The remaining 900 residents who are pressure ulcer free are followed weekly. At the end of 1 week, 9 residents develop a pressure ulcer. The cumulative incidence at 1 week is 9/900, or 1%. Another survey is conducted at the end of 4 weeks and 11 more new pressure ulcers are observed. The cumulative incidence at 4 weeks is 20/900, or 2.2%. If the 100 residents with the prevalent pressure ulcers are still residents in the facilities (and assuming no more residents were admitted with pressure ulcers), the total prevalent cases at the end of 4 weeks is 120 for a prevalence of 120/1000, or 12%.

guidelines of some state and federal agencies have reinforced the belief that pressure ulcers reflect negatively on quality of care.

Prevalence and incidence are confusing terms and are frequently used interchangeably or incorrectly (Baumgarten, 1998; Frantz, 1997; Lake, 1999). Prevalence and incidence assess the frequency of a condition. Prevalence, a cross sectional measure, indicates the proportion of a population that has a given condition at a specific time. For the condition under study, such as pressure ulcers, prevalence includes old and new conditions.

Cumulative incidence is a longitudinal measure and indicates the probability of developing a condition over a specific period of time. Incidence is the number of *new* conditions that devleop during a specific time period in a population at risk for the condition. Therefore when measuring incidence, patients are initally free of the condition being measured and then followed over time to determine how many develop the condition. Box 11-1 outlines the differences between these two measurements.

Prevalence

Prevalence measures the burden of a condition at a particular point in time. It is useful for planning human, material, and financial resources necessary to manage the condition of interest. Reported prevalence varies widely according to country, patient population, and methodology. For example, international studies report a prevalence of 8.85% to 10% (Clark et al, 1978; Hawthorne, Jefferson, and Paduano, 1989; Weststrate and Bruining, 1996). Adult patients in critical care may have higher prevalence with ranges from 13.6% for short stay to 42.1% for long stay (Weststrate and Bruining, 1996). In general, these studies include all inpatients and outpatients receiving care on one specific day and exclude all maternity patients, ambulatory patients, psychiatric patients, and physically mobile mentally retarded patients.

In the United States, the Fourth National Pressure Ulcer Prevalence Study reported a prevalence in acute care at 10.1%; findings have remained constant over time (Barczak et al, 1997; Meehan, 1990). Some acute care facilities have reported prevalence as high as 15% to 21% (Langemo et al, 1991; Moore and Wise, 1997) or examined specific groups of patients such as those who experienced prolonged surgery with a prevalence of 8.1% (Aronovitch, 1998). This discrepancy in rates can be attributed to the fact that some studies include intact pressure-damaged skin (stage 1), whereas other studies exclude such lesions. Lower prevalence rates are reported when intact pressure-damaged skin is excluded from the sample (Allman et al, 1986; Shannon and Skorga, 1989). However, prevalence can also be overestimated by erroneous inclusion of patients with ordinary hyperemic responses, such as pressure-damaged intact skin. The prevalence of pressure ulcers in dark-skinned persons may also be missed (Lyder et al, 1998). Some skin changes, such as candidiasis or herpetic lesions, may be misclassified as pressure ulcers (Pieper et al, 1997b). Thus it is imperative that data collectors accurately distinguish between pressure ulcers and other causes of erythema and skin ulcerations.

Eckman (1989) reported a 23.6% prevalence of pressure ulcers among a unique sample of 1378 subjects in 130 funeral homes. Based on these findings, Eckman extrapolated that dermal ulcers were present in 500,000 of the 2.13 million people who died in the United States in 1987.

Some populations, such as the elderly and the spinal cord injured, are at especially high risk for pressure ulcers. The most common group for pressure ulcers is persons 65 to 80 years of age (Barczak et al, 1997; Margolis, 1995; Meehan, 1990). The prevalence of pressure ulcers in nursing homes or long-term care ranges from 12% to 35% (Brandeis et al, 1995; Langemo et al, 1991; Reed and Weksler, 1998; Spector and Fortinsky, 1998). There are 200,000 persons with spinal cord injury in the United States, and each year 25% of them develop a pressure ulcer; 85% of them will develop a pressure ulcer at some point in life (Niazi et al, 1997).

Children may also develop pressure ulcers, primarily in the occipital region for infants and toddlers and the sacrum for children (Quigley and Curley, 1996). Pressure ulcer prevalence has been studied in home care with rates estimated around 20% (Kanj, Wilking, and Phillips, 1998; Langemo et al, 1991). Surgical patients are often immobile during the perioperative experience. The prevalence of pressure ulcers in patients with surgeries 3 hours or longer is 8.5% (Aronovitch, 1998).

Incidence

Cumulative incidence measures new conditions (e.g., pressure ulcers) and is therefore considered more reflective of quality of care within that setting. It is a measure used to evaluate the effects of preventive and therapeutic interventions. Determining the incidence of pressure ulcers is inherently difficult because such studies require longitudinal observations. As with prevalence, incidence will vary by setting. Among home care patients, the incidences of pressure ulcers is reported as 17% (Ramundo, 1995). In long-term care or nursing homes, the incidence may range from 5% to 23% (Bergstrom et al, 1996, 1998; Brandeis et al, 1995; Xakellis et al, 1998). Critically injured survivors of serious trauma have a reported pressure ulcer incidence of 30.6% (Baldwin and Ziegler, 1998).

There are considerable methodologic issues that surround the calculation of incidence. For example, defining who is at risk (the number used in the denominator of the incidence formula) can have a significant influence on the resulting value, which may actually overestimate or underestimate the true frequency of the condition. Consequently, variation in reports of incidence may reflect a real difference in frequency of the condition or simply different data-collection techniques, definitions, and methods. The reader is encouraged to seek additional references for further discussion of this topic before conducting an incidence study. However, although differences in methodology make it difficult to compare incidence from one setting or report with another, it remains an important measure. Health care institutions, facilities, and agencies are encouraged to be consistent in data collection, maintain data collection for comparisons, and share information with others (Gallagher, 1997).

Summary

In summary, several factors contribute to the difficulty in accurately determining the size and scope of the pressure ulcer problem. Variations in patient populations and study designs, inappropriate attempts to generalize findings from small population samples, and frequently the expertise of the researchers make data comparisons difficult. Other problems include the lack of a uniform classification system (i.e., staging or grading), confusion in the use of the terms prevalence and incidence (see Box 11-1), inconsistencies in the definition of *pressure ulcer,* variation in the inclusion of stage 1 pressure ulcers, difficulty in assessing dark skin, and misdiagnosis of a skin change as a pressure ulcer.

Some large scale studies have been done in the United States (Aronovitch, 1998; Bergstrom et al, 1996, 1998; Brandeis et al, 1995; Langemo et al, 1991). In addition, patients now are older and sicker; they are hospitalized for shorter periods of time and are discharged to home or to intermediate or long-term care facilities at a more acute stage of illness. These changes in the patient population can be expected to increase the number of people at risk for pressure ulcers, increase the number of high-risk patients in extended care and home care settings, and potentially alter the incidence and prevalence of pressure ulcers in each setting.

TERMINOLOGY

Over the years, several terms have been used to describe pressure ulcers: bedsore, decubitus ulcer, decubiti, and pressure sore. *Pressure ulcer* is the accepted term because it is more accurate and descriptive.

The origin of the term *bedsore* is not known but predates the term *decubitus. Decubitus,* a Latin word referring to the reclining position (Fox and Bradley, 1803), dates from 1747 when the French used it to mean 'bedsore' (Arnold, 1983). This term, however, is inaccurate because it does not convey the tissue destruction associated with these lesions and because these lesions result from positions other than the lying position (such as sitting). Additionally, although *decubiti* is used as the plural form of decubitus, it also is incorrect. *Decubitus* is a fourth-declension Latin noun, and "fourth declension nouns form their plural with the ending –us . . ." (Arnold, 1983). Therefore the plural of *decubitus* is *decubitus;* the English plural *decubitus ulcers* is better.

Several definitions for *pressure ulcers* have been proposed in the literature (Cherry and Ryan, 1983; Parish, Witkowski, and Crissey, 1983), and all commonly describe impaired blood supply. *Pressure ulcers* is defined as localized areas of tissue necrosis that tend to develop when soft tissue is compressed between a bony prominence and an external surface for a prolonged period of time (NPUAP, 1989; Panel for the Prediction and Prevention of Pressure Ulcers in Adults, 1992).

Pressure ulcers occur most commonly over a bony prominence such as the sacrum, ischial tuberosity, trochanter, and calcaneus; however, they may develop anywhere on the body (e.g., underneath a cast, splint, or cervical collar). Approximately 60% of pressure ulcers develop in the area of the pelvis (Barczak et al, 1997). The most common locations for pressure ulcers in adults are the sacrum (30% to 49%) and heels (19% to 36%) (Aronovitch, 1998; Barczak et al, 1997; Clark and Cullum, 1992; Kemp et al, 1993; Meehan, 1990; Vyhlidal et al, 1997). Figure 11-1 demonstrates the typical locations for pressure ulcers and the frequency of ulcer formation at each site.

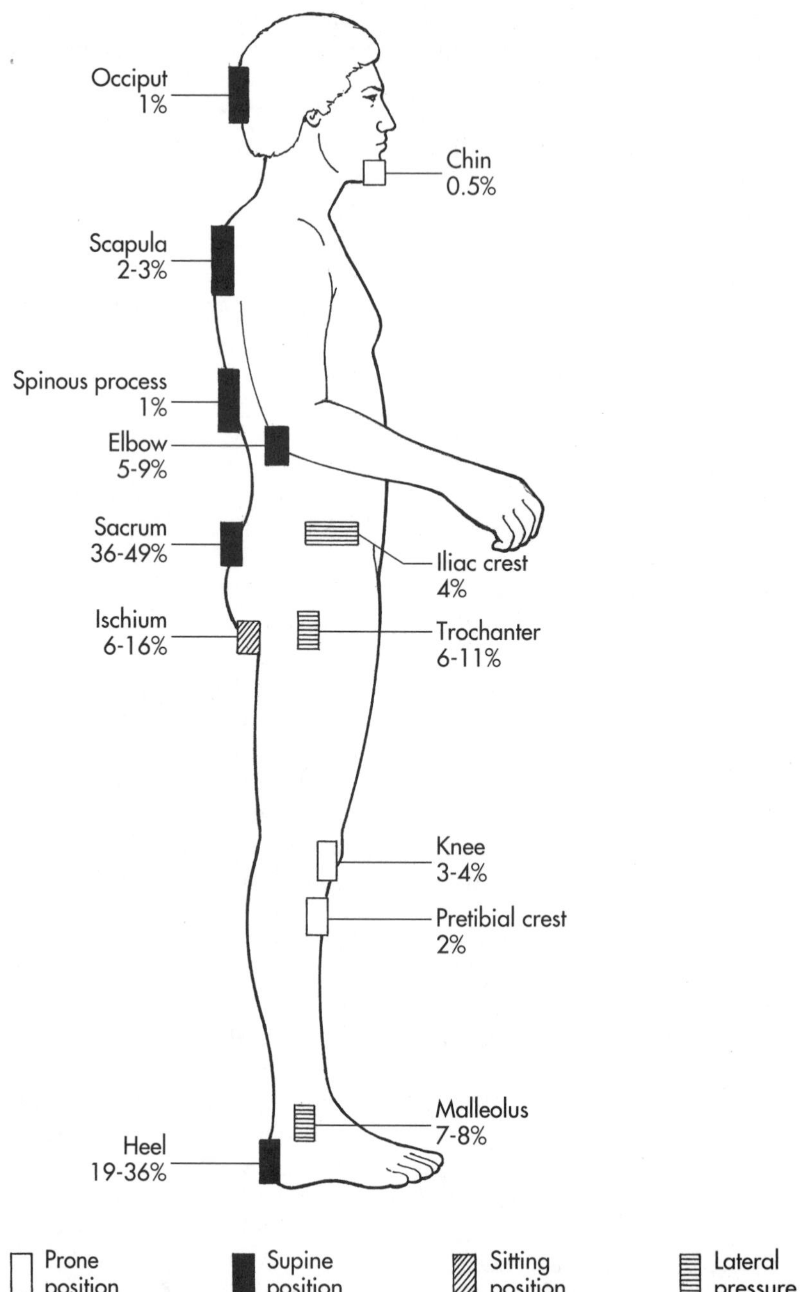

Figure 11-1 Common sites for pressure ulcers and frequency of ulceration per site. (Data from Agris J, Spira M: Pressure ulcers: prevalence and treatment, *Clin Symp* 31(5):21, 1979.; Aronovitch SA: Intraoperative acquired pressure ulcer prevalence: a national study, *Adv Wound Care* 11(3 suppl):8, 1998; Barczak CA et al: Fourth national pressure ulcer prevalence survey, *Adv Wound Care* 10(4):18, 1997; Clark M, Cullum N: Matching patient need for pressure sore prevention with the supply of pressure redistributing mattresses, *J Adv Nurs* 17:310, 1992; Meehan M: Multisite pressure ulcer prevalence survey, *Decubitus* 3:14, 1990.)

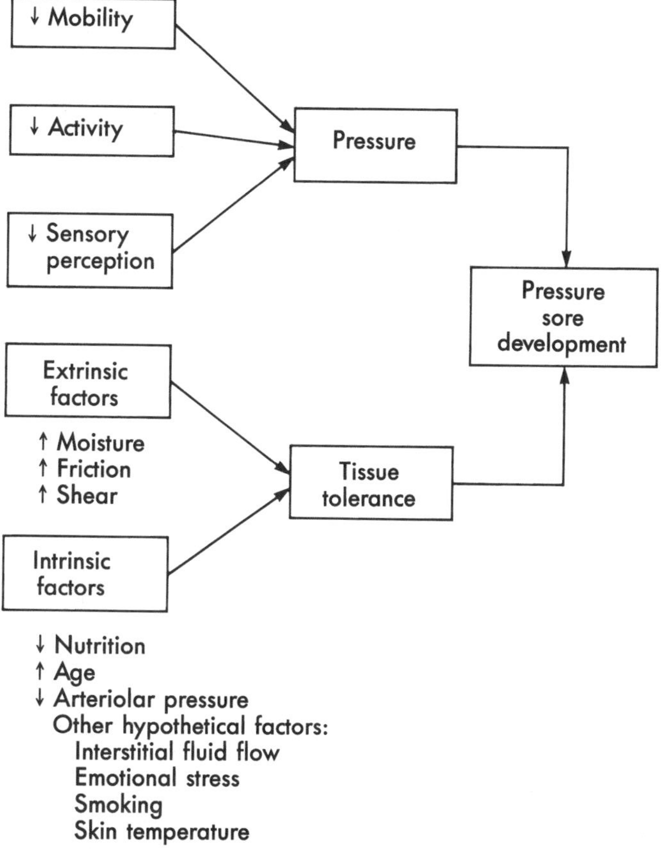

Figure 11-2 Factors contributing to the development of pressure ulcers. (From Braden B, Bergstrom N: A conceptual schema for the study of the etiology of pressure sores, *Rehabil Nurs* 12(1):8, 1987.)

Bony locations are the areas most prone to pressure ulcer formation because a person's body weight is concentrated on these areas when resting on an unyielding surface. Those who have atrophy of the subcutaneous and muscle tissue layers are at even greater risk for the "mechanical load" of pressure and thus increased soft tissue and capillary compression. The coccyx, sacrum, and heel are particularly vulnerable because less soft tissue is present between the bone and skin.

ETIOLOGY

Pressure

Pressure is the major causative factor in pressure ulcer formation. However, several factors play a role in determining whether pressure is sufficient to create an ulcer. The pathologic effect of excessive pressure on soft tissue can be attributed to 1) intensity of pressure, 2) duration of pressure, and 3) tissue tolerance (the ability of both the skin and its supporting structures to endure pressure without adverse sequelae). Two models describe how these factors, in addition to the three major factors that cause pressure ulcers (shear, friction, and nutritional debilitation), contribute to pressure ulcer development (Figures 11-2 and 11-3).

Intensity of Pressure. To understand the importance of intensity of pressure, it is important to review the terms *capillary pressure* and *capillary closing pressure.* Capillary pressure tends to move fluid outward through the capillary membrane (Guyton and Hall, 1996). Exact capillary pressure is

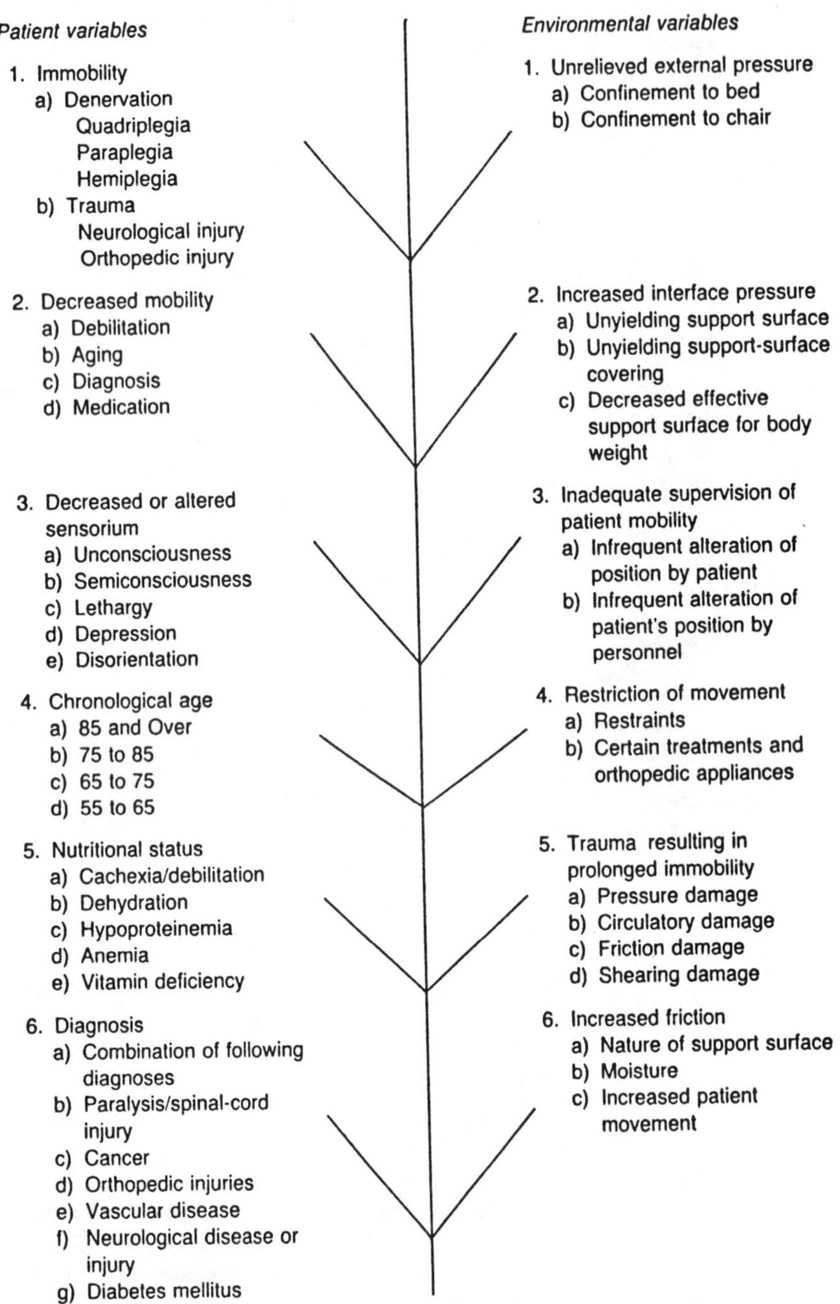

Figure 11-3 Etiologic (causal) model of pressure sore production. (From Shannon ML: Pressure sores. In Norris CM: *Concept clarification in nursing*, Rockville, Md, 1982, Aspen.)

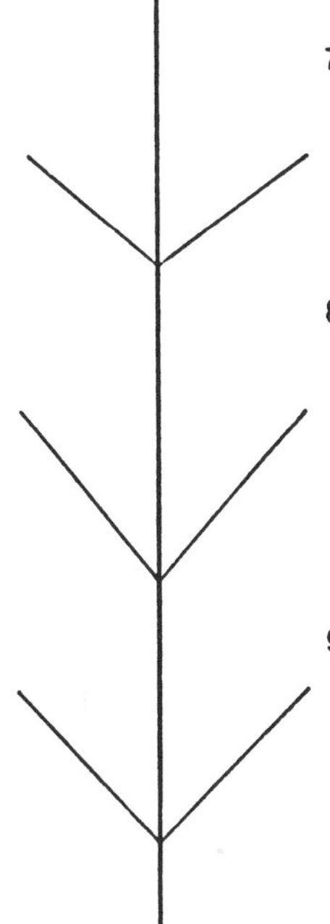

7. Musculoskeletal alterations
   a) Loss of subcutaneous tissue
   b) Loss of muscle mass
   c) Increasing prominence of bony support surfaces

7. Shearing force
   a) Pulling patients up in bed without lifting them clear of mattress
   b) Elevating head of bed

8. Soft-tissue changes
   a) Medication-induced changes, as with steroids
   b) Disease-associated changes, as with amyotrophic lateral sclerosis
   c) Race-related changes

8. Lack of adequate nutritional management
   a) IV fluids only
   b) Formula feedings
   c) Inadequate oral intake

9. Incontinence
   a) Bladder
   b) Bowel

9. Failure to maintain dry environment
   a) Wet or soiled bed linens
   b) Skin maceration due to wetness and chemical irritation

10. Major surgery
    a) Any procedure lasting 4 or more hours
    b) Orthopedic procedures of hip and femur

11. Medications
    a) Narcotics
    b) Sedatives
    c) Analgesics
    d) Soporifics
    e) Steroids

12. Infection
    a) Severe generalized infection
    b) Localized infection in pressure-supporting areas
    c) Sustained elevated body temperature

The greater number of patient and environmental variables present and interacting, the greater the risk of pressure sore formation.

↓

Pressure sore formation

Figure 11-3, cont'd.

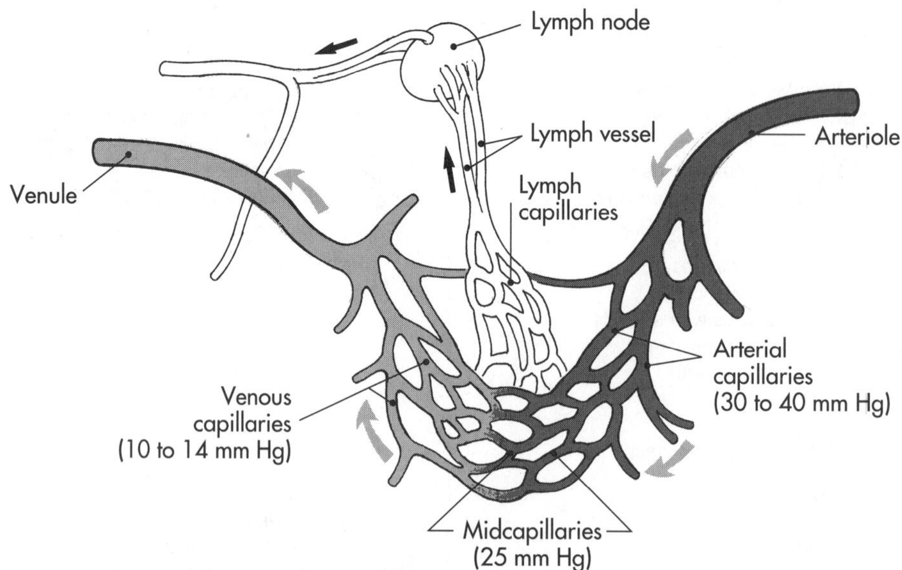

Figure 11-4 Capillary pressure within the capillary bed.

not known because of the difficulty of obtaining the measurement. Various methods have been used to estimate capillary pressure.

One method used to measure capillary pressure is by direct cannulation of the capillary with a microscopic glass pipet. A manometer is then attached to the pipet, and a pressure reading is obtained. Capillary pressures have been obtained in animals and in the fingernails of humans using this method. Using such techniques, capillary pressures have been reported as follows: 32 mm Hg in the arteriolar limb, 12 mm Hg in the venous limb, and 20 mm Hg in the midcapillary (Landis, 1930) (Figure 11-4). More commonly, capillary pressures are reported as 30 to 40 mm Hg at the arterial end, 10 to 14 mm Hg at the venous end, and about 25 mm Hg in the middle of the capillary.

Two indirect methods to measure capillary pressure have been reported and result in a pressure termed the *functional capillary pressure,* or the pressure (17 mm Hg) believed necessary to keep the capillary system open and functional (Guyton and Hall, 1996). Indirect measurements are probably closer to the normal value of capillary pressure than the micropipet measurements (Guyton and Hall, 1996).

The term *capillary closing pressure,* or *critical closing pressure,* describes the minimal amount of pressure required to collapse a capillary (Burton and Yamada, 1951). Tissue anoxia develops when externally applied pressure causes vessels to collapse. It is believed that the amount of pressure required to collapse capillaries must exceed capillary pressure. It is common to use capillary pressures of 12 to 32 mm Hg as the numerical "standard" for capillary closing pressure.

To quantify the intensity of pressure being applied externally to the skin, one measures the interface pressures. Numerous studies have been conducted to measure interface pressures (Kosiak, 1961; Kosiak et al, 1958; Lindan, 1961). These studies have shown that the interface pressures attained while one is in the sitting or supine position commonly exceed capillary pressures (Bennett et al, 1984).

In 1961, Lindan used an experimental "bed" to calculate the pressure distribution over the skin of a healthy adult male in the supine, prone, side lying, and sitting positions. The range of interface pressures was from 10 to 100 mm Hg. Interface readings as high as 300 mm Hg have been obtained over the ischial tuberosity of healthy, able-bodied male subjects when sitting in an unpadded chair (Kosiak, 1961).

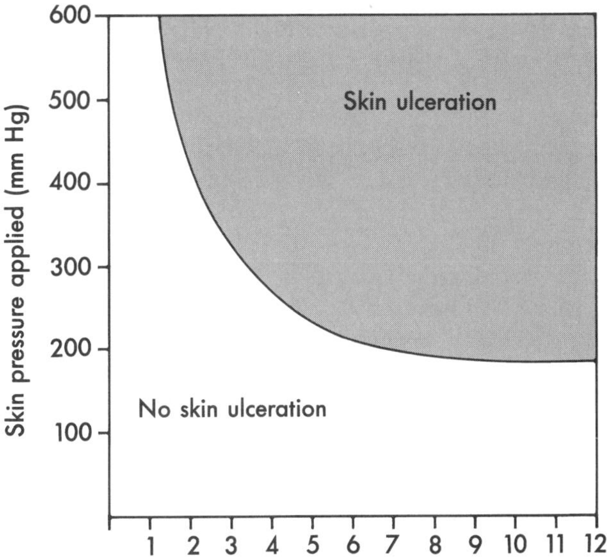

Figure 11-5 Graph demonstrating relationship between intensity and duration of pressure. (From Kosiak M: Etiology of decubitus ulcers, *Arch Phys Med Rehabil* 42:191, 1961.)

Fortunately, interface pressures in excess of capillary pressure will not routinely result in ischemia. Healthy people with normal sensation regularly shift their weight in response to the discomfort associated with capillary closure and tissue hypoxia. Unfortunately, pathologic processes such as spinal cord injury or sedation impair a person's ability to recognize or respond to this discomfort. Tissue hypoxia can then develop and progress to tissue anoxia and cellular death.

Duration of Pressure. Duration of pressure is an important fact that influences the detrimental effects of pressure and must be considered in tandem with intensity of pressure. An inverse relationship exists between duration and intensity of pressure in creating tissue ischemia (Brooks and Duncan, 1940; Kosiak, 1961; Trumble, 1930). Specifically, low-intensity pressures over a long period of time can create tissue damage just as high-intensity pressure can over a short period of time (Figure 11-5).

Husain (1953) underscored the significance of the relationship between duration and intensity of pressure. Husain found that a 100 mm Hg pressure applied to rat muscle for 2 hours was sufficient to produce only microscopic changes in the muscle. The same pressure applied for 6 hours, however, was sufficient to produce complete muscle degeneration.

Tissue Tolerance. Tissue tolerance is the third factor that determines the pathologic effect of excessive pressure and describes the condition or integrity of the skin and supporting structures that influence the skin's ability to redistribute the applied pressure. Compression of tissue against skeletal structures and the resulting tissue ischemia can be avoided by effective redistribution of pressure.

The concept of tissue tolerance was first discussed in the literature in 1930 by Trumble, who recognized the need to identify how much pressure skin could "tolerate." Later, Husain (1953) introduced the concept of sensitizing the tissue to pressure and consequently to ischemia. Rat muscle was sensitized with a pressure of 100 mm Hg applied for 2 hours. Seventy-two hours later, a mere 50 mm Hg pressure applied to the same tissue caused muscle degeneration in only 1 hour. This muscle destruction resulted during the second application of pressure, even though the intensity and duration of pressure were lower than the initial intensity and duration. This finding has significant implications for the patient population at risk for pressure ulcers. It indicates that episodes of deep tissue ischemia can occur without cutaneous manifestations and that such episodes can sensitize the patient's skin. Small increments of pressure, even if only slightly above normal capillary pressure ranges, may then result in breakdown.

Tissue tolerance is influenced by the ability of the skin and underlying structures (e.g., blood vessels, interstitial fluid, collagen) to "work together as a set of parallel springs that transmit load from the surface of the tissue to the skeleton inside" (Krouskop, 1983). Several factors can alter the ability of the soft tissue to perform this task (see Figure 11-2).

Shear

Shear was first described in 1958 as a contributing element in pressure ulcers (Reichel, 1958). Shear is caused by the interplay of gravity and friction. It exerts force parallel to the skin and is the result of both gravity pushing down on the body and resistance (friction) between the patient and a surface, such as the bed or chair. For example, when the head of the bed is elevated, the effect of gravity on the body is to pull the body down toward the foot of the bed. However, the resistance generated by the bed surface tends to try to hold the body in place. What is actually held in place is the skin, whereas the weight of the skeleton continues to pull the body downward.

Because the skin does not move freely, the primary effect of shear occurs at the deeper fascial level of the tissues overlying the bony prominence. Blood vessels, which are anchored at the point of exit through the fascia, are stretched and angulated when exposed to shear. This force also dissects the tissues "in the plane of greater concentration which is observed clinically as a large area of undermining which extends circumferentially" (Reichel, 1958).

Shear causes much of the damage often observed with pressure ulcers. In fact, some lesions that may result solely from shear are misinterpreted to be pressure ulcers. According to Bennett and Lee (1988), as many as 40% of injuries that could actually be shear injury are reported as pressure ulcers. Vascular occlusion is enhanced if shear and pressure are together (Kanj, Wilking, and Phillips, 1998). For example, when the head of the bed is elevated more than 30 degrees, shear force occurs in the sacrococcygeal region. The sliding of the body transmits pressure to the sacrum and the deep fascia; the outer skin is fixed because of friction with the bed. The vessels in the deep superficial fascia angulate with thrombosis and undermining of the dermis.

Friction

Friction is a significant factor in pressure ulcer development because it acts in concert with gravity to cause shear. Alone, its ability to cause skin damage is confined to the epidermal and upper dermal layers. In its mildest form, friction abrades the epidermis and dermis similar to that of a mild burn, and such skin damage is often reported as a "sheet burn." This type of damage most frequently develops in patients who are restless. To avoid friction when moving up in bed, a patient who can lift himself or herself should do so with a lift device or with use of the hands and arms. A patient who is dependent in care may need two caregivers to assist with moving up in bed while using a lift sheet to prevent the body from dragging.

When friction acts with gravity, however, the effect of the two factors is synergistic and the outcome is shear. It is not possible to have shear without friction. However, it is possible to have friction without significant shear (such as moving the palm of the hand repeatedly against a bed sheet).

Moisture

Moisture, specifically incontinence, is frequently cited in the literature as a predisposing factor to pressure ulcer development (Braden and Bergstrom, 1987). The mechanism may be that moisture alters the resiliency of the epidermis to external forces. According to Adams and Hunter (1969) both shear and friction are increased in the presence of mild to moderate moisture. However, it appears that shear and friction actually decrease in the presence of profuse moisture. Contrary to earlier beliefs, studies have shown that the high-moisture environment created by urinary incontinence is not a major factor in the production of pressure ulcers (Allman et al, 1986; Shannon and Skorga, 1989).

Nutritional Debilitation

Approximately 3% to 50% of hospitalized patients suffer from malnutrition; in the general population, 25% of older Americans are malnourished (Wellman, 1997). A nutritional assessment helps to identify the presence of malnutrition, assess its severity, and determine baseline data to evaluate nutritional interventions (Evans-Stoner, 1997). The nutritional assessment should include anthropometric data (weight and body mass index), biochemical data (serum albumin, serum transferrin, total lymphocyte count, nitrogen balance, serum prealbumin, and serum retinol-binding protein), clinical data, and dietary history (Flanigan, 1997; Strauss and Margolis, 1996). Serum albumin and body weight are valuable gauges of nutrition, yet their decreases may indicate poor health rather than poor nutritional intake (Evans-Stoner, 1997; Wellman, 1997). Nutrition assessment tools and dietary consultation are helpful in documenting nutritional status.

Although good nutrition is necessary for wound healing, the role of significant nutritional debilitation in producing pressure ulcers is often less appreciated. In hospitals and long-term care facilities, impaired nutritional intake, lower dietary protein intake, impaired ability to self-feed, and recent weight loss have been identified as independent predictors of pressure ulcer development (Allman et al, 1995; Bergstrom and Braden, 1992; Brandeis et al, 1990; Berlowitz and Wilking, 1989; Chernoff, 1996). Research is needed to determine if improving dietary intake reduces the incidence of pressure ulcers.

Severe protein deficiency renders soft tissue more susceptible to breakdown when exposed to local pressure because hypoproteinemia alters oncotic pressure and causes edema formation. Oxygen diffusion and transport of nutrients in ischemic and edematous tissue are compromised. Additionally, there is a decreased resistance to infection with low protein levels because of the effect on the immune system (Thomas, 1997c). Malnutrition has also been associated with altered tissue regeneration and inflammatory reaction; increased postoperative complications; increased risk of infection, sepsis, and death; and increased length of stay (Strauss and Margolis, 1996; Thomas, 1997c).

Certain vitamin deficiencies, particularly vitamins A, C, and E, may also contribute to pressure ulcer development. Vitamin A has a role in epithelial integrity, collagen synthesis, and humoral and cell-mediated protective mechanisms against infection (Flanigan, 1997; Thomas, 1997b). Vitamin A deficiency delays reepithelialization, collagen synthesis, and cellular cohesion. Vitamin C plays a part in collagen synthesis, wound repair, and immune function (Flanigan, 1997). Vitamin C deficiency compromises collagen production and immune system function and results in capillary fragility. Vitamin E deficiency may decrease cell-mediated immunity and may also increase tissue damage from toxic free radicals. All nutrients have a positive role. Still there are questions regarding how much supplementation of nutrients will positively affect outcomes (Thomas, 1996). Using creative methods, nutrition should be maintained or enhanced as long as possible (Bergstrom, 1997).

Other Factors

Other factors that have been identified as important in the development or predisposition to pressure ulcer formation include advanced age, low blood pressure, smoking, and elevated body temperature.

Advanced Age. Several changes occur in the skin and its supporting structures with aging. A flattening of the dermoepidermal junction occurs; there is less nutrient exchange and less resistance to shear force. Skin tears occur more commonly. There is a loss of dermal thickness; the skin appears paper thin and nearly transparent. Aging skin experiences decreased epidermal turnover, decreased surface barrier function, decreased sensory perception, decreased delayed and immediate hypersensitivity reaction, increased vascular fragility, loss of subcutaneous fat, and clustering of melanocytes. With these changes, the ability of the soft tissue to distribute the mechanical load without compromising blood flow is impaired (Braden and Bergstrom, 1987; Krouskop, 1983). These changes combine with many other age-related changes that occur in other body systems to make the skin more vulnerable to pressure, shear, and friction (Jones and Millman, 1990). For example, studies have shown that the blood flow in the area of the ischial tuberosity while one is sitting on an unpadded surface is lower in paraplegic and geriatric populations than in normal patients.

Low Blood Pressure. When Trumble (1930) identified the need to study tissue tolerance, he looked at the amount of external pressure needed to create skin "pain" in relationship to the patient's blood pressure instead of capillary pressure. He postulated that "skin pressure tolerance varies slightly with blood pressure."

In fact, systolic blood pressures below 100 mm Hg and diastolic pressures below 60 mm Hg have been associated with pressure ulcer development (Bergstrom, 1997; Gosnell, 1973; Moolten, 1972). Hypotension may shunt blood flow away from the skin to more vital organs, thus decreasing the skin tolerance for pressure by allowing capillaries to close at lower levels of interface pressure.

Psychosocial Status. Psychosocial issues such as motivation, emotional energy, and emotional stress have been associated with pressure ulcer formation (Rintala, 1995). Cortisol may be the trigger for lowered tissue tolerance when a person is under stress. One stress for older adults is relocation to a long-term care facility. Cortisol is the primary glucocorticoid secreted when a person is exposed to a stressor and lacks appropriate coping mechanisms to mediate the stress-related hormonal response (Braden, 1990; Krouskop, 1983).

There are two mechanisms by which cortisol might decrease the ability of the skin to absorb mechanical load:

1. Cortisol may alter the mechanical properties of the skin by disproportionately increasing the rate of collagen degradation over collagen synthesis (Cohen, Diegelmann, and Johnson, 1977; Rodriquez et al, 1989). Loss of skin collagen has been associated with the development of pressure ulcers among patients with spinal cord injury.
2. Glucocorticoids may trigger structural changes in connective tissue and may affect cellular metabolism by interfering with the diffusion of water, salt, and nutrients between the capillary bed and the cells.

Some research has reported that a causal relationship between cortisol and pressure ulcers cannot be inferred (Braden, 1998). Many factors affect cortisol, such as advanced age, immobility, body fat, recent surgery, stroke, and malnutrition.

Smoking. Smoking may be a predictor of pressure ulcer formation (Salzberg et al, 1998). Cigarette smoking has been reported to correlate positively with the presence of pressure ulcers in a group of patients with spinal cord injury (Lamid and El Ghatit, 1983). The incidence and extent of existing ulcers was greater in those patients with higher pack-per-year histories. In addition, patients who smoke have been reported to have higher recurrence rates of pressure ulcers.

Elevated Body Temperature. Elevated body temperature has been associated with pressure ulcer development (Allman et al, 1986; Braden and Bergstrom, 1987; Gosnell, 1973). Although the mechanism of this association between elevated body temperature and pressure ulcer development is not proven, it may be related to increased oxygen demand in already anoxic tissue.

Miscellaneous Factors. Other conditions, such as those that create sluggish blood flow, anemia, blood dyscarias, or poor oxygen perfusion, may also be significant intrinsic factors jeopardizing tissue tolerance (Kanj, Wilking, and Phillips, 1998; Schmid-Schönbein, Rieger, and Fischer, 1980; Niazi et al, 1997). For example, greater tissue damage has been associated with increased blood viscosity and high hematocrit level. This may explain why dehydration is sometimes mentioned as a contributing factor to pressure ulcer development. The Minimum Data Set Plus has been examined for items associated with pressure ulcer prevalence in newly institutionalized elderly patients (Zulkowski, 1998). Strongly associated factors were serum albumin, dependence for transfer, bowel incontinence, history of resolved or healed pressure ulcer, and absence of Alzheimer's disease or non-Alzheimer's dementia.

PATHOPHYSIOLOGIC CHANGES

Clinical Presentation

The pathophysiologic tissue changes that occur with pressure ulcer formation are a predictable series of events (Parish, Witkowski, and Crissey, 1983). Clinical presentation can vary from nonblanching erythema to ecchymosis and then to frank necrosis.

Obstruction of capillary blood flow by externally applied pressure creates tissue ischemia (hypoxia). If the pressure is removed in a short period of time, blood flow returns and the skin can be seen to flush. This phenomenon, known as *reactive hyperemia*, is a compensatory mechanism whereby blood vessels in the pressure area dilate in an attempt to overcome the ischemic episode. Reactive hyperemia by definition is transient and may also be described as blanching erythema. Blanching erythema is an area of erythema that becomes white (blanches) when compressed with a finger. The erythema promptly returns when the compression is removed. The site may be painful for the patient with intact sensation. Blanching erythema is an early indication of pressure and will usually resolve without tissue loss if pressure is reduced or eliminated.

When the hyperemia persists, deeper tissue damage should be suspected. Nonblanching erythema is a more serious sign of impaired blood supply and is suggestive that tissue destruction is imminent or has already occurred; it results from damage to blood vessels and extravasation of blood into the tissues. The color of the skin can be an intense bright red to dark red or purple. Many people misdiagnose pressure-induced nonblanching erythema as a hematoma or ecchymosis. When deep tissue damage is also present, the area is often either indurated or boggy when palpated. Nonblanching erythema attributable to ischemia is seldom reversible.

Cellular Response

When pressure occludes capillaries, a complex series of events is set into motion. Surrounding tissues become deprived of oxygen, and nutrients and metabolic wastes begin to accumulate in the tissue. Damaged capillaries become more permeable and leak fluid into the interstitial space to cause edema. Because perfusion through edematous tissue is slowed, tissue hypoxia worsens. Cellular death ensues, and more metabolic wastes are released into the surrounding tissue. Tissue inflammation is exacerbated, and more cellular death occurs (Figure 11-6).

Muscle Response

Muscle damage may occur with pressure ulcers and is more significant than the cutaneous damage. Pressure is highest at the point of contact between the soft tissue (such as muscle or fascia) and the bony prominence (Kosiak, 1961). This cone-shaped pressure gradient indicates that deep pressure ulcers initially form at the bone–soft tissue interface, not the skin surface, and extend outward to the skin (Figure 11-7) (Shea, 1975). Thus deep tissue damage may occur with relatively little initial superficial evidence of damage to alert caregivers of its extensiveness. The skin damage seen in pressure ulcers is often referred to as the "tip of the iceberg" because a larger area of necrosis and ischemia is expected at the tissue-bone interface.

It has been further suggested that muscle damage is more extensive than skin damage because the muscle is more sensitive to the effects of ischemia (Cherry et al, 1980). In addition, atrophied, scarred, or secondarily infected tissue has an increased susceptibility to pressure (Yarkony, 1994). An understanding of the structure of the vascular system allows one to form a rationale for this enhanced muscle damage.

The vascular circulation can be divided into three sections: segmental, perforator, and cutaneous (Daniel and Kerrigan, 1979). The segmental system is composed of the main arterial vessels arising from the aorta. The perforator system supplies the muscles but also serves as an interchange supply to the skin. The cutaneous system consists of arteries, capillary beds, and veins draining at different levels of the skin and serves to provide thermoregulation and limited nutritional support. This indicates that occlusion of the perforator system may initiate muscle damage and may also create some of the cutaneous ischemia. The significance of the perforator blood flow to skin damage has been demonstrated when musculocutaneous flaps have been elevated surgically.

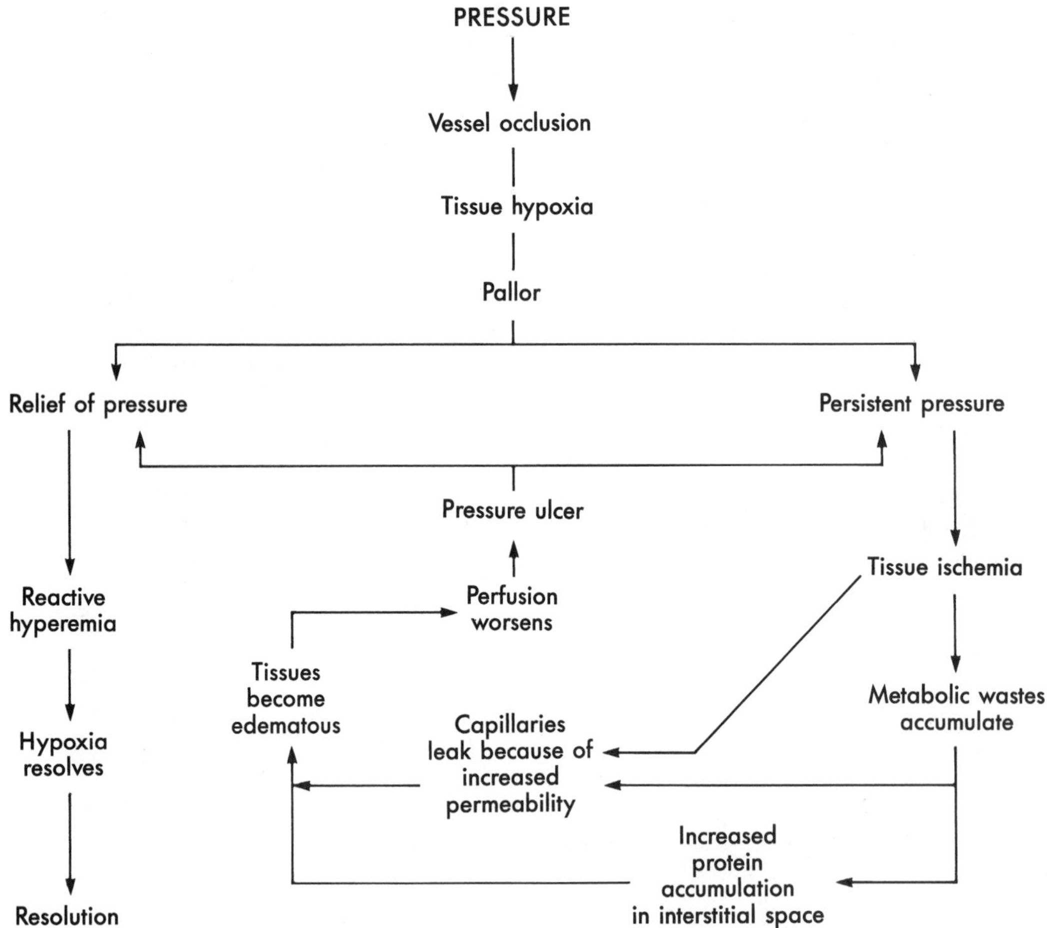

Figure 11-6 Cellular response to pressure.

"Interruption of the blood supply to the muscle can lead to skin necrosis, emphasizing the importance of the relationship of the physiological blood supply to the skin from underlying muscle. It is reasonable to suspect that the same type of tissue breakdown or necrosis could result from pressure-induced muscle ischemia in bedridden patients, and that in some cases the cutaneous lesions are secondary to the impaired muscle circulation" (Daniel and Kerrigan, 1979).

Because the skin receives its blood supply from both the perforator and the cutaneous systems, the skin actually receives more blood than necessary to meet metabolic needs (Parish, Witkowski, and Crissey, 1983). It is possible that the occlusion of "perforators" may be of more significance than the occlusion of the cutaneous system and may produce more extensive tissue damage.

Variables Influencing Extent of Tissue Damage

If pressure is not relieved, ischemic changes occur as a consequence of decreased perfusion; however, the occlusion also triggers a cascade of events that further intensifies the extent of tissue ischemia. Hence the tissue damage typically seen with pressure is precipitated by pressure but then worsened by events such as venous thrombus formation, en-

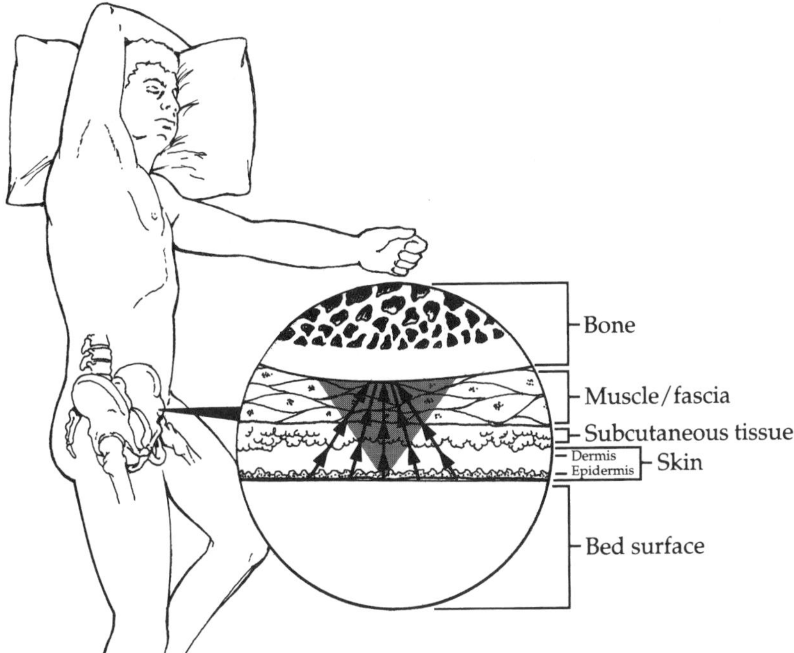

Figure 11-7 Diagram of extent of tissue damage at muscle and skin levels.

dothelial cell damage, redistribution of blood supply in ischemic tissue, alteration in lymphatic flow, and alterations in interstitial fluid composition.

Externally applied high pressures, even when applied for a short duration, damage the blood vessels directly, which in turn causes tissue ischemia. In 1961, Kosiak described the changes in larger vessels and the formation of venous thrombi, which impair the normal reactive hyperemia that should occur once pressure is removed. Thus tissue remains ischemic even after the pressure has been alleviated.

Compression of the capillary wall also damages the endothelium (Cherry, Ryan, and Ellis, 1974). Once pressure is removed and reperfusion begins, the damaged endothelial cells are shed into the bloodstream and proceed to occlude the blood vessel. As the endothelium is shed, platelets are activated by the underlying collagen and clot formation is triggered. Furthermore, damaged endothelial cells lose their usual anticoagulant characteristics and release thrombogenic substances that exacerbate vessel occlusion and ultimately cause increased tissue ischemia.

The redistribution of the blood supply that occurs in ischemic skin further aggravates pressure-induced tissue hypoxia. Because of the externally applied pressure, blood flow to surface capillaries is reduced, and such reduction renders them more vulnerable and more permeable than before. The extent of ischemia created can be further worsened when neutrophils are present in the tissue because their resting oxygen demands are 30 times greater than those of resting epithelial cells (Ryan, 1980).

Alteration in the lymphatic flow and the composition of the interstitial fluid also affects pressure-induced ischemia (Reuler and Cooney, 1981). Lymphatic flow in pressure-damaged skin ceases. Likewise, the normal movement of interstitial fluid is inhibited by both the pressure and the ischemia. Consequently, protein is retained in the interstitial tissues, causing increased interstitial oncotic pressure, edema formation, dehydration of the cells, and tissue irritation.

In summary, extensive or extended pressure occludes blood flow, lymphatic flow, and interstitial fluid movement. Tissues are deprived of oxygen and nutrients, and toxic metabolic products accumulate. Interstitial fluids retain proteins that dehydrate cells and irritate tissues. The ensuing tissue acidosis, capillary permeability, and edema contribute to cellular death.

An essential component in the reduction or elimination of pressure ulcers is the understanding of risk factors. With an in-depth review of the etiology of pressure ulcer formation and the pathophysiologic process involved, those factors that place a patient at risk for developing a pressure ulcer become apparent.

PREVENTION OF PRESSURE ULCERS

The Agency for Health Care Policy and Research (AHCPR; currently known as the Agency for Healthcare Research and Quality [AHRQ]) convened a panel of private sector and multidisciplinary health care members to create a research-based practice guideline for the prediction and prevention of pressure ulcers (Bergstrom, 1997; Panel for the Prediction and Prevention of Pressure Ulcers in Adults, 1992). The Panel performed a comprehensive literature search, wrote guidelines, sponsored a review conference, held an open forum to hear testimony, and pilot tested the guideline. This guideline, *Pressure Ulcer Prediction and Prevention in Adults*, has four components: risk assessment, skin care and early treatment, mechanical loading and support surfaces, and education (Panel for the Prediction and Prevention of Pressure Ulcers in Adults, 1992). Each component contains from 3 to 10 recommendation statements (see Appendix C for the 1992 AHCPR *Pressure Ulcer Prediction and Prevention Guideline*). A formal, comprehensive pressure ulcer prevention program is essential to effectively prevent pressure ulcers. Such a program is best developed and implemented with a multidisciplinary team who can provide a holistic approach. Typically, members of this team should consist of representatives from nursing, medicine, physical therapy, occupational therapy, and nutritional support. An algorithm for pressure ulcer prediction and prevention is presented in Figure 11-8.

Background

Pressure ulcer prevention programs establish guidelines that allocate resources and describe activities aimed at decreasing the probability that a patient will develop a pressure ulcer. When allocating resources for pressure ulcer prevention, nurses have three options:

1. Assume that all patients are at risk and use preventive resources on all patients.
2. Depend on their clinical judgment and intuitive sense to identify those patients at risk.
3. Use a risk assessment tool to identify patients who are at risk.

The assumption that all patients are at risk and thus that preventive measures should be universally applied is difficult to defend in most settings and likely represents an extremely inefficient use of resources. To treat all patients in such settings as being at risk is a tremendously wasteful approach to care. However, such an approach is probably acceptable practice in neurologic centers, especially spinal cord rehabilitation, where the degree of immobility is so profound that all patients should be considered at risk.

The accuracy of clinical judgment and intuitive sense in identifying those at risk has not been studied extensively, but Bergstrom, Demuth, and Braden (1987) found that using a risk-assessment tool more accurately identified those patients who would develop a pressure ulcer than the nurse's "best guess." Furthermore, clinical judgment is likely to be much less reliable (consistent) than risk scales because it will be based on highly variable individual experience and knowledge. Hergenroeder, Mosher, and Sevo (1992) noted a relationship between nurses judgment of risk and the Braden Scale but only for patients at moderate to high risk. Risk scales should be both more reliable and more accurate than clinical judgment, and they may also enhance the judgment of the novice nurse and focus the attention of the expert nurse.

The most cost-efficient method of implementing a pressure ulcer prevention program is to use a risk-assessment scale so that those patients who are most in need of preventive care can be targeted. Unfortunately, risk assessment has been reported to be underused for some patients (Stotts et al, 1998). Therefore risk assessment becomes an essential ingredient in a pressure ulcer prevention program. Such a program should provide guidelines that 1) identify patients at risk for developing pressure

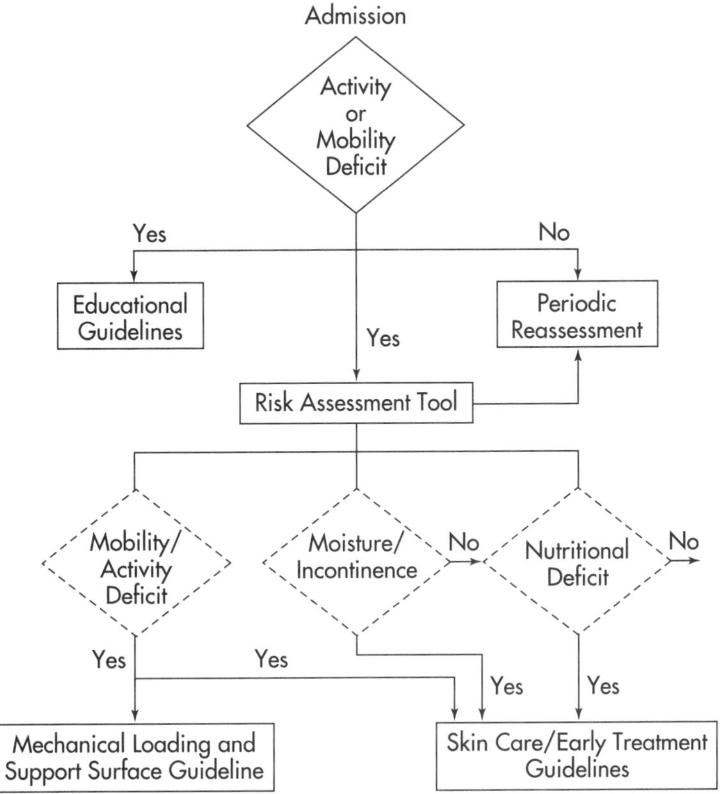

Figure 11-8 Algorithm for pressure ulcer prediction and prevention (AHCPR).

ulcers and 2) minimize the negative effects of identified risk factors. From these guidelines, policies or standards of care can be established.

Identifying Patients at Risk

Screening tests or risk-assessment tools are the backbone of any pressure ulcer prevention program. Screening tests facilitate prevention primarily by distinguishing those who are at risk for developing pressure ulcers from those who are not, thus allowing for judicious allocation of resources. The second function of this type of assessment is to identify the extent to which a person exhibits a specific risk factor, thus prompting the nurse to initiate individualized preventive interventions.

Features of Risk-Assessment Tools. Screening tests vary in terms of cost, invasiveness, use (ease of use, time required), reliability, and predictive validity. Although the cost-benefit ratio of a screening tool can be a particularly difficult determination, it should be considered. How high a cost can be tolerated for detection on a per case basis? What kind of costs are either incurred or avoided based on the outcome of the test? How often would a test have to be repeated to effectively identify those at highest risk?

The selection of screening tests requires practical and ethical considerations. For example, interface pressure might be an excellent predictor of pressure ulcer risk yet be impractical for routine screening (Wasson et al, 1985). Although the serum albumin level might be moderately predictive of pressure ulcer risk, it may be more invasive and expensive than could be justified in certain settings, such as nursing homes and home care.

The rating scale is the most common screening tool used by nurses to identify patients at risk for pressure ulcer development. Although rating scales have the advantage of being low cost and noninvasive, a critical evaluation of their performance is necessary. Specifically, information concerning

TABLE 11-1 Definitions of Measures of Validity for Screening Tools to Predict Development of Pressure Sores (PS+/PS−)

	PS+	PS−	
Positive test	TP (true positive)	FP (false positive)	PVP
Negative test	FN (false negative)	TN (true negative)	PVN
	Sensitivity $= \frac{TP}{TP + FN}$	Specificity $= \frac{TN}{TN + FP}$	

Sensitivity: Answers the question: How well does the tool predict disease? Interpreted as: Of those who became PS+, the percentage who had a positive test.
Specificity: Answers the question: How accurately does the tool rule out people who will not develop disease. Interpreted as: Of those who remained PS−, the percentage who had a negative test.
Predictive value of positive results (PVP): Answers the question: How well does the tool predict who will develop the disease? Interpreted as: Of those who had a positive test, the percentage who became PS+.
Predictive value of negative results (PVN): Answers the question: How well does the tool predict who will not develop the disease? Interpreted as: Of those who had a negative test, the percentage who remained PS−.

reliability and validity is crucial. Does the tool accurately predict the development of a pressure ulcer (validity)? When rating the same patient simultaneously, do different raters consistently assign the same rating (reliability)? Additionally, several related questions should be considered. Does the educational background (registered nurse [RN], licensed practical nurse [LPN], nurse aide [NA]) of the rater or the shift during which the rater worked affect reliability? Is the scale consistent in predicting pressure ulcer development regardless of age? Does patient population (such as nursing home, acute care, or critical care) affect the predictive ability of the scale? Does the timing of the assessment influence the predictive validity?

Common measures of predictive validity are sensitivity, specificity, predictive power of positive results, and predictive power of negative results (Table 11-1) (Baumgarten, 1998; Frantz, 1997). Sensitivity and specificity are the two measures that best reflect predictive validity; these measures are less likely to be influenced by the pressure ulcer prevalence of different patient populations (Baumgarten, 1998; Eager, 1997; Frantz, 1997). Sensitivity addresses the following question: Of the patients who developed pressure ulcers, what percentage were identified by the screening tool as being at risk (true positives). Specificity addresses the following question: Of the patients who did not develop a pressure ulcer, what percentage were identified by the screening tool as being at no risk (true negatives)?

Rating scales can also create false-positive and false-negative results. Patients who were predicted to develop a pressure ulcer but do not are referred to as *false positives*, whereas patients who are predicted to remain pressure ulcer free and do not are referred to as *false negatives*. Both sensitivity and the predictive value of negative results are influenced by the number of false negatives; the number of false positives influences specificity and the predictive value of positive results.

The ideal screening test would be 100% sensitive and 100% specific, but this is rarely achieved, even by tests intended for diagnosis rather than screening. This ideal is still less likely to be achieved when one is attempting to predict a condition that is preventable. Nevertheless, these measures of predictive validity are invaluable when one compares the results of various instruments for screening (Table 11-2).

Several instruments designed to predict the risk of pressure ulcers have been reported in the literature. These instruments use summative rating scales based on contributing factors and specify critical scores for identifying patients are risk. An example of the Gosnell scale, Braden scale, and Norton scale can be found in Appendix B.

Norton Scale. Doreen Norton developed the first pressure ulcer risk assessment scale (Norton,

TABLE 11-2 Reliability and Validity Data on Selected Risk-Assessment Tools

	Reliability Studies with Interrater Reliability		Validity Studies						
	% AGREEMENT	RATERS	SETTING	*n*	RANGE	AGE	STANDARD DEVIATION	% SENSITIVE	% SPECIFIC
Norton scale									
Roberts and Goldstone (1979)	NR	RNs	Orthopedic wards	59	NR	(Over age 60)		92	57
Goldstone and Goldstone (1982)	NR	NR	Orthopedic wards	40	NR	(Over age 60)		89	36
Lincoln et al (1986)	39.7	RNs	Acute Med-surg	50	65-89	72.2	15.8	0	94
Pang and Wong (1998)	99	RN and trained assessor	Medical and orthopedic rehabilitation hospital in Hong Kong	106	45-92	—	—	81	59
Gosnell scale									
Gosnell (1973)	NA	—	Extended care	30	65-91	78.8	NR	50	73
Gosnell and Pontius (1988)	90	RNs							
Braden scale									
Bergstrom et al (1987)	88	RNs	Med-surg	99	18-92	57.2	16.8	100	90
Bergstrom et al (1987)	15	LPN, NA	Stepdown	100	14-102	50.5	24.0	100	64
Bergstrom, DeMuth, and Braden (1987)	NA	—	Adult ICU	60	21-84	58.5	14.5	83	64
Bergstrom et al (1998)	95	RN	Six settings in three U.S. cities	843	19-102	63	16	72-81 (Skilled nursing facility)	60-73
								70 (VAMC)	79
								38-88 (Tertiary care)	68-92
Capobianco and McDonald (1996)	—	RN	Medical-surgical	50	20-95	66.9	19.3	29-93	67-97
Pang and Wong (1998)	99	RN and trained assessor	Medical and orthopedic in a rehabilitation hospital in Hong Kong	106	45-92	—	—	91	62
Ramundo (1995)	80	RN	Homecare	48	—	—	—	100	34

NR, Not reported; *NA*, not applicable.

Differences in outcome criteria and timing of assessment exist between studies and interfere with comparisons. Some adjustments were made for these differences when reporting was adequate.

1996). The Norton scale has been studied extensively (Goldstone and Goldstone, 1982; Goldstone and Roberts, 1980; Lincoln et al, 1986, Roberts and Goldstone, 1979; Haalboom, den Boer, and Buskens, 1999) and consists of five parameters: physical condition, mental state, activity mobility, and incontinence. Each parameter is rated on a scale of 1 to 4, with one- or two-word descriptors for each rating. The sum of the ratings for all five parameters yields a score that can range from 5 to 20, with lower scores indicating increased risk. Norton found an almost linear relationship between the scores of the elderly patients and the incidence of pressure ulcers, with a score of 14 indicating the "onset of risk" (although subsequent publications would place risk at 15 or 16 [Norton, 1996]) and a score of 12 or below indicating a high risk for pressure ulcer formation.

A summary of reliability and validity data from three studies can be found in Table 11-2 (Goldstone and Goldstone, 1982; Lincoln et al, 1986; Pang and Wong, 1998; Roberts and Goldstone, 1979). Only one study reported interrater reliability, which was a low-percentage agreement among RN raters. This study also reported disagreement among experts concerning face validity. When tested with other scales, the Norton scale was able to predict the development of pressure ulcers (Haalboom et al, 1999).

Gosnell Scale. In 1973, Gosnell adapted the Norton scale by adding nutrition and deleting physical condition. The Gosnell scale consists of five parameters (mental status, continence, mobility, activity, and nutrition), which were further clarified by descriptors. Additionally, two- or three-sentence descriptive statements were added for each rating on each parameter. Gosnell also studied several additional variables, such as body temperature, blood pressure, skin tone and sensation, medication, and medical diagnoses. However, these variables were given no weight in the score.

The range of possible scores for the Gosnell scale is 5 to 20. Although early studies (Gosnell, 1973) reported that lower scores denoted higher risk (16 was the critical cutoff score), a later revision (Gosnell, 1988) shows the scoring to be reversed (high scores denote high risk). Testing to determine the cutoff score is in progress. Since all ratings have historically been done by the investigator, early reports did not address interrater reliability. Most recent testing demonstrates a percentage agreement of 90% when used by RNs (Gosnell, 1989). A review of the reliability and validity of the Gosnell scale is summarized in Table 11-2.

Braden Scale. A third instrument, the Braden scale (Bergstrom, Demuth, and Braden, 1987; Bergstrom et al, 1987, Braden and Bergstrom, 1989) is composed of six subscales that conceptually reflect degrees of sensory perception, skin moisture, physical activity, nutritional intake, friction and shear, and ability to change and control body position. All subscales are rated from 1 to 4, except for the friction and shear subscale, which is rated from 1 to 3. Each rating is accompanied by a brief description of criteria for assigning the rating. Potential scores range from 4 to 23, and an hospitalized adult patient with a score of 16 or below is considered at risk (Bergstrom et al, 1987). Research in three types of settings has identified the critical cutoff score as 18 (Bergstrom et al, 1998). A score of 18 results in higher overprediction but decreases the number of false negatives (Bergstrom et al, 1998). In a small study, Lyder and colleagues (1998) concluded that the Braden scale did not predict pressure ulcer risk in African-American and Hispanic elders and identified a need for further research.

This instrument has undergone testing in three settings (critical care, acute care, and extended care), and validity has been established by expert opinion. Raters have been RNs, LPNs, and NAs. Data demonstrate that the Braden scale is highly reliable when used by RNs, as shown in Table 11-2 (Aronovitch, 1998; Bergstrom et al, 1998; Bergstrom, Demuth, and Braden, 1987; Bergstrom et al, 1987; Braden and Bergstrom, 1989; Capobianco and McDonald, 1996; Pang and Wong, 1998; Ramundo, 1995).

Implementing Risk Assessment

When implementing the risk-assessment component of a pressure ulcer prevention program, one must make several decisions. It must first be determined what caregiver can perform the assessment. Since only RNs have been found to reliably use any of these scales, it seems wise to specify that assessments be performed by RNs whenever possible.

The one test of interrater reliability, in which raters were LPNs and NAs, tested personnel untrained in use of the tool and found an unacceptably low percentage agreement. Therefore in settings where LPNs or NAs are the predominant bedside caregivers, the RN must "train" these personnel in the correct use of the tool. Furthermore, the assessment of the RN should be validated until there is consistently no more than one point difference in the total score assigned to any patient.

Another decision involves the timing of risk assessment. Admission assessment is important because it allows the nurse to identify those at highest risk; however, the nurse is rarely able to learn enough during the admission assessment to accurately identify lesser degrees of risk. For this reason, as well as the propensity for this patient's condition to change, risk assessment should be repeated 24 to 48 hours after admission and repeated when the patient's condition changes. In establishing a protocol, it is wise to specify an interval for reassessment that reflects how quickly the patient's condition changes in that setting. For example, one might set the interval at daily in the intensive care unit (ICU), every 48 hours on medical-surgical floors, weekly in skilled nursing facilities, and monthly in intermediate care facilities. It has been demonstrated that within the extended care facility, most patients who develop a pressure ulcer do so within the first 2 weeks of admission (Bergstrom and Braden, 1992; Vyhlidal, 1997). Kemp and colleagues (1993) reported that 61% of the individuals who developed a pressure ulcer did so within 10 days of admission. These reports reinforce the importance of reassessment at properly timed intervals. None of these tools requires more than 30 seconds to complete when the nurse is familiar with the patient, and so frequent assessment should not be burdensome.

In summary, risk assessment involves more than simply determining the patient's score on an assessment tool. It involves synthesizing risk factors identified through use of an assessment tool with knowledge of additional contributing factors as well as nursing judgment based on experience. The nurse should be aware that a risk score on an assessment tool is important data but that knowledge of the score without recognition of the specific deficits contributing to that score is insufficient for determining a program of prevention.

Minimizing Negative Effects of Risk Factors

Identification of factors (intrinsic and extrinsic) that place the patient at risk for developing a pressure ulcer is, in itself, insufficient to prevent pressure ulcers. Risk assessment must serve as a basis to identify measures that will alleviate, reduce, or minimize the negative effects of identified risk factors.

Assessment. The nurse must first determine which risk factors are present for an individual patient. Because pressure is the causative factor of pressure ulcers, reduction or elimination of the interface pressure is essential. Positions that may result in pressure ulcer formation, such as supine, sitting, or an operative position, must be determined. For example, patients who spend much of their time sitting in a chair are prone to pressure ulcer formation over the ischial tuberosities. Pressure relief or reduction in the bed will not be beneficial for these patients; pressure reduction in the chair is imperative. The activity, mobility, and sensory perception subscale score on the Braden scale risk-assessment tool can also be used to provide an indication of specific risk so that risk-reduction strategies can be better tailored to meet that individual's needs (Vyhlidal et al, 1997).

Systematic skin assessments should also be conducted (and documented) at least once per day on people at risk. Skin inspection may be done when bathing, dressing, or assisting a patient.

Coexisting factors predisposing to pressure-ulcer formation must also be assessed. Reduction of pressure alone is not sufficient if the patient is subjected to shear, friction, or fungal infection, for example. Interventions appropriate for prevention of these types of skin damage are discussed in detail in Chapter 6.

During the assessment process, it is also important to ascertain the effectiveness of the current plan, such as the turning frequency or the support surface. For example, an every-2-hour turning schedule for a hemodynamically unstable patient may not be appropriate. Likewise, although the support surface may be appropriate, it may be performing suboptimally because of improper inflation

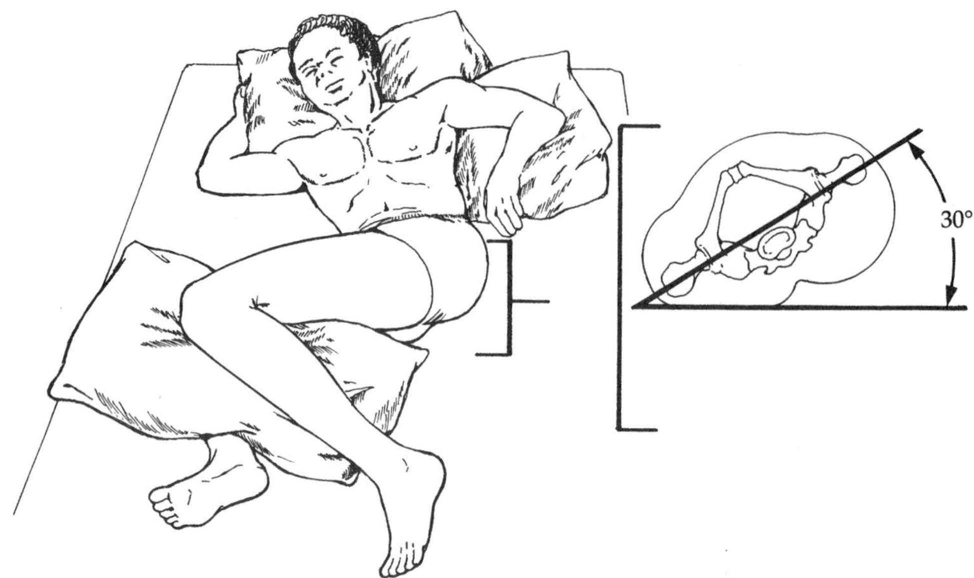

Figure 11-9 Thirty-degree lateral position at which pressure points are avoided.

or a change in the patient's condition. Vyhlidal and colleagues (1997) reported that of 40 patients already on quality support surfaces, 17 still developed a pressure ulcer. Kemp and colleagues (1993) reported a total of 33 new pressure ulcers in 57 patients despite the presence of a support surface.

Interventions

Positioning. For many years, frequent repositioning of the patient has been recommended to prevent capillary occlusion, tissue ischemia, and pressure ulceration (Kosiak, 1959; Scales, 1976; Trumble, 1930). Although repositioning does not reduce intensity of pressure, it does reduce the duration, which is the more critical element of pressure ulcer formation. In 1961, Kosiak recommended the frequency of repositioning to be hourly to every 2 hours based on the interface pressure readings from healthy, able-bodied subjects. Currently, the AHCPR (Panel for the Prediction and Prevention of Pressure Ulcers in Adults, 1992) recommends repositioning at least every 2 hours. Turning is necessary even when pressure-reducing or pressure-relieving overlays, mattresses, or special beds are used (Bergstrom, 1997; Patterson and Bennett, 1995). The effectiveness of small shifts in body weight, such as by placing a small folded towel under different parts, remains to be demonstrated (Bergstrom, 1997).

Unfortunately, because capillary closing pressures vary among persons and pressure points, the frequency of repositioning required to prevent ischemia is variable and unknown. Furthermore, there are many other factors that impinge on the frequency of repositioning, such as pain, hemodynamic instability, staffing. Therefore frequent repositioning alone may not be sufficient to prevent tissue ischemia.

Additionally, one should avoid the 90-degree side-lying position when repositioning (Bergstrom, 1997; Schmid-Schönbein, Rieger, and Fischer, 1980), because this position exerts such intense pressure directly over the trochanter. Instead, the 30-degree lateral position as described by Seiler and Stahelin (1985) should be used alternately with the supine position (Figure 11-9). Keeping the head of the bed at an angle of 30 degrees or less prevents shear.

Because heels have a small surface area and a large underlying bony surface, they are a prime site for pressure ulcer development. Some practices, such as wrapping heels with gauze or floating heels on water-filled gloves, have not been shown to be effective (Cheneworth et al, 1994; Williams, 1993). Heels can be protected from pressure when they are kept off the bed with a pillow under the lower leg or by use of specially designed heel protectors. Some commercial heel products may not fit the foot and leg well and may increase the risk for pressure ulcers (Tymec, Pieper, and Vollman, 1997). Commercial products need to be carefully evaluated for proper fit and effectiveness in preventing pressure ulcers. Because support surfaces vary in their ability to reduce interface pressure under the heels, heel protection may be indicated in combination with the support surface.

A posted turning schedule is a reminder to a nurse or caregiver of the time to turn a patient and the position to use. A patient's bony prominences should not touch; thus additional pillows to place between the legs and/or a positioning wedge may be needed. Unfortunately, positioning products and a turning schedule have been found to be lacking for patients at risk for pressure ulcers (Pieper et al, 1997a, 1998).

Patients who sit in a chair must also change position. A person who is dependent in care should have his or her position changed in a chair at least every hour (Panel for the Prediction and Prevention of Pressure Ulcers in Adults, 1992). Those who are capable should shift their weight every 15 minutes. A patient should be properly positioned in a chair for postural alignment, distribution of weight, and balance and stability (Panel for the Prediction and Prevention of Pressure Ulcers in Adults, 1992). A pressure-reducing chair cushion should be used.

Incontinence. Patients who are incontinent should be cleaned as soon as possible and at intervals. Soap is a powerful degreaser that emulsifies fats and removes lipids, thus causing dryness. Soap also alters the skin's acid mantle, an effective antimicrobial. Specialized incontinence skin cleaners or soaps that are neutral in pH and contain a moisturizer are a better choice (Skewes, 1996). Barrier ointments help to protect the skin from incontinence episodes. Incontinence may increase the risk of perineal candidiasis or fungal infections. The skin exposed to incontinence should be assessed daily so that proper treatment can be determined.

Outdated interventions. Many devices used to prevent pressure in the past are now known to be deleterious. For example, foam or rubber rings (i.e., donuts) are never indicated to relieve pressure because they concentrate the intensity of the pressure to the surrounding tissue (Agris and Spira, 1979). Furthermore, sheepskin has no effect on pressure and so is inappropriate for pressure prevention.

Support Surfaces

A cornerstone in the reduction or elimination of interface pressures is the use of support surfaces. These products reduce tissue interface pressures over the bony prominences by maximizing contact and redistributing weight over a large area (Bergstrom, 1997; Tallon, 1996; Whittemore, 1998). However, proper support surface use is one of many components of a quality pressure ulcer prevention program. It is critical that support surfaces be used in conjunction with the other risk reduction inteventions as outlined by the AHCPR (see Appendix C).

Many support surfaces are available, and numerous claims are made about their effectiveness and efficacy. Unfortunately, few clinical trials are available to support most claims. Very few randomized prospective clinical trials exist that evaluate the effectiveness of support surfaces in terms of outcome such as pressure ulcer incidence (Kemp et al, 1993; Vyhlidal et al, 1997). Support surfaces are available in a variety of sizes and shapes that are appropriate for beds, chairs, examining tables, and operating room tables. The construction of the support surface and the process for selecting a support surface for an individual is similar regardless of the size or shape needed. Unfortunately, the use of support surfaces for the chair or operating room is frequently overlooked.

In addition to pressure reduction or relief, many support surfaces also provide shear and friction reduction, moisture control, or kinetic therapy. To use support surfaces efficiently and effectively, the nurse must be knowledgeable of their indications, contraindications, advantages, and disadvantages. Once a plan for reducing or eliminating pressure is developed and the plan is implemented, the effectiveness of the intervention (turning, support surface, etc.) should be evaluated.

Tissue Interface Pressure. The capillary closing pressure (12 to 32 mm Hg) is used as a measurement of the effectiveness of support surfaces. It is implied that as the skin-resting surface interface pressure nears capillary closing pressures, the support surface is more effective and less likely to interrupt or occlude capillary blood flow. However, this overreliance on capillary pressure values as absolutes when making determinations about pressure prevention equipment is questioned for several reasons:

1. Capillary closing pressure was measured in the fingertips of young healthy males.
2. Lower capillary pressures have been reported in older patients.
3. It is an assumption that skin-resting interface pressures actually reflect pressure at the bone-tissue interface. Skin-resting pressures do not necessarily ensure that blood flow through the capillaries is unimpeded.

Because skin-resting surface interface pressure is the method currently used to evaluate support surfaces and their ability to reduce pressure, it is important to understand how interface pressure is calculated. Interface pressure is a measurement obtained by placement of a sensor between the skin and the resting surface. When one is interpreting the significance of reported pressure readings, it is important to consider the following issues (Reger et al, 1988):

1. The range of pressure readings obtained per site and the number of readings conducted per site should be reported instead of one single pressure reading per site.
2. The procedure used to acquire the pressure reading should be described.
3. The population tested should be described (i.e., healthy subjects versus patients).
4. Researchers should state how often equipment was recalibrated because the sensors are fragile and may malfunction.
5. Factors known to affect the results of interface pressure measurements should be disclosed (transducer size and shape, the load shape and its interaction with the support material, the method of equilibrium detection, and the uniformity of the measurement technique).

BOX 11-2 Categories of Support Surfaces

A. Management of pressure
   1. Pressure reduction
   2. Pressure relief
B. Air or fluid support
   1. Dynamic
   2. Static
C. Type of device
   1. Overlay
   2. Replacement mattress
   3. Specialty bed

The importance of the shape of the load is exemplified by the fact that a healthy person with normal muscle mass will support and distribute weight more effectively than a debilitated person. As a result, the healthy subject will usually demonstrate lower pressure readings than the debilitated subject. Uniformity of the measurement technique is necessary because the skill of the person taking the readings may make a difference.

As noted previously, in addition to reducing tissue interface pressure, many support surfaces also reduce shear, friction, and moisture. Products that have a slick surface, such as low air-loss beds, are believed to decrease friction and shear. Surfaces with porous cover material through which air flows help reduce moisture between the body and support surface, thus preventing maceration.

Categories of Support Surfaces. Support surfaces can be categorized many ways (Box 11-2).

1. They can be described as a pressure-reducing or pressure-relieving device. *Pressure-relieving devices* are those that consistently reduce pressure below capillary closing pressure (Fletcher, 1997). The indications for use are to prevent skin breakdown in people who cannot be turned, prevent further skin breakdown, promote healing in the patient who already has skin breakdown involving multiple surfaces, or reduce mechanical stress in the patient who has had a myocutaneous flap or skin graft on the trunk or pelvis within the last 60 days. These products conform closely to the patient's body

for support and are responsive to a patient's movement regardless of the patient's position (Fletcher, 1997). Products include the Medicare Group 2 powered air-flotation bed and Group 3 air-fluidized bed (Weaver and McClausland, 1998). *Pressure-reducing devices* are those that lower pressure as compared with a standard hospital mattress or chair surface but do not consistently reduce pressure to less than capillary closing pressure. The product redistributes pressure over a greater area, thus reducing the amount of pressure at any given point (Fletcher, 1997). Pressure-reducing devices therefore must be used with a turning schedule that is tailored for the individual patient. The turning schedule is determined by evaluation of the status of the skin after progressive lengthening of the interval between position changes.

2. Support surfaces can be categorized according to whether support is dynamic or static. Dynamic systems typically use electricity to alter inflation and deflation and thus decrease tissue interface pressure, such as alternating pressure pad. Static devices reduce pressure by spreading the load over a larger area. A constant inflation is maintained by use of a material that molds to the body surface, such as foam, gel, water, and some air-filled overlays.
3. Support surfaces can be categorized as overlays, replacement mattresses, and specialty beds. Overlays are products that are applied on top of the hospital mattress and use foam, air, water, gel or any combination of these modalities to distribute the load and reduce pressure. Replacement mattresses are complete hospital mattresses designed to reduce pressure as compared with the standard hospital mattress. Specialty beds are entire units that are used in place of the hospital bed. This category includes low-air-loss, high-air-loss, and kinetic therapy beds. Kinetic therapy is continuous passive motion designed to counteract the negative effects of immobility.

Overlay. Overlay mattresses are devices that are applied over the surface of the hospital mattress; most overlays provide pressure reduction. Overlay mattresses require a one-time charge, a setup fee, a daily rental fee, or a combination (such as one-time charge of mattress and daily rental of pump). Because overlay mattresses are applied over an existing hospital mattress, the height of the bed is increased, and such an increase may complicate patient transfers in and out of bed and alter the fit of linens. Overlays may be static (foam, gel, water, air filled, low air loss) or dynamic (alternating air). Most overlay mattresses are single-patient-use items that present environmental issues relative to disposal of the product. Gel, water, and some air-filled overlays are reusable (multiple-patient use). Because moisture entrapment against the skin is a problem with certain patient populations, some air-filled, low-air-loss, and alternating air-filled overlays provide air movement designed to reduce moisture buildup.

Static overlays

Foam. Foam overlays have been used for many years and are probably the most universally used overlay. Foam is a static system and provides pressure reduction. Several characteristics of foam are important for effective pressure reduction: base height, density, indentation load deflection (ILD), and contours (Krouskop and Garber, 1987; Krouskop et al, 1985, 1986). *Base height* refers to the height of the foam from the base to where the convolutions begin (not to the peak of the convolution). Density is the weight per cubic foot, is a measurement of the amount of foam in the product, and reflects the foam's ability to support the person's weight. ILD is a measurement of the firmness of the foam and is determined by the number of pounds required to indent a sample of foam with a circular plate to a depth of 25% of the thickness of the foam.

For example, because 25% of a 4-inch foam is 1 inch, the 25% ILD would measure the number of pounds required to make a 1-inch indentation in the 4-inch foam. If this takes a 30-pound weight, the ILD would be stated as 25% ILD of 30 pounds. Likewise, 60% ILD of a 4-inch foam measures the number of pounds required to make a 2.4-inch depression in the foam (60% of 4 inches is 2.4 inches). ILD describes the foam's compressibility and conformability and indicates the ability of the foam to distribute the mechanical load. A low ILD is desirable. A relationship of 60% ILD to 25% ILD is an important characteristic in a therapeutic foam because it reflects the relationship between support and conformability. This ratio is recommended to be 2.5 or greater. Practically speaking, because the desired 25% ILD is 30 pounds, the 60% ILD should be at least 75 pounds (2.5 × 30). This indicates that 30 pounds would make a 1-inch depression in the 4-inch foam, whereas at least 75 pounds would be needed to make a 2.4-inch depression in the same foam.

Contours describe the surface of the foam pad (e.g., egg crate, slashed, smooth, etc.). Benefits of one surface over another are largely subjective currently. However, Kemp and colleagues (1993) reported statistically fewer pressure ulcers in acute care and long-term care at-risk patients using a solid foam overlay versus a convoluted foam overlay.

The base height of foam overlays varies widely. A foam overlay with a 2-inch base does not significantly reduce pressure when compared with a standard hospital mattress (Krouskop et al, 1985; Whittemore, 1998). Therefore it is appropriately used only as a comfort device for persons at low risk for skin breakdown. A summary of research noted that a 2-inch foam overlay only slightly lowers tissue interface pressure as compared with a standard hospital mattress, whereas a 4-inch foam significantly lowers interface pressure (Whittemore, 1998). Foam products may be only marginally efficacous for high-risk persons; its use may best be restricted to moderate-risk patients (Whittemore, 1998).

In summary, the following features in a therapeutic foam overlay are recommended (Krouskop, 1989; Krouskop and Garber, 1987; Whittemore, 1998):

- Base height of 3 to 4 inches
- Density of 1.3 to 1.6 pounds per cubic foot
- ILD of about 30 pounds
- Ratio of 60% ILD to 25% ILD of 2.5 or greater

The manufacturer's guidelines will state the amount of body weight that the foam product will support and its length of use. When used for long-term pressure reduction, the staff or family must examine the product at intervals and replace the foam when effectiveness appears reduced. Advantages and disadvantages of foam overlays are listed in Box 11-3.

BOX 11-3 Foam Overlays: Advantages and Disadvantages

Advantages

One-time charge
No setup fee
Cannot be punctured by needle or metal traction
Light weight
Available in many sizes (bed, operating tables, chairs)
Requires no maintenance
No electric fee for use; readily available

Disadvantages

May be hot and trap perspiration
Washing removes flame-retardant coating
Foam has a limited life
Plastic protective sheet necessary for protection from incontinent episodes
Lack of firm edge, so patient feels unsure when tranferring on and off surface
Discarded when wet with drainage or incontinence
Adds height to bed

Water. Water-filled overlays and waterbeds have long been used to reduce interface pressure (Siegel, Vistness, and Laub, 1973). Several studies have demonstrated that the waterbed provides significantly lower interface pressure than a hospital mattress does (Sloan, Brown, and Larson, 1977; Wells and Geden, 1984). According to Berecek (1975), pressure points are eliminated because the function of the waterbed is based on Pascal's law: "The weight of a body floating on a fluid system is evenly distributed over the entire supporting system." Unfortunately, the waterbed presents three concerns: leaks, maintenance of bed warmth, and appropriate filling. Although water-filled devices are popular for the home, their many disadvantages make them inappropriate for acute care or long-term care settings. Advantages and disadvantages are listed in Box 11-4.

Gel. Gel-flotation pads are constructed of Silastic (silicone elastomer), silicone, or polyvinyl chloride (Berecek, 1975). These surfaces provide flotation with pressure reduction, may be for single-patient

BOX 11-4 Water Overlays: Advantages and Disadvantages

Advantages

Readily available in community
Baffle system available to control motion effects
Easy to clean

Disadvantages

Requires water heater to maintain comfortable water temperature
Fluid motion makes procedures difficult (e.g., positioning or cardiopulmonary resuscitation)
Patient transfers may be difficult
Inadvertent needle punctures will create leaks
Water leaks can create safety hazards
Maintenance is needed to prevent microorganism growth
Heavy
Cannot raise head of bed unless mattress has compartments
Can be overfilled or underfilled

or multiple-patient use, require minimal maintenance, are available in a variety of sizes and shapes, and have a surface that is easy to clean. These features make them attractive for use in long-term care settings and operating rooms. However, gel-filled overlays tend to be expensive and heavy and lack air-flow for moisture control. Friction control is variable depending on the surface of the gel. Gel-filled pads are particularly useful in wheelchairs.

Gels may be combined with foam to create a mattress. Foam sections are removed, and the gel pad is inserted where the pressure-reducing effect of the gel is desired. A list of advantages and disadvantages of gel-filled overlays is listed in Box 11-5.

Air filled. Static air-filled overlays consist of interconnected bulbous cells that are inflated with an air blower to an appropriate pressure level. These overlays are available in a chair size, in a bed size, and as operating room pads. They are probably the most widely used pressure-reduction surface. Static air-filled overlays are considered pressure reducing and should be used for patients who can reposition themselves.

BOX 11-5 Gel-Filled Overlays: Advantages and Disadvantages

Advantages

Low maintenance
Easy to clean
Multiple-patient use
Impermeable to punctures with needles

Disadvantages

Heavy
Expensive
Limited research on effectiveness

BOX 11-6 Static Air-Filled Overlays: Advantages and Disadvantages

Advantages

Easy to clean
Multiple-patient use products available
Low maintenance
Repair of some products is possible
Durable

Disadvantages

Can be damaged by sharp objects
Requires regular monitoring to determine proper inflation and need for reinflation
Adds height to bed
Lacks a firm edge, so transfer on and off surface may be difficult

Numerous investigators have examined static air overlays and documented pressure-reduction capabilities and significant lower mean tissue interface pressures as compared with a standard hospital mattress (Whittemore, 1998). Air-filled overlays may not be effective in preventing pressure ulcers if the inflation is not checked daily and reinflation is not performed or if the overlay is punctured by a sharp object. Static air-filled overlays may be used with moderate- and high-risk patients as long as the product is maintained (Whittemore, 1998). Advantages and disadvantages of static air-filled overlays are listed in Box 11-6.

BOX 11-7 Low-Air-Loss Overlays: Advantages and Disadvantages

Advantages

Easy to clean
Maintains a constant inflation
Deflates to facilitate transfers, cardiopulmonary resuscitation, and so on
Setup provided by company
Moisture control

Disadvantages

Can be damaged by sharp objects
Noisy
Requires electricity

BOX 11-8 Alternating Air-Filled Overlay: Advantages and Disadvantages

Advantages

Easy to clean
Pump is reusable
Quick deflation for emergencies

Disadvantages

Assembly required
Sensation of inflation and deflation may bother patient
Requires electricity
Motor may be noisy
Excessive or sudden surface movement may disturb sleep

Low-air-loss overlay. Low-air-loss overlays are attached to motorized pumps that maintain a constant inflation and provide slight air movement against the skin to prevent moisture buildup. The fabric covering for these overlays is air permeable, bacteria impermeable, and waterproof and reduces shear and friction. Low-air-loss overlays may have kinetic features. Advantages and disadvantages of low-air-loss overlays are listed in Box 11-7.

Dynamic overlays.

Alternating air-filled overlay. The objectives for use of an alternating air-pressure overlay are to prevent constant pressure against the skin and to enhance blood flow by creating high-pressure and low-pressure areas. These pressure-reducing dynamic systems consist of a configuration of chambers through which air is pumped at regular intervals to provide inflation and deflation. These products constantly change pressure points and create pressure gradients that enhance blood flow (McLeod, 1997; Whittemore, 1998). Typically, interface pressures are lower than capillary closing pressure when the cylinders are deflated; interface pressures are then higher than capillary closing pressure when the cylinders are inflated. Interface pressures in the trochanter area commonly remain high during both phases; however, because interface pressures are significantly less than a standard hospital bed for the sacrum, scapula, and trochanter, pressure reduction in these areas is attained (Krouskop et al, 1985). Studies may only include the minimum pressure reading in statistical analyses (Whittemore, 1998). Additional research about alternating air-filled mattresses is needed since new equipment may have pressure-adjustable controls, automatic pressure settings for a patient, and a number of cells inflating and deflating (McLeod, 1997). Advantages and disadvantages for this overlay are listed in Box 11-8.

Replacement mattress. Replacement mattresses are designed to reduce interface pressures and replace the standard hospital mattress. Replacement mattresses vary in design; most are made of foam and gel combinations or layers of different foam densities (i.e., very firm, high-density foam for the periphery or bottom layer and low-density, more comfortable foam for the upper layer) (Bergstrom, 1997; Krouskop et al, 1985; Weaver and Jester, 1994). Some replacement mattresses have removable foam shapes, and some have a replaceable foam core. Other replacement mattresses are a series of air-filled chambers covered with a foam structure. All replacement mattresses are covered with a conformable bacteriostatic cover that can be maintained with standard terminal cleaning.

Important features of a replacement mattress include a water-repellent, antimicrobial top cover; flame retardency; and a waterproof antibacterial bottom cover, and when foam is a component of the mattress, it should have an appropriate foam ILD with high resiliency and be antimicrobial.

Maintenance of replacement mattresses varies with type of design. Although some mattresses have to be turned (or flipped) regularly to maintain efficacy, others cannot be turned because of their design. This feature is significant to the institution because it may reduce the employee's risk of low back injuries resulting from such activities. Another feature of some replacement mattresses is air flow to reduce moisture build-up against the skin.

Evidence is increasing that replacement mattresses are superior to a standard hospital mattress and may be more effective than some overlays (Vyhlidal et al, 1997). Weaver and Jester (1994) examined the tissue interface pressures of different brands of replacement mattresses. The products lower interface pressures, but there is variation in brands. Replacement mattresses are effective for moderate-risk patients, but their effectiveness with high-risk patients is not known.

Purchase of these mattresses entails a significant initial expense and is probably most justifiable in settings with a large number of at-risk patients or when a large number of overlays is used. Because some third-party payers limit reimbursement for overlays (particularly Medicaid and Medicare), institutions with a large percentage of Medicare and Medicaid patients who are at risk for pressure ulcer development may find that replacement is a more cost-effective alternative. However, the use of specialty beds may not be reduced by use of replacement mattresses. The years of use of hospital replacement mattresses is not fully known; some may begin to deteriorate before the expected warranty time. Advantages and disadvantages are listed in Box 11-9.

Specialty beds. Air-fluidized and low-air-loss beds were developed to allow deformation of the bed surface to the body contours, thereby reducing tissue interface pressure below capillary closure. In addition to providing pressure relief, these specialty beds also eliminate shear and friction and decrease moisture (Counsell et al, 1990). Specialty beds replace hospital beds and are the most costly of all support surfaces. Electricity (or a battery pack) is required for a specialty bed to function.

BOX 11-9 Replacement Mattresses: Advantages and Disadvantages

Advantages

Reduce use of overlay mattresses
Reduce staff time
Do not add height to mattress
Provide certain level of pressure reduction automatically
Multiple-patient use
Easy to clean
Use standard hospital linens
Low maintenance

Disadvantages

Initial expense high
Some mattresses have removable sections, which may be misplaced
May not control moisture
Potential for excessive delay in using other support surface
No objective method for determining when or if product loses effectiveness
Life of product is not known

Investigators have examined the pressure-relief capacity of both types of air-loss beds. With proper adjustment, the pressure-relief and redistribution characteristics of air-fluidized and low-air-loss specialty beds do not differ (Krouskop, Williams, and Krebs, 1984).

Air-fluidized beds. Air fluidized beds, initially developed to treat persons with burns, consist of a bed frame containing silicone-coated beads and incorporating both air and fluid support (Tallon, 1996). Fluidization of the beads occurs when air is pumped through the beads, making them behave like a liquid. The person "floats" on a sheet with one third of the body above the surface and the rest of the body immersed in the warm, dry, fluidized beads (Viner, 1986). High-air-loss beds have bactericidal properties because of their temperature, alkalinity (pH 10), and entrapment of the microorganisms by the beads (Thomson et al, 1980). When the air-fluidized bed is turned off, it quickly becomes firm enough for cardiopulmonary resuscitation or for repositioning the patient for dressing changes.

Although some evidence indicates that air-fluidized beds enhance pressure ulcer healing rates (Parish and Witkowski, 1980), occipital and calcaneous skin-resting surface interface pressures may remain sufficient to occlude capillary perfusion. Occipital and calcaneous ulcers have been reported to develop in patients while on the air-fluidized bed surface (Parish and Witkowski, 1980).

Air-fluidized beds have also been compared with the standard hospital mattress in wound-healing studies (Allman et al, 1987; Greer et al, 1988; Jackson et al, 1988). Researchers generally agree that ulcers decrease significantly in size and that fewer ulcers develop in the patients placed on an air-fluidized bed.

Air-fluidized beds are recommended for patients with burns or multiple stage 3 or 4 pressure ulcers. They may be used to rewarm a person with hypothermia, since they can quickly narrow the gap between the core and peripheral temperatures, thus reducing vasoconstriction and improving peripheral circulation. This may reduce shivering and the subsequent increased oxygen demand. Patients with severe debilitating pain are often more comfortable on this bed because of the "cocooning" effect and decreased need to be turned. Furthermore, appetite is reported to improve with air-fluidized therapy, which may correlate with the pain control provided by the bed (Jackson et al, 1988). Air-fluidized beds are not recommended for patients with pulmonary disease or unstable spines or for patients who are ambulatory. Advantages and disadvantages are listed in Box 11-10.

Low-air-loss beds. A low-air-loss bed consists of a bed frame with a series of connected air-filled pillows. The amount of pressure in each pillow is controlled and can be calibrated to provide maximum pressure reduction for the individual patient. The low-air-loss bed deflates quickly for cardiopulmonary resuscitation.

As with air-fluidized beds, low-air-loss beds are also indicated for patients who need pressure relief (i.e., patients who cannot be frequently repositioned or who have skin breakdown on more than one surface). These beds have the added features of a regular hospital bed frame. Low-air-loss beds are contraindicated for patients with an unstable spine. Some low-air-loss beds include pulsation therapy, and although this is believed to enhance cutaneous blood flow and to reduce edema, further research is needed. Bennett and colleagues (1998) examined use of a low-air-loss hydrotherapy bed with incontinent hospitalized patients. Some patients developed hypothermia, and staff, patients, and family members expressed some dissatisfaction with it. Not enough patients with pressure ulcers were fol-

BOX 11-10 Air-Fluidized Specialty Beds: Advantages and Disadvantages

Advantages

Less frequent repositioning required
Improved patient comfort
Traction can be applied
Procedures can be facilitated by turning the bed off
Quickly become firm for cardiopulmonary resuscitation and procedures
Reduce shear, friction, and edema to site
May facilitate management of copious wound drainage or incontinence
Sales force can provide setup, monitoring, and on-call services

Disadvantages

Continuous circulation of warm, dry air may dehydrate patient
Bed may be hot or make room hot
Additional wound care measures are necessary to prevent wound desiccation
Coughing is less effective in mobilizing secretions
Leakage of beads (microspheres) may irritate the eyes and respiratory tract and make floor slippery
Width of bed may preclude care to obese patients or patients with a contracture
Height of bed makes some nursing care difficult, and a step is needed to facilitate care
Transfer of patient out of bed is difficult
Bed is heavy and not easily transferrable
Some patients become disoriented or complain of feeling weightless
Dependent drainage of catheters may be compromised because the patient is immersed in the bed
Head of the bed cannot be raised; semi-Fowler's position is achieved by use of a series of foam wedges or a movable sling-type device
Size and weight may be too large for most homes

BOX 11-11 Low-Air-Loss Specialty Bed: Advantages and Disadvantages

Advantages

Head and foot of bed can be raised and lowered
Transfers in and out of bed easily accomplished
Portable motor available to maintain inflation during bed transfers
Less frequent turning schedules required
Sales force provides setup, monitoring, and on-call services

Disadvantages

Portable motors are noisy
Bed surface material is slippery, and caution must be used so that patients do not slide down or out of bed when being transferred

lowed long enough to assess the effect on pressure ulcer healing (Bennett et al, 1998). Low-air-loss beds have been combined with an air-fluidized component in the lower half of the bed. This bed is similar in size to a hospital bed, and the head is readily adjustable, but it is lighter than a total air-fluidized system. Advantages and disadvantages are listed in Box 11-11.

Kinetic therapy. Some specialty beds provide kinetic therapy. These beds are designed to counteract the effects of immobility by continuous passive motion or oscillation therapy. Some beds are a combination of oscillation therapy and low air loss. Oscillation therapy is believed to 1) provide mobilization of respiratory secretion, thus decreasing the incidence of atelectasis and pneumonia and improving oxygenation of blood; 2) prevent urinary stasis, thus reducing the risk of urinary tract infection; and 3) reduce venous stasis and risk of deep vein thrombosis and pulmonary emboli. Thus kinetic therapy may have a significant positive effect on multiple body systems.

Kinetic therapy is available with a low-air-loss surface or with a firm, slightly padded surface. A kinetic treatment table has a firm, slightly padded surface. By rotating slowly side to side, the treatment table alternates pressure points; however, it does not reduce shear or moisture. Access to body parts is possible by opening special hatches without affecting body alignment. This device is primarily indicated to stabilize the spine or for victims of major trauma requiring traction. It is not used if a patient is hemodynamically unstable or for the patient with severe claustrophobia.

Kinetic therapy with low-air-loss support is indicated for patients who need pressure relief and will also benefit from kinetic therapy. This type of specialty bed is contraindicated for patients in cervical or skeletal traction.

Selecting Support Surfaces for Institution or Agency

Selecting a pressure-relief or pressure-reduction device for a specific patient and for the institution or agency presents many challenges. Generally, one product alone is not sufficient for an institution, and a range of products is more appropriate. Several factors should be considered when determining what support surfaces to have available in an institution or agency.

1. What are the common needs for the patient population typically served? For example, an institution that has many high-risk patients for pressure ulcer development may find replacement mattresses to be effective at reducing their number of overlays. An institution with a variety of acutely ill patients will have different patient needs and may need a range of products such as an overlay mattress, a specialty bed, and a kinetic therapy product. Rehabilitation centers or nursing homes, on the other hand, will need access to mattress overlays, replacement mattresses, or a select combination of both, as well as wheelchair overlays. Settings where many grafts or flaps are performed will need access to specialty beds and appropriate "stepdown" support surfaces. Additionally, the type of surgical procedures performed within the institution should be assessed. Duration and type of surgical procedures are becoming increasingly recognized as factors contributing to pressure ulcer formation.
2. The cost of the support surface should be considered. Some devices are available on a rental basis, whereas others have a one-time

fee. The cost of the device should be considered with the length of time the product will be used, goals for use, and length of product efficacy.

Indirect costs associated with the use of support surfaces, such as the time commitment of the staff to use the product, must also be considered. How long does it take the staff to set up the device? Will the staff need to provide some degree of maintenance or frequent checks to ensure effective inflation? The ease with which the product can be used and maintained is important to minimize staff time required by the device. A device that requires daily maintenance is probably not appropriate in a low staffing situation.

The electrical costs for a product used in the home should be considered. For home care, the reimbursement for support surfaces is affected by the *Coverage and Payment Policy for Support Surfaces* published by the Medicare Part B Durable Medical Equipment Regional Carriers (DMERCs) (Weaver and McClausland, 1998). Support surfaces are placed in three categories:

- *Group 1.* Products for patients at risk for pressure ulcers and those with lower-staged ulcers. This includes nonpowered static overlays; mattress replacements made of foam, air, water, or gel; and powered alternating air-pressure pass and pumps.
- *Group 2.* Products for patients with higher-staged wounds or those with flaps. This includes non-powered, adjustable-zone, pressure-reducing air mattress overlay; powered air overlay for a mattress; alternating pressure mattress; and powered air-flotation bed.
- *Group 3.* Products for the most severely compromised patients, including the air-fluidized bed (Weaver and McClausland, 1998). Medicare will pay 80% of the allowed charge on a rental surface (Weaver and McClausland, 1998). A detailed description of the patient's wound, activity level, and state of health is important in obtaining reimbursement for the support surface.

3. Company performance and service should also be assessed. Services such as setup, maintenance, storage, and disposal may be provided. The company should be examined for its shipping and delivery policy and guarantee. Some companies provide in-service programs for the staff. A trial of the product may be possible. Talking with other nurses who have used the product may help identify the advantages and disadvantages of a company and the product.

   Product disposal is becoming a critical environmental issue. If it is costly for the hospital to dispose of trash, a rented, reusable overlay may be more cost effective than a disposable overlay. Storage of the standard hospital bed while a specialty bed is in use is also a concern in some facilities where space is limited.
4. Do effectiveness studies exist for this particular product? Ideally, clinical trial results should be available describing the effects of the particular support surface on outcomes such as incidence, comfort, cost, satisfaction, etc. There should be available independently written literature that describes the range and standard deviation of interface pressures for the product. The method of recording interface pressures, the age and health of the study sample, and the size of the sample should be considered. The size of the sensor measuring the pressure is important, since a small sensor may be misplaced and not even obtain the highest reading. Test data should be published in a reputable scientific journal, not in literature produced by the manufacturer's marketing department.

   It would be less than ideal to select a support surface without efficacy studies or based on the results of one study (especially if the study used a limited sample). For example, many studies regarding interface pressures are done on healthy, young adults; generalizability of these measurements to an older person and ill population is not known. A small sample size may increase the risk of saying that a product makes a significant difference when it does not. Sample sizes need to be large enough to account for the type of statistical analysis performed and ability to predict a significant effect. When limited research on products of interest is available, the nurse should design and conduct a test to evaluate the product's effectiveness (Berecek, 1975).

Selecting Support Surface for Individual Patient

Once a decision is made as to what products to have available in the agency or institution, attention must turn to educating the staff as to appropriate use of the products. Guidelines for selecting a support surface for a specific patient are necessary to enable appropriate staff decision making and proper use (Jay, 1997; Tallon, 1996; Whittemore, 1998). Although no universal decision tree exists, several factors should guide the selection process:

1. *Does the patient need pressure reduction or relief?* The patient who cannot be repositioned or who has pressure ulcers involving multiple surfaces requires pressure relief.
2. *Is this support system needed on a short-term or a long-term basis?* For example, an acutely ill patient may need pressure relief during an illness crisis but by discharge may not require any support surface. A patient in a nursing home or with a chronic disease may require long-term pressure reduction. Surgical patients may need pressure relief during the surgery and only mild pressure reduction or no pressure reduction postoperatively. Some patients confined to a chair need no pressure relief in bed but need pressure reduction while in the chair.
3. *Is the patient, staff, or family compliant with repositioning?* Because most overlays or replacement mattresses do not eliminate the need for a turn schedule, they may be inappropriate for patients who are hemodynamically unstable. Likewise, the patient has to cooperate and stay repositioned. The family of a bed-bound patient has to be able to turn the patient at appropriate intervals, understand the importance of repositioning, and provide consistency and follow through.
4. *Will the support surface interfere with the patient's independent functioning?* For example, the height of an overlay can add to the height of the mattress, and its soft edge may affect a persons stability with transfer; thus complicating a rehabilitation patient's ability to transfer. A high-air-loss bed would not be indicated for a patient who is getting in and out of bed.
5. *What is financially feasible?* Institutions cannot afford to have all support systems available. Many institutions establish contractual relationships with companies to control costs and to provide access to a specific range of products. Reimbursement for products in the home or nursing home setting is limited and should be explored before a decision is made (Weaver and McClausland, 1998). Families need to be aware of the electrical costs to run products with a motor and if there are safety features in case of a power failure (Weaver and McClausland, 1998).
6. *What mechanism is needed to ensure appropriate functioning of the support surface?* Air- or water-filled overlays must be checked on a regular basis to ascertain appropriate flotation. Many low-air-loss overlays and specialty beds have service people to monitor this; however, staff or family still require some degree of familiarity with features and functions.
7. *The patient's surrounding environment needs to be examined.* Are there adequate outlets for electrical equipment in the patient's room, or would an overlay that does not use electricity be a better choice? How noisy is the product, and can the patient tolerate this additional noise? Some products generate heat, which may also be poorly tolerated by some patients and poorly dissipated in some environments. How heavy is the equipment?
8. *Are there other therapeutic effects needed in addition to pressure reduction or relief?* For example, a patient with a closed head injury may need a support surface that reduces pressure but also controls moisture.
9. *How durable is the product?* Is it subject to puncture? Can it be cleaned, or must it be discarded when wet with incontinence or drainage?
10. *What is the person's body weight and build?* Most products have a maximum weight that they are capable of supporting. An obese

patient may be too heavy for some products. Persons with thin body builds may have higher tissue interface pressures on a product (Whittemore, 1998).

11. *Is the patient comfortable on the product?* Some persons may not be accustomed to sleeping on a soft surface. If the product negatively affects sleep or increases pain, then a patient may not tolerate it (Fletcher, 1997).

Once a product is selected, its effectiveness for that particular patient needs to be reevaluated at regular intervals. As the patient recuperates, a less aggressive support surface may be warranted. Conversely, if the patient is deteriorating, a more aggressive support surface or a product with more features may be indicated.

Summary

Selecting the most appropriate support surface involves many considerations. The primary goal for use of a support surface is to prevent and manage pressure ulcers; thus products are examined in terms of their therapeutic effects.

The state of the art for determining therapeutic effectiveness of support surfaces is advancing:

1. There is a lack of consensus as to what constitutes capillary closing pressure.
2. The tools and methods for accurate measurement of tissue interface pressures need to continue to evolve.
3. There is an assumption that skin-resting surface interface pressures reflect the more important muscle-bone interface pressures.

The process of selecting support surfaces will continue to be refined as new products are developed and as more is learned about measuring effectiveness. The nurse should keep abreast of these changes so products can be used in an effective, efficient fashion.

MANAGEMENT OF PRESSURE ULCERS

Wound management should be based on scientific principles. A holistic approach to effective wound management must be based on four principles of wound care:

1. Relieve or eliminate the source
2. Optimize the microenvironment
3. Support the host
4. Provide education

Although optimizing the microenvironment through topical wound care and supporting the host with nutritional interventions are important components of pressure ulcer management, effective elimination or reduction of skin-resting interface pressure is imperative and cannot be overemphasized. Optimizing the wound environment and supporting the host can be marginally successful, if at all, in the presence of continued pressure. Interventions for interface pressure management and wound care have been discussed. The AHRQ has published the clinical practice guidelines, *Treatment of Pressure Ulcers* (Bergstrom et al, 1994). The guidelines address six areas: assessment, managing tissue loads, ulcer care, managing bacterial colonization and infection, operative repair, and education and quality improvement (see Appendix C for the guideline). This section highlights nuances of wound care that are specific to ulcers precipitated by pressure.

Optimizing the Microenvironment

Historically, pressure ulcers have been managed with a variety of poorly researched or scientifically unsubstantiated treatment modalities. The heat lamp, antacids, honey, insulin, and maggots are just a few therapies that should be put to rest. Likewise, the practice of massaging pressure points, which for many years was believed to stimulate circulation to areas injured by pressure, should be critically evaluated. Buss, Halfens, and Abu-Saad (1997) examined the research literature about massage. Although not significant, massage increased and decreased skin temperature, and studies about pressure ulcer development lacked statistical significance (Buss, Halfens, and Abu-Saad, 1997). Furthermore, extended massage may further injure ischemic, fragile capillaries. Massage cannot be recommended in preventing pressure ulcers.

Before selecting topical therapy, the pressure ulcer should be carefully examined for undermining or tunneling. Because of the shear force that often contributes to pressure ulcer formation, undermining of the ulcer edges is common. This is particularly true in the sacrococcygeal area. A cotton-tipped applicator can be used to ascertain the extent of undermining or the presence of tunnels. Assessment of tunnels with a cotton-tipped applicator needs to be done carefully so as to not traumatize poorly visible tissue. A tunneling pressure ulcer may communicate with a joint space or deep viscera or be close to a major blood vessel. The topical therapy selected must include a method of filling this dead space created by undermining or tunneling.

As with all wounds, careful, accurate wound assessment and documentation of wound status at regular intervals is critical for evaluation of the progress of wound repair. Regular reevaluation of topical therapy based on these assessments is also essential to ensure appropriateness of interventions. Appropriate topical therapy means using dressings that are best indicated for the ulcer, therapy that is manageable by those providing the care, and therapy that is consistent with the patient's health status, prognosis, and care objectives. For example, the patient who is being managed with twice-daily dressing changes requires a reevaluation before being discharged to home care. The goal is to develop a care plan that can be effectively implemented by the caregivers or home care nurses. It is important to remember that topical wound care is not static; it must be reevaluated and changed as the wound changes and as the patient's needs change.

When measurable improvement in the wound has not been observed for a significant period of time (such as 2 to 4 weeks), the patient should be reevaluated for the presence of factors that would prevent healing (such as pressure, shear, malnourishment); these must be corrected. Adaptations to the topical therapy should also be made. If intrinsic factors are uncorrectable, the goals for the ulcer healing must be reconsidered.

Supporting the Host

Once the pressure has been eliminated, attention must be given to the patient's nutritional status. Protein, calories, vitamins, and minerals are essential to support the wound-repair process and prevent extension of the ulcer. Nutritional support may be in the form of snacks, oral supplements, adjunctive tube feedings, or parenteral nutrition. The method selected is guided by the extent of the patient's nutritional needs.

Local or systemic infection must be controlled or eliminated. Because necrotic tissue harbors bacteria, aggressive debridement of necrotic wounds that appear clinically infected is indicated. The method of debridement is determined by the type of wound, amount of necrotic tissue, condition of the patient, care setting, and nurse's experience (Sieggreen and Maklebust, 1997). Systemic antibiotics are commonly used to control the release of toxins during and immediately after debridement.

Osteomyelitis must also be considered in infected or nonhealing pressure ulcers. Osteomyelitis may be difficult to diagnosis. When osteomyelitis is suspected, a bone scan or magnetic resonance imaging (MRI) should be done (Kanj, Wilking, and Phillips, 1998). Osteomyelitis is unlikely if the these are normal, but if they are abnormal, a bone biopsy and culture are needed to determine bone infection and causative organisms (Kanj, Wilking, and Phillips, 1998)

Pressure Ulcer Healing. Measuring healing of pressure ulcers requires accurate measurement with tools that are consistent, reliable, and easily used by staff (Thomas, 1997a; Xakellis and Frantz, 1996). Measurement may include wound dimensions, photography, exudate characteristics, and predominant tissue in the ulcer (Eager, 1997; Ovington, 1997; Xakellis and Frantz, 1996). Some instruments include scored wound descriptors, such as the Pressure Sore Status Tool (PSST), the Sussman Wound Healing Tool, the Sessing Scale, the Wound Healing Scale, and the Pressure Ulcer Scale for Healing (PUSH) (Bates-Jensen, 1997; Ferrell, 1997b; Krasner, 1997; PUSH Task Force, 1997; Sussman and Swanson, 1997; Thomas, 1997a).

Pressure ulcer staging should not be used to indicate pressure ulcer healing, and the pressure ulcer should never be "downstaged" or reverse staged (Cuddigan, 1997). Pressure ulcer healing is complicated by many comorbid conditions and outcomes may be unpredictable. Some intermediate outcomes of healing may also be included, such as resolution of infection, decreased pain, enhanced quality of life, treatment costs, or change in caregiver burden (Allman and Fowler, 1995).

The time to heal a pressure ulcer is variable. Stage 2 pressure ulcers have a mean or median time to heal ranging from 8.7 to 38 days (van Rijswijk, 1995). The median time to heal a stage 3 or 4 pressure ulcer has been reported as 69 days with the percentage reduction in ulcer area after 2 weeks of treatment as an independent predictor of time to heal (van Rijswijk, 1995). Healing rates are lower for stage 3 and 4 ulcers than for stage 2 ulcers in all health care settings (Allman, 1995). Complete wound closure may not be a practical way to assess healing because of prolonged healing time, patient's loss to follow-up, and changing care goals (Ferrell, 1997a).

Quality of Life. Pressure ulcers may affect quality of life in terms of occurrence, reoccurrence, ulcer characteristics, and ulcer demands. Most quality-of-life research is about persons with spinal cord injury (Rintala, 1995). Quality-of-life research studies are small, and additional research is needed (Rintala, 1995). Mental, functional, and financial status should also be considered with quality of life.

Pain. Little is known about pain associated with pressure ulcers. Krasner (1996) examined nurses' reflections about patients' pressure ulcer pain and identified three patterns.

1. Nursing expertly included reading the pain, attending to the pain, and acknowledging and empathizing.
2. Denying the pain included assuming that it does not hurt, not hearing the cries, and avoiding failure.
3. Confronting the challenge of pain included coping with frustration and being with the patient.

Dallam and colleagues (1995) studied pressure ulcer pain among hospitalized patients. Some type of pain was reported by 59% of persons who could respond. They concluded that patients with pressure ulcers experience pain, most do not receive analgesics for pain relief, patients who cannot respond should not be considered pain free, and stage 4 pressure ulcers are associated with more pain than other pressure ulcer stages (Dallam et al, 1995).

There are several etiologies for pressure ulcer pain, such as the release of noxious chemicals from damaged tissue, erosion of tissue planes with destruction of nerve terminals, regeneration of nociceptive nerve terminals, infection, dressing changes, and debridement (Rook, 1997). The cause of pain needs to be determined and corrected. Pain assessment scales should be used with patients when possible. Analgesics should be used to treat pressure ulcer pain. Besides medications, pain may be treated with physical and occupational therapy to decrease muscle spasms, decrease contractures, and aid in wound debridement and cleansing (International Committee on Wound Management, 1994; Rook, 1997). Proper seating, positioning, and adaptive equipment may also help to decrease pain.

Quality Improvement. Continuous quality improvement looks for problems that exist in care delivery and attempts to correct them. Pressure ulcers are often viewed as a quality-of-care marker in health care settings. Quality of care may be examined by reviewing medical records to determine if care delivered was acceptable or appropriate as well as the use of standards and guidelines (Ferrell, 1995). The method to collect quality data needs to be reliable and valid. The use and recording of prevention methods or risk assessment may be found to be lacking (Motta, 1996; Pieper et al, 1997b). Educational programs and decision charts may assist health care workers to enhance quality of care (Kiernan, 1997; Kynes, 1986; Letourneau and Jensen, 1998; Moore and Wise, 1997; Suntken et al, 1996; Xakellis, 1997). Education about pressure ulcers should be integrated into medical and nursing school curricula. The health professional's knowledge about pressure ulcers needs to be updated (Pieper and Mattern, 1997; Pieper and Mott, 1995).

Legal Concerns. An issue in medical malpractice is whether the practitioner met the standard of care, namely that exercised by other practitioners in the same line of practice under the same or similar circumstances (Murphy, 1996). Pressure ulcers may be viewed as an indicator of neglect (Hoffman, 1997). Documentation is critical and should be done in detail. Concerns are raised when there are numerous and varying descriptions of the pressure ulcer, lack of evidence of ordered care, and not matching or monitoring a treatment protocol. Photographs document many aspects of wound assessment and may be used during litigation (Kutcher and Arnell, 1992). Health professionals must constantly ask if prevention and/or treatment are effective. If not, what are criteria for changing care? It is important to document whenever interventions are performed, patient instructions are given, or a patient refuses care.

Provide Education

Pressure ulcer care and prevention is not a passive process for the patient or caregivers. Teaching provides information and enhances skill development. The patient or primary caregivers must understand the cause of pressure ulcer formation, the significance of factors contributing to pressure injury, preventive measures, the significance of nutrition in wound repair, and the indicators of wound healing (Bergstrom, 1997; Panel for the Prediction and Prevention of Pressure Ulcers in Adults, 1992). Teaching materials about pressure ulcer prevention and treatment should be left at the bedside. All health care personnel providing care to the patient need to appreciate the role that they play in preventing pressure ulcers.

Formal patient education programs are common for patients with a spinal cord injury in rehabilitation centers. These could serve as a model for similar educational programs for patients with any chronic disease that limits mobility as the disease progresses and increases risk for pressure injury (e.g., multiple sclerosis, terminal cancer). Family members should be included in such programs (Bergstrom, 1997; Panel for the Prediction and Prevention of Pressure Ulcers in Adults, 1992). Requesting that caregivers come to the hospital to work with a nurse before a patient's discharge may be helpful for learning techniques of care. Likewise, high-risk patients should be routinely assessed, specifically for indications of pressure damage. Education of the patient, staff, caregivers, and family members is the key to effective prevention of pressure ulcers and to successful management of existing pressure ulcers (Xakellis et al, 1998).

Resources for Wound Care. Research about the prevention and treatment of pressure ulcers continues to evolve and affect patient care. Resources are available on the World Wide Web. These services may allow the nurse to learn about specific treatments, chat with wound care experts, read articles about wound care, and provide information about conferences and courses (Ayello, 1997). Dermatology resources are also available, such as professional and general public information, clinical databases, dermatologic images, and patient-support resources (Korn, 1997). The World Wide Web can provide rapid access to information but does not replace text and journal information. Many professional organizations provide information. These include but are not limited to the Wound, Ostomy, and Continence Nurses Society, the Association for the Advancement of Wound Care, the Dermatology Nurses' Association, the American Academy of Dermatologists, and the NPUAP.

SUMMARY

Pressure ulcers are a national health concern because, for the most part, they are a preventable and costly complication. Pressure ulcers develop as a consequence of the occlusion of capillaries because of unrelieved pressure. The extent of tissue damage is influenced by numerous variables.

Prevention of pressure is a critical element in managing pressure ulcers and requires judicious use of interventions such as support surfaces. Regardless of the presence or absence of tissue damage, interface pressure must be reduced. Appropriate topical therapy must be initiated to enhance the wound repair. When the nurse is familiar with the pathologic process of tissue destruction caused by unrelieved pressure, appropriate interventions can be derived.

SELF-ASSESSMENT EXERCISE

1. Define *prevalence* and *cumulative incidence.*
2. Why are the data describing the prevalence of pressure ulcer formation in hospitals, nursing homes, and high-risk populations so varied?
3. Define *pressure ulcer.*
4. What is the role of muscle in preventing pressure ulcers?
   a. Muscle redistributes pressure load
   b. Muscle provides the blood supply to the skin
   c. Muscle enables blood vessels to resist shear injury

   d. Muscle concentrates pressure over the bony prominence

5. State the three factors that play a role in determining the negative effects of pressure.

6. What is the common range of capillary closing pressure?
   a. 5 to 15 mm Hg
   b. 12 to 32 mm Hg
   c. 10 to 20 mm Hg
   d. 15 to 45 mm Hg

7. Capillary closing pressure is the:
   a. Pressure required to keep a capillary patent
   b. Difference in pressures between the arteriolar end of the capillary and the venous end
   c. Pressure needed to occlude the capillary blood flow
   d. Mean capillary pressure

8. Explain why it is difficult to accurately assign a numerical value to capillary closing pressure.

9. Tissue interface pressure is believed to be an indirect measure of:
   a. Capillary closing pressure
   b. Mean capillary pressure
   c. Pressure being exerted on a capillary
   d. Pressure required to keep a capillary patent

10. Explain the relationship between tissue interface pressure and capillary closing pressure.

11. Describe how intensity of pressure and duration of pressure affect tissue ischemia.

12. Which of the following are major factors that contribute to pressure ulcer development?
   a. Shear, smoking, friction
   b. Age, smoking, blood pressure
   c. Nutrition, moisture, shear
   d. Shear, friction, nutritional debilitation

13. Which of the following statements about blanching erythema is false?
   a. It resolves once pressure is removed
   b. It indicates deep tissue damage
   c. It is an area of erythema that turns white when compressed
   d. It implies that pressure is not adequately relieved or reduced

14. State four variables that influence the extent of tissue damage associated with pressure.

15. State at least two variables that contribute to cellular death in a pressure-damaged area.

16. Describe the pressure gradient in pressure ulcer formation.

17. The undermining that is commonly observed with pressure ulcers may be the result of which process?
   a. Shear
   b. Friction
   c. Maceration
   d. Advanced age

18. Differentiate between specificity and sensitivity.

19. Identify at least two differences among the three pressure sore risk-assessment scales.

20. List therapeutic features that are provided by various support surfaces.

21. Tissue interface pressures are frequently used as indicators of support surface effectiveness. Identify at least three factors that may affect the accuracy of tissue interface readings.

22. Define the following terms:
   a. Overlay
   b. Replacement mattress
   c. Specialty bed

23. List the criteria for a therapeutic foam overlay.

24. Explain why water overlays are more appropriate for long-term and home care use than for acute care settings.

25. Compare and contrast static and dynamic air overlays.

26. Which of the following are considered to be pressure-relieving devices?
   a. Low-air-loss beds
   b. Therapeutic foam overlays
   c. Alternating pressure pads and water mattresses
   d. Replacement mattresses

27. Explain the rationale for selection of a pressure-relief versus a pressure-reducing device.

28. List factors to be considered in selecting an appropriate support surface for an individual patient.

REFERENCES

Adams T, Hunter WS: Modification of skin mechanical properties by eccrine sweat gland activity, *J Appl Physiol* 26:417, 1969.

Agris J, Spira M: Pressure ulcers: prevalence and treatment, *Clin Symp* 31(5):21, 1979.

Allman RM: Outcomes in prospective studies and clinical trials, *Adv Wound Care* 8(4):28, 1995.

Allman RM: The impact of pressure ulcers on health care costs and mortality, *Adv Wound Care* 11(3 Suppl):2, 1998.

Allman RM, Damiano AM, Strauss MJ: Pressure ulcer status and post-discharge health care resource utilization among older adults with activity limitations, *Adv Wound Care* 9(2):38, 1996.

Allman RM, Fowler E: Expected outcomes for the treatment of pressure ulcers, *Adv Wound Care* 8(4):28, 1995.

Allman RM et al: Air-fluidized beds or conventional therapy for pressure sores, *Ann Intern Med* 107:641, 1987.

Allman RM et al: Pressure sores among hospitalized patients, *Ann Intern Med* 105:3371, 1986.

Allman RM et al: Pressure ulcer risk factors among hospitalized patients with activity limitations, *JAMA* 273:865, 1995.

Allman RM et al: Pressure ulcers, hospital complications, and disease severity: impact on hospital costs and length of stay, *Adv Wound Care* 12(1):22, 1999.

Arnold HL: Decubitus: the word. In Parish LC, Witkowski JA, Crissey JT: *The decubitus ulcer,* New York, 1983, Masson Publishing.

Aronovitch SA: Intraoperative acquired pressure ulcer prevalence: a national study, *Adv Wound Care* 11(3 suppl):8, 1998.

Ayello EA: Wound care on the web, *Adv Wound Care* 10:24, 1997.

Baldwin, KM, Ziegler SM: Pressure ulcer risk following critical traumatic injury, *Adv Wound Care* 11(4):168, 1998.

Barczak CA et al: Fourth national pressure ulcer prevalence survey, *Adv Wound Care* 10(4):18, 1997.

Bates-Jensen BM: The pressure sore status tool a few thousand assessments later, *Adv Wound Care* 10(5):65, 1997.

Baumgarten M: Designing prevalence and incidence studies, *Adv Wound Care* 11(6):287, 1998.

Beckrich K, Aronovitch SA: Hospital-acquired pressure ulcers: a comparison of costs in medical versus surgical patients, *Adv Wound Care* 11(3 suppl):2, 1998.

Bennett LM et al: Skin stress and blood flow in sitting paraplegic patients, *Arch Phys Med Rehabil* 65:1861, 1984.

Bennett LM, Lee BY: Vertical shear existence in animal pressure threshold experiments, *Decubitus* 1:18, 1988.

Bennett RG et al: Low airloss hydrotherapy versus standard care for incontinent hospitalized patients, *J Am Geriatr Soc* 45:569, 1998.

Berecek KH: Treatment of decubitus ulcers, *Nurs Clin North Am* 10:1711, 1975.

Bergstrom NI: Strategies for preventing pressure ulcers, *Clin Geriatr Med* 13(3):437, 1997.

Bergstrom NI, Braden B: A prospective study of pressure sore risk among institutionalized elderly, *J Am Geriatr Soc* 40:747, 1992.

Bergstrom NI, Demuth PJ, Braden B: A clinical trial of the Braden Scale for predicting pressure sore risk, *Nurs Clin North Am* 22(2):4171, 1987.

Bergstrom NI et al: Multi-site study of incidence of pressure ulcers and the relationship between risk level, demographic characteristics, diagnoses, and prescription of preventive interventions, *J Am Geriatr Soc* 44:22, 1996.

Bergstrom NI et al: Predicting pressure ulcer risk: a multisite study of the predictive validity of the Braden Scale, *Nurs Res* 47(5):261, 1998.

Bergstrom NI et al: The Braden Scale for predicting pressure sore risk, *Nurs Res* 36(4):2051, 1987.

Bergstrom NI et al: *Treatment of pressure ulcers.* Clinical Practice Guideline #15, Rockville, Md, 1994, USDHHS, PHS, AHCPR, Pub. No. 95-0652.

Berlowitz DR et al: Effect of pressure ulcers on the survival of long-term care residents, *J Gerontol* 52A(2):M106, 1997.

Berlowitz DR, Wilking SVB: Risk factors for pressure sore: a comparison on cross-sectional and cohort-derived data, *J Am Geriatr Soc* 37:1043, 1989.

Braden BJ: *Emotional stress and pressure sore formation among the elderly recently relocated to a nursing home: key aspects of recovery: improving mobility, rest, and nutrition,* New York, 1990, Springer.

Braden BJ: The relationship between stress and pressure sore formation, *Ostomy Wound Manage* 44(3A):26S, 1998.

Braden BJ, Bergstrom N: A conceptual schema for the study of the etiology of pressure sores, *Rehabil Nurs* 12(1):81, 1987.

Braden BJ, Bergstrom N: Clinical utility of the Braden Scale for predicting pressure sore risk, *Decubitus* 2(3):441,1989.

Brandeis GH et al: Pressure ulcers: the minimum data set and the resident assessment protocol, *Adv Wound Care* 8(6):18, 1995.

Brandeis GH et al: The epidemiology and natural history of pressure ulcers in elderly nursing home residents, *JAMA* 264(22):2905, 1990.

Brooks B, Duncan W: Effects of pressure on tissues, *Arch Surg* 40:696, 1940.

Burton AC, Yamada S: Relation between blood pressure and flow in the human forearm, *J Appl Physiol* 4:3291, 1951.

Buss IC, Halfens RJG, Abu-Saad HH: The effectiveness of massage in preventing pressure sores: a literature review, *Rehabil Nurs* 22(5):229, 1997.

Capobianco ML, McDonald DD: Factors affecting the predictive validity of the Braden Scale, *Adv Wound Care* 9(6):32, 1996.

Cheneworth CC et al: Portrait of practice: healing heel ulcers, *Adv Wound Care* 7(2):44, 1994.

Chernoff R: Policy: Nutrition standards for treatment of pressure ulcers, *Nutr Rev* 54(1):S43, 1996.

Cherry GW et al: Functional microcirculatory changes after flap elevation: possible factor in flap failure, *Plast Surg Forum* 3:2061, 1980.

Cherry GW, Ryan TJ: Pathophysiology. In Parish LC, Witkowski JA, Crissey JT: *The decubitus ulcer,* New York, 1983, Masson Publishing.

Cherry GW, Ryan TJ, Ellis J: Decreased fibrinolysis in reperfused ischemic tissue, *Thromb Diathesis Haemorrhag* 32:659, 1974.

Clark MO et al: Pressure sores, *Nursing Times* 74(9):363, 1978.

Clark MO, Cullum N: Matching patient need for pressure sore prevention with the supply of pressure redistributing mattresses, *J Adv Nurs* 17:310, 1992.

Cohen IK, Diegelmann RF, Johnson MJ: Effect of corticosteroids on collagen synthesis, *Surgery* 82(1):151, 1977.

Counsell C et al: Interface skin pressures on four pressure-relieving devices, *J Enterostom Ther* 17(4):150, 1990.

Cuddigan J: Pressure ulcer classification: what do we have? what do we need? *Adv Wound Care* 10:13, 1997.

Dallam L et al: Pressure ulcer pain: assessment and quantification, *J Wound Ostomy Continence Nurs* 22:211, 1995.

Daniel RK, Kerrigan CL: Skin flaps: an anatomical and hemodynamic approach, *Clin Plast Surg* 6:181, 1979.

Eager CA: Monitoring wound healing in the home health arena, *Adv Wound Care* 10(5):54, 1997.

Eckman KL: The prevalence of dermal ulcers among persons in the U.S. who have died, *Decubitus* 2:36, 1989.

Evans-Stoner N: Nutritional assessment: a practical approach, *Nurs Clin North Am* 32:637, 1997.

Ferrell BA: Assessment of healing, *Clin Geriatr Med* 13(3):575, 1997a.

Ferrell BA: Outcomes in quality improvement activities, *Adv Wound Care* 8(4):28, 1995.

Ferrell BA: The Sessing Scale for measurement of pressure ulcer healing, *Adv Wound Care* 10(4):78, 1997b.

Flanigan KH: Nutritional aspects of wound healing, *Adv Wound Care* 10(3):48, 1997.

Fletcher J: Pressure-relieving equipment: criteria and selection, *Br J Nurs* 6(6):323, 1997.

Fox J, Bradley R: *A new medical dictionary,* London, 1803, Darton & Harvey.

Frantz RA: Measuring prevalence and incidence of pressure ulcers, *Adv Wound Care* 10(1):21, 1997.

Gallagher SM: Outcomes in clinical practice: pressure ulcer prevalence and incidence studies, *Ostomy Wound Manage* 43(1):28, 1997.

Goldstone LA, Goldstone J: The Norton score: an early warning of pressure sores? *J Adv Nurs* 1:4191, 1982.

Goldstone LA, Roberts BV: A preliminary discriminant function analysis of elderly orthopaedic patients who will or will not contract a pressure sore, *Int J Nurs Stud* 17(5):171, 1980.

Gosnell DJ: An assessment tool to identify pressure sores, *Nurs Res* 22(1):551, 1973.

Gosnell DJ: Pressure sore risk assessment: a critique, *Decubitus* 2(3):321, 1989.

Gosnell DJ, Pontius C: A model of quality assurance for decubitus ulcer monitoring, *Decubitus* 1(4):24, 1988.

Greer DM et al: Cost effectiveness and efficacy of air-fluidized therapy in the treatment of pressure ulcers, *J Enterostom Ther* 15:247, 1988.

Guyton AC, Hall JE: *Textbook of medical physiology,* Philadelphia, 1996, W.B. Saunders.

Haalboom JR, den Boer J, Buskens E: Risk-assessment tools in the prevention of pressure ulcers, *Ostomy Wound Manage* 45(2):20, 1999.

Hawthorne MH, Jefferson JW, Paduano DJ: The prevalence of dermal wounds, *Decubitus* 2:64, 1989.

Hergenroeder P, Mosher C, Sevo D: Pressure ulcer risk assessment–simple or complex? *Decubitus* 5:47, 1992.

Hoffman DR: The Federal effort to eliminate fraud and ensure quality, *Adv Wound Care* 10:36, 1997.

Husain T: An experimental study of some pressure effects on tissues, with reference to the bedsore problem, *J Pathol Bacteriol* 66:3471, 1953.

International Committee on Wound Management: Wound management and quality of life in the elderly, *Wounds* 6:94, 1994.

Jackson BS et al: The effects of a therapeutic bed on pressure ulcers: an experimental study, *J Enterostom Ther* 15:220, 1988.

Jay R: Other considerations in selecting a support surface, *Adv Wound Care* 10(7):37, 1997.

Jones PL, Millman A: Wound healing and the aged patient, *Nurs Clin North Am* 25:2631, 1990.

Kanj LF, Wilking SVB, Phillips TJ: Pressure ulcers, *J Am Acad Dermatol* 38(4):517, 1998.

Kemp MG et al: The role of support surfaces and patient attributes in preventing pressure ulcers in elderly patients, *Res Nurs Health* 16:89, 1993.

Kiernan M: Pressure sores: adopting the principles of risk management, *Br J Nurs* 6(6):329, 1997.

Korn K: Dermatology on the internet, *J Am Acad Nurse Pract* 9:487, 1997.

Kosiak M: Etiology and pathology of ischemic ulcers, *Arch Phys Med Rehabil* 40:62, 1959.

Kosiak M: Etiology of decubitus ulcers, *Arch Phys Med Rehabil* 42:191, 1961.

Kosiak M et al: Evaluation of pressure as a factor in the production of ischial ulcers, *Arch Phys Med Rehabil* 39:623, 1958.

Krasner D: Using a gentler hand: reflections on patients with pressure ulcers who experience pain, *Ostomy Wound Manage* 42:20, 1996.

Krasner D: Wound healing scale, version 1.0: a proposal, *Adv Wound Care* 10(5):82, 1997.

Krouskop TA: A synthesis of the factors that contribute to pressure sore formation, *Med Hypotheses* 11(2):2551, 1983.

Krouskop TA: *Scientific aspects of pressure relief,* Lecture presented at the 1989 International Association for Enterostomal Therapy annual conference, Washington, DC, June 8, 1989.

Krouskop TA et al: Effectiveness of mattress overlays in reducing interface pressure during recumbency, *J Rehabil Res* 22:7, 1985.

Krouskop TA et al: Factors affecting the pressure-distributing properties of foam mattress overlays, *J Rehabil Res* 23(3):331, 1986.

Krouskop TA, Garber SL: The role of technology in the prevention of pressure sores, *Ostomy Wound Manage* 16:45, 1987.

Krouskop TA, Williams R, Krebs M: The effectiveness of air flotation beds in lowering the pressures under the recumbent body, *CARE, Sci Pract* 4(2):9, 1984.

Kutcher J, Arnell I: Documentation of skin using photography, *Ostomy Wound Manage* 38:23, 1992.

Kynes P: A new perspective on pressure sore prevention, *J Enterostom Ther* 13(2):421, 1986.

Lake NO: Measuring incidence and prevlaence of pressure ulcers for intergroup comparison, *Adv Wound Care* 12:31, 1999.

Lamid S, El Ghatit AZ: Smoking, spasticity and pressure sores in spinal cord injured patients, *Am J Phys Med* 62(6):300, 1983.

Landis EM: Micro-injection studies of capillary blood pressure in human skin, *Heart* 15:209, 1930.

Langemo DK et al: Incidence and prediction of pressure ulcers in five patient care settings, *Decubitus* 4(3): 25, 1991.

Letourneau S, Jensen L: Impact of a decision tree on chronic wound care, *J Wound Ostomy Continence Nurs* 25(5):240, 1998.

Lincoln R et al: Use of the Norton pressure sore risk assessment scoring system with elderly patients in acute care, *J Enterostom Ther* 13:171, 1986.

Lindan O: Etiology of decubitus ulcers: an experimental study, *Arch Phys Med Rehabil* 42:774, 1961.

Lyder CH et al: Validating the Braden Scale for the prediction of pressure ulcer risk in Blacks and Latino/Hispanic elders: a pilot study, *Ostomy Wound Manage* 44(3A):42, 1998.

Margolis DJ: Definition of a pressure ulcer, *Adv Wound Care* 8(4):28, 1995.

McLeod R: Other considerations in selecting a support surface, *Adv Wound Care* 10(7):37, 1997.

Meehan M: Multisite pressure ulcer prevalence survey, *Decubitus* 3:14, 1990.

Moolten SE: Bedsores in the chronically ill patient, *Arch Phys Med Rehabil* 53:4301, 1972.

Moore SM, Wise L: Reducing nosocomial pressure ulcers, *J Nurs Adm* 27(10):28, 1997.

Motta GJ: Documentation and reimbursement by clinical setting, *Ostomy Wound Manage* 42:18, 1996.

Murphy RN: Legal and practical impact of clinical practice guidelines on nursing and medical practices, *Adv Wound Care* 9:31, 1996.

National Pressure Ulcer Advisory Panel: Pressure ulcers prevalence, cost and risk assessment: consensus development conference statement, *Decubitus* 2(2):241, 1989.

Niazi ZBM et al: Recurrence of initial pressure ulcer in persons with spinal cord injuries, *Adv Wound Care* 10(3):38, 1997.

Norton D: Calculating the risk: reflections on the Norton Scale, *Adv Wound Care* 9(6):38, 1996.

Ovington LG: What is needed to monitor healing in the outpatient clinic setting? *Adv Wound Care* 10(5):58, 1997.

Panel for the Prediction and Prevention of Pressure Ulcers in Adults: *Pressure ulcers in adults: prediction and prevention. Clinical practice guideline,* AHCPR Pub. No. 92-0047, 1992.

Pang SM, Wong TK: Predicting pressure sore risk with the Norton, Braden, and Waterlow Scales in a Hong Kong rehabilitation hospital, *Nurs Res* 47(3):147, 1998.

Parish LC, Witkowski JA: Clinitron therapy and the decubitus ulcer: preliminary dermatologic studies, *Dermatology* 19:517, 1980.

Parish LC, Witkowski JA, Crissey JT: *The decubitus ulcer,* New York, 1983, Masson Publishing.

Patterson JA, Bennett RG: Prevention and treatment of pressure sores, *J Am Geriat Soc* 43:919, 1995.

Pieper B, Mattern J: Critical care nurses' knowledge of pressure ulcer prevention, *Ostomy Wound Manage* 43(3):22, 1997.

Pieper B, Mott M: Nurses' knowledge of pressure ulcer prevention, staging and description, *Adv Wound Care* 8(3):34, 1995.

Pieper B et al: Presence of pressure ulcer prevention methods used among patients considered at risk versus those considered not at risk, *J Wound Ostomy Continence Nurs* 24:191, 1997a.

Pieper B et al: Risk factors, prevention methods, and wound care for patients with pressure ulcers, *Clin Nurse Spec* 12:7, 1998.

Pieper B et al: The occurrence of skin lesions in ill persons, *Dermatol Nurs* 9(2):91, 1997b.

Powers J: A multidisciplinary approach to occipital pressure ulcers related to cervical collars, *J Nurs Care Qual* 12(1):46, 1997.

PUSH Task Force: Pressure ulcer scale for healing: derivation and validation of the PUSH Tool, *Adv Wound Care* 10(5):96, 1997.

Quigley SM, Curley MAQ: Skin integrity in the pediatric population: preventing and managing pressure ulcers, *J Soc Pediatr Nurs* 1(1):7, 1996.

Ramundo JM: Reliability and validity of the Braden Scale in the home care setting, *J Wound Ostomy Continence Nurs* 22(3):128, 1995.

Reed MJ, Weksler ME: Wound repair in older patients: preventing problems and managing the healing, *Geriatrics* 53(5):88, 1998.

Reger SI et al: Correlation of transducer systems for monitoring tissue interface pressures, *J Clin Engineering* 13(5):365, 1988.

Reichel SM: Shearing force as a factor in decubitus ulcers in paraplegics, *JAMA* 166:762, 1958.

Reuler JB, Cooney TG: The pressure sore: pathophysiology and principles of management, *Ann Intern Med* 94(5):6611, 1981.

Rintala DH: Quality of life considerations, *Adv Wound Care* 8(4):28, 1995.

Roberts BV, Goldstone LA: A survey of pressure sores in the over sixties on two orthopaedic wards, *Int J Nurs Stud* 16:3551, 1979.

Rodriquez G et al: Collagen metabolite excretion as a predictor of bone and skin-related complications in spinal cord injury, *Arch Phys Med Rehabil* 70(6):4421, 1989.

Rook JL: Wound care pain management, *Nurse Pract* 22:122, 1997.

Ryan TJ: Microvascularization in psoriasis, blood vessels, lymphatics and tissue fluid, *Pharmacol Ther* 10:27, 1980.

Salzberg CA et al: Predicting and preventing pressure ulcers in adults with paralysis, *Adv Wound Care* 11(5):237, 1998.

Scales JT: Pressure on the patient. In Kenedi RM, Cowden JM, editors: *Bedsore biomechanics*, London, 1976, University Park Press.

Schmid-Schönbein H, Rieger H, Fischer T: Blood fluidity as a consequence of red cell fluidity: flow properties of blood and flow behavior of blood in vascular diseases, *Angiology* 31:3011, 1980.

Seiler WO, Stahelin HB: Decubitus ulcers: preventive techniques for the elderly patient, *Geriatrics* 40(7):531, 1985.

Shannon ML: Pressure sores. In Norris CM: *Concept clarification in nursing*, Rockville, Md, 1982, Aspen.

Shannon ML, Skorga P: Pressure ulcer prevalence in two general hospitals, *Decubitus* 2:38, 1989.

Shea JD: Pressure sores: classification and management, *Clin Orthop* (112):891, 1975.

Siegel RJ, Vistness LM, Laub DR: Use of water bed for prevention of pressure sores, *Plast Reconstr Surg* 51:81, 1973.

Sieggreen MY, Maklebust J: Debridement: choices and challenges, *Adv Wound Care* 10:32, 1997.

Skewes SM: Skin care rituals that do more harm than good, Am J Nurs 96:33, 1996.

Sloan DR, Brown RD, Larson DL: Evaluation of a simplified water mattress in the prevention and treatment of pressure sores, *Plast Reconstr Surg* 60(4):5961, 1977.

Spector WD, Fortinsky RH: Pressure ulcer prevalence in Ohio nursing homes, *J Aging Health* 10(1):62, 1998.

Stotts NA et al: Underutilization of pressure ulcer risk assessment in hip fracture patients, *Adv Wound Care* 11(1):32, 1998.

Strauss EA, Margolis DJ: Malnutrition in patients with pressure ulcers: morbidity, mortality, and clinically practical assessment, *Adv Wound Care* 9:37, 1996.

Suntken G et al: Implementation of a comprehensive skin care program across care settings using the AHCPR pressure ulcer prevention and treatment guidelines, *Ostomy Wound Manage* 42(2):20, 1996.

Sussman C, Swanson G: Utility of the Sussman Wound Healing Tool in predicting wound healing outcomes in physical therapy, *Adv Wound Care* 10(5):74, 1997.

Tallon RW: Support surfaces: therapeutic and performance insights, *Nurs Manage* 27(9):57, 1996.

Thomas DR: Existing tools: are they meeting the challenges of pressure ulcer healing? *Adv Wound Care* 10(5):86, 1997a.

Thomas DR: Nutritional factors affecting wound healing, *Ostomy Wound Manage* 42:40, 1996.

Thomas DR: Specific nutritional factors in wound healing, *Adv Wound Care* 10(4):40, 1997b.

Thomas DR: The role of nutrition in prevention and healing of pressure ulcers, *Clin Geriatr Med* 13(3):497, 1997c.

Thomson CW et al: Fluidized-bead bed in the intensive-therapy unit, *Lancet* 1:568, 1980.

Trumble HC: The skin tolerance for pressure and pressure sores, *Med J Aust* 2:7241, 1930.

Tymec AC, Pieper B, Vollman K: A comparison of two pressure-relieving devices on the prevention of heel pressure ulcers, *Adv Wound Care* 10:39, 1997.

van Rijswijk L: Frequency of reassessment of pressure ulcers, *Adv Wound Care* 8:28, 1995.

Viner C: Floating on a bed of beads, *Nuring Times* 82:62, 1986.

Vyhlidal S et al: Mattress replacement or foam overlay? a prospective study on the incidence of pressure ulcers, *Appl Nurs Res* 10(3):111, 1997.

Wasson JH et al: Clinical prediction rules: applications and methodological standards, *N Engl J Med* 313:7931, 1985.

Weaver V, Jester J: A clinical tool: updated readings on tissue interface pressures, *Ostomy Wound Manage* 40:34, 1994.

Weaver V, McClausland D: Revised medicare policies for support surfaces: a review, *J Wound Ostomy Continence Nurs* 25:26, 1998.

Wellman NS: A case manager's guide to nutrition screening and intervention, *J Case Manage* 3:12, 1997.

Wells P, Geden E: Paraplegic body-support pressure on convoluted foam, waterbed, and standard mattresses, *Res Nurs Health* 7:127, 1984.

Weststrate JTM, Bruining HA: Pressure sores in an intensive care unit and related variables: a descriptive study, *Intensive Crit Care Nurse* 12(5):280, 1996.

Whittemore R: Pressure-reduction support surfaces: a review of the literature, *J Wound Ostomy Continence Nurs* 25:6, 1998.

Williams C: Using water filled gloves for pressure relief on heels, *J Wound Care* 2(6):345, 1993.

Xakellis GC: Quality assurance programs for pressure ulcers, *Clin Geriatr Med* 13(3):599, 1997.

Xakellis GC, Frantz RA: Pressure ulcer healing: what is it? what influences it? how is it measured? *Adv Wound Care* 10(5): 20, 1997.

Xakellis GC, Frantz RA: The cost of healing pressure ulcers across multiple health care settings, *Adv Wound Care* 9(6):18, 1996.

Xakellis GC et al: Cost-effectiveness of an intensive pressure ulcer prevention protocol in long-term care, *Adv Wound Care* 11(1):22, 1998.

Yarkony GM: Pressure ulcers: a review, *Arch Phys Med Rehabil* 75: 908, 1994.

Zulkowski K: MDS+ RAP items associated with pressure ulcer prevalence in newly institutionalized elderly: Study 1, *Ostomy Wound Manage* 44(11):40, 1998.

CHAPTER

12 Lower-Extremity Ulcers of Vascular Etiology

DOROTHY B. DOUGHTY, JOANN WALDROP, & JANET RAMUNDO

OBJECTIVES

1. Differentiate between arterial and venous ulcerations in terms of causative factors, pathophysiology, usual location and appearance, and principles of management.
2. Differentiate among intermittent claudication, nocturnal pain, and rest pain.
3. Identify critical elements of the history and physical examination for the patient with an arterial ulcer or a venous ulcer.
4. Describe the indications and procedure for obtaining an ankle-brachial index (ABI) or an ankle-arm index (AAI).
5. Explain how the intact and competent venous system and muscle pumps within the leg work together to prevent venous hypertension.
6. Compare and contrast the types of therapeutic compression devices.
7. Describe contraindications for compression therapy.
8. Describe the pathophysiologic process of lymphedema as it relates to leg ulcerations.

Lower-limb ulcers of vascular etiology represent a very problematic type of chronic wound; they may be extremely painful, they affect the patient's mobility and quality of life (Franks and Moffatt, 1998), and they are frequently refractory to treatment and prone to recurrence. In addition to ulcers that are clearly of arterial, venous, or mixed etiology, there are atypical leg ulcers that may "mimic" vascular ulcers (Kerstein, 1996; Margolis, 1995) and that are equally difficult to treat. It is difficult to accurately determine the prevalence and incidence of these ulcers since ulceration represents a complication of a systemic process and may not be reported separately. However, these ulcers are associated with significant morbidity, and they represent a costly aspect of disease management.

The first priority in management of any wound is the identification and correction (or control) of the causative and contributing factors. Therefore the nurse managing patients with lower-extremity ulcers must be knowledgeable regarding the various pathologic processes and must use this knowledge as a basis for differential assessment and management. The nurse must remember that many patients have "mixed" disease. For example, a patient with an ulcer caused by chronic venous insufficiency (CVI) may have coexisting arterial disease that precludes standard compression therapy and that further compromises the patient's ability to heal. Similarly, the diabetic patient with neuropathy may present with an ulcer caused by painless trauma but complicated by a coexisting ischemia. The wound care nurse must also remain alert to the possibility that a particular ulcer falls into the "atypical" category, especially when the ulcer fails to respond to initial management. This chapter provides a review of the pathology, presentation, and management of arterial and venous ulcers as well as a brief discussion of lymphedema. More "atypical" leg ulcers are discussed in Chapter 6.

ARTERIAL ULCERS

Arterial ulcers are much less common than ulcers of venous origin; however, they are frequently more difficult to treat because of the underlying disease process. These ulcers occur as a result of severe tissue ischemia and are therefore extremely painful. Even more important, an ischemic ulcer represents potential limb loss. These lesions are generally refractory to healing unless tissue perfusion can be improved, and they are prone to progress to invasive infection and/or gangrene, which may necessitate amputation (Fry, Marek, and Langsfeld, 1998; Hilleman, 1998). Effective management of the ischemic limb frequently requires significant modifications in the patient's lifestyle, which may be difficult for the patient to incorporate (Cantwell-Gab, 1996; Cooke and Ma, 1995). Effective management of these patients is therefore multifaceted and includes measures to maximize perfusion, strategies to minimize the risk of infection, ongoing assessment for deterioration in wound or tissue status, interventions to reduce pain, and patient education regarding care options and needed lifestyle changes.

Epidemiology

The incidence of peripheral arterial disease (PAD) increases with age and is greater among men. The prevalence of clinically evident disease (i.e., intermittent claudication) is less than 2% among men less than 50 years of age but increases to 5% to 6% among those 70 years of age or older (Hilleman, 1998; Meijjer et al, 1998; Verhaeghe, 1998). Prevalence for women follows the same pattern but with a 10-year delay (i.e., the prevalence does not reach 5% to 10% among women until they reach 80 years of age). The prevalence of asymptomatic disease among individuals 55 years of age and older is about 19%, or three to four times that of symptomatic disease (Meijjer et al, 1998; Verhaeghe, 1998).

Fortunately, arterial ulceration is uncommon even among individuals with symptomatic disease. Severe ischemia (Table 12-1) develops in less than 25% of individuals with symptomatic arterial insufficiency (i.e., intermittent claudication), and less than 3% to 5% of the symptomatic population requires amputation (Cooke and Ma, 1995; Hilleman, 1998; Rockson and Cooke, 1998; Verhaeghe, 1998). Severe ischemia portends a poor outcome unless aggressive intervention is employed to interrupt and/or reverse the pathologic processes. This level of disease is associated with an annual mortality rate of 20%, with half of the deaths caused by coronary heart disease (Verhaeghe, 1998).

TABLE 12-1 Classification of Severity of Limb Ischemia

CATEGORY	FINDINGS
Critical ischemia	Nonpalpable pulses ABI < 0.4 $TcPo_2 < 20$ mm Hg
Borderline perfusion	Diminished but palpable pulses ABI between 0.4 and 0.6

Etiology

The most common cause of PAD and arterial ulceration among older adults is atherosclerosis involving the peripheral circulation. In the young adult population, PAD is typically due to premature atherosclerotic disease or to thromboangiitis obliterans (Buerger's disease, or arteriosclerosis obliterans). Both of these processes are uncommon and occur almost exclusively in heavy smokers (Joyce, 1996). Arterial ulcers may also occur as a result of arterial trauma, entrapment syndromes, or acute embolic syndromes; however, these are uncommon etiologic factors (Hilleman, 1998; Rockson and Cooke, 1998).

Pathology of Atherosclerosis

Atherosclerotic disease can occur in any vessel in the body. In the peripheral circulation, it usually occurs between the abdominal aorta and the distal vessels and is most common at bifurcation sites (Golledge, 1997). The pathology of atherosclerotic disease is not yet completely understood but is known to involve cumulative damage caused by a complex interplay among etiologic factors. The initial triggering event is thought to be lipid accumulation and endothelial injury, which is followed by a series of biochemical changes that result in plaque formation and enlargement. Contributing factors include increased blood viscosity and coagulability and increased smooth muscle tone within the involved vessels (Blann, Bignell, and McCollum, 1998; Boneu, Leger, and Arnaud, 1998; DiCorleto et al, 1996; Killewich et al, 1998; Lowe, 1998; Rockson and Cooke, 1998). The result is a chronic reduction in blood flow to the tissues and a loss of the ability to respond to increased metabolic demands with increased blood flow (Philipp et al, 1997; Reininger, Graf, and Reininger, 1996; Smith et al, 1998). In ad-

BOX 12-1 Effects of Nicotine and Cotinine

Primary Endothelial Injury
- Sloughing of endothelial cells
- Hyperplastic response → thickening of arterial wall

Growth of Arthromatous Lesions
- Increased levels of circulating lipids and free fatty acids
- Increased concentrations of the "arthero-genic" lipoproteins (LDL and VLDL)
- Increased production of growth factors and collagen → plaque enlargement
- Increased levels of carbon monoxide → increased endothelial permeability
- Altered production of factors affecting platelet adhesion → increased platelet aggregation

Increased Smooth Muscle Tone (vasoconstriction)
- Increased production of vasconstrictive agents (thromboxane A_2)
- Decreased production of vasodilator agent (prostacyclin, or PGI_2)

Increased Blood Viscosity
- Elevated hematocrit, WBC, and fibrinogen levels → increased blood viscosity and decreased rate of blood flow

LDL, Low-density lipoprotein; *VLDL*, very low-density lipoprotein; *WBC*, white blood cell.

dition, acute vessel occlusion may occur as a result of sudden plaque enlargement or plaque rupture (Rockson and Cooke, 1998).

Risk Factors for Peripheral Arterial Disease

Risk factors for PAD are the same as those for coronary artery disease (Cooke and Ma, 1995). Tobacco use is most predictive of PAD; 80% to 90% of individuals with symptomatic PAD report a history of tobacco use. Nicotine and its primary metabolite, cotinine, have been shown to adversely affect the vasculature in a number of ways (Box 12-1).

Some epidemiologic studies indicate that hypertension, particularly systolic hypertension, is the second most predictive risk factor for PAD. The link between hypertension and PAD is currently thought to be the vessel wall changes associated with hypertension, which are outlined in Box 12-2 (Altemose and Wiener, 1998; Cooke and Ma, 1995). Elevated cholesterol levels, especially elevated low-density lipoproteins (LDLs), play an important pathogenic role in the development of atherosclerosis and are therefore an important risk factor for the development of atherosclerosis and PAD (Cooke and Ma, 1995; DiCorleto et al, 1996).

BOX 12-2 Vessel Wall Changes Associated with Hypertension

- Increased production of vascular smooth muscle
- Activation of the renin-angiotension-aldosterone system
- Increased arteriolar sodium transport
- High intracellular calcium levels
- Increased production of factors contributing to vasoconstriction
- Increased interaction between the endothelium and the circulating blood elements

Diabetes mellitus is another important risk factor and an important prognostic variable for the progression to severe ischemia. Specific pathologic features associated with diabetes that contribute to PAD include increased plaque formation, increased red blood cell (RBC) rigidity, increased blood viscosity and coagulability, hypertrophy of the vascular smooth muscle, and increased vascular resistance (Altemose and Wiener, 1998; Levin, 1996). Hyperinsulinemia and insulin resistance may also contribute to hypertrophy of vascular smooth muscle since insulin is known to be a vascular growth factor. Elevated insulin levels may also help to explain the development of PAD among non-diabetic patients (Price, Lee, and Fowkes, 1996). Diabetics with PAD typically exhibit much more severe and advanced disease at earlier ages, and their risk of ischemic ulceration, gangrene, and amputation are significantly increased (Levin, 1996).

The differences in the presentation and progression of PAD among diabetics as compared with nondiabetics are highlighted in Box 12-3 (Ghirlanda and Citterio, 1997; Levin, 1996). The

BOX 12-3 PAD in the Diabetic Population Versus the Nondiabetic Population

- Onset at earlier age
- Faster progression to critical ischemia/increased risk of limb loss
- Most commonly involved vessels are infrapopliteal (i.e., tibial and peroneal)
- Multisegmental occlusions and multivessel disease common
- Disease usually bilateral as opposed to unilateral
- Poor candidates for angioplasty because of small size of vessels (tibial and peroneal)

diabetic with PAD is at particular risk for ischemia and gangrene of the toes as a result of one or more of the following: advanced atherosclerosis with thrombosis; microthrombi formation resulting from infection; reduced blood flow secondary to vasopressor medications; and/or cholesterol emboli resulting in "blue toe syndrome" or in painful petechiae and livedo reticularis. Homocystinuria is a rare autosomal dominant disease associated with early onset of severe atherosclerotic disease known to contribute to endothelial injury and platelet aggregation. The abnormal metabolism of homocysteine (a thiol-containing amino acid) can be easily normalized through administration of vitamin B_6, vitamin B_{12}, and/or folic acid (Robinson, Mayer, and Jacobsen, 1994).

Pathology of Thromboangiitis Obliterans (Buerger's Disease)

Thromboangiitis obliterans, also known as *Buerger's disease* and *arteriosclerosis obliterans,* is a rare condition almost exclusively limited to young adults (under 50 years of age) who are heavy smokers (Joyce, 1996). The disease typically involves the distal veins and arteries in both the upper and lower extremities. The lesions cause significant pain (claudication), and there is a high incidence of digit or limb amputation but no increase in mortality. The cause of the disease is not known but does not involve plaque formation or hypercoagulability; instead the lesions appear to be inflammatory in origin, which suggests an autoimmune process (Joyce, 1996; Rockson and Cooke, 1998).

Patients may present with complaints of cold sensitivity, rest pain, pedal claudication, digital ulceration, or gangrene. Ulceration may occur spontaneously but more commonly is precipitated by minor trauma. The disease process is always bilateral and frequently involves all four limbs. The most effective management is elimination of tobacco, which provides consistent interruption of the disease process.

Pathology of Arterial Ulceration

The exact pathologic mechanisms producing ulceration in the ischemic limb have not been clearly defined. Ulceration is believed to result from 1) progressive occlusion; 2) minor trauma, which leads to increased oxygen demands; and/or 3) external occlusive pressures (e.g., heel pressure in a bedbound patient).

Assessment Parameters

The goals of assessment are to determine the severity of the PAD, to identify potential contributing factors that may affect treatment decisions, and to evaluate the potential for healing of any ulceration. The components of assessment for any patient presenting with signs or symptoms of PAD include the patient history, physical examination, and simple noninvasive vascular studies. Selected patients require more complex vascular studies.

Patient History. The patient interview should include queries regarding any past illnesses or surgical procedures, general state of health, and any medications being taken (prescription and over-the-counter). Specific questions should be posed regarding any cardiovascular symptoms or "problems with circulation," presenting signs and symptoms, risk factors, ulcer characteristics (if present), and pain (Box 12-4).

Pain is typically the first indication of PAD. The patient should therefore be questioned regarding the presence of pain and its location and characteristics. There are three categories of ischemic pain:

1. *Intermittent claudication* is pain that occurs only with moderate to heavy activity and is relieved by approximately 2 to 5 minutes of rest.

BOX 12-4 Arterial Ulcer: Components of a Focused Patient History

1. Risk factors for arterial insufficiency
   - Past and present tobacco use (to include type and amount)
   - History of hypertension or treatment with medications
   - Diabetes mellitus (include type, onset, past and present management)
   - History of high cholesterol levels and management
   - History of angina, myocardial infarction, or cerebrovascular accident
2. Pain
   - Location
   - Characteristics of the pain (cramping versus constant deep aching pain)
   - Exacerbating and relieving factors
3. Ulcer history
   - Onset
   - Precipitating factors (e.g., minor trauma, bedrest)
   - Past and present management
   - Progress or regression in healing

This type of pain typically occurs when the involved vessel is approximately 50% occluded (Cantwell-Gab, 1996).

2. *Nocturnal pain* develops as the occlusion worsens. This type of pain occurs when the patient is in bed and is caused by the combination of leg elevation and reduced cardiac output.
3. *Rest pain* refers to pain that occurs in the absence of activity and with the legs in a dependent position; rest pain signals advanced occlusive disease (Cantwell-Gab, 1996; Rockson and Cooke, 1998).

Pain location and characteristics suggest the level and severity of the occlusion. In general, pain occurs one joint distal to the occlusion as outlined in Table 12-2. Intermittent claudication is typically described as "cramping," whereas rest pain is usually perceived as a "constant deep aching pain." Some patients interpret claudication as the "leg giving out" or "leg fatigue" rather than pain; therefore it is important to ask questions concerning activity

TABLE 12-2 Correlation between Site of Occlusion and Location of Pain

SITE OF OCCLUSION	LOCATION OF PAIN
Ileofemoral arteries	Thighs and buttocks; calves
Superficial femoral artery	Calf
Infrapopliteal	Foot

Data from Rockson S, Cooke J: Peripheral arterial insufficiency: mechanisms, natural history, and therapeutic options, *Adv Intern Med* 253, 1998.

tolerance. Exacerbating and relieving factors help to verify the etiology of the pain and also the severity of the occlusion (e.g., nocturnal pain that is relieved by dependency is characteristic of ischemic pain involving marked vessel occlusion). In contrast, leg pain that is relieved by elevation is more consistent with a venous etiology, and the diabetic patient who complains of leg pain relieved by walking is probably experiencing neuropathic pain (Cantwell-Gab, 1996; Rockson and Cooke,1998; Rubano and Kerstein, 1998).

Physical Assessment. The physical assessment must include a careful assessment of the lower extremities to determine perfusion status. Data to be gathered include the following:

General appearance of the limb. Limb appearance should be compared with the contralateral limb to identify or rule out trophic changes (e.g., thinning of the epidermis, loss of hair growth) or changes in skin color (e.g., pallor in the individual with fair skin, greyness in the patient with dark skin). However, trophic changes alone are *not* diagnostic of arterial insufficiency; positive findings must be interpreted cautiously (Cantwell-Gab, 1996; McGee and Boyko, 1998; Rockson and Cooke, 1998).

Color changes with limb elevation and dependence. The patient is placed supine, and the leg is raised to a 60-degree angle for 15 to 60 seconds while the examiner observes for a visible color change (pallor in fair-skinned individuals, grey hues in dark-skinned individuals). The leg is then placed in a dependent position, and the examiner observes for the development of rubor (a purple-red discoloration of the lower limb that is thought to be caused by pooling of the blood within the chronically dilated arterioles). Pallor occurring within 25 seconds of elevation generally indicates severe occlusive disease, as does dependent rubor. Pallor usually develops within 30 seconds in the patient with moderately severe occlusive disease and within 45 to 60 seconds in the patient with mild disease (Cantwell-Gab, 1996; Rockson and Cooke, 1998).

Venous filling time. To conduct this test, the examiner elevates the limb to provide for venous drainage and then places the leg in a dependent position. The amount of time (in seconds) required for venous filling is then recorded. Prolonged venous filling time is independently predictive of PAD. A filling time of more than 20 seconds usually indicates fairly severe occlusive disease (McGee and Boyko, 1998; Rockson and Cooke, 1998).

Auscultation for bruits. All major pulses should be auscultated for evidence of bruits, which may be an indication of occlusion (Cantwell-Gab, 1996; McGee and Boyko, 1998).

Palpation of pulses. Pulses should be compared with the contralateral pulse and should be assessed in a proximal-to-distal approach (Figure 12-1). Diminished or absent pedal pulses are independently predictive of PAD; however, both the dorsalis pedis and the posterior tibialis pulses must be evaluated before documenting significantly diminished or absent pedal pulses. Palpation of a normal pulse at either location is considered indicative of normal pedal pulses. The absence of *both* a normal dorsalis pedis pulse *and* a normal posterior tibialis pulse is evidence of PAD (McGee and Boyko, 1998; Rockson and Cooke, 1998). A handheld Doppler probe should be used to auscultate when both pulses are nonpalpable, and findings should be documented. A Doppler probe that generates the correct frequency (in megahertz, or MHz) for assessment of skin level vessels is an 8 to 10 MHz probe (Cantwell-Gab, 1996).

Capillary refill. Capillary refill is measured by pressing against the toe pad firmly to empty the surface vessels and then monitoring the time required for the tissue to regain normal color. Normal "refill" time is considered to be less than 3 seconds. However the patient with PAD may have normal capillary refill because the emptied vessels may refill in a retrograde manner from surrounding veins even if arterial inflow is markedly impaired or absent (Cantwell-Gab, 1996; McGee and Boyko, 1998).

Palpation of skin temperature. Skin temperature of one extremity should be compared with that of the contralateral limb by palpating lightly with the palmar surface of the fingers and hands, moving from proximal to distal and comparing right leg with left leg and right foot with left foot. Significant findings include unilateral coolness, which has been found to have positive positive predictive value, and a sudden marked change from proximal to distal (Cantwell-Gab, 1996; McGee and Boyko, 1998).

Ankle-brachial index. The ankle-brachial index (ABI), also known as the *ankle-arm index*, is a simple bedside comparison of perfusion pressures in the lower leg with those in the upper arm (Figure 12-2). This noninvasive test is used to screen patients for evidence of significant arterial insufficiency and to identify patients who require further workup. The procedure for conducting an ABI is outlined in Box 12-5. Table 12-3 provides guidelines for interpretation of ABI results. ABI measurements provide only an indirect measure of peripheral perfusion and cannot be considered accurate in patients with noncompressible vessels (e.g., the diabetic patient with vessel calcification). Therefore diabetic patients who have clinical evidence of ischemia but normal or elevated ABI measurements should be referred for more definitive testing (Rockson and Cooke, 1998).

An alternative to the ABI is the toe-brachial index (TBI), also known as the *toe-arm index*. Toe pressures are generally more accurate in the presence of vessel calcification because these vessels are much less likely to be calcified. This procedure is performed in exactly the same manner as the ABI test, except a toe cuff is placed around the great toe and the Doppler probe is placed against the distal toe surface to monitor the pulse signal. A normal TBI value is >0.6 (Rockson and Cooke, 1998).

Ulcer characteristics. The physical examination must include a comprehensive assessment of any ulcers (assessment is discussed in Chapter 4).

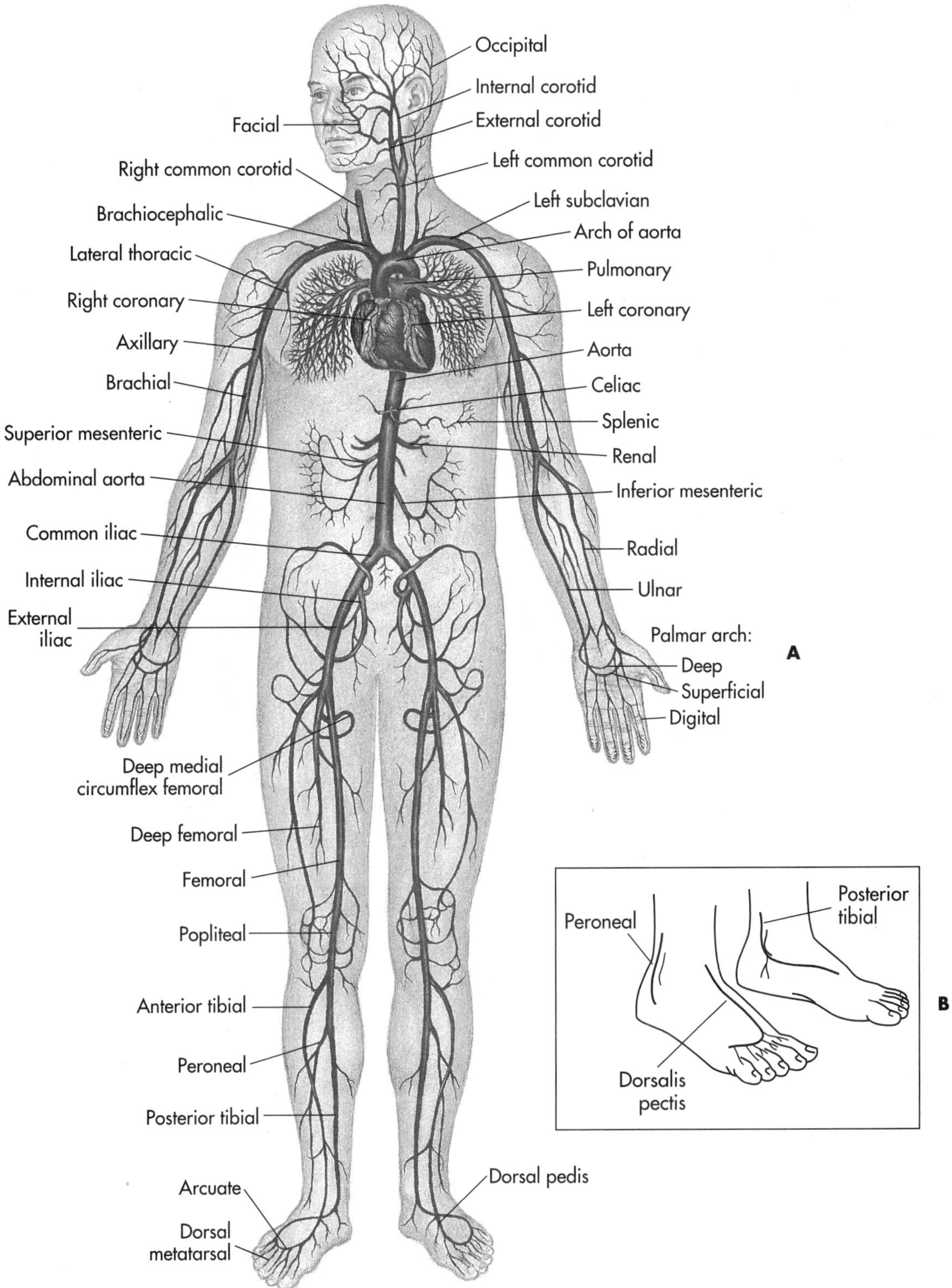

Figure 12-1 A, Arterial structure of lower extremity. Note location of peroneal artery, posterior tibialis, and dorsalis pedis. B, Note location of peroneal artery, posterior tibialis, and dorsalis pedis. (**A** from Seidel HM et al: *Mosby's guide to physical examination*, ed 4, St Louis, 1999, Mosby.)

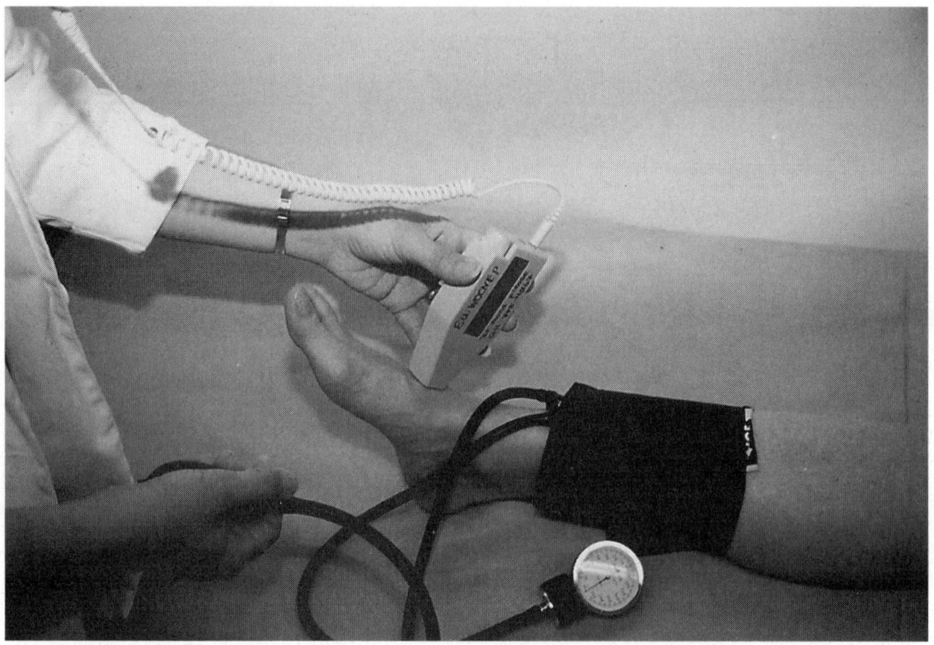

Figure 12-2 A handheld Doppler probe being used to obtain an ankle-brachial index.

Classic arterial ulcer characteristics are listed in Box 12-6 (see also Plates 19 and 21). It is particularly important to determine the presence of any sinus tracts or undermined areas, which are common in the diabetic patient with foot ulcers. The nurse must also assess for signs of infection, which is common but frequently manifest only by very subtle signs (caused by the attenuated vascular response) (Rockson and Cooke, 1998). Finally, the nurse must assess verbal and nonverbal indicators of pain. Because these lesions are typically quite painful, topical and oral analgesics are frequently required before wound care.

Vascular Studies. Vascular studies may be warranted to further assess adequacy of perfusion and consists of noninvasive and invasive studies. Noninvasive studies include pulse volume recordings, segmental pressure analysis, transcutaneous oxygen measurements, and color-flow duplex imaging (Gahtan, 1998; Rockson and Cooke, 1998).

Pulse volume recordings. A pulse volume recording provides an accurate reflection of actual perfusion volume. This test is typically performed using a machine with pneumatic cuffs. The cuff is inflated to a preset level, and the machine provides a tracing that reflects the change in blood volume occurring within that limb segment over the course of the cardiac cycle. A similar tracing may be obtained using a Doppler probe that records the change in blood volume and is commonly referred to as a *Doppler waveform.* Pulse volume recordings and Doppler waveform studies of normal vessels are described as *triphasic* (Figure 12-3, *A*). They clearly demonstrate a systolic peak, a dicrotic notch representing blood flow reversal during early diastole, and a diastolic wave. With moderately severe occlusive disease, the waveform becomes monophasic (Figure 12-3, *B*), and with advanced disease the waveform is severely blunted (Figure 12-3, *C*) (Gahtan, 1998; Rockson and Cooke, 1998).

Segmental pressure recordings. These recordings are used to determine the level of occlusion. Cuffs are placed at thigh level, below the knee, and just above the ankle. A Doppler probe is used to lo-

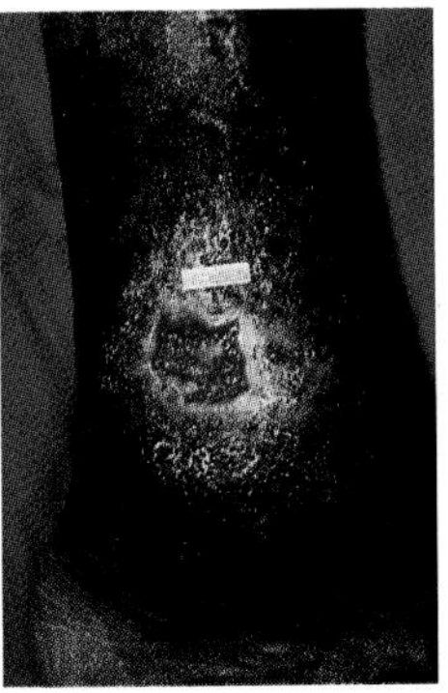

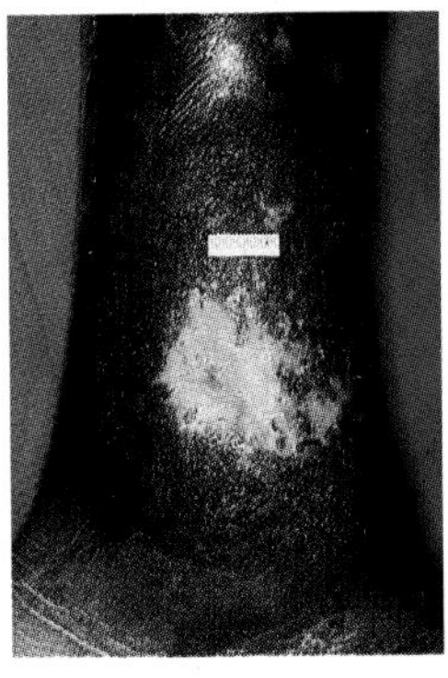

Plate 1 Partial-thickness venous ulcer healing by epithelialization. Resurfaced venous ulcer lacks normal dark pigmentation because of depth of damage (below basement membrane).

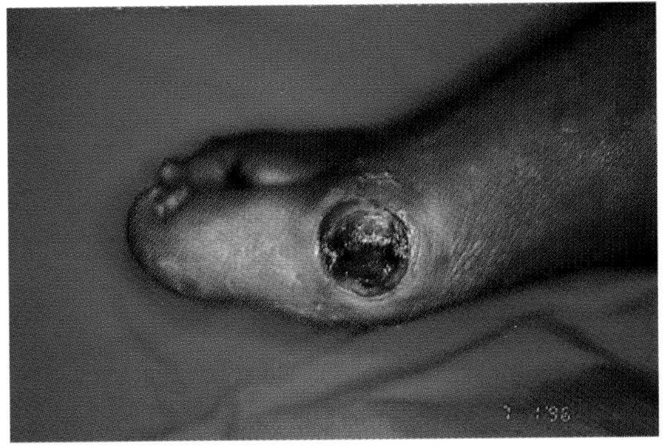

Plate 2 Full-thickness tissue destruction over bunion on patient with diabetes.

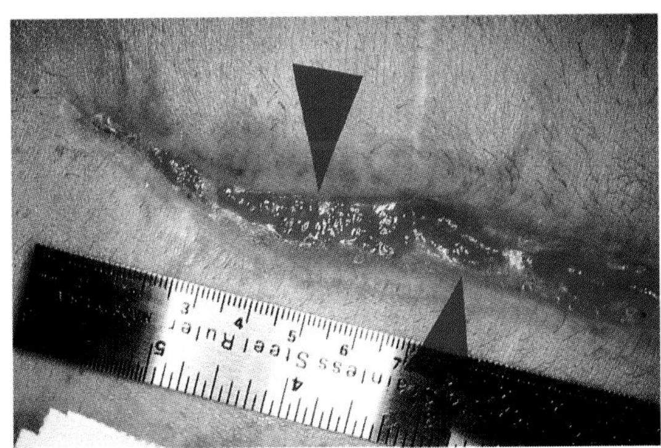

Plate 3 Surgical incision with epithelialization and healing ridge present.

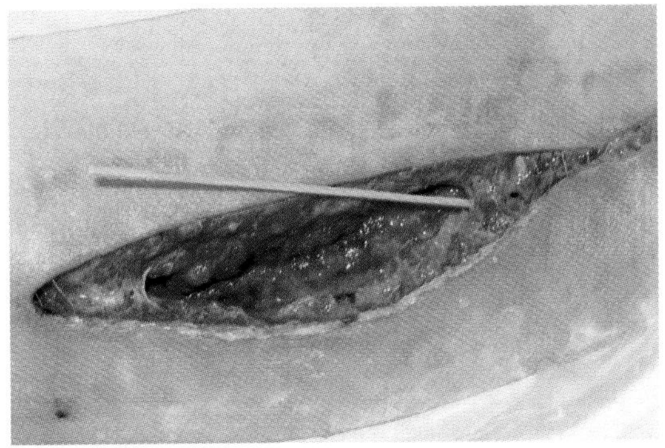

Plate 4 Dehisced surgical incision that has tunneling present. Wound bed does not provide any indication of healing; wound edges are not attached along left lateral aspect.

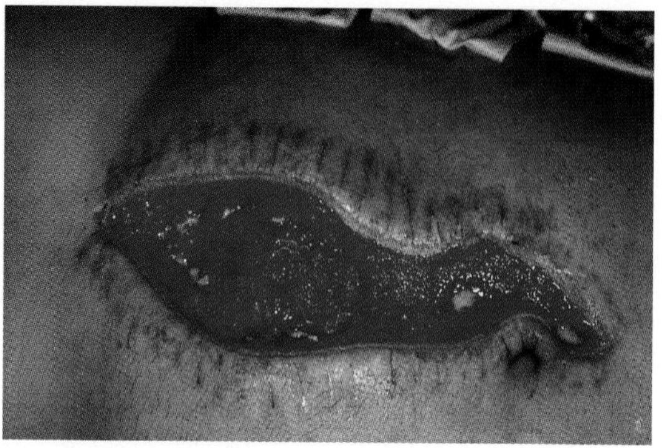

Plate 5 Abdominal wound with beefy red granulation tissue present and attached wound edges.

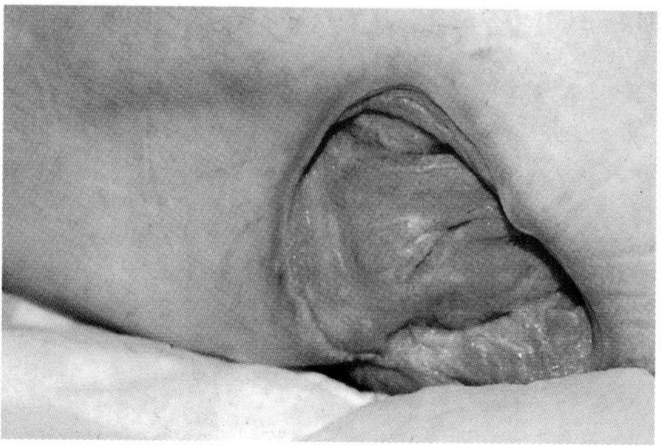

Plate 6 Stage 4 pressure ulcer with pale wound bed.

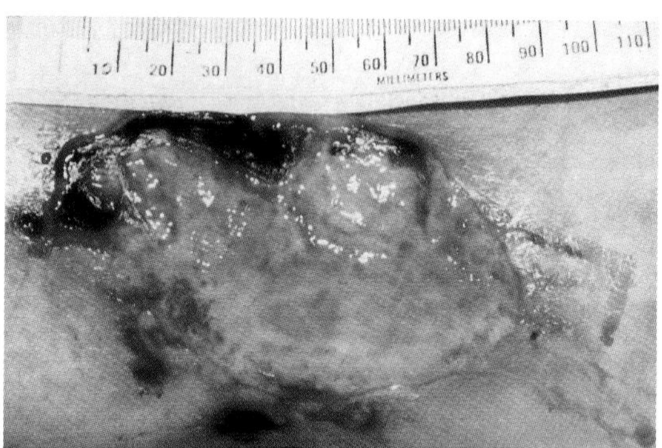

Plate 7 Highly exudative venous ulcer with slough present in wound bed and eschar present along superior aspect.

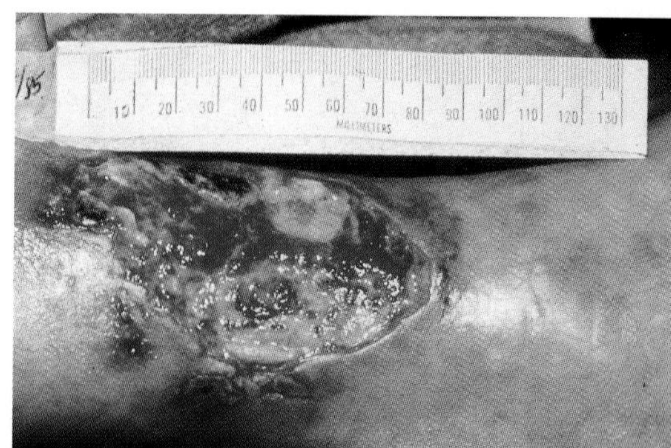

Plate 8 After 1 week of hydrocolloids and compression therapy, autolysis has occurred and venous ulcer has granulation tissue present. Amount of slough and eschar is reduced; remaining eschar is softened.

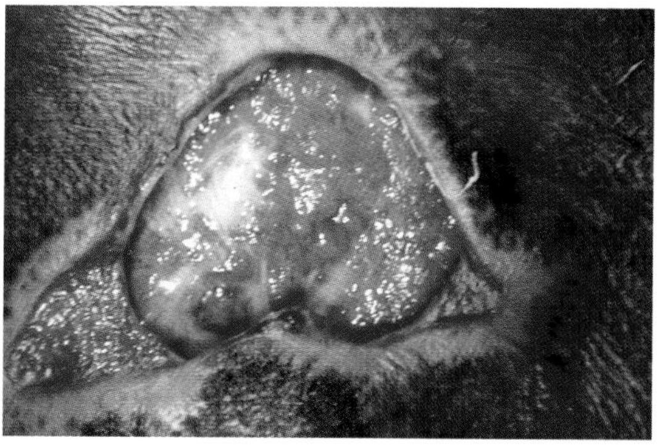

Plate 9 Pressure ulcer with predominantly clean granular wound base. However, epibole (closed wound edges) is present along inferior aspect, which is an impediment to wound closure.

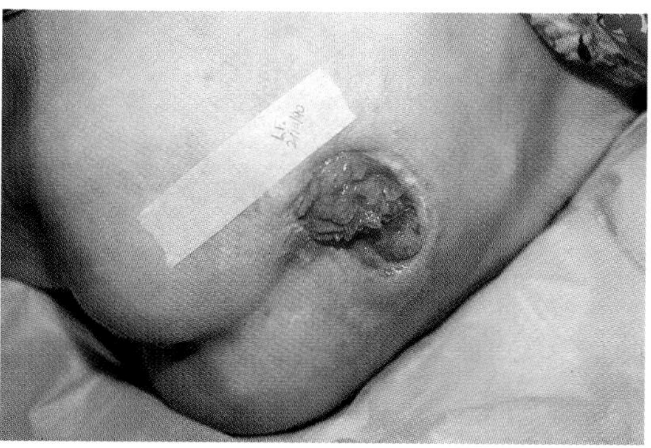

Plate 10 Healing stage 3 pressure ulcer with hyperplasia present in wound bed.

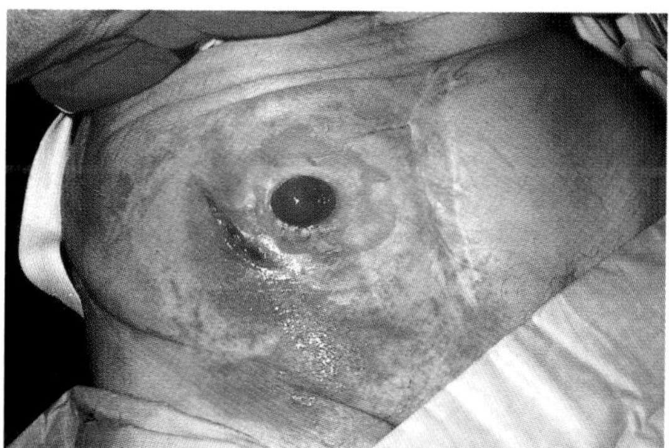

Plate 11 Patient with an ileostomy and incision placed to drain peristomal abscess. Chemical dermatitis present along inferior aspect of incision because of inadequate protection of skin from drainage. Candidiasis also present as indicated by satellite papular lesions and solid plaque-like rash advancing into groin and over suprapubic area.

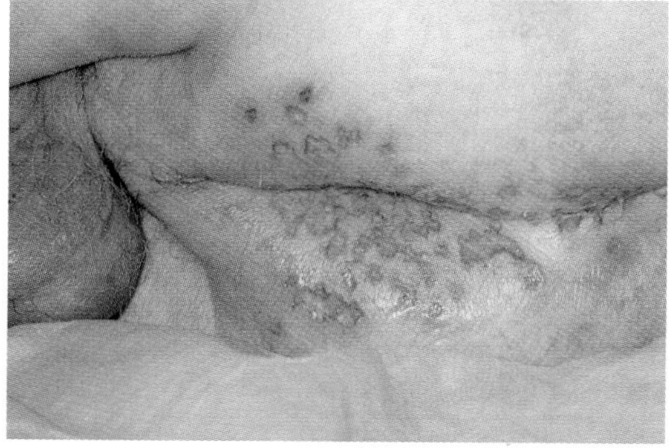

Plate 12 Herpes simples on buttocks. Note cluster of vesicles on erythematous base.

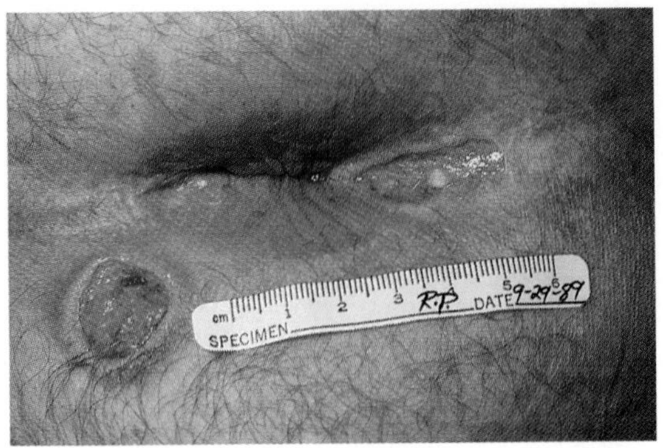

Plate 13 Perianal herpes simplex ulcers.

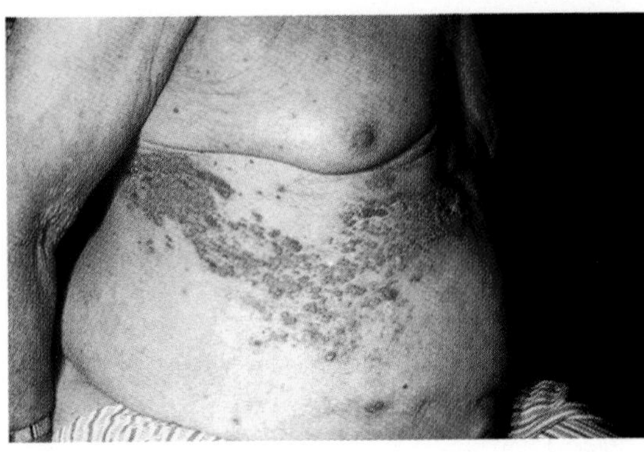

Plate 14 Herpes zoster involving simple thoracic dermatome. Vesicles are cluster and erythematous.

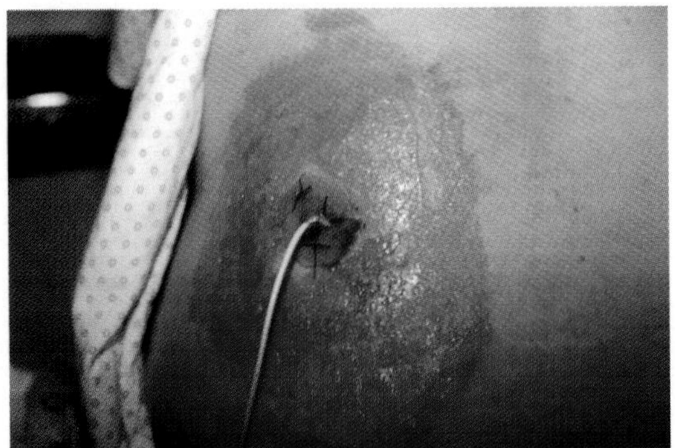

Plate 15 Moist desquamation after an allergic reaction in response to the second application of benzoin to a percutaneous nephrostomy site.

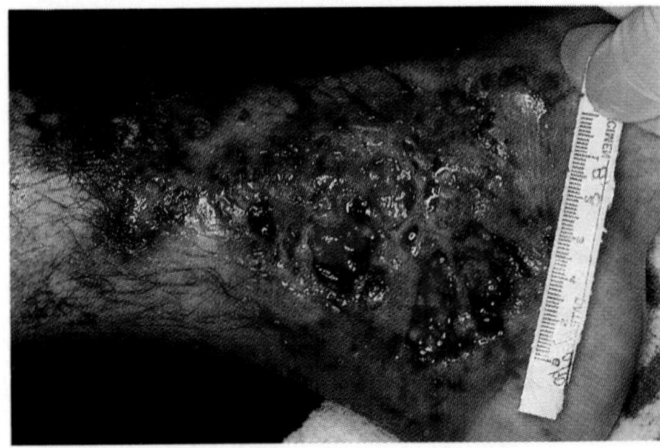

Plate 16 Classical ulceration form of pyoderma gangrenosum. Note violaceous color of skin surrounding ulcerations.

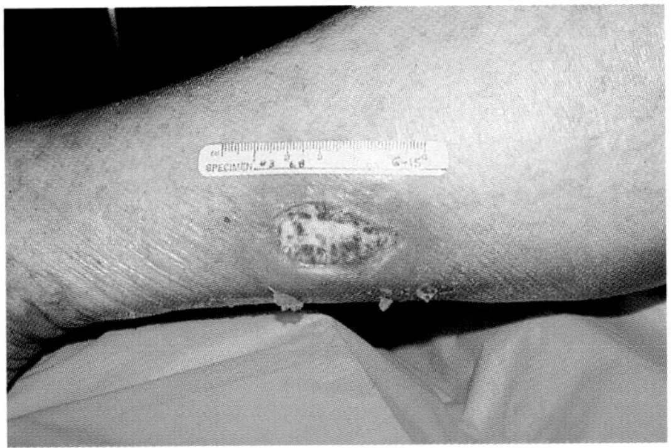

Plate 17 Vasculitic ulcer that developed in patient with rheumatoid arthritis. Wound bed has attached dry slough present, and surrounding skin is slightly erythematous.

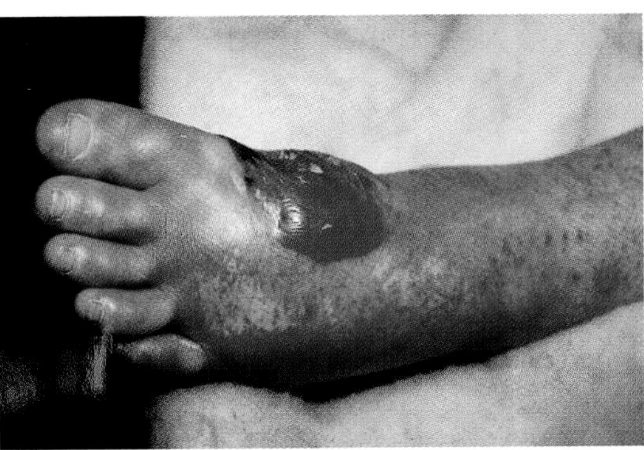

Plate 18 Graft-versus-host disease (GVHD) in patient after allogeneic bone marrow transplantation. Edema, erythema, and bulla formation are present.

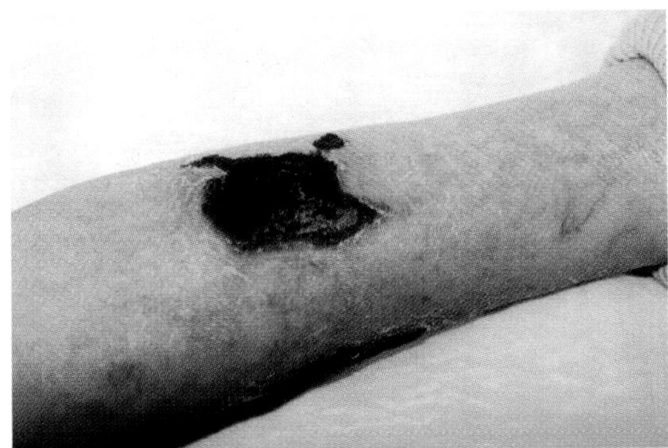

Plate 19 Arterial ulcer with dry stable eschar covering. Note dry condition of leg.

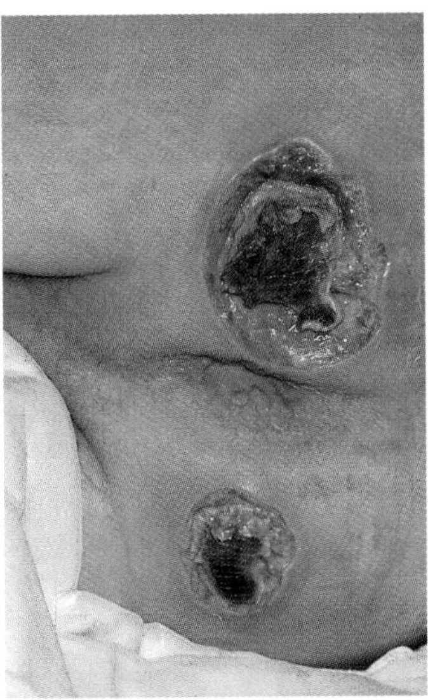

Plate 20 Bilateral ischial tuberosity pressure ulcers with eschar detaching from wound edges and softening in response to topical hydrogels. Cross hatching of eschar was initially performed and is visible in necrotic tissue.

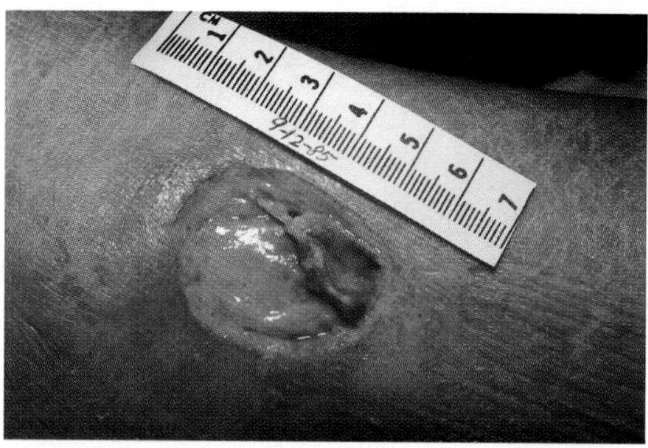

Plate 21 Arterial ulcer with loose and adherent yellow slough present in wound bed. Mild erythema present along left lateral edge.

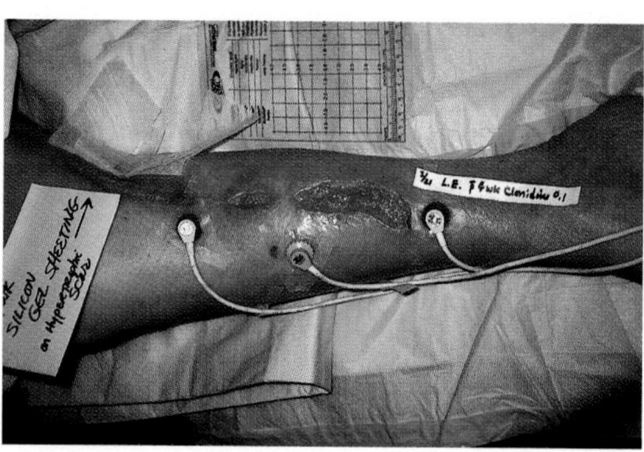

Plate 22 Technique of obtaining $TcPo_2$ in lower leg wounds.

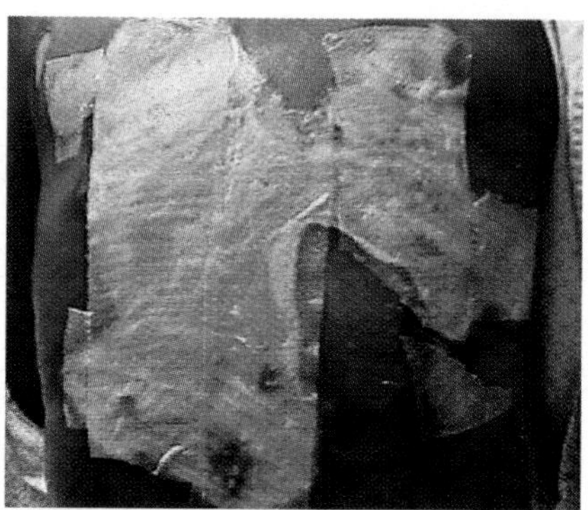

Plate 23 Patient suffered second- and third-degree burns to his back from an oven explosion while trying to heat his home. After debridement the patient was a poor candidate for a successful STSg because of severe malnutrition, so a biosynthetic porcine heterograft (EZ-Derm [Brennen Medical, Inc.]) was applied and an Exu-Dry vest (T.J. Smith and Nephew, Ltd.) was used as cover dressing. The Exu-Dry vest was changed every 4 to 6 days and prn. Pain was relieved, and the patient was able to eat. (Courtesy Ted Tomter, RN, CWOCN, St. Joseph's Candler Health System, Savannah, Ga.)

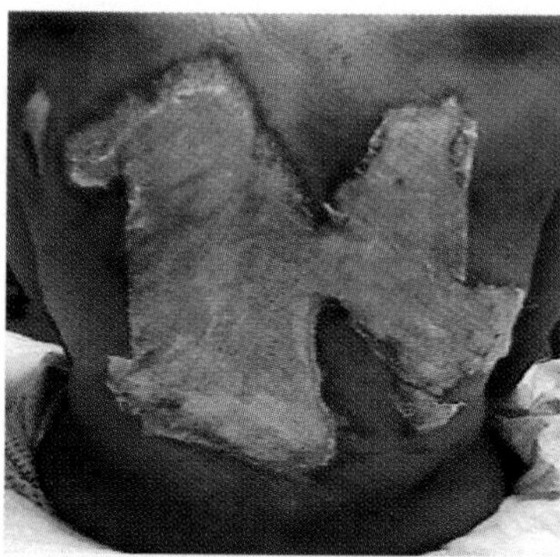

Plate 24 Fourteen days after a porcine skin heterograft, the burn area has decreased in size by 20% and epithelialization is apparent around the wound edges. The heterograft is pulling away from the edges of the wound and becoming desiccated. With improved nutritional status, the wound bed is now appropriate for autologous STSg 15 days after the original debridement. Seven days after STSg, the patient had 100% take of STSg. (Courtesy Ted Tomter, RN, CWOCN, St. Joseph's Candler Health System, Savannah, Ga.)

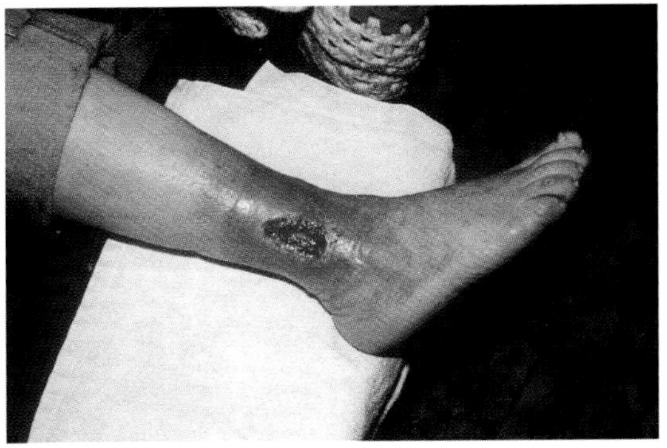

Plate 25 Typical appearance and location of venous ulcer. Surrounding skin has been moisturized to eliminate usual dry skin. Note hemosiderin staining of surrounding skin and ruddy red color of wound bed.

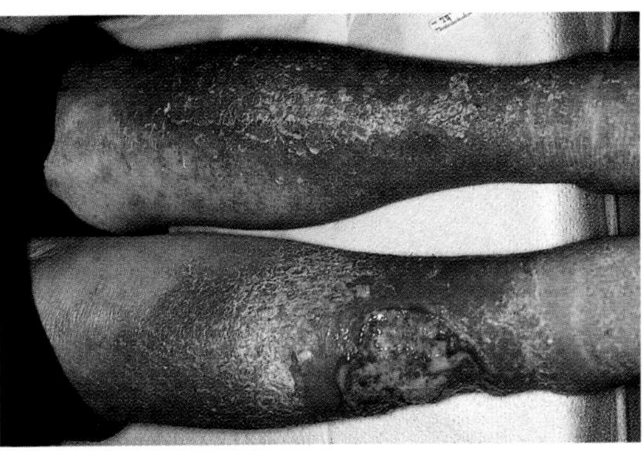

Plate 26 Venous dermatitis of lower leg. Note extensive hemosiderin staining and lipodermatosclerosis.

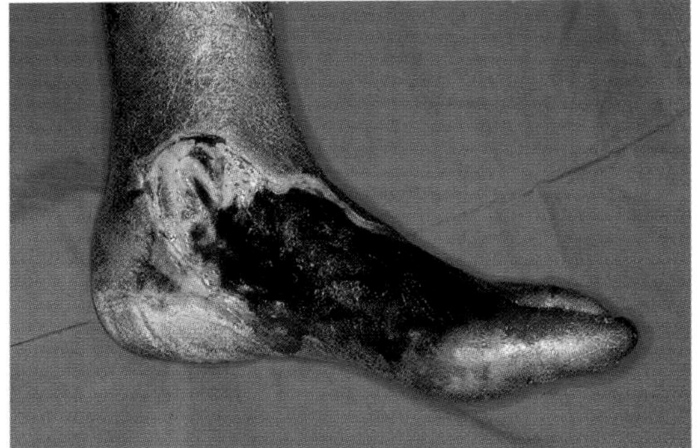

Plate 27 Skin damage as a result of thermal injury in neuropathic foot.

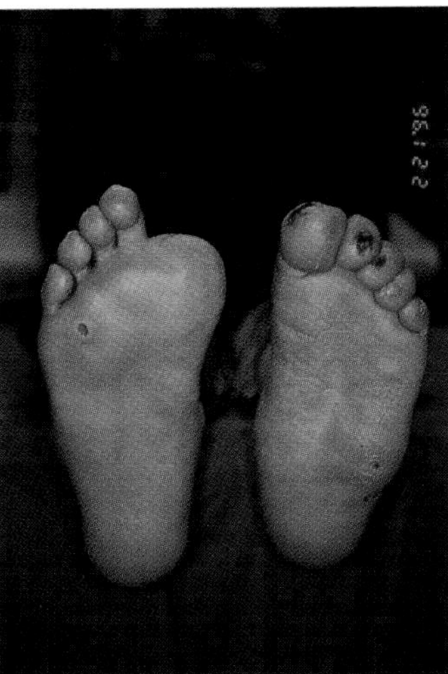

Plate 28 Neuropathic foot with claw toes on right foot and ulcers present on tips of claw toes. Note deformation of lateral plantar surface of the patient's left foot and amputated toe on the patient's right foot.

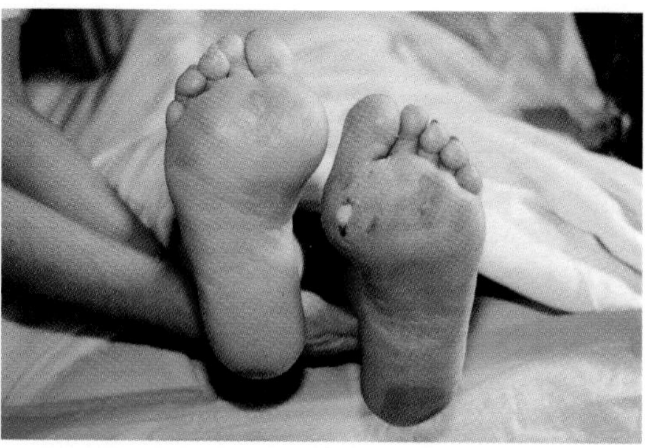

Plate 29 Neuropathic plantar ulcer on first metatarsal head after conservative debridement (packing is present in the ulcer). Note foot and toe deformities and callus formation in this patient with diabetes mellitus. Stage 2 pressure ulcers (blisters) are also present on both heels.

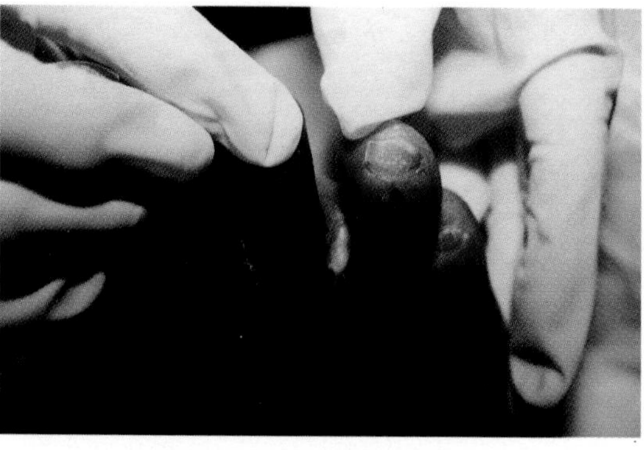

Plate 30 Insignificant-appearing interdigital ulcer in patient with diabetes, peripheral neuropathy, and peripheral vascular disease.

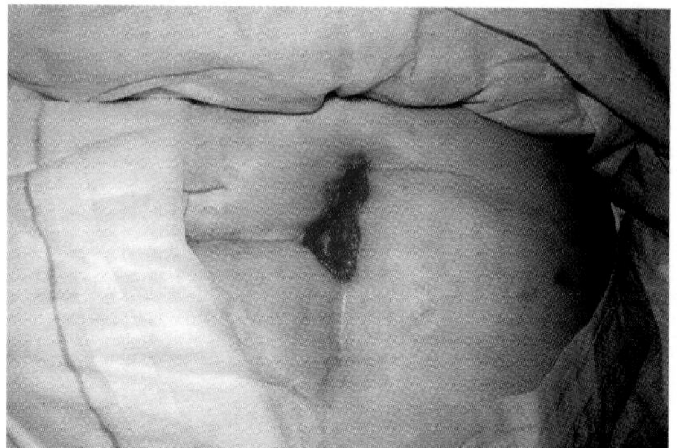

Plate 31 Patient with enterocutaneous fistula with irregular surrounding skin surfaces and depression along fistula-skin junction at inferior aspect and upper left aspect.

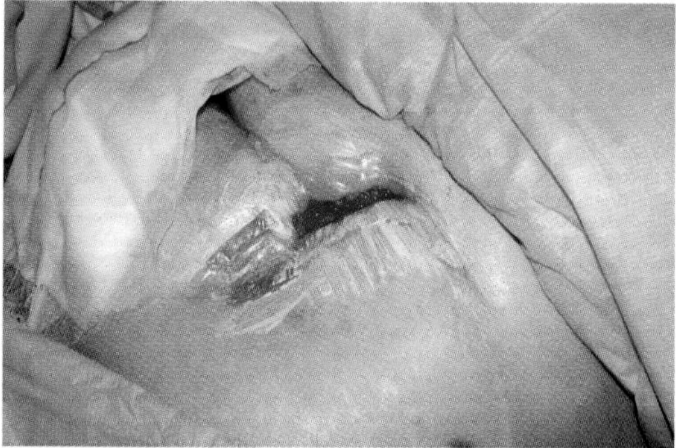

Plate 32 Tapered layers of sold-wafer skin barrier used to help level skin depression at inferior aspect. Skin-barrier paste has been applied to surrounding wound margins and in all three depression (over skin-barrier wafer wedges) to level and protect the skin from effluent. Cement has been painted onto adhesive field (over paste and wedges) to increase adhesion.

BOX 12-5 Procedure for Performing an Ankle-Brachial Index (ABI)

1. Place patient in a supine position for 5 to 15 minutes before the test.
2. Obtain the brachial pressure in *each* arm using standard technique. Record the highest brachial pressure.
3. Place an appropriately sized cuff around the affected lower leg just above the ankle.
4. Apply acoustic gel over the pedal pulse location.
5. Hold the Doppler probe (preferably at a 45-degree angle) touching the skin over the pedal pulse location very lightly.
6. Inflate the cuff to a level 20 to 30 mm Hg higher than the brachial systolic pressure.
7. Slowly deflate the cuff while monitoring for the return of the pulse signal. The point at which the arterial signal returns is recorded as the ankle pressure.
8. Repeat this procedure to obtain the ankle pressure over the other pedal pulse on the affected extremity. The higher of the two values is used to determine the ABI.
9. Calculate the ABI by dividing the higher of the two brachial pressures by the higher of the two pedal pressures on the involved extremity. If only one pedal pressure could be obtained, then that value is used.

calize the most distal pulses (dorsalis pedis and posterior tibialis), and the ankle cuff is inflated until the arterial signal is obliterated. The cuff is then deflated until the arterial signal is again audible. The pressure at which the signal is heard is recorded as the ankle systolic pressure. The procedure is then repeated with inflation of the "below-the-knee" cuff and then with the thigh cuff. Each pressure is then compared with the adjacent pressure. Differences of >20 mm Hg indicate an occlusive lesion located between the two involved cuffs (Gahtan, 1998).

Transcutaneous oxygen pressure measurements ($TcPo_2$). $TcPo_2$ measurements provide information about the adequacy of oxygen delivery to the skin and underlying tissues (see Chapter 9). Values above 40 mm Hg generally indicate sufficient oxygen to support wound repair, values between 20 and 40 mm Hg are considered equivocal in terms of wound healing, and values below 20 mm Hg generally indicate marked ischemia and the inability to heal (Moon, 1998).

Color duplex imaging (CDI). By combining real-time B-mode imaging and Doppler waveform, CDI provides both an anatomic and functional analysis of the arteries in the lower extremities. Data provided include the vessels' structural anatomy (e.g., plaque or thrombus accumulation and any areas of stenosis) and the direction, velocity, and turbulence of blood flow. CDI is a noninvasive alternative to arteriography and can often

TABLE 12-3 Interpretation of Ankle-Brachial Index (ABI) Results

ABI VALUE	INTERPRETATION/CLINICAL SIGNIFICANCE
0.95–1.3	"Normal" range
0.5 to 0.95	Mild to moderate peripheral arterial disease: 0.5 to 0.8 Associated with intermittent claudication Ability to heal wound usually maintained
<0.5	Severe arterial insufficiency; wound healing unlikely unless revascularization can be done.
>1.3	Abnormally high range, typically because of calcification of the vessel wall in the diabetic. Renders ABI test invalid as measure of peripheral perfusion.

Data from Cantwell-Gab K: Identifying chronic peripheral arterial disease, *Am J Nurs* 96(7):40, 1996; McGee S, Boyko D: Physical examination and chronic lower-extremity ischemia: a critical review, *Arch Intern Med* 158(12):1357, 1998; Rockson S, Cooke J: Peripheral arterial insufficiency: mechanisms, natural history, and therapeutic options, *Adv Intern Med* 43: 253, 1998.

BOX 12-6 Classic Characteristics of Arterial Ulcers

Location. Distal aspect of extremity (e.g., tips of the toes), on pressure points of the foot (e.g., heel or lateral foot), and in an area of trauma

Wound size and shape. Relatively small craters; well-defined borders

Wound bed. Pale or necrotic

Volume of exudate. Minimal exudate because of the diminished blood flow to the area

Appearance of surrounding skin. Faint halo of erythema or slight fluctuance suggests infection

Pain. Can be cramping or constant deep aching pain

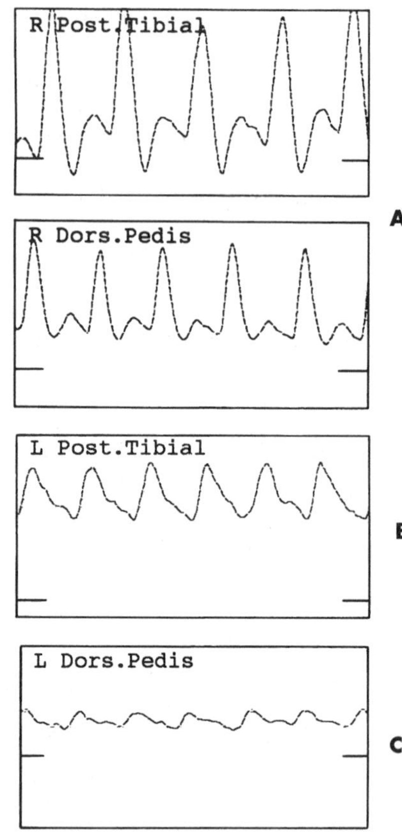

Figure 12-3 A, Normal Doppler waveforms from normal vessels (right posterior tibialis and right dosalis pedis). Signal is triphasic showing systolic peak, dicrotic notch representing blood flow reversal during early diastole, and a diastolic wave. B, Doppler waveform study of vessel with moderately severe occlusive disease as evidenced by a monophasic waveform. C, Doppler waveform study of vessel with advanced occlusive disease. Note that waveform is severely blunted.

safely replace the arteriogram (Aly et al, 1998; Gahtan, 1998).

Arteriography. Arteriography has been the gold standard in assessment of PAD; however, the arteriogram is an invasive procedure that provides anatomic data only and is therefore restricted to patients in whom surgical intervention is planned (Aly et al, 1998; Goldstein et al, 1998).

Management of the Patient with Arterial Ulceration

Correct the Cause: Measures to Improve Perfusion. The prognosis for wound healing is directly correlated with the patient's ability to deliver sufficient volumes of oxygen and nutrients to support the repair process. Therefore the first priority in management is correction of the underlying ischemia. Perfusion and tissue oxygenation can be improved via surgical techniques, pharmacologic agents, lifestyle changes, and the administration of hyperbaric oxygen therapy. The specific interventions selected for the individual patient are determined by the severity of the ischemia, the patient's overall medical status and prognosis for healing, and the patient's preferences and priorities.

Surgical options. The patient with an arterial ulcer and an ABI of <0.5 is very unlikely to heal without surgical revascularization; therefore if the overall goal of care for the patient is wound healing, the patient should be immediately referred for vascular evaluation. Surgical intervention should also be considered for patients with an ABI of >0.5 who are surgical candidates and who fail to respond to pharmacologic and behavioral therapy. Surgical intervention is generally an option as long as preoperative imaging studies demonstrate patent distal vessels. Options include bypass grafting, angioplasty, and placement of stents (Cantwell-Gab, 1996; Cragg and Dake, 1997; Golledge, 1997; Hilleman, 1998; Rockson and Cooke, 1998).

1. *Bypass grafts* are most commonly constructed using the patient's saphenous vein. If the saphenous veins are damaged, an upper extremity vein may be harvested or a synthetic graft may be used (Figure 12-4) (Cantwell-Gab, 1996; Levin, 1996).
2. *Angioplasty* has frequently been advocated as a simpler and less invasive approach to revascularization than bypass grafting. However, angioplasty is not a good option for widespread or extensive occlusive disease or for occlusive lesions >10 cm in length and may not be feasible in smaller vessels. Approximately one third of patients with severe ischemic disease of the lower leg are candidates for angioplasty, and initial results are generally good. Long-term patency rates have been disappointing but can be improved by long-term administration of anticoagulants or antiplatelet agents or by placement of expendable metallic endovascular stents into the stenotic area immediately after angioplasty (Cantwell-Gab, 1996; Cragg and Dake, 1997; Golledge, 1997; Hilleman, 1998).

Amputation is reserved as the "treatment of last resort" and is indicated primarily for patients with irreversible ischemia (i.e., tissue necrosis) and invasive infection (Golledge, 1997; Levin, 1996).

Hyperbaric oxygen therapy. Hyperbaric oxygen therapy increases the amount of oxygen dissolved in the plasma, which results in the delivery of "oxygen-enriched" blood to the tissues. It can be of particular benefit to the patient with an arterial ulcer since oxygen delivery is no longer dependent upon the ability of the red blood cell to traverse the narrowed vessels (Moon, 1998; Stone and Cianci, 1997). Hyperbaric oxygen therapy is discussed in detail in Chapter 20.

Pharmacologic options. The mainstays of pharmacologic therapy for patients with PAD include medications to reduce the risk of thrombotic events (anticoagulants and antiplatelet agents), hemorrheologic agents, and analgesics.

Antithrombotic agents. Antithrombotic agents work primarily by reducing platelet aggregation. The most commonly used antiplatelet agent is low- to medium-dose aspirin (60 to 325 mg/day). Newer antiplatelet drugs include ticlopidine and clopidrogel, which inhibit platelet activation by antagonizing specific receptors (Cooke and Ma, 1995; McNamara, Champion, and Kadowitz, 1998; Rockson and Cooke, 1998).

Hemorrheologics. Specific effects of hemorrheologic agents include reduced concentrations of fibrinogen, which reduces blood viscosity, and reduced rigidity and aggregation of red blood cells, which improves their deformability and ability to pass through narrow vessels. Unfortunately, pentoxifylline (the agent currently approved by the FDA for PAD) has only minimal to moderate beneficial effects in clinical practice, complicated by a fairly high incidence of gastrointestinal side effects. Pentoxifylline should be given for 8 to 12 weeks at a dose of 400 mg tid (with meals) and then evaluated for objective and subjective evidence of improvement. Failure to demonstrate improvement should result in discontinuation (Cooke and Ma, 1995; Rockson and Cooke, 1998).

Analgesics. Opioid analgesics may be required for patients with advanced ischemia to relieve the chronic pain and thus improve quality of life. Pain control also prevents vasoconstriction caused by sympathetic stimulation (Golledge, 1997; Rockson and Cooke, 1998). Systemic vasodilators are generally contraindicated for patients with PAD because the resulting vasodilatation may divert blood from the affected area (McNamara, Champion, and Kadowitz, 1998; Rockson and Cooke, 1998).

Investigational agents. The pharmacologic agents discussed previously have limited ability to improve perfusion and no ability to induce new vessel growth. Therefore they are of limited benefit to patients with advanced ischemic disease and ulceration. Fortunately, there are several investigational agents and procedures (antioxidants, prostaglandin derivatives, selective vasodilators, metabolic agents, and gene transfer therapy) that may prove beneficial in halting and/or reversing the atherosclerotic process, inducing selective vasodilatation, improving oxygen use by ischemic tissues, and promoting growth of new vessels. Clinically, these benefits are manifest by reducing rest pain and promoting ulcer healing (Baumgartner et al, 1998; Capecchi et al, 1997; Cooke and Ma, 1995; McNamara, Champion, and Kadowitz, 1998; Rockson and Cooke, 1998).

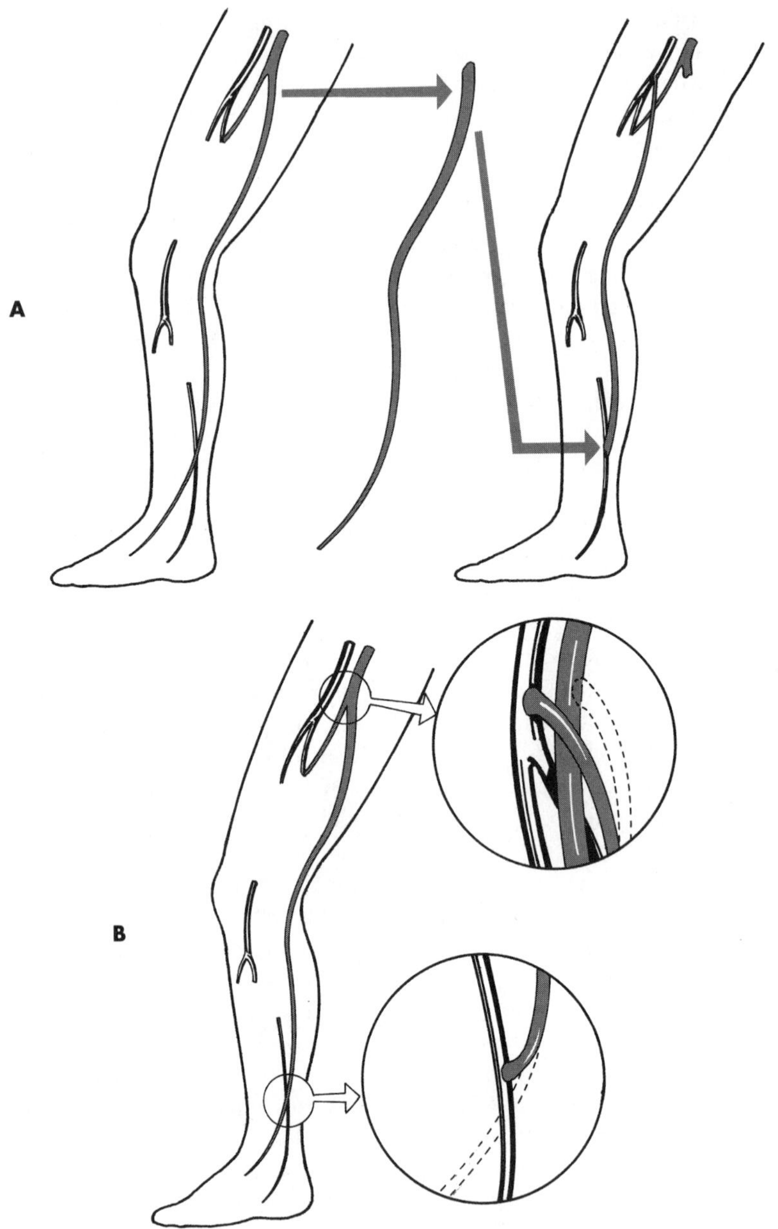

Figure 12-4 Illustration of bypass grafts using an autologous saphenous vein (A) (reversed saphenous vein procedure) and in-situ procedure (B).

Behavioral strategies. Currently, the ability to improve tissue perfusion and to promote wound healing depends on the patient's willingness to make appropriate lifestyle changes. Specifically, the patient must be counseled regarding strategies to modify correctable risk factors (Boxes 12-7 and 12-8), improve tissue perfusion (Box 12-9), and protect the compromised limb (Box 12-10) (Levin, 1996; Rockson and Cooke, 1998). Lifestyle changes may be more difficult for the patient than either a

BOX 12-7 Goals and Strategies for PAD

Goals

- Normalize blood pressure
- Normalize blood glucose levels
- Normalize serum cholesterol levels
- Eliminate tobacco use

Strategies

- Intensify patient education
- Regularly monitor physiologic and laboratory indices
- Aggressively modify the treatment plan to achieve and maintain as "near normal" a state as possible.

BOX 12-8 Interventions to Promote Cessation of Tobacco Use

1. General education concerning the negative effects of tobacco use on health status
2. Specific and consistent advice to eliminate tobacco use from health care team
3. Establishment of patient-provider contracts in which the patient commits to a date on which he or she will eliminate tobacco use
4. Anticipatory guidance (e.g., counseling to help the patient identify triggers for tobacco use and specific strategies for managing triggering events and situations)
5. General stress management and support
6. Appropriate use of adequate doses of nicotine replacement agents (nicotine replacement therapy)
7. Frequent follow-up during the critical weeks after initial termination of tobacco use (either by phone or by office visit)
8. Appropriate counseling after any relapse on recognition that most individuals who successfully stop smoking have one to four relapses

BOX 12-9 Measures to Improve Tissue Perfusion

- Maintenance of hydration (to reduce blood viscosity)
- Avoidance of cold, caffeine, and constrictive garments (to reduce vasoconstriction)
- Weight control (to reduce the workload of the ischemic limb)
- Planned graduated walking program (to improve tissue perfusion and oxygen use)

surgical procedure or drug therapy. Effective introduction of such changes requires in-depth education and supportive, goal-directed patient counseling (Cooke and Ma, 1995; Hilleman, 1998; Rockson and Cooke, 1998; Terry, Berkowitz, and Kerstein, 1998).

The patient should be informed of the benefits of a walking program (Box 12-11) and given a specific "walking prescription." The guidelines for therapeutic walking in the patient with PAD usually address frequency, duration, and rate. A typical walking program involves 30 to 60 minutes of walking 4 to 5 days a week at a rate of 2 miles per hour (Altemose and Wiener, 1998; Cooke and Ma, 1995; Rockson and Cooke, 1998).

Few data are available regarding the effects of graduated walking programs in the patient with critical limb ischemia, and it may have a negative effect on wound repair (Cooke and Ma, 1995; Rockson and Cooke, 1998).

Topical Therapy. Topical therapy of arterial ulcers is based on the principles outlined in Chapter 5, including debridement, identification and elimination of infection, filling of dead space, absorption of excess exudate, maintenance of a moist wound surface, protection from bacterial invasion, protection from mechanical trauma, and insulation. Three issues, however, are unique to the management of ulcers complicated by ischemia: management of a noninfected dry necrotic wound, identification and management of infection, and the use of occlusive dressings.

One aspect of wound management that is different for the ischemic wound is the recommended approach for a dry, noninfected necrotic wound. Although necrotic tissue is clearly a potential medium for bacterial growth, a dry intact eschar can also serve as a bacterial barrier. A closed wound

BOX 12-10 Limb Preservation Strategies

Routine Skin Care
- Application of emollients after bathing to prevent cracking and fissures
- Careful drying between toes to prevent maceration
- Use of lamb's wool or foam toe "sleeves" to prevent interdigital friction and pressure

Measures to Prevent Mechanical Trauma
- Avoidance of "barefoot" walking, even indoors, including consistent use of protective footwear (e.g., closed-toe shoes) to prevent inadvertent cuts or puncture wounds
- Inspection of shoes before wearing
- Careful fitting of shoes to prevent pressure, friction, or shear injuries
- If indicated, use of protective shin guards when working around house or yard
- Professional foot and nail care (or self-care of nails limited to conservative trimming and filing); no "bathroom surgery"

Measures to Prevent Thermal Trauma
- Warm socks to be worn during cold weather to prevent vasoconstriction
- No use of hot water bottles, heating pads, or other thermal devices
- Hand or elbow checks of water temperature before bathing

Measures to Prevent Chemical Trauma
- No use of antiseptic or chemical agents such as corn removers

General Measures
- Daily inspection of feet and legs
- Prompt reporting of any minor injuries

BOX 12-11 Benefits of a Planned Graduated Walking Program

Physiologic Benefits
- Adaptive changes within ischemic tissues, resulting in improved oxygen use at the cellular level (increased cellular levels of oxidative enzymes and L-carnitine)
- Enhanced workload tolerance
- Reduced blood viscosity
- Promotion of weight loss
- Reduction of blood pressure
- General stress reduction
- Improved gait efficiency

Clinical Benefits
- Improved exercise tolerance
- Reduced pain

BOX 12-12 Protocol for Topical Therapy in Dry, Necrotic, Uninfected Arterial Wound

- Inspect for subtle indicators of infection. If any signs or symptoms of infection develop, immediate referral for debridement and initiation of antibiotic therapy is critical.
- Paint with antiseptic solution (e.g., povidone-iodine 10% solution); allow to dry.
- Apply dry gauze dressing and secure with wrap gauze.

surface is advantageous when managing a very poorly perfused wound in which any bacterial invasion is likely to result in clinical infection and limb loss. Therefore current opinion supports maintenance of a closed wound when 1) the involved limb is clearly ischemic with limited or no potential for healing, 2) there are no indications of infection, and 3) the wound surface is dry and necrotic. The maintenance of a dry wound with frequent monitoring for any deterioration in wound status (i.e., any signs of infection) is the current standard. A sample topical therapy protocol is outlined in Box 12-12.

The prompt identification and aggressive treatment of any infection is critical when managing an ischemic wound. Because the ischemic wound is much less able to mount an inflammatory response, these patients are at risk for overlooked infections that can become severe (e.g., cellulitis, necrotizing fasciitis, and deep compartment infections). Therefore the nurse must be alert to subtle

BOX 12-13 Indicators of Wound Infection in Ischemic Limbs

- Increased pain
- Increased necrosis
- Fluctuance of the periwound tissues
- Faint halo of erythema surrounding the wound

indicators of infection as listed in Box 12-13 and intervene promptly and aggressively if limb loss is to be avoided (Fry, Marek, and Langsfeld, 1998). Management of the infected ischemic ulcer is dependent on aggressive and early debridement of all necrotic tissue, elimination of dead space through appropriate wound packing, and culture-based antibiotic therapy. The critically ischemic limb (i.e., the limb with no palpable pulses and an ABI <0.4 to 0.5) should be revascularized if at all possible once the necrotic tissue has been debrided and antibiotic therapy has been initiated. For the patient with critical ischemia in whom revascularization is not possible, amputation may be required if meticulous wound care coupled with antibiotic therapy (and, if possible, hyperbaric oxygenation) is ineffective (Fry, Marek, and Langsfeld, 1998; Levin, 1996).

The last issue in topical therapy unique for ischemic ulcers is the use of occlusive and semiocclusive dressings. Although these dressings provide protection against secondary bacterial invasion, they are usually opaque and are changed two to three times weekly, which precludes frequent assessment of wound status. Therefore the nurse must carefully consider perfusion status, potential for infection, wound depth, volume of exudate, and level of caregiver when selecting topical therapy. A conservative approach is to avoid occlusive and adhesive semiocclusive dressings.

In summary, appropriate management of the patient with an ischemic ulcer is based on an accurate assessment of perfusion status as well as the presence or absence of infection. If the limb falls into the critical ischemia category, revascularization must be pursued if the goal is wound healing. For patients with critical ischemia in whom revascularization is not an option, the goals of care should be prevention of limb-threatening infection and control of ischemic pain. If the limb falls into the borderline perfusion category, meticulous wound care and conservative measures to improve perfusion should be initiated and revascularization options should be explored. These patients may also benefit from hyperbaric oxygen therapy. Failure to respond to conservative therapy mandates revascularization if the goal remains wound healing.

VENOUS ULCERS

Venous ulcers account for approximately 70% to 90% of all leg ulcers (Lopez and Phillips, 1998; Reichardt, 1999). The most common etiologic factor is venous insufficiency, which is precipitated by venous hypertension. Management of venous ulcers requires ongoing treatment of the underlying venous hypertension. Failure to manage the hypertension adequately contributes to the high recurrence rate associated with venous ulcers. Nursing care for patients with venous ulcers must focus on measures to improve venous return, systemic factors to promote wound healing, and provision of a wound environment conducive to healing. Once the ulcer is healed, the emphasis shifts to long-term disease management to prevent recurrence.

Epidemiology

Venous ulcers are prevalent in 1% to 2% of the population and generally correlate with aging and female gender (Douglas and Simpson, 1995; Margolis et al, 1996; Nelzen, Bergqvist, and Lindhagen, 1997; O'Donnell and Welch, 1996). Venous ulcerations significantly affect lifestyle because of chronic pain and/or discomfort, inability to work, social isolation, and frequent hospitalizations or clinic visits (Krasner, 1998). In one study, 68% of the patients reported that the ulcer had a negative effect on their lives, and there was a positive correlation between time spent on ulcer care and feelings of anger and resentment (Phillips, 1994). Venous insufficiency and venous ulcers also have a major economic effect that results from the loss of productivity and the cost of care.

The negative effects associated with venous ulcers is compounded considering the high recurrence rates (57% to 97%) that have been reported for these wounds. This high recurrence rate is a reflection of the chronicity of the underlying condition and of the frequent failure of clinicians and patients to adequately address the primary problem of venous insufficiency (Erikson et al, 1995; Samson and Showalter, 1996).

Etiology

The most common cause of venous ulceration is venous insufficiency. Predisposing conditions for venous insufficiency include processes that trigger venous hypertension, including deep vein thrombosis, multiple pregnancies, edema, ascities, congenital anomalies, severe trauma to the legs, tumors, and a sedentary lifestyle or job. Venous ulcerations are the culmination of a cascade of deleterious events and a failure to effectively manage venous hypertension.

Pathology

To understand the abnormal mechanisms associated with venous insufficiency and ulceration and the principles for management of these disorders, a clear understanding of the anatomy and physiology of the normal venous system is necessary.

Normal Venous Function. The venous system of the lower extremity includes three major components: deep veins, superficial veins, and perforator veins. The deep veins include the posterior and anterior tibial and the peroneal veins, which are encased in a tight muscle-fascial envelope within the calf muscle. The superficial venous system, located in the subcutaneous tissue, is also referred to as the *saphenous system* because it is comprised of the greater and lesser saphenous veins (Figure 12-5). The perforator, or communicating, veins provide conduits between the superficial and the deep venous systems.

All veins are equipped with one-way valves that support a unidirectional flow of blood toward the heart. This valvular system prevents retrograde blood flow and divides the venous system of the leg into smaller segments, making the gravitational pressures more bearable within each segment (Vanhoutte, Corcaud, and de Montrion, 1997).

The primary mechanisms by which venous blood is returned to the heart are the smooth muscle tone within the venous walls, contraction of the skeletal muscles, and the negative intrathoracic pressure created during inspiration (Scanlon and Sanders, 1999; Sumner and van Bemmelen, 1997). Blood from the lower extremity must flow uphill against the forces of gravity. These gravitational forces create a column of hydrostatic pressure that normally equals about 90 mm Hg while standing. The hydrostatic pressure peaks at about 120 mm Hg when the calf muscle contracts (O'Donnell and Welch, 1996; Reichardt, 1999; Scanlon and Sanders, 1999).

The calf muscle pump and deep veins within the calf work together to propel venous blood back toward the heart. This collaborative effort parallels the function of the cardiac cycle. During ambulation, the calf muscle contracts and compresses the blood out of the deep veins much like the ventricles contract and empty during the systolic phase of the cardiac cycle. While blood is being pumped from the deep veins, the one-way valves in the perforator system are closed to prevent backflow of blood into the superficial veins, which is comparable to the heart valves that prevent reflux of blood from the ventricles into the atria of the heart. As the calf muscle relaxes, the valves in the perforator veins open to permit the blood in the superficial system to flow into the deep veins. This is analogous to the refilling of the ventricles with blood from the atria through the open atrioventricular valves during the diastolic phase of the cardiac cycle (O'Donnell and Welch, 1996). Figure 12-6 illustrates venous function and the pressures normally produced within the lower-extremity venous system during muscle contraction and relaxation.

The calf muscle is the most important muscle pump in the lower extremity, but the foot pump and the thigh pump also support venous return to the heart. The foot pump is unique in that no muscle contraction is required to drain the venous plexus of the foot. It is effectively drained as the veins are stretched during weight bearing (Lopez and Phillips, 1998).

In summary, physiologic venous function is dependent on an anatomically intact venous system, a

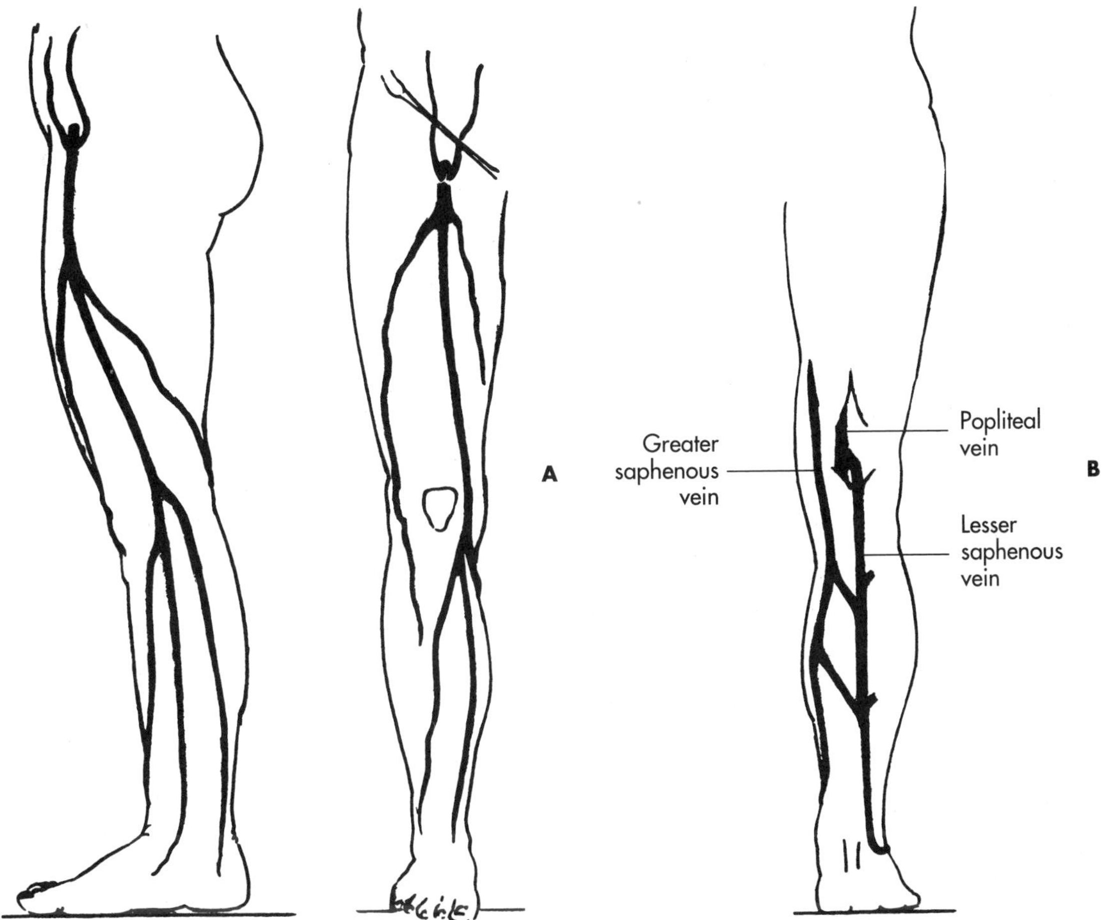

Figure 12-5 A, Anatomy of greater saphenous vein with anterior and posterior branches. B, Anatomy of lesser saphenous vein and its communication with greater saphenous vein and the popliteal vein. (From Young JR, Olin JW, Bartholomew JR: *Peripheral vascular diseases*, ed 2, St Louis, 1996, Mosby.)

competent valvular system, and well-functioning muscle pumps within the lower extremity.

Pathology of Venous Insufficiency. The underlying pathologic mechanism for CVI and ulceration is venous hypertension. Venous hypertension is usually caused by one or more of the following: obstruction, which blocks outflow; valvular incompetence, which permits retrograde flow; or muscle pump failure, which results in incomplete emptying.

The most common cause of outflow obstruction is deep vein thrombosis (DVT), or postphlebitic syndrome. DVT is present in up to 75% of patients with CVI (Franks et al, 1995; Goldstein et al, 1998; O'Donnell and Welch, 1996). Other factors that may impede venous flow include pregnancy, obesity, congestive heart failure, congenital abnormalities, edema, ascites, severe trauma to the leg, or tumors (Cordts and Gawley, 1996; O'Donnell and Welch, 1996). When obstruction occurs and forward flow is impaired, the veins distal to the obstruction become distended and venous pressures rise, resulting in venous stasis. The severity of the venous obstruction and resulting stasis is determined by the anatomic extent of venous obstruction and

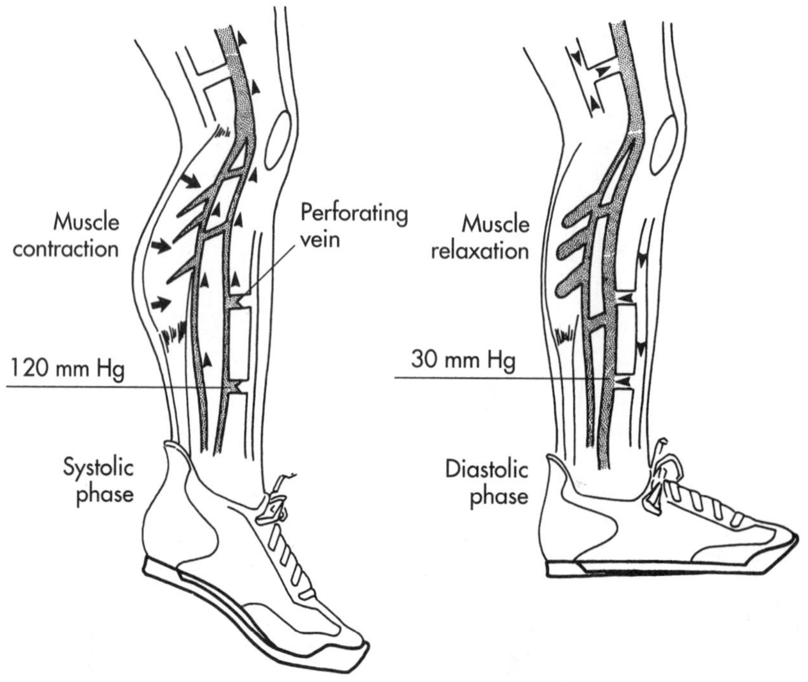

Figure 12-6 Anatomy of the perforating (communicating) veins. During the systolic phase of calf muscle contraction, the one-way valves of the perforating veins are closed, which prevents deep to superficial blood flow. During the diastolic phase the valves of the perforating veins are open, allowing superficial to deep blood flow to refill the deep veins. (From O'Donnell TF Jr, Shepard AD: Chronic venous insufficiency. In Jarrett F, Hirsch SA, editors: *Vascular surgery of the lower extremities,* St Louis, 1996, Mosby.)

the development of collateral circulation (Labropoulos et al, 1996).

The causes of valvular incompetence are not fully understood. It is theorized that valve leaflets are damaged by venous distention, venous hypertension, DVT, or vavlular agenesis (Sales, Rosenthal, and Petrillo, 1998). Valvular impairment allows reflux and pooling of blood in the lower extremities.

The causes of muscle pump failure are also not completely understood but are thought to include inactivity, neuromuscular abnormalities, or musculoskeletal changes associated with aging, arthritis, or a sedentary lifestyle (Back et al, 1995; McRorie, Ruckley, and Nuki, 1998). When the muscle pump fails to completely empty the veins during ambulation, blood begins to pool and venous hypertension ensues.

Pathology of Venous Ulceration. The etiologic factors causing venous insufficiency and venous hypertension are well recognized. Unfortunately, the events leading to dermal disruption are not as clearly understood. Three theories exist: the fibrin cuff theory, the white cell trapping theory, and the trap hypothesis.

Fibrin cuff theory. Browse and Burnand (1982) had initially postulated that venous hypertension leads to capillary bed distention, causing the space between the endothelial cells of the capillaries to widen and permitting leakage of large molecules such as fibrinogen into the dermal tissue. Fibrinogen then polymerized or hardened, forming a fibrin cuff around the dermal capillaries. Several studies confirmed the presence of fibrin cuffs in patients with venous ulcerations, and investigators found a decrease in fibrinolytic activity, which would normally breakdown the cuffs. As a result, fibrin cuffs were thought to persist and become more numerous over time (Margolis et al, 1996). Sclerotic changes in the skin were attributed to the polymerized fibrin. The fibrin cuffs were thought to act as a physical barrier to the diffusion of oxygen and nutrients into the tissues, thus resulting in tissue death and ulceration. However, several studies have demonstrated that transcutaneous oxygen levels are unchanged in the presence of fibrin cuffs and that venous ulcers have been shown to heal in the presence of fibrin cuffs (Falanga et al, 1992; Roszinski and Schmeller 1995). Fibrin cuffs may serve as markers for endothelial cell damage. They may also affect the wound-healing process by inhibiting collagen formation, contributing to a prolonged inflammatory state, or acting as a "trap" or block for growth factors and other molecules needed for healing (Bogensberger et al, 1999; Van de Scheur and Falanga, 1997).

White blood cell trapping theory. Currently, the white blood cell trapping theory is thought to be the best explanation of venous ulcer formation. In the presence of venous hypertension, the velocity of blood flow through the capillary system becomes sluggish, which allows leukocytes to marginate (line up and adhere to the capillary wall) (Saharay et al, 1997; Smith 1996). Some of the leukocytes become trapped, plugging the capillaries and causing tissue ischemia. Others migrate out into the tissues where they become activated and release proteolytic enzymes, oxygen free radicals, and inflammatory mediators that can cause tissue damage (Ono et al, 1998; Van de Scheur and Falanga, 1997). Numerous studies have demonstrated the presence of trapped white blood cells in the lower extremities of patients with venous insufficiency.

Trap hypothesis. Falanga and Eaglstein (1993) formulated a new hypothesis called the *trap hypothesis*. They propose that fibrin and other macromolecules that leak out of the permeable capillary beds bind or trap growth factors and other substances that are necessary for the maintenance of normal tissue and the healing of wounded tissue. Studies have verified that wound fluid from venous ulcers varies from that of acute wounds (Tarnuzzer and Schultz, 1996), favoring inflammation and tissue destruction rather than cell proliferation. Furthermore, venous ulcers have been characterized by leakage of a known binding protein for growth factors known as 2-macroglobulin (Higley et al, 1995; Van de Scheur and Falanga, 1997).

Assessment Parameters

A thorough patient history and physical assessment provides the foundation for further diagnostic evaluation, determination of the origin of the ulcer, and development of an appropriate management plan.

Patient History. The history should include a screen for etiologic factors associated with venous disease, including prior surgeries, pregnancies, leg trauma, cardiac disease, or ulcerations; family history of venous disease; and/or a history of DVT (Goldstein et al, 1998). A family history of venous disease is significant because venous disease carries a strong familial predisposition. The history of the current ulceration should include onset and duration of the ulcer, treatments that have been tried, and their effectiveness. The patient should be specifically asked whether compression therapy has been used and, if so, the type, his or her tolerance, and the response. The patient's lifestyle and occupation should also be assessed because this may affect his or her ability to remain compliant with the management plan. The patient should also be asked about personal habits that may affect wound repair, such as nutrient and vitamin intake and tobacco use.

The nurse should obtain a complete history of all medications being taken by the patient (both prescription and over-the-counter). Medications of particular importance in the management of venous ulcers include oral contraceptives or estrogen replacement therapy and analgesics (Vanhoutte, Corcaud, and de Montrion, 1997).

A thorough pain history should be obtained, including characteristics and location of the pain and factors that initiate, exacerbate, or relieve the painful episodes. Venous ulcers have historically been depicted as "relatively painless" as compared with ulcers caused by arterial insufficiency; however, recent reports have indicated that patients experience significant pain with venous ulcers (Hofman et al, 1997; Krasner, 1998). Commonly, venous insufficiency is characterized by a dull aching sensation accompanied with heaviness, typically worsens during the day as a result of prolonged dependency, and is usually alleviated with limb elevation. Some patients also experience a sudden "bursting" type of pain called *venous claudication*, which is caused by increased venous congestion in response to increased blood flow during exercise. Venous claudication can be mistaken for intermittent claudication (associated with ischemic disease) (O'Donnell and Welch, 1996; Sumner and van Bemmelen, 1997). Venous pain may be worse during warm weather, humid weather, or menses. The common etiologic factor is sodium and water retention, which worsens the edema (O'Donnell and Welch, 1996).

Physical Assessment. The physical assessment should focus on vascular status, with specific attention to manifestations of venous disease (e.g., edema, trophic changes, varicosities), and on characteristics of the ulcer and periulcer skin.

Vascular assessment. Up to 26% of patients with venous ulcers have concomitant arterial disease (Nelzen, Bergqvist, and Lindhagen, 1997). The presence of arterial disease affects the treatment plan and may pose a significant impediment to wound healing. If there is no coexisting arterial disease, the feet are usually warm, pulses are palpable, and the ABI is normal. Even in the absence of arterial disease, severe edema has an obscuring effect on the pedal pulses, making them difficult to palpate. Doppler studies may be helpful in this situation.

Lower-extremity edema is a common finding in the patient with venous disease and can be present to varying degrees. Edema occurs because the elevated venous pressures push fluid through the distended and permeable capillary membrane into the surrounding tissue. Sudden onset (acute) edema is associated with rapidly developing pathologies such as DVT, trauma, cellulitis, or acute lipodermatosclerosis (Bogensberger et al, 1999; Terry, O'Brien, and Kerstein, 1998). In contrast, venous insufficiency is accompanied by a gradual onset of pitting edema that worsens with prolonged standing and diminishes after rest in a recumbent position with the legs elevated. Prolonged venous insufficiency, however, is associated with edema that is persistent despite periods of leg elevation. Furthermore, the initial pitting edema may become "nonpitting" or "brawny" as more fibrin and fluid leak into the tissues. Cumulative deposits of fibrin produce progressive changes in the soft tissues (Margolis et al, 1996).

The combination of chronic edema, polymerized fibrin deposits, and the presence of inflammatory mediators causes lipodermatosclerosis, which involves sclerosing of the dermis and subcutaneous tissues and is indicative of longstanding venous disease (Bogensberger et al, 1999; Goldstein et al, 1998; O'Donnell and Welch, 1996). On palpation, the leg may feel indurated and appear hyperpigmented around the gaiter area. Edema above and below the gaiter area creates the appearance of an inverted bottle, with the sclerosed area representing the neck of the bottle and the edematous portion representing the body of the bottle.

Varicosities, (varicose veins and telangiectasias) are another prevalent finding in venous insufficiency. Dilated, tortuous varicose veins may be observed in the calf area and along the thighs. The exact distribution is determined by the anatomic location of the distended superficial vein. Another common finding is a sunburst pattern of small venous channels inferior and distal to the medial malleolus known as the *ankle venous flare* (Goldstein et al, 1998; Rudolph, 1998).

Skin and tissue changes. Hemosiderosis and venous dermatitis are characteristic skin changes associated with venous disease. Hemosiderosis is a grayish brown hyperpigmentation caused by extravasation of red blood cells into the tissues. The subsequent breakdown of red blood cells causes deposition of hemosiderin, an iron-containing pigment, into the dermis (Lopez and Phillips, 1998; Reichardt, 1999). Venous dermatitis (or stasis dermatitis) is characterized by erythema, edema, scaling, and weeping of the lower leg and may be intensely pruritic.

These changes in the skin create maceration and small breaks in the integrity, which can significantly compromise the skin's barrier function and lead to increased absorption of topically applied substances. Consequently, the patient becomes sensitized and is at an increased risk for developing contact dermatitis or an allergic reaction. This potential for contact dermatitis must be considered when selecting topical therapy. Products should be used sparingly and not indescriminately. In one study,

BOX 12-14 Classic Characteristics of Venous Ulcers

Location. Gaiter area, particularly medial malleolus

Wound edges and depth. Irregular edges may be limited to dermis or shallow subcutaneous tissue

Wound bed. Ruddy red; yellow adherent or loose slough may be present; undermining or tunnels uncommon

Volume of exudate. Typically large amount

Appearance of surrounding skin. Macerated, crusted, and scaling

Pain. Variable; can be severe; dull, aching, or bursting in character

63% of the patients with leg ulcers developed a contact dermatitis in response to products commonly used in leg ulcer treatment (Cameron et al, 1992).

Atrophie blanche is another potential finding that presents as a white, avascular, sclerotic area. Capillaroscopic findings reveal dense loops of glomerulus-like capillaries with microvascular obstructions. This is an area that is prone to ulcer formation as a result of a relative lack of oxygen and nutritive flow (Bollinger et al, 1997; Terry, O'Brien, and Kerstein, 1998).

Ulcer characteristics. Venous ulcers usually exhibit distinct characteristics that are easily identifiable on examination (Box 12-14). The medial malleolus is the "classic" location for venous ulcers. In one study, 95% were located in the gaiter area and 61% were located around the medial malleolus (Nelzen et al, 1997). This location is the point of highest pressure within the venous system because the medial malleolus represents the most distal point along the hydrostatic column of pressure, is distal to the calf pump, and is near the endpoints of the lesser saphenous vein. The typical "ruddy" appearance of the ulcer bed and high volume of exudate reflect the underlying venous congestion (Plate 7).

Diagnostic Evaluation

Although a thorough history and physical assessment usually suggest or support venous insufficiency as the primary etiologic factor for the ulcer, diagnostic testing provides a definitive diagnosis, specifies the functional or anatomic abnormality, and directs therapy in regards to surgical or medical intervention. Specifically, diagnostic evaluation can determine the particular components of the vascular system involved in the disease process (e.g., superficial, deep, or perforating venous systems), the specific pathologic process (e.g., valvular incompetence, outflow obstruction, or calf muscle failure), and the anatomic level of the lesions or dysfunction.

Tourniquet Testing. The tourniquet test is a noninvasive technique used to identify the level of valvular incompetence in *superficial* venous insufficiency and to ascertain whether the deep venous system is involved. The patient lies in a supine position with the leg elevated to empty the venous system. Subsequently, tourniquets are applied to the upper and lower thigh, below the knee, and above the ankle. The patient then stands and the tourniquets are sequentially removed while the examiner observes for distention of the superficial veins at each level. This test can be combined with calf muscle compression to assess the function of the perforator system (O'Donnel and Welch, 1996).

Doppler Ultrasonography. Doppler ultrasonography is a noninvasive test used to verify pulses when the presence of edema renders palpation inaccurate or inconclusive. The Doppler ultrasound device can also be used to auscultate venous reflux and to obtain ABI measurements (Goldstein et al, 1998). An ABI of less than 0.8 is generally considered to be a contraindication to compression therapy because of the risk of worsening the preexisting ischemia.

Photoplethysmography. Photoplethysmography is a noninvasive test using an infrared light source and a transducer probe to provide a measure of venous reflux and venous filling times. In venous hypertension, it takes less than 20 to 25 seconds for the venous system to refill (normally it takes about 35 to 45 seconds) (Goldstein et al, 1998; O'Donnel and Welch, 1996; Rudolph, 1998). Delayed healing is predicted by photoplethysmography-derived venous refill time of 10 seconds or less (Erickson et al, 1995).

Air Plethysmography. Air plethysmography is conducted by placing an air-filled cuff around the calf and measuring the calf muscle dynamics (e.g., calf venous volume, venous reflux and refill, calf muscle pumping capacity, and ambulatory venous pressures). The air-filled cuff is connected to a transducer so that pressure changes during the various test maneuvers can be recorded. Again the patient is placed with the leg elevated to evacuate the venous system. The patient is then instructed to stand with the leg in a dependent position but without weight bearing (to prevent activation of the venous pumps), and data are recorded until a plateau is reached. The patient is then asked to perform a single tip-toe maneuver to activate the calf pump and to again wait for a plateau. At that point the patient performs ten successive tip-toe procedures and returns to a nonweight-bearing, dependent position for the final plateau to be attained. The components of calf muscle function are calculated based on the pressures achieved during different parts of the test (O'Donnell and Welch, 1996; Rudolph, 1998). Normal venous function is characterized by high intravenous "standing pressures" and low intravenous "walking pressures." Venous hypertension is characterized by high walking pressures.

Venography. Venography, an invasive study that requires injection of a radiopaque dye into the lower extremity veins, details the venous system in the leg. Venography studies are commonly obtained before surgical intervention (Lopez and Phillips, 1996; Reichardt, 1999; Roenigk and Young, 1996).

Duplex Imaging. Duplex imaging with or without color has become the standard diagnostic tool for assessing venous disease and has replaced venography in many situations. Duplex scanning is noninvasive and highly sensitive in evaluating both the anatomy and the hemodynamic function of all three venous sytems in the lower extremity. Specifically, duplex imaging produces images of blood flow through vessels, pinpointing the anatomic site of reflux or obstruction (such as a deep vein thrombus); thickened, abnormal vein walls; and the presence and age of a thrombus. Duplex scanning can be used to calculate the superficial venous pressures (based on the length of the saphenous vein) and allows for quantification of venous reflux and valve closure times using the Valsalva maneuver or manual compression to elicit venous reflux (O'Donnel and Welch, 1996; Zamboni et al, 1998).

Multiple techniques can be used to obtain an in-depth assessment of the venous system and to supplement baseline information obtained through a careful history and physical examination. Additional diagnostic techniques include leg volumetry, laser-Doppler flowmetry, or impedance plethysmography. Accurate diagnostic information is critical so that appropriate decisions regarding immediate and long-term management of the patient with a venous ulcer can be made.

Management of Venous Ulcers

The first priority in venous ulcer management is to address the underlying etiology (i.e., to improve venous return). Improving venous return reduces venous hypertension, thereby controlling edema formation and increasing the velocity of blood flow. This in turn reduces white blood cell margination and extravasation into the surrounding tissues. Surgical and nonsurgical strategies for correction of venous insufficiency and ulceration include the following:

1. Surgical obliteration or ligation of veins
2. Valvular repair (valvuloplasty, valve transplantation, valve transposition)
3. Compression therapy
4. Elevation
5. Pharmacologic therapy

More recently, the advent of bioengineered tissue replacements is gaining distinction in the management of venous ulceration (Dolynchuk et al, 1999).

Surgical Management. Operative repair may be the treatment of choice when 1) manifestations of CVI and ulceration are resistant to more conservative therapies, 2) venous obstruction is present, or 3) a more aesthetic outcome is desirable. For patients with primarily superficial venous disease, vein ligation or stripping may minimize superficial venous congestion and hypertension (Akesson and Bjellerup, 1995). In patients with deep vein pathology, valvular procedures only partially correct venous hypertension; however, positive outcomes have been reported by several investigators when valvular incompetence is the primary pathologic condition (Kistner, 1997; Sumner and van Bemmelen, 1997). Likewise, in the presence of combined superficial and deep venous involvement, ligation of the perforating veins may decrease superficial venous congestion but fail to address venous hypertension in the deep venous system (Pierik, van Urk, and Wittens, 1997). However, Padberg and colleagues (1996) found that surgical correction of superficial venous insufficiency significantly improved venous hemodynamics despite the presence of deep vein insufficiency. Operative treatment is one option for resolving venous insufficiency and reducing the risk of recurrence (DePalma and Kowallek, 1996; Padberg et al, 1996).

Compression Therapy. Compression therapy is the application of externally applied pressure or static support to the lower extremity as a means of facilitating normal venous flow. It has long been considered the cornerstone in the prevention and management of CVI and ulceration. A critical factor in the success of compression therapy in venous ulcer healing and prevention of recurrence is patient compliance (Erickson et al, 1995). Multiple options for compression therapy are readily available. An understanding of the mechanisms of action and the advantages and disadvantages of the various types of compression is helpful in selecting the appropriate product for an individual patient (Table 12-4).

Mechanisms of action. Compression therapy provides constant compression to tissues, partially collapses the superficial veins, and provides support to the calf muscle during ambulation. Constant compression causes increased interstitial tissue pressure, which opposes the leakage of fluid out of the capillary system and supports reabsorption of fluid back into the blood stream. In turn, the external pressure partially collapses the superficial dilated veins, which reduces the diameter of the vessels and thereby increases the velocity of blood flow. Increased velocity reduces the tendency of white blood cells to marginate and exstravasate into the tissues (Choucair and Phillips, 1998; Spence and Cahall, 1996). Compression therapy has recently been shown to increase fibrinolytic activity and possibly to inhibit platelet activation and aggregation, thus contributing to management of lipodermatosclerosis (Kessler et al, 1996).

A therapeutic level of compression is commonly considered to be 30 to 40 mm Hg at the ankle, although lower levels of compression have also been found to be beneficial in patients with lesser degrees of venous insufficiency. For example, Brown and Brown (1995) demonstrated the effectiveness of padded, lightweight support socks that provided 6 and 12 mm Hg compression in patients with mild venous insufficiency. The compression should be a gradient compression with the highest sub-bandage pressures at the ankle and decreasing sub-bandage pressures toward the knee, which allows for augmented, unobstructed venous flow. Most compression products provide sub-bandage pressures between 20 and 50 mm Hg (Reichardt, 1999).

Compression dressings can be categorized as either static compression (therapeutic stockings and compression wraps) or dynamic compression (pneumatic pump devices). Static compression devices can be further subdivided into elastic products, including short- and long-stretch wraps (Comprilan [Biersdorf-Jobst] and Profore [T.J. Smith and Nephew, Ltd.], respectively), and inelastic products, including paste bandages and orthotic devices (Unna's boot and Circ-Aid Thera-Boot [Coloplast Corp.], respectively). Products with elasticity deliver sustained compression whether the patient is ambulatory or sedentary, whereas inelastic devices work by compressing the calf during ambulation and are therefore most effective for ambulatory patients. The orthotic device, which is considered inelastic, provides both sustained compression and calf pump support.

Long-stretch elastic wraps (such as Ace bandages) and antiembolism hose provide "sub-therapeutic" levels of compression and are *not* considered therapeutic compression. Elastic wraps are very user dependent, and the stretch, or "give," of an elastic bandage does not offer calf muscle support during ambulation. Additionally, when the patient is resting, they remain tight and subsequently cause high resting pressures.

Compression

Support stockings. Therapeutic support stockings are most commonly used in patients with stable venous insufficiency to prevent ulceration (either initial or recurrent). They may also be used for patients with an existing ulcer once the edema has been controlled and the limb circumference has stabilized. They offer various levels of compression,

TABLE 12-4 Comparison of Types of Compression Therapy

TYPE OF COMPRESSION THERAPY	MECHANISM OF ACTION	ADVANTAGES	DISADVANTAGES	COMMENTS
Therapeutic support stockings Static-short stretch (Biersdorf-Jobst)	• Support calf muscle pump with ambulation • Compress superficial system to minimize edema	• Available in varying degrees of compression at the ankle • Custom fit for different types of legs • Can be removed frequently for wound care and assessments • Patient or caregiver can apply	• Difficult to apply and remove; stocking donners and slickers are available • Success is heavily dependent on compliance, which cannot be closely monitored	• Must be premeasured • Need to be replaced at appropriate intervals • Variable levels of compression Light 14–17 mm Hg Medium 25-35 mm Hg Strong 25-35 mm Hg
Orthotic device Static-inelastic (Circ-Aid [Thera-Boot, Coloplast Corp.])	• Supports calf muscle pump with ambulation • Provides sustained compression	• Very easy for patient to apply • Custom fit • Easy removal for wound care and assessments • Sustained pressures • Can be adjusted for patient comfort and as edema decreases • Good patient compliance because of some control over adjusting velcro closures for comfort	• Somewhat bulky with multiple velcro closure straps	• Must be premeasured
Zinc paste bandage Static-inelastic (Unna's Boot) (Dome paste bandage)	• Supports calf muscle pump • Prevents edema buildup	• Comfortable and soothing to skin • Provides protection from scratching • Serves as a dressing in addition to providing compression	• Known sensitivity to some dressing components • May not accommodate highly exudative wounds • Pressure changes over time as edema decreases • Not as effective for a nonambulatory patient	• Can add a self-adherent elastic wrap to continue providing active compression as leg size changes • Should add outer wrap to protect clothing from the moist dressing • Must be applied by trained physician, nurse, or physical therapist

Four-layer bandage system Static-layers 1 and 2 inelastic; layers 3 and 4 elastic (Profore [T.J. Smith and Nephew, Ltd.]) (Dynaflex [Johnson and Johnson Medical] 3-layer bandage system: layer 1: inelastic; layers 2 and 3: elastic)	• Provides support for calf muscle pump with ambulation • Provides continuous compression during rest to increase interstitial tissue pressures and partially collapse superficial venous system	• Sustained pressure for up to 1 week • Good for highly exudative wounds • Can be adjusted to leg shape with additional padding • Very comfortable • Profore 4-layer system has a wide range of safe and therapeutic compression at variable stretch (40% to 70%)	• Somewhat bulky and hot	• Needs to be applied by trained physician, nurse, or physical therapist
Limited-stretch wraps Static-elastic (Comprilan [Biersdorf-Jobst], Setopress [Convatec])	• Supports calf muscle pump • Prevents edema buildup	• Markers indicate correct degree of stretch • Can be washed and reused multiple times • Can be applied by caregiver with appropriate training	• Sometimes difficult to stay on because of decreased elasticity • Potential risk for moisture maceration • Potential risk for pressure necrosis • May not be effective in a nonambulatory patient	• Can add a self-adherent elastic wrap to secure in place • May need to add an absorbent dressing for a highly exudative wound
Compression pumps Dynamic • Intermittent pneumatic compression (IPC) • Sequential compression • A-V impulse (Kendall)	• Enhances venous return by propelling and/or milking blood out of the lower extremity	• Good for patients unable to tolerate static devices • IPC shown to stimulate fibrinolysis • A-V impulse can be used safely in patients with arterial ischemia • Treatments can be done in home setting • Calf pump function not necessary • Promotes lymphatic flow	• Daily rental charge may become expensive • Requires 2 to 4 hours per day of immobility during treatments	• Must monitor closely for acute pulmonary edema

from mild to high, and are available in a variety of sizes, colors, and styles. To determine the correct size for a therapeutic support stocking, the leg is measured at the ankle, at the calf, and from the ankle to the knee. Noncompliance is a major issue with support stockings. Reasons cited by patients include the cost, difficulty of application, comfort issues (e.g., "too hot"), and simply forgetting to put them on (Erickson et al, 1995; Samson and Showalter, 1996). Stocking donners and slick sleeves are available to facilitate application by the patient (Figure 12-7). Compression stockings will become nontherapeutic because of loss of elasticity over the course of 3 to 6 months. Patients should be fit with two pair of support stockings so that they can wear one pair while the other is being cleaned. Stockings are removed when going to bed and reapplied as soon as they awaken and before dangling the legs over the side of the bed. The adequacy of the stocking should be evaluated with every clinic or home visit, and the importance of routine replacement should be emphasized (Reichardt, 1999).

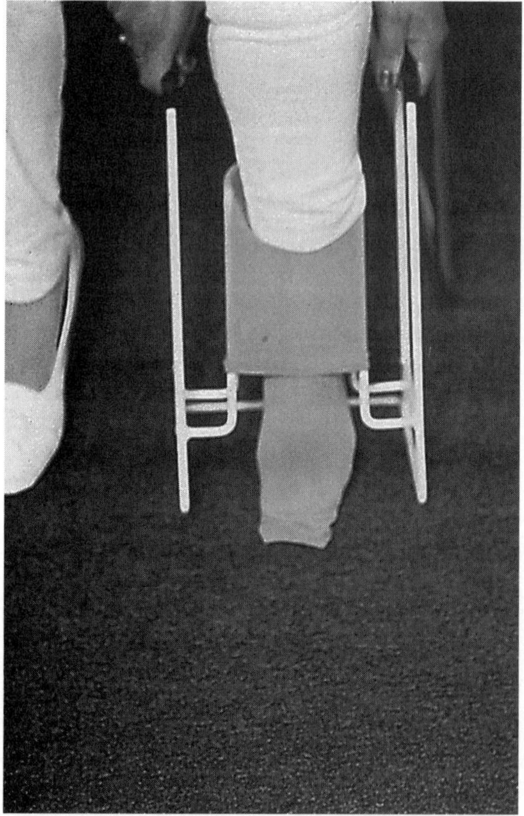

Figure 12-7 Applying a therapeutic support stocking with "stocking donner."

Orthotic device. The Circ-Aid Thera-Boot (Coloplast Corp.) is an orthotic device that works by augmenting calf pump function in addition to providing a level of continuous compression (Figure 12-8). It consists of multiple velcro straps that can be adjusted by the patient for comfort. The ability to adjust the product and the ease of removal and application may improve compliance among motivated individuals who respond positively to having some control over their own therapy. In addition, the ability to remove and reapply the device permits more frequent bathing and wound care (Choucair and Phillips, 1998).

Bandages. Compression bandages include the Unna's boot, layered systems, and short-stretch bandages. LaPlace's law of physics provides the foundation for the therapeutic benefits provided by these systems. LaPlace's law states that pressure is a function of tension, thickness, circumference, and width (Figure 12-9). Sub-bandage pressure is directly proportional to the tension and thickness of the bandage and inversely proportional to leg circumference and bandage width. In other words, sub-bandage pressure is equal to the stretch (tension) applied to the wrap, multiplied by the number of layers (thickness), divided by the circumference of the leg and the width of the bandage (Moffatt and O'Hare, 1995).

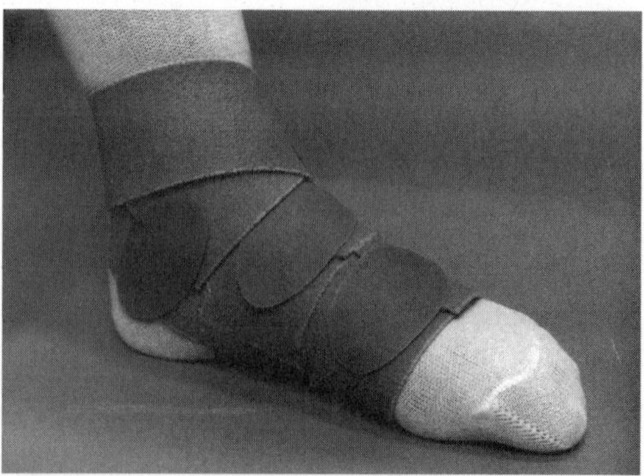

Figure 12-8 Orthotic compression device: the Circ-Aid Thera-Boot. (Courtesy Coloplast Corp., Marietta, Ga.)

Unna's boot. There are several zinc-based paste wrap products used to create a conformable inelastic "boot" around the lower extremity. The generic term for these dressings is *Unna's boot* in recognition of the physician who originated the concept (Dr. P.G. Unna). Most of these products are comprised of wrap gauze bandages that are impregnated with zinc oxide and glycerine. Some contain additional ingredients such as calamine, sorbitol, and magnesium silicate (Choucair and Phillips, 1998).

The bandage should be applied from the ball of the foot to 1 inch below the knee in a spiral fashion with 50% to 75% overlap and consistent slight tension (Figure 12-10). An outer wrap of elastic bandage or self-adherent wrap (Coban, 3M Co.) should be applied over the paste bandage from the base of the toes to the knee. This provides a component of active compression (as a result of added tension) and layers as limb size changes and also prevents soiling of clothes. A procedure for paste bandage application is provided in Box 12-15.

$$\text{Sub-bandage pressure} = \frac{\text{Tension} \times \text{Number of layers}}{\text{Leg circumference} \times \text{Width of bandage}}$$

Figure 12-9 LaPlace's law of physics as it applies to compression bandaging. La Place's law demonstrates how compression therapy is a function of tension, number of layers, leg circumference, and bandage width. Increases in tension and/or layering increase sub-bandage pressure, whereas increases in leg circumference and/or bandage width decrease sub-bandage pressure.

In reference to LaPlace's law, if tension, thickness, and width are constant, the reduced circumference at the ankle will yield a higher sub-bandage pressure. As the wrap is continued up the leg, the sub-bandage pressure will gradually decrease as the circumference of the leg becomes progressively greater, producing a gradient pressure dressing.

Unna's boot is most appropriate for ambulatory patients because it works primarily by providing static support of the calf muscle pump. The Unna's boot should be changed when the patient detects a loosening of the boot or a rubbing point. As edemas diminishes and limb circumference decreases, the boot loses its therapeutic effect as a result of its inability to continue to conform to the leg. Regular boot changes can occur weekly and in some situations every 2 weeks.

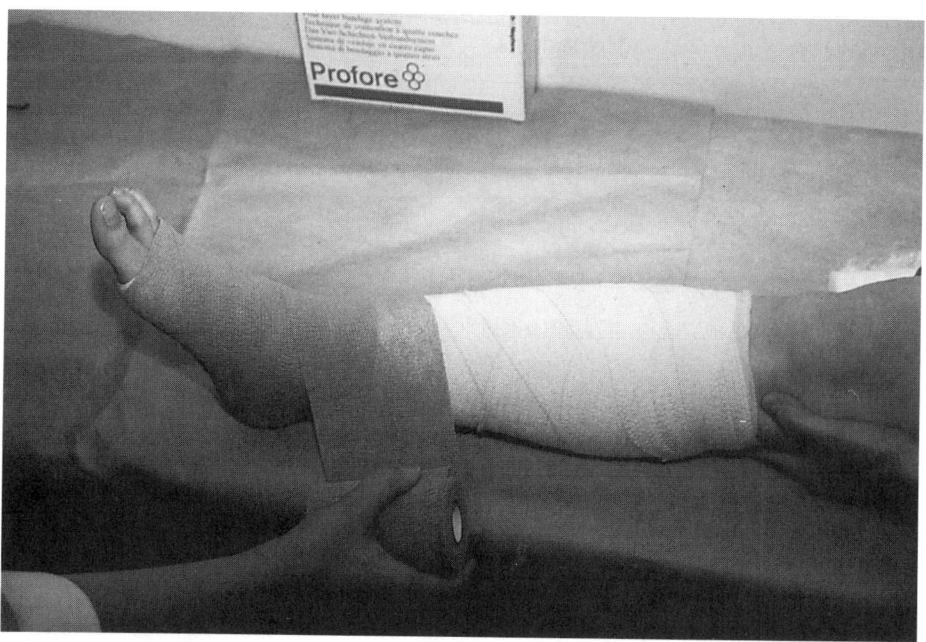

Figure 12-10 Compression wraps: Unna's boot with nonadhesive stretch cover-wrap.

BOX 12-15 Procedure for Paste Bandage Application

1. Apply gloves.
2. Gently wash extremity and dry.
3. Place patient in supine position with affected leg elevated. Foot and leg should be at a 90-degree angle.
4. Open all paste bandage wrappers and cover wrap. Estimate at least two layers of paste bandaging on the leg.
5. Holding paste bandage, roll in nondominant hand. Begin to apply bandage at base of toes.
6. Wrap twice around toes without using tension.
7. Continue wrapping bandage around foot, ankle, and heel using a circular technique, with each strip overlapping the previous strip approximately 50% to 80%.
8. Smooth paste bandage as applying, and remove any wrinkles and folds.
9. Wrap up to knee and finish smoothing.
10. Remove gloves.
11. Apply cover wrap using the same technique.
12. Remove twice weekly, weekly, or every other week as indicated by leakage, hygiene, or anticipated decrease in edema.

Layered bandage systems. Layered bandage systems combine inelastic and elastic layers to provide calf muscle support and sustained compression. The Profore system (Convatec) consists of two inner inelastic layers that provide protective padding and absorption and two elastic outer layers that provide compression and support. The first two layers are spiral wrapped from the base of the toes to 1 inch below the knee. The third layer is applied in a figure-eight fashion with 50% stretch and 50% overlap. The final layer (Coban, 3M Co.) is applied in a spiral wrap with 50% tension and 50% overlap (Figure 12-11). The combined effects of layering and tension, with circumference and width being relatively constant, afford effective sub-bandage pressures that can be maintained for up to 1 week (Choucair and Phillips, 1998).

The Dyna-Flex system (Johnson and Johnson Medical) consists of an inelastic layer covered by two elastic compression layers. This system is applied in a similar fashion to the four-layer system, with the first layer providing padding and absorption. The Dyna-Flex system (Johnson and Johnson Medical) provides a visual indicator that guides the nurse in achieving the correct amount of tension.

Short-stretch bandages provide sustained compression and calf muscle support. They are advantageous in that they can be washed and reused multiple times. In addition, caregivers can be taught to apply the short-stretch bandages, which permits more frequent bathing and/or dressing changes.

Problems encountered with short-stretch bandages occur because they are relatively inelastic, which means that they are less conformable and more likely to slip out of place. In one study, a self-adherent elastic wrap was used to maintain the short stretch bandage in position (Scriven et al, 1998). Short-stretch bandages also have the potential to create pressure injuries over the tibial surfaces of patients with very small limbs; thus they must be applied carefully and may require padding over the bony prominences of very slender patients.

Dynamic compression devices. Dynamic compression therapy consists of powered devices that are applied to the lower extremity to propel venous blood upward. Intermittent pneumatic pumps, sequential gradient compression devices, and the A-V impulse device (Kendall) are examples of dynamic therapy. Most of the dynamic devices consist of a limb sleeve with one or more cells that inflate intermittently and/or sequentially to create a positive pressure gradient that propels blood out of the extremity and back to the heart (Figure 12-12) (O'Donnel and Welch, 1996). Intermittent pneumatic compression has also been shown to have a positive effect on fibrinolytic activity (Margolis et al, 1996).

The A-V impulse device is a single-cell unit that wraps around the foot and promotes venous return by activating the venous plexus on the plantar surface of the foot. This device can be safely used in the presence of ischemic disease.

Dynamic compression devices are effective in reducing edema in the lower extremity, but the patient must commit 2 to 4 hours a day for therapy.

Contraindications and considerations associated with compression therapy. Contraindications for compression therapy include arterial insufficiency,

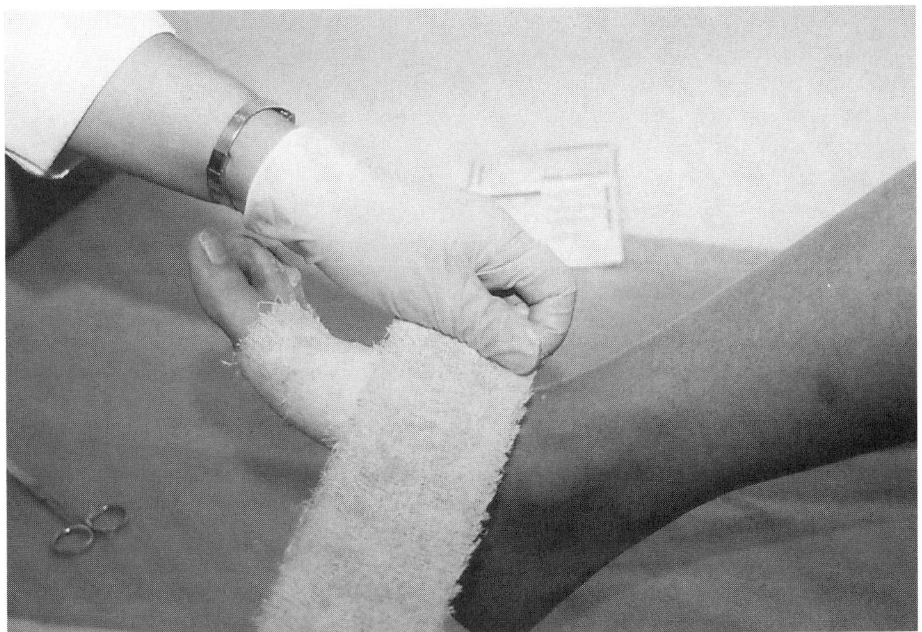

Figure 12-11 Compression wraps: Layered bandage system (Profore [T.J. Smith and Nephew, Ltd.]).

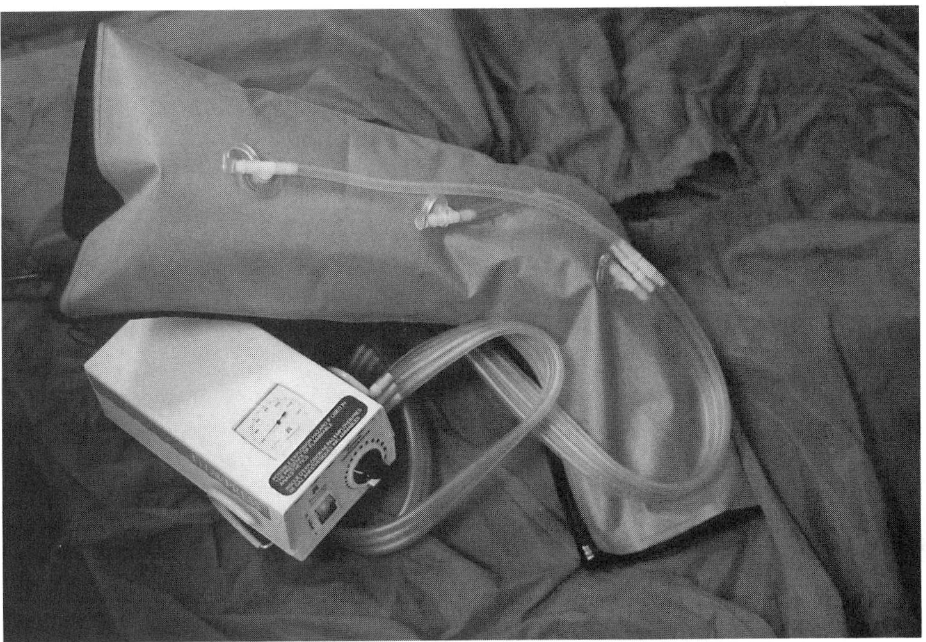

Figure 12-12 Dynamic compression device: sequential compression therapy.

uncompensated congestive heart failure (CHF), and active thrombus (O'Donnell and Welch, 1996). It is critical to ascertain that the ABI is >0.8 before initiation of compression therapy when there is any question as to the adequacy of arterial perfusion. Caution must also be used in patients with uncompensated CHF because there is the risk of causing fluid volume overload by shifting fluid out of the tissues into the vascular system and potentially contributing to acute pulmonary edema. This is of particular concern when using the dynamic devices because fluid shifts can occur rapidly. Also, compressing an extremity with an active thrombus can result in dislodgment and free embolism.

A consistent concern in the use of compression products is the importance of correct measurement and application. Improper application of a compression wrap or inaccurate measurement for a compression stocking may result in dangerously high pressures, producing iatrogenic ischemia, or in pressures too low to adequately support venous return. Application or measurements should be done in the morning or midmorning hours (i.e., before the development of significant edema).

One of the most critical aspects of effective compression therapy is the associated patient education and monitoring. After the compression device is applied, the patient should be monitored for signs of ischemia and should be taught to immediately report any numbness, tingling, discoloration of toes, or increase in pain. Studies indicate that the effects of compression on arterial perfusion are manifest in the tissues distal to the compression device (e.g., the toes) as opposed to the tissues beneath the bandage itself (Mayrovitz, Delgado, and Smith, 1997). These findings reinforce the importance of screening for concomitant arterial disease and providing patient education concerning the signs of ischemia and appropriate response.

Limb Elevation. Limb elevation is a simple but effective strategy for improving venous return by the use of gravitational forces. Patients should be instructed to elevate the feet above the thighs while sitting and to elevate the legs above the heart when lying down.

Pharmacologic Therapy. Several medications have been studied for their hypothesized ability to reduce edema, enhance fibrinolysis, or promote anticoagulation. These include stanozolol and various plant extracts and bioflavinoids such as horse chestnut seed extract (Diehm et al, 1996; Kirsner et al, 1993; Mayberry, Moneta, and Porter, 1997; Smith, 1996). To date, no drug has demonstrated significant benefit; however, research continues into the possibility of agents to address the pathology of venous insufficiency.

The hemorrheologic agent pentoxifylline (Trental) has shown the most promising result in venous ulcer therapy. It decreases blood viscosity and white cell adhesion while increasing fibrinolysis (Mayberry, Moneta, and Porter, 1997). Several studies report that dosages of 400 to 800 mg, taken orally three times a day, can accelerate the healing of venous ulcers (Falanga, 1999).

Aspirin, heparin, ifetroban (a thromboxane receptor agonist), and prostaglandin E1 have been studied for a potential role in venous wound healing but have failed to demonstrate significant benefit. Topical growth factors have not shown effective in venous ulcerations.

At this time, the role of pharmacologic agents in venous ulcer management seems to be limited to the use of antibiotics (for infected wounds), topical and systemic corticosteroids (for the control of venous dermatitis), and anticoagulants (for the management of recurrent thrombosis). Further research into the pathologic mechanisms of venous disease may provide insight into other pharmaceutical agents of potential benefit. At present, however, compression therapy remains the indisputable gold standard in venous ulcer management (Cullum et al, 1999).

Topical Therapy. Topical therapy for venous ulcers should follow the same principles of topical therapy for any chronic wound and be based on wound needs. Debridement and infection control are of utmost importance. Beyond this, topical therapy should provide exudate absorption, maintenance of a moist environment, protection, and insulation.

Venous ulcers may be covered with a layer of yellow fibrinous tissue or slough that will need to be removed for wound healing to occur. Special attention should be paid to the periwound skin status for signs of maceration or other trophic changes commonly seen in CVI. A skin sealant can be used to protect the surrounding skin from wound exudate. Dermatitis, scaling, and pruritus may need to be treated with topical steroid creams or ointments to prevent further tissue damage from scratching.

Bioengineered Tissue. Because human skin equivalents are capable of producing growth factors and cytokines, they may prove beneficial in venous ulcers by converting the chronic wound microenvironment to an acute wound microenvironment (Dolynchuk et al, 1999; Sabolinski et al, 1996). One human skin equivalent, Apligraf (Organogenesis, Canton, Mass.; Novartis Pharmaceuticals Canada, Inc., Dorval, Quebec, Canada), has been FDA approved specifically for venous ulcers, and studies to date indicate improved healing (Falanga et al, 1998; Falanga, 1999).

Summary

Venous ulcerations are a chronic problem that will continue to present challenges to nurses as the age wave continues. Positive outcomes are achievable with appropriate assessment and management but require long-term attention by a multidisciplinary team to control venous insufficiency and encourage patient compliance to prevent recurrence (Akesson and Bjellerup, 1995; Erickson et al, 1995).

LYMPHEDEMA

In contrast to CVI, which is fairly common, lymphedema is relatively rare, especially in industrialized societies. However, it is important for the nurse that deals with CVI to have sufficient knowledge regarding lymphedema to appropriately differentiate between the two pathologic entities.

The lymphatic system operates in conjunction with the arterial and venous systems to maintain normal plasma volume. Approximately 2 to 4 liters of the protein-rich fluid that moves out of the bloodstream into the interstitial space on a daily basis fails to return. This fluid is "picked up" by the lymphatic capillaries and eventually returned to the blood stream, thus providing an important "salvage" operation (Villavicencio and Pikoulis, 1997).

The lymphatic system also has important secondary functions that include the removal of toxic substances and damaged cells from the tissues, protection against infection, and defense against the spread of malignancy (Villavicencio and Pikoulis, 1997). Lymph nodes, which are located at various points along the larger lymphatic channels, contain large numbers of lymphocytes. These lymphocytes "clear" the lymph of toxins, pathogens, and malignant cells. Lymphedema occurs when there is a tremendous increase in the volume of lymph produced and/or a major reduction in the capacity for lymph transport. The characteristics and associated conditions for the two types of lymphedema are listed in Table 12-5 (International Society of Lymphology Executive Committee, 1995; Terry, O'Brien, and Kerstein, 1998; Villavicencio and Pikoulis, 1997).

The resulting accumulation of protein-rich fluid in the tissues manifests as progressive edema that begins in the most distal portion of the extremity (e.g., the foot); the edema responds poorly to

TABLE 12-5 Lymphedema: Classification, Characteristics, and Associated Conditions

CLASSIFICATION	CHARACTERISTICS	ASSOCIATED CONDITIONS
High output	Massive increase in the volume of lymph produced	Cirrhosis Nephrosis Severe venous insufficiency
Low output	Failure of lymph transport	Filariasis Congenital lymphatic insufficiency Surgical manipulation or excision of lymphatic channels Irradiation of lymphatic channels

TABLE 12-6 Lymphedema: Treatment Components

INTERVENTION	DESIRED EFFECT	ACTION	CAUTIONS
Complex decongestive physiotherapy	Mobilization of retained lymph	Therapeutic massage to mobilize lymphatic fluid in channels adjacent and proximal to involved site, followed by massage of affected area Compression bandages applied immediately after treatment	Performed only by therapists trained in the technique Usually requires one to two treatments daily for 1 to 3 weeks
Sequential compression therapy	Mobilization of retained lymph	Dynamic compression pumps with limb sleeves compress lymphatics and mobilize lymph	Risk of displacing fluid to proximal leg or genitalia
Limb elevation	Edema reduction	Counters the effect of gravity on lymph flow	Effective only in early phase of disease
Compression bandaging	Critical component of maintenance therapy Inelastic or short stretch bandages and custom-fitted sleeves or stockings most effective	Applies pressure to tissues to facilitate compression of lymph channels and movement of lymph from interstitial space into channels	Should provide 40 to 60 mm Hg sub-bandage pressure Replace regularly to prevent loss of therapeutic effectiveness
Exercises	Maintenance of lymph reduction	Stimulate the intact lymphatics to increase rate of lymph transport	Encouraged to exercise involved limb with compression bandage or garment in place
Skin and nail care	Infection control during restorative and maintenance phases	Keeps skin supple and prevents breaks in skin to reduce risk of infection	May have standing prescription for antibiotics to be filled if signs of infection develop

Based on Casley-Smith F et al: Treatment for lymphedema of the arm-the Casley-Smith method: a noninvasive method produces continued reduction, *Cancer* 83(12 suppl):2843, 1998; Boris M, Weindorf S, Lasinski B: The risk of genital edema after external pump compression for lower limb lymphedema, *Lymphology* 31(1):15, 1998; International Society of Lymphology Executive Committee: Consensus Document. The diagnosis and treatment of peripheral lymphedema, *Lymphology* 28:113, 1995; Ko D et al: Effective treatment of lymphedema of the extremities, *Arch Surg* 133(4):452, 1998; Villavicencio J, Pikoulis E: Lymphedema. In Raju S, Villavicencio JL, editors: *Surgical management of venous disease,* Baltimore, 1997, Williams & Wilkins.

elevation. The edema is generally nonpitting or minimally pitting and may produce a "hump" on the dorsal aspect of the foot. As the condition worsens, the progressive accumulation of lymph within the tissues can result in severe distortion of the limb and destruction of the elastic components of the skin, a condition known as *elephantiasis*. The protein deposits within the tissues also cause a progressive thickening of the skin and fibrosis of the soft tissues, which increases the risk of skin breakdown (International Society of Lymphology Executive Committee, 1995; Terry, O'Brien, and Kerstein, 1998; Villavicencio and Pikoulis, 1997).

Because the compromised lymphatic system is much less able to handle any bacterial challenge, even minor breaks in the skin can precipitate acute cellulitis (International Society of Lymphology Executive Committee, 1995; Terry, O'Brien, and Kerstein, 1998). Any traumatic or infectious event causes additional inflammation and fibrosis, which further damages the compromised lymphatic system.

Effective management of the patient with lymphedema is dependent on an accurate diagnosis. A careful history and physical assessment usually provide the data to distinguish lymphedema from venous edema. When the diagnosis is unclear, imaging studies (lymphoscintigraphy) may be performed to elucidate the structure and function of the lymphatic system.

Management of lymphedema is directed toward mobilization of the "trapped" lymph with elimination of the edema and restoration of normal limb contours, maintenance of the "restored" state, and prevention of infection. Therapy can be divided into two main phases: restorative, or "volumetric reduction," and maintenance. The components of treatment are listed in Table 12-6.

Research is ongoing into surgical techniques to improve lymphatic return via techniques such as the establishment of venolymphatic anastomoses; however, surgical intervention is currently limited to patients who require reduction of redundant tissue (International Society of Lymphology Executive Committee, 1995; Ko et al, 1998).

In summary, lymphedema is a chronic condition that at present has no known cure. Effective management requires a comprehensive lifelong program and is most effectively provided in a lymphedema center.

SUMMARY

Ulcerations on the lower extremities can present a confusing array of intervening characteristics. Although at first glance it seems easy to distinguish between an arterial ulcer and a venous ulcer based on the characteristics of the ulcer and the extremity, coexisting pathologic conditions and other less common maladies (such as vasculitic disorders and pyoderma gangrenosum) can cloud the assessment. The wound care nurse must be cognizant of appropriate diagnostic tests to confirm ulcer etiology and current management approaches for the key conditions that may manifest as leg ulcers. Treatment must address systemic needs and reflect a long-term commitment to the patient. A multidisciplinary and individualized approach is a key factor in successful management of the leg ulcer patient.

SELF-ASSESSMENT EXERCISE

1. Rest pain is indicative of:
   - a. Mild occlusive disease, such as with 25% occlusion
   - b. Moderate occlusive disease, such as with 50% occlusion
   - c. Advanced occlusive disease, such as with 90% occlusion
   - d. Need for amputation
2. Risk factors for PAD include:
   - a. Alcoholism
   - b. Hypertension
   - c. Elevated HDL levels
   - d. Diabetes insipidus
3. Claudication is the type of pain that:
   - a. Exists without precipitating activity
   - b. Develops when the patient elevates the legs
   - c. Is triggered by moderate to heavy activity
   - d. Worsens with rest
4. Which of the following ABI values is indicative of calcification of vessel wall in a person with diabetes?
   - a. 0.95-1.3
   - b. 0.5-0.95

   c. <0.5
   d. >1.3
5. List the classic characteristics of an arterial ulcer.
6. Maintenance of an eschar-covered arterial ulcer is preferred when:
   a. The involved limb is ischemic and can be revascularized
   b. The wound suface is exudative
   c. The wound is infected
   d. Indications of an infection are absent and there is limited potential for healing
7. Describe how the intact and competent venous system and muscle pumps within the leg work together to prevent venous hypertension.
8. Which of the following scenarios is most likely indicative of coexisting arterial disease in a patient with a venous ulcer?
   a. Pedal pulses are not palpable and legs are edematous
   b. Feet are warm
   c. ABI value is 0.70
   d. Presence of dull aching pain in the ulcerated limb
9. Distinguish between elastic and inelastic static compression products.
10. Lipodermatosclerosis is associated with:
   a. Ankle venous flare
   b. Hardening of the dermis and subcutaneous tissue
   c. Presence of varicose veins
   d. Venous disease of recent origin
11. Summarize the value and mechanical action of compression therapy.

REFERENCES

Akesson H, Bjellerup M: Leg ulcers: report on a multidisciplinary approach, *Acta Derm Venereol* 91:133, 1995.

Altemose G, Wiener D: Control of risk factors in peripheral vascular disease: management of hypertension, *Surg Clin North Am* 78(3):69, 1998.

Aly S et al: Comparison of duplex imaging and arteriography in the evaluation of lower limb arteries, *Br J Surg* 85:1099, 1998.

Back TL et al: Limited range of motion is a significant factor in venous ulceration, *J Vasc Surg* 22:519, 1995.

Baumgartner I et al: Intramuscular gene transfer promotes collateral vessel development in patients with critical limb ischemia, *Circulation* 97(12):1114, 1998.

Blann A, Bignell A, McCollum C: von Willebrand factor, fibrinogen, and other plasma proteins as determinants of plasma viscosity, *Atherosclerosis* 139:317, 1998.

Bogensberger G et al: Lipodermatosclerosis, *Wounds* 11(suppl A):2A, 1999.

Bollinger A et al: Microvascular changes in venous disease: an update, *Angiology* 48(1):27, 1997.

Boneu B, Leger P, Arnaud C: Haemostatic system activation and prediction of vascular events in patients presenting with stable peripheral arterial disease of moderate severity, *Blood Coagul Fibrinolysis* 9(2):129, 1998.

Boris M, Weindorf S, Lasinski B: The risk of genital edema after external pump compressionfor lower limb lymphedema, *Lymphology* 31(1):15, 1998.

Brown JR, Brown AM: Nonprescription, padded, lightweight support socks in treatment of mild to moderate lower extremity venous insufficiency, *J Am Osteopath Assoc* 95(3):173, 1995.

Browse NL, Burnand KG: The cause of venous ulceration, *Lancet* 2(8292):243, 1982.

Cameron J et al: Contact dermatitis in leg ulcer patients, *Ostomy Wound Manage* 38(9):8, 1992.

Cantwell-Gab K: Identifying chronic peripheral arterial disease, *Am J Nurs* 96(7):40, 1996.

Capecchi PL et al: Carnitines increase plasma levels of adenosine and ATP in humans, *Vasc Med* 2(2):77, 1997.

Casley-Smith F et al: Treatment for lymphedema of the arm—the Casley-Smith method: a noninvasive method produces continued reduction, *Cancer* 83(12 suppl):2843, 1998.

Choucair M, Phillips TJ: Compression therapy, *Dermatol Surg* 24:141, 1998.

Cooke J, Ma A: Medical therapy of peripheral arterial occlusive disease, *Surg Clin North Am* 75(4):569, 1995.

Cordts PR, Gawley TS: Anatomic and physiologic changes in lower extremity venous hemodynamics associated with pregnancy, *J Vasc Surg* 24:763, 1996.

Cragg A, Dake M: Treatment of peripheral vascular disease with stent-grafts, *Radiology* 205:307, 1997.

Cullum N et al: Compression bandages and stockings in the treatment of venous leg ulcers (Cochrane Review). In *The Cochrane Library*, Issue 2, 1999. Oxford: Update Software.

DePalma RG, Kowallek DL: Venous ulceration: a cross-over study from nonoperative to operative treatment, *J Vasc Surg* 23:78, 1996.

DiCorleto P et al: Pathogenesis of atherosclerosis. In Young J, Olin J, Bartholemew J, editors: *Peripheral vascular diseases*, ed 2, St Louis, 1996, Mosby.

Diehm C et al: Comparison of leg compression stocking and oral horse-chestnut seed extract therapy in patients with chronic venous insufficiency, *Lancet* 347(8997):292, 1996.

Dolynchuk K et al: The role of apligraf™ in the treatment of venous leg ulcers, *Ostomy Wound Manage* 45(1):34, 1999.

Douglas WS, Simpson NB: Guidelines for the management of chronic venous leg ulceration: report of a multidisciplinary workshop, *Brit J Dermatol* 132:446, 1995.

Erickson CA et al: Healing of venous ulcers in an ambulatory care program: the roles of chronic venous insufficiency and patient compliance, *J Vasc Surg* 22:629, 1995.

Falanga V: Care of venous leg ulcers, *Ostomy Wound Manage* 45(suppl 1A):33S, 1999.

Falanga V, Eaglstein WH: The "trap" hypothesis of venous ulceration, *Lancet* 341:1006, 1993.

Falanga V et al: Pericapillary fibrin cuffs in venous ulceration: persistence with treatment and during ulcer healing, *J Dermatol Surg Onc* 18(5):409, 1992.

Falanga V et al: Rapid healing of venous ulcers and lack of clinical rejection with an allogeneic cultured human skin equivalent, *Arch Dermatol* 134:293, 1998.

Franks PJ et al: Risk factors for leg ulcer recurrence: a randomized trial of two types of compression stocking, *Age Ageing* 24:490, 1995.

Franks PJ, Moffatt C: Quality of life issues in patients with chronic wounds, *Wounds* 10(suppl E):1E, 1998.

Fry D, Marek J, Langsfeld M: Infection in the ischemic lower extremity, *Surg Clin North Am* 78(3):465, 1998.

Gahtan V: The noninvasive vascular laboratory, *Surg Clin North Am* 78(4):507, 1998.

Ghirlanda G, Citterio F: Lower limb ischemia, *Rays* 22(4):535, 1997.

Goldstein D et al: Differential diagnosis: assessment of the lower extremity ulcer—is it arterial, venous, neuropathic? *Wounds* 10(4):125, 1998.

Golledge J: Lower-limb arterial disease, *Lancet* 350:1459, 1997.

Higley HR et al: Extravasation of macromolecules and possible trapping of transforming growth factor-B in venous ulceration, *Brit J Dermatol* 132:79, 1995.

Hilleman D: Management of peripheral arterial disease, *Am J Health Syst Pharm* 55(19 suppl 1): S21, 1998.

Hofman D et al: Pain in venous leg ulcers, *J Wound Care* 6(5):222, 1997

International Society of Lymphology Executive Committee: Consensus Document. The diagnosis and treatment of peripheral lymphedema, *Lymphology* 28:113, 1995.

Joyce J: Thromboangiitis obliterans (Buerger's disease). In Young J, Olin J, Bartholemew J, editors: *Peripheral vascular diseases*, ed 2, St Louis, 1996, Mosby.

Kerstein M: The non-healing leg ulcer: peripheral vascular disease, chronic venous insufficiency, and ischemic vasculitis, *Ostomy Wound Manage* 42(10A suppl):19S, 1996.

Kessler CM et al: Intermittent pneumatic compression in chronic venous insufficiency favorably affects fibrinolytic potential and platelet activation, *Blood Coagul Fibrinolysis* 7:437, 1996.

Killewich L et al: Progressive intermittent claudication is associated with impaired fibrinolysis, *J Vasc Surg* 27(4):645, 1998.

Kirsner RS et al: The clinical spectrum of Lipodermatosclerosis, *J Am Acad Dermatol* 28:623, 1993.

Kistner RL: Venous valve surgery: an overview. In Raju S, Villavicencio JL, editors: *Surgical management of venous disease* Baltimore, 1997, Williams & Wilkins.

Ko D et al: Effective treatment of lymphedema of the extremities, *Arch Surg* 133(4):452, 1998.

Krasner D: Painful venous ulcers: themes and stories about living with the pain and suffering, *J Wound Ostomy Continence Nurs* 25(3):158, 1998.

Labropoulos N et al: The role of venous reflux and calf muscle pump function in nonthrombotic chronic venous insufficiency: correlation with severity of signs and symptoms, *Arch Surgery* 131(4):403, 1996.

Levin M: Diabetic foot lesions. In Young J, Olin J, Bartholemew J, editors: *Peripheral vascular diseases*, ed 2, St Louis, 1996, Mosby.

Lopez AP, Phillips TJ: Venous ulcers, *Wounds* 10(5):149, 1998.

Lowe GD: Etiopathogenesis of cardiovascular disease: hemostasis, thrombosis, and vascular medicine, *Ann Periodontol* 3(1):121, 1998.

Margolis DJ: Management of unusual causes of ulcers of lower extremities, *J Wound Ostomy Continence Nurs* 22(2):89, 1995.

Margolis DJ et al: Fibrinolytic abnormalities in two different cutaneous manifestations of venous disease, *J Am Acad Dermatol* 34:204, 1996.

Mayberry JC, Moneta GL, Porter JM: Conservative management of chronic lower extremity venous insufficiency. In Raju S, Villavicencio JL, editors: *Surgical management of venous disease*, Baltimore, 1997, Williams & Wilkins.

Mayrovitz HN, Delgado M, Smith J: Compression bandaging effects on lower extremity peripheral and subbandage skin blood perfusion, *Wounds* 9(5):146, 1997.

McGee S, Boyko D: Physical examination and chronic lower-extremity ischemia: a critical review, *Arch Intern Med* 158(12):1357, 1998.

McNamara D, Champion H, Kadowitz P: Pharmacologic management of peripheral vascular disease, *Surg Clin North Am* 78(3):447, 1998.

McRorie E, Ruckley C, Nuki G: The relevance of large-vessel vascular disease and restricted ankle movement to the aetiology of leg ulceration in rheumatoid arthritis, *Brit J Rheumatol* 37(12):1295, 1998.

Meijjer W et al: Peripheral arterial disease in the elderly: the Rotterdam Study, *Arterioscler Thromb Vasc Biol* 18:185, 1998.

Moffatt CJ, O'Hare L: Venous leg ulcerations: treatment by high compression bandaging, *Ostomy Wound Manage* 41(4):16, 1995.

Moon R: Use of hyperbaric oxygen in the management of selected wounds, *Adv Wound Care* 11(7):332, 1998.

Nelzen O, Bergqvist D, Lindhagen A: Long-term prognosis for patients with chronic leg ulcers: a prospective cohort study, *Eur J Vasc Endovasc Surg* 13:500, 1997.

O'Donnell TF Jr, Shepard AD: Chronic venous insufficiency. In Jarrett F, Hirsch SA, editors: *Vascular surgery of the lower extremities*, St Louis, 1996, Mosby.

O'Donnell TF Jr, Welch HJ: Chronic venous insufficiency and varicose veins. In Young JR, Olin JW, Bartholomew

JR, editors: *Peripheral vascular diseases*, ed 2, St Louis, 1996, Mosby.

Ono T et al: Monocyte infiltration into venous valves, *J Vasc Surg* 27:158, 1998.

Padberg FT Jr et al: Hemodynamic and clinical improvement after superficial vein ablation in primary combined venous insufficiency with ulceration, *J Vasc Surg* 24:711, 1996.

Philipp C et al: Association of hemostatic factors with peripheral vascular disease, *Am Heart J* 134(5 Pt 1):978, 1997.

Phillips T et al: A study of the impact of leg ulcers on quality of life: financial, social, and psychologic implications, *J Am Acad Dermatol* 31(1):49, 1994.

Pierik EG, van Urk H, Wittens CH: Efficacy of subfascial endoscopy in eradicating perforating veins of the lower leg and its relation with venous ulcer healing, *J Vasc Surg* 26(2):255, 1997.

Price J, Lee A, Fowkes F: Hyperinsulinaemia: a risk factor for peripheral arterial disease in the non-diabetic general population, *J Cardiovasc Risk* 3(6):501, 1996.

Reichardt LE: Venous ulceration: compression as the mainstay of therapy, *J Wound Ostomy Continence Nurs* 26(1):39, 1999.

Reininger C, Graf J, Reininger A: Increased platelet and coagulatory activity indicate ongoing thrombogenesis in peripheral arterial disease, *Thrombosis Res* 82(6):523, 1996.

Robinson K, Mayer E, Jacobsen DW: Homocysteine and coronary artery disease, *Cleve Clin J Med* 61(6):438, 1994.

Rockson S, Cooke J: Peripheral arterial insufficiency: mechanisms, natural history, and therapeutic options, *Adv Intern Med* 43:253, 1998.

Roenigk H, Young J: Leg ulcers. In Young J, Olin J, Bartholomew J, editors: *Peripheral vascular disease*, ed 2, St Louis, 1996, Mosby.

Roszinski J, Schmeller W: Differences between intracutaneous and transcutaneous skin oxygen tension in chronic venous insufficiency, *J Cardiovasc Surg* 36:407, 1995.

Rubano J, Kerstein M: Arterial insufficiency and vasculitides, *J Wound Ostomy Continence Nurs* 25(3):147, 1998.

Rudolph DM: Pathophysiology and management of venous ulcers, *J Wound Ostomy Continence Nurs* 5(5):248, 1998.

Sabolinski ML et al: Cultured skin as 'smart material' for healing wounds: experience in venous ulcers, *Biomaterials* 17(3):311, 1996.

Saharay M et al: Leukocyte activity in the microcirculation of the leg in patients with chronic venous disease, *J Vasc Surg* 25:265, 1997.

Sales CM, Rosenthal D, Petrillo KA: The valvular apparatus in venous insufficiency: a problem of quantity? *Ann Vasc Surg* 12:153, 1998.

Samson RH, Showalter DP: Stockings and the prevention of recurrent venous ulcers, *Dermatol Surg* 22:373, 1996.

Scanlon VC, Sanders T: *Essentials of anatomy and physiology*, ed 3, Philadelphia, 1999, F.A. Davis.

Scriven JM et al: A prospective randomised trial of four-layer versus short stretch compression bandages for the treatment of venous leg ulcers, *Ann R Coll Surg Engl* 80:215, 1998.

Seidel HM et al: *Mosby's guide to physical examination*, ed 4, St Louis, 1999, Mosby.

Smith F et al: Smoking, hemorheologic factors, and progression of peripheral arterial disease in patients with claudication, *J Vasc Surg* 28:129, 1998.

Smith PC: The microcirculation in venous hypertension, *Cardiovasc Res* 32:789, 1996.

Spence RK, Cahall E: Inelastic versus elastic leg compression in chronic venous insufficiency: a comparison of limb size and venous hemodynamics, *J Vasc Surg* 24:783, 1996.

Stone J, Cianci P: The adjunctive role of hyperbaric oxygen therapy in the treatment of lower extremity wounds in patients with diabetes, *Diabetes Spectrum* 10(2):118, 1997.

Sumner DS, van Bemmelen PS: Hemodynamics of the venous system: calf pump and valve function. In Raju S, Villavicencio JL, editors: *Surgical management of venous disease*, Baltimore, 1997, Williams & Wilkins.

Tarnuzzer RW, Schultz GS: Biochemical analysis of acute and chronic wound environments, *Wound Rep Regen* 4:321, 1996.

Terry M, Berkowitz H, Kerstein MD: Tobacco: Its impact on vascular disease, *Surg Clin North Am* 78(3):409, 1998.

Terry M, O'Brien SP, Kerstein MD: Lower-extremity edema: evaluation and diagnosis, *Wounds* 10(4):118, 1998.

Van de Scheur M, Falanga V: Pericapillary fibrin cuffs in venous disease, *Dermatol Surg* 23:955, 1997.

Vanhoutte PM, Corcaud S, de Montrion C: Venous disease: from pathophysiology to quality of life, *Angiology* 48(7):559, 1997.

Verhaeghe R: Epidemiology and prognosis of peripheral obliterative arteriopathy, *Drugs* 56(suppl 3):1, 1998.

Villavicencio J, Pikoulis E: Lymphedema. In RajuS, Villavicencio JL, editors: *Surgical management of venous disease*, Baltimore, 1997, Williams & Wilkins.

Zamboni P et al: In vitro versus in vivo assessment of vein wall properties, *Ann Vasc Surg* 12:324, 1998.

CHAPTER 13

Vascular and Neuropathic Wounds: The Diabetic Wound

LAUREL A. WIERSEMA-BRYANT & BRUCE A. KRAEMER

OBJECTIVES

1. Describe three types of neuropathy that may occur in the diabetic patient in terms of risk for ulcer formation.
2. Identify risk factors for the development of a diabetic foot ulcer.
3. Identify critical factors to be included in the history and physical examination of the patient with a neuropathic ulcer.
4. Identify patients who require referral for vascular assessment, nutritional assessment, orthotics, or diabetes management.
5. Identify key components of a patient education program for the patient with diabetic neuropathy.

In 1998, history was made when the first recombinant human platelet derived growth factor, REGRANEX (becaplermin) gel 0.01%, was approved for use in the management of diabetic foot ulcers. This product is an adjunct in the management of neuropathic foot ulcers and is discussed in this chapter. However, before a discussion of the management strategies for diabetic foot ulcers, this chapter discusses the etiology and pathogenesis of peripheral neuropathy, which can accompany diseases such as diabetes mellitus and Hanson's disease. Diabetic peripheral neuropathy is the focus of this discussion.

The patient with neuropathy often presents with multiple problems, including ulcerations, foot deformities, and circulatory changes. The challenges facing the patient and nurse provide a perfect opportunity for the multidisciplinary team approach to management. Although this approach may be costly, the potential for early recognition of problems with rapid referral for proper management proves cost effective in improved healing, limb salvage, continued patient ambulation, and a decrease in ulcer recurrence. Members of several disciplines may be involved in the care of the patient with a neuropathic foot, including the wound care nurse, advanced practice nurse, diabetologist/endocrinologist, orthopedic surgeon, vascular surgeon, orthotist/pedorthist, dermatologist, and physical therapist.

After the discussion of peripheral neuropathy, prevention strategies for maintaining skin integrity of the neuropathic extremity are covered. These prevention opportunities are also applicable once the ulcer is healed. Finally, management strategies for the diabetic foot ulcer are discussed. Management of the ulcer must extend beyond the actual topical management if successful healing is to be achieved and maintained. The wound care specialist is often asked to recommend or provide the newest and presumed greatest dressing or medication. However, in the absence of glycemic control and in the absence of adequate management of tissue load (pressure), even the newest and greatest interventions will be defeated.

EPIDEMIOLOGY AND COST

Peripheral neuropathy can accompany diseases such as diabetes mellitus and Hanson's disease. The exact cause of diabetic peripheral neuropathy is unknown but is probably multifactorial. Diabetic peripheral neuropathy tends to be bilateral and symmetric. Patients complain of pain, paresthesias, and paradoxically, a diminished or absent ability to feel pain and temperature. Neuropathic pain, however, must be distinguished from ischemic pain and can be determined when the patient is asked if the pain is relieved by walking. Neuropathy is the presumed cause when pain is relieved by ambulation. The neuropathic foot is often termed the *insensate foot.*

Neuropathy is the most important risk factor leading to ulceration and is present in more than 80% of diabetic patients with foot ulceration (Levin, 1995). Of the estimated 16 million individuals with diabetes in the United States, approximately 15% will develop a foot ulcer (Reiber, Boyke, and Smith, 1995). Diabetics are 15 times more likely than nondiabetics to develop an ulcer, which will lead to amputation, and the incidence of amputation increases with increasing age. Approximately 50,000 diabetic patients per year have lower-extremity amputations, and of these individuals, approximately 50% will develop an infected ulcer of the contralateral limb within 18 months. Approximately 50% to 60% of patients having a lower extremity amputation will have an amputation involving the contralateral limb within 3 to 5 years of the first amputation (Reiber, Boyke, and Smith, 1995). The 3-year mortality after the first amputation is as high as 50% (LeFrock and Joseph, 1995).

As a result of these statistics, clinical care must be aggressive and comprehensive. A study by Apelqvist, Larsson, and Agardh (1993) evaluated foot ulcer recurrence and cumulative amputation and mortality rates in patients with previous foot ulcers. The study included evaluation of patient care by a multidisciplinary foot care team including a diabetologist, orthopedic surgeon, orthotist, podiatrist, and diabetes nurse. Patients were followed from 6 months to 7 years. Findings indicate that patients with primary healing were generally younger and those who healed after amputation were older and had poorer distal perfusion and signs of neuropathy. New ulcers were slightly more common among patients with a previous amputation during the first 4 years of observation. In both age- and gender-matched populations; mortality rates were twice as high in patients with diabetes.

There is a high cost both financially and in human suffering associated with diabetic neuropathy and ulceration. Financially, approximately $300 million per year in direct hospital costs is incurred in the treatment of diabetic foot infections. The average cost to heal a single diabetic ulcer in a traditional health care setting using traditional therapies is $36,000 (Glover et al, 1997). Primary amputation has been estimated to cost from $25,000 per procedure to more than $40,000 per procedure (LeFrock and Joseph, 1995). Rehabilitation after amputation may take as long as 6 to 9 months to maximize walking ability. During the rehabilitation phase, the patient may experience missed work, costs related to rehabilitation services, and social and emotional effects. The long-term costs, although difficult to quantify, include prevention and treatment of new ulcers, treatment of complications, and the costs of disability from previous and recurrent ulcers. During the 3-year study period reported by Apelqvist, Larsson, and Agardh in 1995, the calculated costs for the patient who healed with minor amputation were $43,100 and the averaged costs for the patient with a major amputation were $63,100. The findings of increased cost for both minor and major amputations further emphasize the need for a long-term prevention program for patients at risk. This program must include screening to identify those truly at risk because the insidious nature of the neuropathy may mean that a patient does not realize that he or she cannot feel a hidden danger.

The high financial cost and the high cost in human suffering through ulcer occurrence, recurrence, amputation, and decreased long-term survival rates indicate that there has been little improvement in preventing morbidity from foot ulcers in the past few decades (Reiber, 1992). There are data to support the use of meticulous, scientifically based wound care and patient education strategies to reduce lower-extremity amputation rates by reducing the frequency and severity of foot ulcers (NIH and NIDDK, 1998). Most clinicians agree that a multidisciplinary approach is important in managing these patients most effectively. Furthermore, new approaches, such as growth factors, that have a more direct physiologic effect on wound healing are becoming increasingly studied for the management of chronic wounds (Mast and Schultz, 1996).

PATHOLOGY

Neuropathy is the impairment of nerve function and is one of the most frequently reported complications of diabetes. The incidence of neuropathy appears to be related to the duration of diabetes and, to some extent, the degree of glycemic control. Two hypotheses have been proposed to explain the cause of neuropathy:

1. Hyperglycemia leads to intracellular accumulation of sorbitol and other metabolites. This subsequently leads to reduced myoinositol, reduced Na^+ - K^+ATPase activity, and ultimately nerve damage (Catanzariti, Blitch, and Karlock, 1995; Veves and Sarnow, 1995).
2. Microvascular disease is implicated. The presence of microvascular disease has been shown to result in endoneural hypoxia and subsequent nerve fiber loss. It is likely that both metabolic changes and vascular changes contribute (Page and Chen, 1997).

Three types of neuropathy occur: sensory, motor, and autonomic. These can occur in isolation or together.

Sensory Neuropathy

Sensory neuropathic changes are the most disastrous because the loss of sensation puts the patient at risk for mechanical, chemical, and thermal trauma. The soles of the feet, thickened from a daily regimen of abuse, provide feedback to the surrounding cells, structures, and brain only after a weight of 250 mg/mm^2 is applied (Christman, 1971). When slides of color-coded feet are reviewed, the way a healthy person with intact sensation puts feet to the ground changes radically with continued walking. At the beginning a long hike, the feet are placed heel-toe, heel-toe, but at the end of the hike, the foot is lifted and set down as one unit, all adjustments having been made subconsciously. Muscular fatigue does not cause the shifts. Instead, pain cells in the toes, heels, and lateral bones are intermittently informing the brain. A patient with neuropathy, having lost this intercellular conversation, will walk without changing gait or shifting weight. The same pressure strikes the same cells with unrelenting force, and ulcers develop. This individual simply "walks through their skin" (Brand and Yancey, 1984).

There are additional unfortunate and preventable injuries to the foot from stepping on nails, using a heating pad to warm cold feet, using chemical callus and corn removers, or wearing new shoes that are too tight. Thermal injury causes additional damage because the extremity with peripheral vascular disease (PVD) can maintain a resting blood flow. However, when presented with an increased demand, the system cannot respond and tissue malnourishment, or even death, occurs (Plate 27). Levin and Sicard (1987) provides the following cogent scenario:

> At an ambient foot temperature of 70° F, a patient requires one milliliter of blood flow per 100 grams of tissue per minute. A patient with even moderate PVD can manage this. Soaking the foot in hot water can quickly raise the skin temperature to 104° F. This requires an increase of 10 times the flow of blood. A patient with PVD cannot achieve this. The results are blistering, ulceration, infection and/or gangrene, and often amputation.

Motor Neuropathy

Motor neuropathy from impairment of the nerves controlling musculature results in muscular atrophy in the foot and creates two basic problems. The most common example is muscle atrophy in the toes, which causes the toes to remain in a state of constant flexion (claw toes). As a result, the tips or tops of the toes may rub against the shoes, leading to ulceration (Plate 28). Foot deformities such as cocked-up toes, or hammer toes, develop and the patient's gait changes. These gait changes cause repetitive stresses on areas of the foot, usually a metatarsal head, rather than distributing the stresses of walking more uniformly. Adding to the pressure on the metatarsal head is the thinning of the protective fat pads, which results in even higher pressures. Callus build-up is the first sign of repetitive stress and will progress to ulceration if the weight is not properly redistributed with special shoes (orthotics) (Coleman, 1988) (see Figures 13-4 to 13-7). These ulcers are sometimes referred to as *neuropathic, neurotrophic, trophic, perforating,* or *malperforans* ulcers (Plate 29).

Autonomic Neuropathy

Autonomic neuropathy is the third category of peripheral neuropathy. A principal symptom is distal anhydrosis, the absence of sweating. Anhydrosis results in xerosis (dry skin) and predisposes the patient to develop cracks and fissures. A chronically dry or moist interdigital environment on the foot favors selective bacterial or fungal flora (Plate 30). These bacteria or fungi that gain entry to soft tissues through the cracks and fissures penetrate further into the soft plantar tissues with repetitive stresses of ambulation and may cause infection, gangrene, and amputation. Additional symptoms of autonomic neuropathy are the loss of skin temperature regulation and autosympathectomy. The increased blood flow to the lower limb as a result of autosympathectomy leaves a patient with a warm, insensitive foot at risk for neuropathic ulceration. These individuals may be mistakenly reassured of good circulation as the dorsal veins become dilated and the foot has rubor without increased warmth (Murray and Boulton, 1995).

PATHOLOGY OF ULCERATION

It is likely that a long history of uncontrolled or poorly controlled diabetes will lead to peripheral neuropathy, retinopathy with vision loss, and nephropathy. This results in trauma as depicted in Figure 13-1. Ulcerations are the result of repetitive stress, unrelieved pressure, and trauma in an insensate foot.

ASSESSMENT

Risk Assessment

Several risk factors have been associated with the presence of ulceration. Although there is general agreement on the significance of most risk factors, the strength of association of the risk factors varies in the literature. It may be more significant for the clinician to evaluate the number of risk factors with which a patient presents rather than attempting to weigh the individual factors (Box 13-1). Lavery and colleagues (1998) found a linear relationship between level of risk and number of risk factors present (i.e., level of risk increased as the number of risk factors present increased). In their study, three categories of risk were analyzed:

1. Loss of protective sensation
2. Presence of deformity
3. History of amputation

Relative risk of ulceration was 1.7 for patients with only loss of protective sensation, 12.1 for patients with loss of protective sensation and deformity, and 36.4 for patients with all three risk categories present.

Limited joint mobility as a risk factor for ulceration is essential to understand (Thomson et al, 1991). In the diabetic, limited motion of the small joints in the foot increases abnormal pressures at the

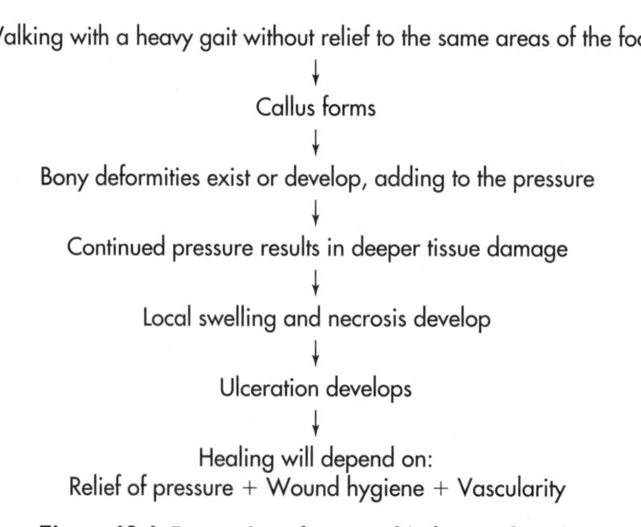
Walking with a heavy gait without relief to the same areas of the foot
Callus forms
Bony deformities exist or develop, adding to the pressure
Continued pressure results in deeper tissue damage
Local swelling and necrosis develop
Ulceration develops
Healing will depend on:
Relief of pressure + Wound hygiene + Vascularity

Figure 13-1 Progression of neuropathic foot to ulceration.

base of those joints, further leading to callus formation. The glycosylation of collagen causes thickening and cross-linking of collagen bundles, causing the skin to become thick, waxy, and tight with resulting restriction of both large and small joint movements (Murray and Boulton, 1995). This stiffness limits movement in the subtalar joint, contributing to elevated plantar pressures in the foot and susceptibility to ulceration. Shearing forces are subsequently increased under stiff joints, resulting in rubbing and skin breakdown. There are additional risk factors that also contribute to the formation of ulcers, including the elderly who live alone or with an equally elderly and infirmed partner, those with mental confusion, those with no support system, or those who have economic difficulties.

Physical Examination

A thorough examination includes visual inspection of both feet, a vascular assessment for ischemia, and neurosensory testing. Examination should also include a basic history and physical as well as a diet history and evaluation of glycemic control. However, these components of the examination are beyond the scope of this chapter and are not discussed.

The physical examination conducted by the wound care nurse should emphasize an examination of the foot so that the origin of the problem can be identified and appropriate corrective actions can be taken. Box 13-2 lists parameters to be included in a foot examination. Signs of elevated pressure can be detected by visual inspection of the feet and include callus. The presence of callus is very important as ulcers are often found under them. Callus is a firm, thickened area on the foot from repeated pressure or shear. It worsens the problem of pressure in the insensate foot because the area of callus itself adds a pressure point that the individual is unaware of walking on. Structural deformities such as hammer toes and claw toes may also contribute to increased pressure and facilitate ulceration (Plate 28). A bunion, if present, further makes shoe fitting difficult and can lead to ulceration (Plate 2). This is an area that is also subject to pressure in the bed-bound individual.

Neuroosteoarthropathy, or Charcot's joint, is a progressive destruction of the bone joint that results in bony protrusions in the foot, which in turn lead to pressure-induced ulceration (Grunfeld, 1991; Murray and Boulton, 1995). The patient with the early stages of Charcot's joint presents with a hot, red, and swollen foot with bounding pulses and prominent veins. Early presentation of Charcot's joint may be mistaken for cellulitis. Over time, metatarsals and bones of the ankle fragment, the arch collapses, and the result is a rocker-bottom configuration of the foot. This subjects the arch of the foot, which is least capable of handling pressure, to maximum pressure, resulting in tissue breakdown and ulceration of the arch (Levin, 1993).

BOX 13-1 Risk Factors Associated with Ulceration in the Patient with Neuropathy

Peripheral neuropathy
Structural foot abnormality
Limited joint mobility
Elevated, sustained pressure
Previous history of ulcers
History of amputation
Retinopathy
Nephropathy
Duration of diabetes
Suboptimal glycemic control
Increased age (elderly)
Vascular insufficiency
Inadequate footwear

BOX 13-2 Examination of the Foot

1. Risk factor assessment
2. Visual inspection for rubor, pallor, callus, dry skin, edema, foot deformity, amputation, ingrown toenails, fissures, etc.
3. Vascular assessment for pulses, dorsal vein distention, temperature
4. Sensory assessment for pressure, touch, vibration
5. Motor assessment to observe for joint rigidity, muscle wasting, gait disturbance

TABLE 13-1 Wagner Classification of Diabetic Foot Ulcers

GRADE	CHARACTERISTICS
0	Preulcerative lesions Healed ulcers Presence of bony deformity
1	Superficial ulcer without subcutaneous tissue involvement
2	Penetration through the subcutaneous tissue involvement
3	Osteitis, abscess, or osteomyelitis
4	Gangrene of digit
5	Gangrene of the foot requiring disarticulation

A vascular assessment is also indicated in the patient with diabetes and an insensate extremity. The presence or absence of palpable pulses should be assessed. The nurse needs to consider that the presence of warmth and distended dorsal veins may be falsely reassuring of adequate blood flow, yet it may be a result of autosympathectomy. (A complete discussion of assessment for ischemia is presented in Chapter 12.)

Neurosensory testing should be part of the examination of the foot. An easy and inexpensive device to establish neuropathy is the Semmes-Weinstein monofilament (Caputo et al, 1994). The device has hairlike filaments of different diameters that are touched to various areas of the plantar surface of the foot, avoiding areas of heavy callus build-up. Inability to sense the 5.07 monofilament correlates with neuropathy. Because the development of neuropathy is gradual and insidious, the patient does not know that he or she has it and the presence of neuropathy will not be detected unless the nurse tests for it.

If an ulcer is found, then its dimensions (size, depth) and the degree of the involvement of underlying tissues should be noted. If no deep skin breakdown is apparent but there are signs of pressure on the periwound epidermis, the patient should be advised to change shoe gear so that continued pressure does not lead to deep ulceration (van Rijswijk, 1997). The standard scale most commonly used for grading diabetic ulcers is based on a system developed by Wagner (1981) and outlined in Table 13-1. The system describes five grades of ulcer based on appearance and depth. In general, grades 1 to 3 occur in patients with neuropathic feet without vascular disease, and grades 4 and 5 occur most frequently in patients with neuropathy and vascular disease (Boulton, 1991).

An additional component of assessment is an evaluation of the patient's gait and footwear. Watching the patient walk into the office or examination room allows the nurse to observe for gait disturbance. The individual with sensory neuropathy walks with a heavier, more plodding gait as the feedback mechanism allowing awareness of contact with the floor is diminished or absent. The footwear also reveals unusual wear patterns, which may indicate where areas of increased pressure are located. In the individual with special shoes or inserts, it is important to assess for signs of wear, which indicate both wear patterns and clues as to how often a shoe is being worn.

MANAGEMENT

When managing ulcers on the lower extremity, it is essential that the nurse be able to distinguish between ulcers caused by trauma in the patient with peripheral neuropathy and those caused by arterial insufficiency (Table 6-2). Furthermore, the nurse should understand the effects that peripheral neuropathy has on PVD. According to Levin (1990), three times more patients with diabetes are admitted to a hospital for foot ulcers caused by an insensitive, neuropathic foot than patients admitted because of ischemic pain.

The ulcer of neuropathic origin may be in a well-perfused extremity; but if PVD coexists, the diminished blood supply prevents oxygen and antibiotics from reaching the ulcer, which retards or prevents healing. In summary, the signs and symptoms of ischemia must be differentiated from peripheral neuropathy caused by diabetes. However, the nurse must keep in mind that it is entirely possible for the patient to have a combination of both PVD and neuropathy.

The goals of management of the patient with diabetic neuropathy are listed in Box 13-3. These

BOX 13-3 Goals for Patient with Diabetic Neuropathy

1. Identify risk factors for prevention and complicating management
2. Identify ulcer etiology
3. Locally manage the wound environment
4. Obtain or maintain glycemic control
5. Prevent recurrence
6. Identify referrals needed for assistance with the plan

goals are established as a team with the patient as a member of the team.

Foot Protection

Trauma from chemical, thermal, and mechanical sources must be avoided when the patient has neuropathy because this insensate state has diminished protective sensation in the diabetic patient, a disease known to impair wound repair. Box 13-4 provides a guide to enhance recognition of common sources of trauma and hence facilitate prevention.

BOX 13-4 Patient Instruction for Care of the Diabetic Foot

1. Do not smoke.
2. Inspect the feet daily for blisters, cuts, and scratches. A mirror can aid in seeing the bottom of the feet. Always check between the toes.
3. Wash feet daily. Dry them carefully, especially between the toes.
4. Avoid temperature extremes. Test water with elbow before bathing.
5. If feet feel cold at night, wear socks. Do not apply hot water bottles or heating pads. Do not soak feet in hot water.
6. Do not walk on hot surfaces such as sandy beaches or on the cement around swimming pools.
7. Do not walk barefoot.
8. Do not use chemical agents to remove corns and calluses. Do not use corn plasters. Do not use strong antiseptic solutions on the feet.
9. Do not use adhesive tape on the feet.
10. Inspect the inside of shoes daily for foreign objects, nail points, torn linings, and rough areas.
11. If your vision is impaired, have a family member inspect your feet daily, trim the nails, and buff down calluses.
12. Do not soak feet.
13. For dry feet, use a very thin coat of lubricating oil such as baby oil. Apply the oil after bathing and drying the feet. Do not put oil or cream between the toes. Consult your physician or diabetes nurse educator for detailed instructions.
14. Wear properly fitting stockings. Do not wear mended stockings. Avoid stockings with seams. Change stockings daily.
15. Do not wear garters.
16. Shoes should be comfortable at the time of purchase. Do not depend of shoes to stretch out. Shoes should be made of leather. Running shoes may be worn after checking with your physician.
17. Do not wear shoes without stockings.
18. Do not wear sandals with thongs between the toes.
19. In winter, take special precautions. Wear wool socks and protective footgear, such as fleece-lined boots.
20. Cut nails straight across.
21. Do not cut corns and calluses. Follow special instructions from your diabetes nurse educator, physician, or podiatrist.
22. Avoid crossing your legs. This can cause pressure on the nerves and blood vessels.
23. See your physician regularly and be sure that your feet are examined at each visit.
24. Notify your diabetes nurse educator, physician, or podiatrist at once if a blister or sore has developed on your feet.
25. Be sure to inform your podiatrist that you are a diabetic.

It is critical that the patient be taught to visually examine the feet on a regular basis. If the patient has a corresponding retinopathy, a family member or other person of the patient's choosing may be instructed to assist. The patient should also be advised against walking barefoot and to feel inside the shoe before putting it on. Recently one patient presented with a new foot ulcer having recently recovered from a contralateral limb amputation. She described her inability to locate her glasses all day, and when she removed her shoe that evening, the glasses had been in her shoe all day.

Avoidance of trauma when the patient has arterial insufficiency is not difficult because the pain in the extremity serves as a reminder to be cautious. However, in the presence of peripheral neuropathy, ischemic tissues may not always be painful. The hospitalized patient with neuropathy serves as an excellent example. A patient with diabetes and coexisting peripheral neuropathy who is in bed, in surgery, or otherwise supine for a period of time (recuperating from an illness) will not sense the discomfort of pressure-induced ischemia to the heels and hence the need for a position change. If PVD is also present, tissue damage can be swift and limb threatening.

Providing complete pressure relief by the heels entirely off the mattress is essential. Care should be taken to avoid elevating the heels too high because such a position would compromise blood flow. Furthermore, it should be reinforced that heel protectors do not reduce pressure. Operating room staff and radiology staff should be alerted to the role that they play in preventing trauma so that they may position and transfer the patient safely.

The neuropathic extremity is also more vulnerable to trauma because neuropathy makes temperature sensation difficult, if not impossible. Although the patient with arterial insufficiency may complain of cold legs or feet, the patient with neuropathy may not feel temperature changes. Patients with diabetes should never use hot-water bottles, heating pads, or foot soaks to "warm-up" the feet because warmth increases the demand for blood. Although the discussion of neuropathy has been primarily directed to the foot, the nurse needs to also assess the upper extremities. It is not uncommon to see burns on the fingers from hot beverages or a cigarette with hand glove neuropathy. If neuropathy is present with arterial insufficiency and this increased demand for blood cannot be met, tissue injury results.

Debridement

Existing wounds should be evaluated for the need for surgical debridement. Surgical debridement is an effective and rapid method to remove all devitalized tissue and callus, and in the presence of neuropathy it may be possible to accomplish with no or minimal anesthesia. Small ulcers can be debrided in the patient's home, at the bedside, or during an office visit. Steed and colleagues evaluated 118 patients with diabetic foot ulcers being treated as a part of a multicenter study of growth factor (Steed, 1995). It was discovered that the site with the lowest debridement rate also had the lowest healing rate. Surgical debridement allowed a more thorough examination of the wound base for hidden pockets of pus and the removal of senescent cells (Steed et al, 1996).

Alternatives to surgical debridement include mechanical debridement with high-pressure water spray jets to remove loose debris. Some nurses use wet-to-dry dressings; however, this technique may result in the removal of periwound skin stuck to the dressing (Kennedy and Tritch, 1997). Several other products and dressing materials have been developed to induce debridement either through enzymes or by allowing enzymes in the body's serum to lyse tissue. These alternative methods to surgical debridement have not been proven through research and should be used judiciously with defined end-points in place. Although necrotic tissue is in place, the normal process of liquefaction is occurring under the surface. If trapped by an adherent cover, it will flow along fascial planes, causing additional damage to the structures of the foot.

Offloading of Pressure and Stress

As neuropathic bone and muscle changes develop and callus tissue forms, the foot becomes increasingly vulnerable to ulcerations. Inappropriate footwear is the most common factor leading to foot ulcer in the patient with neuropathy and is the easiest

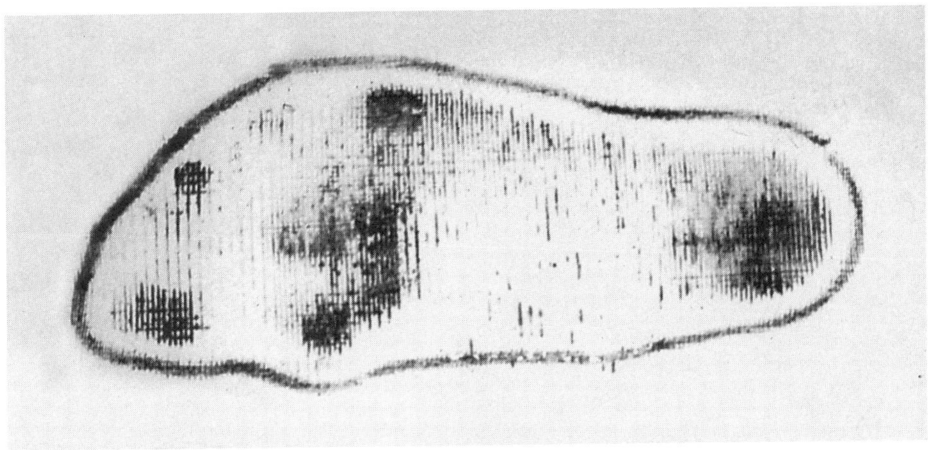

Figure 13-2 Harris mat pressure map and tracing can be performed to identify where pressure is being directed. (Courtesy David M. Osterman)

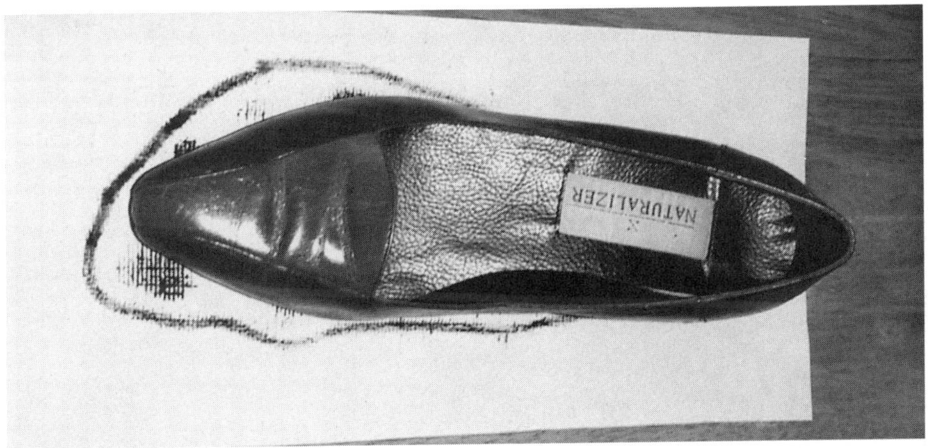

Figure 13-3 Tracing of foot in contrast with patient's shoe demonstrates disparity. (Courtesy David M. Osterman)

to correct. Ill-fitting, tight, or shallow shoes increase pressure and shear on the foot. Ulcers may develop on the sole of the foot, along the side of the foot, or on top of the foot under the laces. Patients may be inadvertently wearing a shoe that is tight fitting in an attempt to "feel" the shoe on their foot. A very simple tool in helping patients realize that their shoe size has changed is to trace the foot on a piece of paper while the patient is standing (Figure 13-2). Cut out the tracing and place the patient's shoe over the tracing (Figure 13-3). Any disparity in fit will become readily apparent. Interventions for offloading include orthotics and contact casting.

Orthotics are specially fit shoes that are indicated to redistribute the weight of the foot, thus preventing mechanical trauma from shear and repetitive stress to the foot (Coleman, 1988; Levin, 1990). The orthotist uses a variety of visualizations, molds, and pressure mappings to appreciate where the pressure is being focused (see Figure 13-2). This

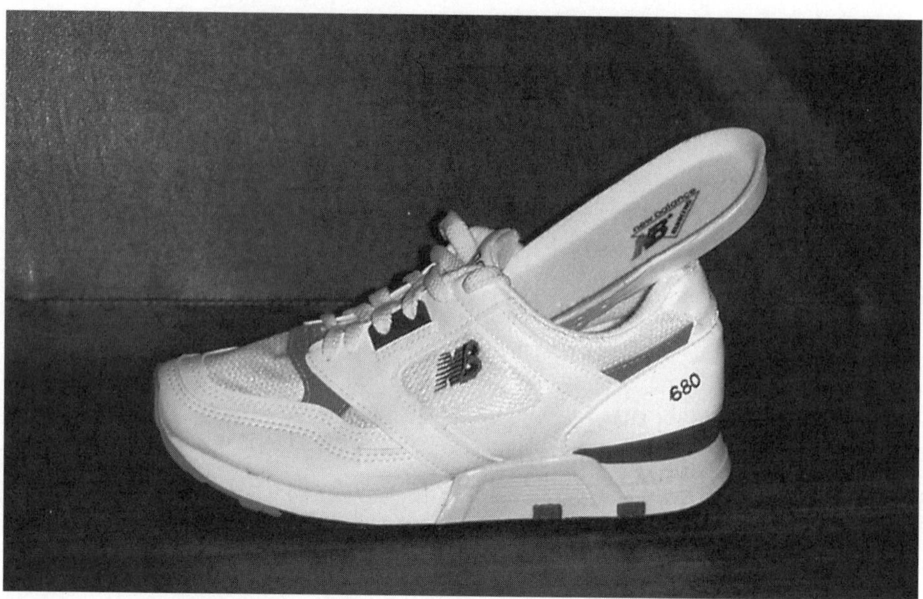

Figure 13-4 A type of orthotic: an extra-depth shoe with an insert.

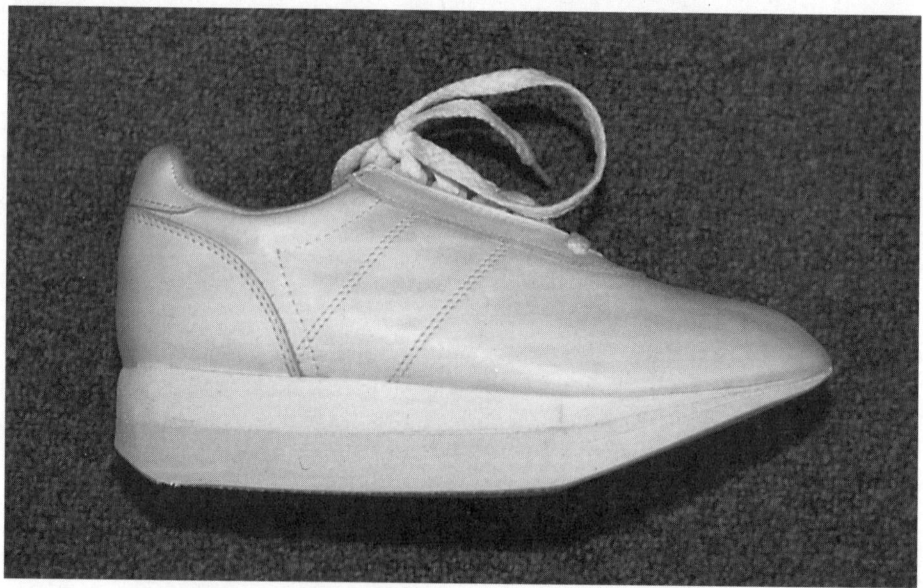

Figure 13-5 An orthotic shoe used to decrease pressure to the forefoot.

helps design the appropriate shoe or insert to best redistribute the pressure across the surface area of the foot and lower leg (Figures 13-4 to 13-7).

Total contact casting is a temporary intervention that redistributes the weight of the foot and increases the surface area of contact when an ulcer is present (Coleman, Brand, and Birke 1984). Originally the contact cast was used for the insensate foot of patients with Hansen's disease (leprosy). Unfortunately, the insensate foot lacks the sensory

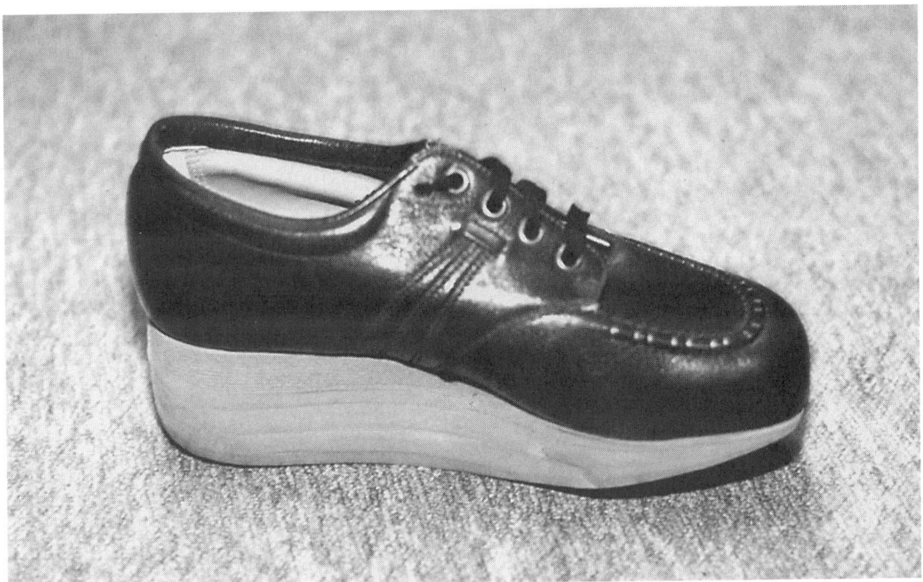

Figure 13-6 An orthotic shoe.

signals that prompt the person to shift gait pattern, remove a rock from the shoe, or rest. Consequently, ulcers that are largely the result of repetitive stress and shear develop on the plantar or dorsal surface of the foot. Because the contact cast reduces the pressure of walking to an insignificant amount, it can be applied when the patient already has a plantar ulcer (Figures 13-8 and 13-9).

To apply the cast, the ulcer should be debrided, any callus tissue should be removed, and the edema should be allowed to resolve. Contact casting is contraindicated in the presence of cellulitis, sinus tracts, or profuse drainage and in patients with an inconsistent pattern of keeping follow-up appointments.

With the patient in a prone position and the leg bent so that the foot is in the air, the cast material is wrapped carefully around the leg. Application begins at the toes, encloses the toes, and continues up the foot and leg to the knee. Wrapping should be loose and without wrinkles. Loose application allows the plaster to be molded over prominences and into uneven skin surfaces. Once applied and as the cast is drying, the plaster is massaged to enhance conformance to the shape of the extremity. To prevent the soiling of clothing from the plaster as it dries, self-

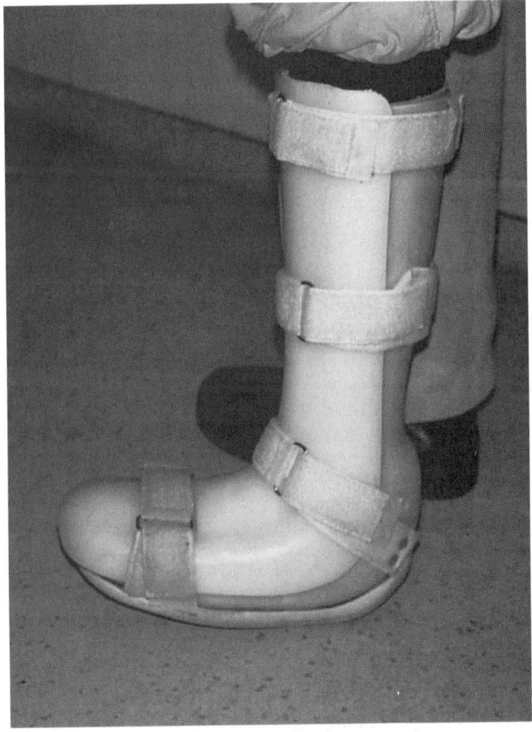

Figure 13-7 An orthotic shoe with rocker bottom.

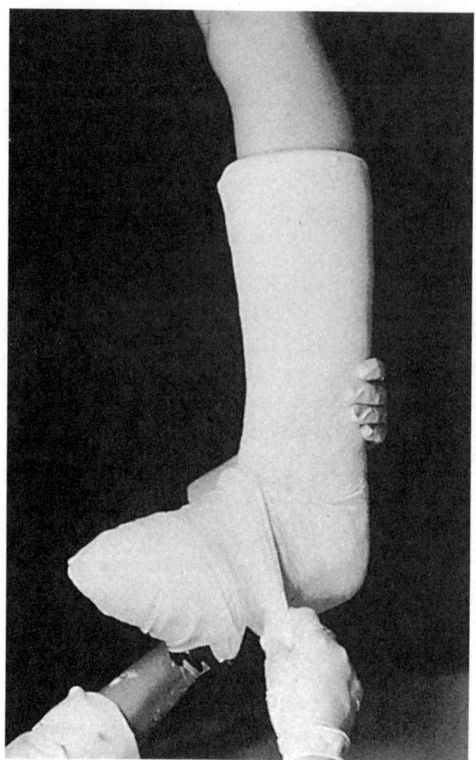

Figure 13-8 Contact cast is applied to foot and lower leg; stockinette can then be applied to protect other leg. (From Levin ME, O'Neal LW, Bowker JH: *The diabetic foot,* ed 5, St Louis, 1995, Mosby.)

adherent tape can be applied to the surface of the cast once it is in place. Contact casts are left on for 3 to 7 days depending on the amount of drainage from the wound. Patients can walk with the cast in place, once it dries, after approximately 24 hours.

A nonadherent dressing and topical antiseptics have been used to cover the wound in preparation for the cast. To prevent interdigital maceration, cotton padding or lamb's wool is applied between the toes.

Local Wound Care

Local wound care should consist of cleansing to remove local contaminants and debris and covering with a dressing that will maintain a moist wound environment without allowing wound desiccation or overhydration (Rodeheaver, 1997). The topical dressing should not be so bulky as to provide an additional source of externally applied pressure. Several dressing products exist that can assist the nurse with local management. There are no known studies that clearly identify one type of product as superior to another in wound healing. Considering the propensity for wound infection to occur in the diabetic foot, occlusive dressings should be used cautiously if at all.

Currently, bioengineered tissue is being used in the clinical research arena as a possible method of treatment of the diabetic foot ulcer. At this writing, Apligraf is the only bioengineered tissue approved for clinical use; however, it is approved in the United States for venous ulcers, not diabetic foot ulcers. Dermagraft is currently being researched for the diabetic foot ulcer; however, it is not yet approved.

REGRANEX gel is the first prescription therapy clinically proven to actively help promote healing in diabetic neuropathic foot ulcers. The mechanism of action of most growth factors is primarily local. This is important because REGRANEX gel is applied topically. REGRANEX gel is the first recombinant platelet-derived growth factor (PDGF) approved by the FDA for the treatment of deep diabetic neuropathic foot ulcers (it is not blood-derived). Binding of the PDGF to its receptor initiates signaling for a range of molecular and cellular responses, such as chemotaxis, mitogenesis, and synthesis, which are necessary for wound healing to occur. When used as an adjunct to good wound care, including sharp debridement, pressure relief, and infection control, REGRANEX gel increases the incidence of complete healing of diabetic ulcers. The gel is applied in a thin layer to a clean wound bed and covered with a gauze dressing dampened with normal saline. Care should be taken to prevent the ulcer from drying out and not adding too much bulk to the gauze dressing. Approximately 12 hours after the initial application, the wound should be gently rinsed and a dressing dampened with normal saline should be applied. If the ulcer size does not decrease by approximately 30% after 10 weeks of treatment or complete healing has not occurred in 20 weeks, continued treatment with REGRANEX gel should be reassessed.

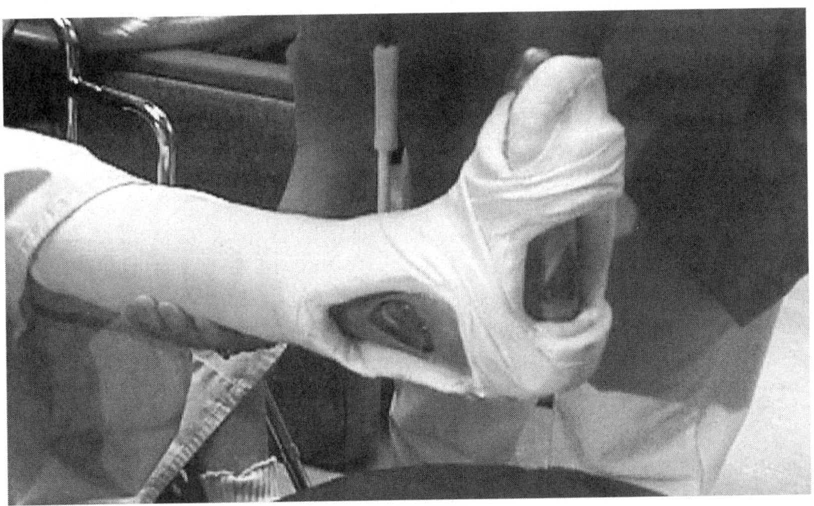

Figure 13-9 Modified total contact cast applied to offload pressure from neuropathic plantar ulcer that developed after prolonged use of a multi-podus boot (L'nard splint). By creating a window in the cast over the pressure ulcer located near the medial malleolus and a window over the plantar neuropathic ulcer, topical dressings can be reapplied without removing the cast. The cutout portion or window of the cast can then be reapplied over the dressing and secured with self-adhering tape (Coban [3M, Co.]) to restore the integrity of the cast. (Courtesy Ted Tomter, RN, CWOCN, St. Joseph's Candler Health System, Savannah, Ga.)

COMPLICATIONS

Foot infections are a frequent cause of limb loss and morbidity in the diabetic. Increased blood glucose levels lead to reduced resistance to infections and increased blood viscosity, further decreasing blood flow (Ehrlichman, 1991). Impaired neutrophil function in combination with peripheral vascular abnormalities cause a hypoxic wound, which increases the potential for a necrotizing infection. An infection can develop in any open wound, breaking the skin's defense against bacteria. Once in the wound of a diabetic, bacteria are able to multiply in an environment optimal for their survival: blood flow is diminished, WBCs may have suboptimal function, and oxygenation is poor. The microbiology of infections of the diabetic foot tends to be complex and usually polymicrobial. It is important to identify the offending organisms accurately to select the most appropriate antimicrobial agent. There are insufficient data to support the use of swab-type cultures because they may identify colonizers and not the source of infection (Robson, 1991). A deep tissue specimen is the most reliable method for identifying the source of infection (Swartz, 1995). For additional information, see Chapter 8.

Lower-extremity amputations in the diabetic result from the contribution of a combination of causes. Pecoraro, Reiber, and Burgess (1990) described causal pathways responsible for 80 consecutive initial lower-extremity amputations in diabetic patients over a 30-month period. The investigators identified a critical triad of minor trauma resulting in cutaneous ulceration and that a subsequent failure of wound healing preceded 72% of the amputations. The seven factors contributing to amputation are ischemia, gangrene, infection, neuropathy, faulty wound healing, initial minor trauma, and ulceration (Pecoraro, Reiber, and Burgess, 1990).

PATIENT EDUCATION

Patient education is an important component of management. Education needs to be relevant, simple, and complete in an attempt to assist patients to their highest level of functioning. Education, however, does not equal knowledge. It often takes the presentation of material multiple times by different members of the health care team to achieve understanding.

In general, issues to be covered in a patient education program should include concepts related to glycemic control, smoking cessation (when applicable), and how and when to contact the physician or other health care provider. Patients should also be advised on how to avoid trauma to their feet, proper foot hygiene, and proper shoe selection, including where to obtain appropriate footwear and the importance of daily foot inspection. It may be necessary to explore resources available in the patient's community that will allow the patient to follow the educational plan.

The patient is being instructed in a large number of things and may be overwhelmed by the teaching plan. Key aspects of the plan require behavior change on the part of the patient, and behavior change is possible but not necessarily easy. The patient needs to be encouraged to make appropriate choices, adopt behavior changes, and believe that doing so is both possible and will translate into an improved outcome. It is also important to impart that the responsibility for the change belongs to the patient. The nurse is responsible for providing the education; however, the patient makes the decision to accept or reject the information.

SUMMARY

Peripheral neuropathy places the patient at risk for ulceration attributable to mechanical, thermal, or chemical trauma. Management of ulcers in the neuropathic or insensate foot has many similarities to the management of ulcers on the extremity with arterial insufficiency. However, the neuropathic foot also has some unique care requirements, which primarily focus on prevention of injury through diligent foot care and orthotics.

Peripheral neuropathy may occur with or without arterial insufficiency. Effective management can occur only when the dangers of neuropathy are appreciated and the status of arterial perfusion is appropriately evaluated.

SELF-ASSESSMENT EXERCISE

1. Identify three types of diabetic neuropathy and the effects of each on skin integrity.
2. True or False: When culturing diabetic foot lesions, needle aspiration provides more accurate results than a swab culture.
3. Which of the following findings are suggestive of osteomyelitis in the patient with a diabetic foot ulcer?
   a. Abnormal bone scan
   b. Nonhealing ulcer
   c. Abnormal x-ray film findings
   d. All of the above
4. Identify factors other than topical therapy that must be addressed in the management plan of a diabetic foot ulcer.
5. Identify routine precautions that one should include in the teaching of the patient with neuropathy.
6. Identify members of the health care team and their roles in the management of the patient with neuropathy.

REFERENCES

Apelqvist J, Larsson J, Agardh C: Long-term prognosis for diabetic patients with foot ulcers, *J Intern Med* 233:485, 1993.

Boulton AJM: Clinical presentation and management of diabetic neuropathy and foot ulceration, *Diabet Med* 8:S52, 1991.

Brand P, Yancey P: *In His image,* Grand Rapids, Mich, 1984, Zondervan.

Caputo G et al: Assessment and management of foot disease in-patients with diabetes, *N Engl J Med* 331:854, 1994.

Catanzariti A, Blitch E, Karlock L: Elective foot and ankle surgery in the diabetic patient, *J Foot Ankle Surg* 34:23, 1995.

Christman R: *Sensory experience,* Scranton, Penn, 1971, Intext Educational Publishers.

Coleman WC: Footwear in a management program of injury prevention. In Levin M, O'Neal L, editors: *The diabetic foot,* ed 4, St Louis, 1988, Mosby.

Coleman WC, Brand PW, Birke JA: The total contact cast: a therapy for plantar ulceration on insensitive feet, *J Am Podiatr Assoc* 74(11):5481, 1984

Glover J et al: A 4-year outcome-based retrospective study of wound healing and limb salvage in-patients with chronic wounds, *Adv Wound Care* 10:33, 1997.

Grunfeld C: Diabetic foot ulcers: etiology, treatment and prevention, *Adv Intern Med* 37:103, 1991.

Kennedy K, Tritch D: Debridement. In Krasner D, Kane D, editors: *Chronic wound care: a clinical source book for healthcare professionals,* Wayne, Penn, 1997, Health Management Publications.

Lavery LA et al: Practical criteria for screening patients at high risk for diabetic foot ulceration, *Arch Intern Med* 158(2):157, 1998.

LeFrock J, Joseph W: Bone and soft-tissue infections of the lower extremity in diabetics, *Clin Podiatr Med Surg* 12:87, 1995.

Levin ME: Diabetic foot lesions: pathogenesis and management, *J Enterostom Ther* 17(7):29, 1990.

Levin ME: Pathogenesis and management of diabetic foot lesions. In Levin M, O'Neal L, Bowker J, editors: *The diabetic foot,* ed 5, St Louis, 1993, Mosby.

Levin ME: Preventing amputation in the patient with diabetes, *Diabetes Care* 18:1383, 1995.

Levin ME, Sicard G: Evaluating and treating peripheral vascular disease. Part I, *Clin Diabetes* 62, 1987.

Mast B, Schultz G: Interactions of cytokines, growth factors, and proteases in acute and chronic wounds, *Wound Rep Reg* 4:411, 1996.

Murray J, Boulton A: The pathophysiology of diabetic foot ulceration, *Clin Podiatr Med Surg* 12:1, 1995.

National Institutes of Health, National Institute of Diabetes and Digestive and Kidney Diseases: Prevention and early intervention for diabetes foot problems. In *Feet can last a lifetime,* Bethesda, Md, 1998, NIDDK.

Page J, Chen E: Management of painful diabetic neuropathy—a treatment algorithm, *J Am Podiatr Med Assoc* 87:370, 1997.

Pecoraro RE, Reiber GE, Burgess EM: Pathways to diabetic limb amputation: basis for prevention, *Diabetes Care* 13(5):513, 1990.

Reiber GE: Diabetic foot care: financial implications and practice guidelines, *Diabetes Care* 15(suppl 1):29, 1992.

Reiber GE, Boyke E, Smith D: Lower extremity foot ulcers and amputations in diabetes. In National Insitutes of Health: *Diabetes in America,* ed 2, Bethesda, Md, 1995, NIH, NIH Pub. No. 95-1468.

Robson M: Wound healing and wound closure. In Heggers J, Robson M, editors: *Quantitative bacteriology: its role in the armamentarium of the surgeon,* Boca Raton, Fla, 1991, CRC Press.

Rodeheaver G: Wound cleansing, wound irrigation, wound disinfection. In Krasner D, Kane D, editors: *Chronic wound care: a clinical source book for healthcare professionals,* ed 2, Wayne, Penn, 1997, Health Management Publications.

Steed D: Clinical evaluation of recombinant treatment of lower extremity diabetic ulcers, *J Vasc Surg* 21:71, 1995.

Steed D et al: Effect of extensive debridement and treatment on the healing of diabetic foot ulcers, *J Am Coll Surg* 183:61, 1996.

Thompson FJ et al: A team approach to diabetic foot care: the Manchester experience, *Foot* 2:75, 1991.

Van Rijswijk L: Wound assessment and documentation. In Krasner D, Kane D, editors: *Chronic wound care: a clinical source book for healthcare professionals,* ed 2, Wayne, Penn, 1997, Health Management Publications.

Veves A, Sarnow M: Diagnosis, classification, and treatment of diabetic peripheral neuropathy, *Clin Podiatr Med Surg* 12:19, 1995.

Wagner FW: The dysvascular foot: a system for diagnosis and treatment, *Foot Ankle* 2:64, 1981.

CHAPTER

14

Management of Drain Sites and Fistulas

BONNIE SUE ROLSTAD & RUTH A. BRYANT

OBJECTIVES

1. Identify factors contributing to fistula formation.
2. List three complications that contribute to mortality from fistulas.
3. Describe three ways to classifiy fistulas.
4. Identify the four phases of medical management for the patient with a draining wound or fistula.
5. List factors known to impede spontaneous closure of fistula tracts.
6. Describe surgical procedures commonly used to close or bypass fistula tracts.
7. List eight goals for nursing management of the patient with a fistula.
8. Describe four factors to be considered when assessing the patient with a draining wound or fistula.
9. Explain the role of four different types of skin barriers, including their indications for use.
10. Identify features to be considered when selecting a fistula pouch.
11. Briefly describe the "bridging" technique, and identify indications for use.
12. Identify options for odor control in a wound managed with dressings and in a wound managed with pouching.

The presence of a draining site or fistula can be a frustrating and disheartening experience to the patient and family because it represents a major catastrophe. It can also be a difficult experience for the nurse; however, management can be quite rewarding when effluent is successfully contained, odor is controlled, the patient is comfortable, and realistic resolution is observed. Caring for this patient population requires astute assessment skills, knowledge of pathophysiology, competent technical skills, and knowledge of equipment alternatives.

INCIDENCE AND ETIOLOGY

The incidence of fistula formation is difficult to determine because it varies widely according to the involved organs, precipitating factors, and referral patterns of the surgeon and institution. However, in most series as much as 90% of enterocutaneous fistulas arise immediately after a surgical procedure and are the result of anastomotic breakdown (Chamberlain, Kaufman, and Danforth, 1998; Fischer, 1983; Reber et al, 1978; Sansoni and Irving, 1985).

Several factors are recognized as contributing to the development of a fistula in the immediate postoperative period:

1. Presence of a foreign body close to the suture line
2. Tension on the suture line
3. Improper suturing technique
4. Distal obstruction
5. Hematoma or abscess formation in the mesentery at the anastomotic site
6. Presence of tumor or disease in the area of anastomosis
7. Inadequate blood supply to the anastomosis

Many of these contributing factors are preventable with basic surgical principles of anastomotic construction (Wong and Buie, 1993).

Fistulas may also develop spontaneously, associated with either intrinsic intestinal disease (such as Crohn's disease, diverticulitis, malignancy, small bowel obstruction, and irradiation) or external trauma (Hollender et al, 1983; Sansoni and Irving, 1985). Patients who have been treated for a gynecologic malignancy are particularly vulnerable for fistula formation because of the increasingly aggressive nature of the treatment (Jones, Woodhouse, and Hendry, 1984; Smith, Pierce, and Lewis, 1984).

An inadequate blood supply can be a consequence of surgical procedures and of radiation therapy. Because surgical procedures require dissection and disruption of vascular structures, tissues can be left somewhat devitalized. Irradiation triggers occlusive vasculitis, fibrosis, and impaired collagen synthesis, a process termed *radiation-induced endarteritis.* Unfortunately, because this endarteritis persists, complications may develop immediately after radiation or years later. Irradiation-induced fistulas most commonly occur when coexisting processes (e.g., atherosclerosis, hypertension, diabetes mellitus, pelvic inflammatory disease, and previous pelvic surgery) already compromise capillary perfusion (Devereux, Sears, and Ketcham, 1980; Smith et al, 1985).

The patient with a fistula experiences a 6% to 20% chance of death despite improvements made in intraoperative technique, sepsis diagnosis and management, perioperative care, and nutritional support (Berry and Fischer, 1996; Fischer 1983; Moser and Roslyn, 1998). In a recent study, Schein and Decker (1991) reported a 37% mortality rate in high-output, postoperative, enterocutaneous fistulas. This wide range in mortality rates is reflective of the differences in patient populations. Complications that contribute to this mortality rate have long been recognized to be the result of electrolyte imbalance, malnutrition, and sepsis (Chamberlain, Kaufman, and Danforth, 1998; Edmunds, Williams, and Welch, 1960).

TERMINOLOGY

Definitions

A fistula is an abnormal passage between two or more structures or spaces. This can involve a communication tract from one body cavity or hollow organ to another hollow organ or to the skin (Figures 14-1 to 14-3). A draining wound, drain site, or wound dehiscence should not be misinterpreted as a fistula.

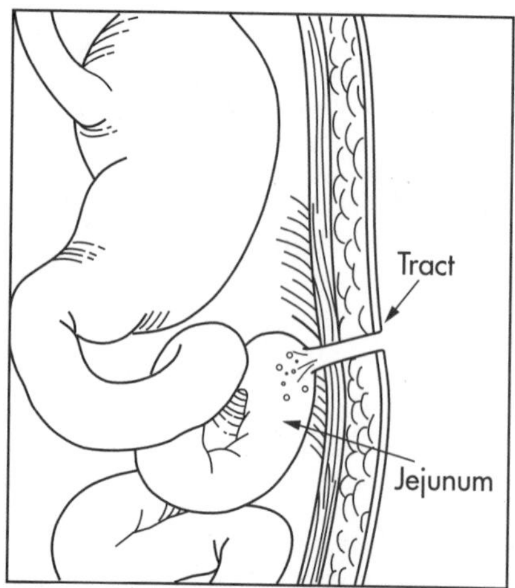

Figure 14-1 Simple enterocutaneous fistula.

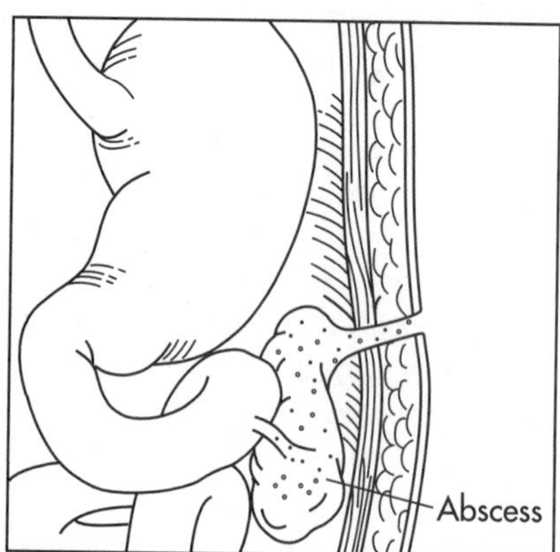

Figure 14-2 Complex type 1 fistula with associated abscess.

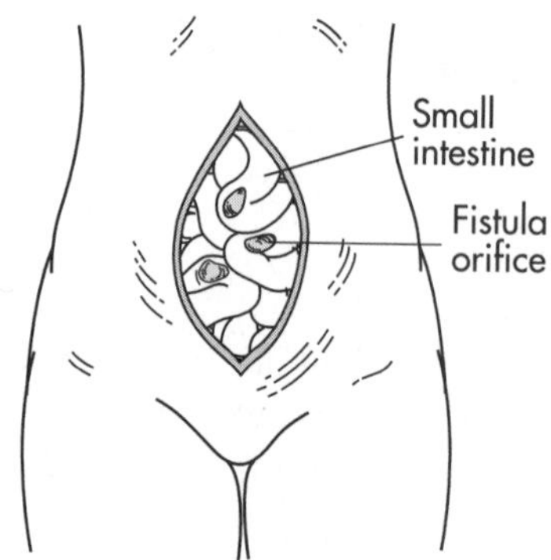

Figure 14-3 Complex type 2 fistula with multiple openings associated with large abdominal wall defect.

BOX 14-1 Classification of Fistulas by Complexity

Simple
- Short, direct tract
- No associated abscess
- No other organ involvement

Complex

Type 1
- Associated with abscess
- Multiple organ involvement

Type 2
- Opens into base of disrupted wound

TABLE 14-1 Fistula Classification

Location	Internal	Tract contained within body
	External	Tract exits through skin
Involved structures	Colon	Colon
	Entero-	Small bowel
	Vesico-	Bladder
	Vaginal	Vagina
	Cutaneous	Skin
	Recto-	Rectum
Volume	High output	Over 200 ml per 24 hours
	Low output	Under 200 ml per 24 hours

Modified from Boarini J, Bryant R, Irrgang S: Fistula management, *Semin Oncol Nurs* 2:287, 1986.

Classification

Fistulas may be classified as simple or complex (Box 14-1) or according to location, involved structures, or volume of output (Table 14-1). These classifications are useful in predicting the morbidity rate, mortality rate, and potential for spontaneous closure (Wong and Buie, 1993). An internal fistula is one where the fistula tract is located inside the body, whereas an external fistula exits cutaneously or within the vagina or rectum. More specific nomenclature is used to identify the involved structures (such as enterocutaneous or rectovaginal); thus the name specifies the structures that adjoin the fistula tract. Examples of such terminology are listed in Table 14-2.

TABLE 14-2 Fistula Terminology

FROM	TO	NAME	INTERNAL/ EXTERNAL
Pancreas	Colon	Pancreatico-colonic	Internal
Jejunum	Rectum	Jejunorectal	External
Intestine	Skin	Enterocutaneous	External
Intestine	Colon	Enterocolonic	Internal
Intestine	Bladder	Enterovesical	Internal
Intestine	Vagina	Enterovaginal	External
Colon	Skin	Colocutaneous	External
Colon	Colon	Colocolonic	Internal
Colon	Bladder	Colovesical	Internal
Rectum	Vagina	Rectovaginal	External
Bladder	Skin	Vesicocutaneous	External
Bladder	Vagina	Vesicovaginal	External

Modified from Irrgang S, Bryant R: Management of the enterocutaneous fistula, *J Enterostom Ther* 11:211, 1984.

Fistula output is a direct reflection of the fistula's site of origin. Large bowel fistulas typically have low output, whereas small bowel fistulas can have either high or low output. *High-output fistulas* are most commonly defined as those producing more than 200 ml/24 hr (Soeters, Ebeid, and Fischer, 1979), although some authors use 500 ml/24 hr as the demarcation (Fazio, Coutsoftides, and Steiger, 1983; McIntyre et al, 1984; Rombeau and Rolandelli, 1987). This type of fistula is associated with higher morbidity and mortality rates and a lower spontaneous closure rate (Sitges-Serra, Jaurrieta, and Sitges-Creus, 1982; Soeters, Ebeid, and Fischer, 1979).

Manifestations

The passage of gastrointestinal secretions or urine through an unintentional opening onto the skin heralds the development of a cutaneous fistula. Manifestations of a fistula exiting through the vagina (i.e., rectovaginal or vesicovaginal) include passage of gas, feces, or urine through the vagina. Irradiation-induced rectovaginal fistulas are often preceded by diarrhea, the passage of mucus and blood rectally, a sensation of rectal pressure, and a constant urge to defecate (Rothenberger and Goldberg, 1983). Typically a rectovaginal fistula produces an odorous vaginal discharge. Fistulas between the intestinal tract and the urinary bladder (such as colovesical) present with passage of gas or stool-stained urine through the urethra.

MEDICAL MANAGEMENT

Goal of Management

The ultimate goal when managing the patient with a fistula is closure of the fistula either spontaneously or surgically. Such a goal requires patience, astute assessment skills, and the cooperation of many health care specialists. Comprehensive and effective medical management of the patient with a fistula requires attention to five objectives: fluid and electrolyte replacement, perifistular skin protection, infection control, adequate nourishment, and measures to enhance closure (Kurtz, Heimann, and Aufses, 1981; Reber and Austin, 1989).

Phases of Management

For convenience and practicality the medical management of patients with fistulas is divided into four phases: stabilization, investigation, conservative treatment, and definitive therapy (Wong and Buie, 1993). Within each phase, attention to fluid and electrolyte balance, skin protection, infection control, nutritional support, and closure plans is necessary.

Stabilization. Approximately 5 to 9 liters of fluid rich in sodium, potassium, chloride, and bicarbonate are secreted into the gastrointestinal tract daily. The loss of fluid and electrolytes that accompanies the presentation of a high-output fistula may result in hypovolemia and circulatory failure. Such blood-volume imbalances must be corrected before further treatments can be instituted. Adequate tissue perfusion and urine output must be maintained. Potential electrolyte imbalances should be anticipated and can be inferred when one knows the electrolyte composition of the gastrointestinal secretions.

There are additional components to the patient's medical profile that must be stabilized. Immediate surgery is imperative when 1) a septic focus has been identified, 2) uncontrolled hemorrhage has developed, or 3) an evisceration is present. The presence of systemic or local sepsis must be evaluated and treated with surgical drainage and antibiotics. Effective drainage can be accomplished by use of surgical or radiographic techniques; the specific approach depends on abscess location, patient status, and available resources. Antibiotics are necessary only in the presence of an infection. Causative organisms of sepsis are commonly of bowel origin: coliform, bacteroides, and enterococci. Staphylococci may also be present. Sepsis is the major cause of death in patients with enteric fistulas (Moser and Roslyn, 1998; Fischer, 1989), and these bacteria proliferate rapidly in the poorly vascularized tissue typically surrounding fistulas. Finally, intestinal output must be minimized. This can be achieved by placing the patient on NPO (nothing by mouth) status (to decrease luminal contents and decrease gastrointestinal stimulation and pancreaticobiliary secretion) and by administering H_2 antagonists (to prevent stress ulcerations and decrease gastric secretions) and somatostatin analogs (to inhibit secretions from the stomach, pancreas, biliary tract, and small intestine). Somatostatin's most encouraging results are with postoperative, high-output small bowel fistulas; spontaneous closure rates increased from 50% to 90% (Nubiola et al, 1989). It is less effective with intrinsic bowel diseases such as ulcerative colitis or Crohn's disease (Hild et al, 1986).

Investigation. After stabilization, the fistula must be examined to ascertain 1) the origin of the fistulas tract, 2) the condition of adjacent bowel, 3) the presence of additional abscess pockets, and 4) the presence of distal obstruction or bowel discontinuity. Water-soluble contrast agents (i.e., Renografin, Hypaque, or Gastrografin) are preferred to visualize the fistula tract and administered through a soft-tip catheter. A computerized tomography (CT) scan is indicated only when the patient is not responding to conservative treatment. If other organs are involved, additional tests such as a cystoscopy or intravenous pyelogram are indicated (Wong and Buie, 1993).

Conservative Treatment. Malnutrition is a significant complication that most patients with a fistula experience. Several factors contribute to the fistula patient's poor nutritional status. Often the patient is malnourished before the fistula develops.

There are many factors contributing to malnutrition and negative nitrogen balance, including reduced protein intake, inefficient nutrient use, excessive losses of protein-rich fluids (especially from pancreatic and proximal jejunal fistulas), and muscle protein breakdown that occurs with sepsis.

Adequate nutritional support is achieved when the patient is maintained in a state of positive nitrogen balance and receives adequate vitamin and trace mineral replacement. The amount of calories and protein required will depend on the patient's preexisting status, sepsis, and fistula output. Caloric needs range from 30 to 40 cal/kg/24 hr; the goal should be a calorie-nitrogen ratio of 150:1. Protein requirements are estimated at 1.5 to 1.75 g/kg/24 hr (Fischer, 1983) or 0.25 to 0.35 g of nitrogen/kg body weight/24 hr (Wong and Buie, 1993). It is important to initiate nutritional support without delay because the caloric deficit alone accumulates at the rate of 1800 to 2700 cal/day (Fischer, 1989). Trace elements, multivitamins, and vitamin K must be given twice weekly; large gastrointestinal losses are associated with low levels of magnesium (Wong and Buie, 1993).

The route of nutritional support is contingent upon the patient's ability to ingest sufficient quantities, the location of the fistula tract, the absorptive capacity of the bowel mucosa, and patient tolerance. The preferred route of nutritional support is always the gastrointestinal tract. Continued use of the gastrointestinal tract has been shown to maintain the normal structure of the intestine and prevent atrophy of the villi (Moran and Greene, 1997). Enteral nutrition is appropriate when fistulas are located in the most proximal or distal portion of the gastrointestinal tract; however, the gastrointestinal tract must be functional and the patient cooperative. Many types of enteral solutions are available, and a dietician should be consulted to recommend the most appropriate solution and administration procedure so that those negative sequelae, such as osmolar diarrhea, can be avoided.

Fibrin glue, cyanoacrylate glue, and prolamine have been applied endoscopically at the origin of the fistula to seal the fistula (Eleftheriadis et al, 1990; Hwang and Chen, 1996; Lange et al, 1990). Fibrin glue appears to be the most successful to date. In a report by Eleftheriadis and colleagues (1990), no complications were noted and patients required an average of 2.4 applications. Hwang and Chen (1996) report no adverse reactions to fibrin glue; all 13 patients with a low-output enterocutaneous fistula healed within 4 days and only 2 required a second infusion. The mechanism of action is theorized as the fibrin inducing a cellular response to injury and assisting in neovascularization and fibroblast proliferation (Wong and Buie, 1993). The role of fibrin glue is yet to be determined relative to the complexity of the fistula and timing of the procedure.

Ultimately, conservative treatment can facilitate spontaneous fistula closure in at least 60% to 70% of all enteric fistulas (depending on the etiology and anatomy) when sepsis is controlled (Berry and Fischer, 1996; Fischer, 1983; Rombeau and Rolandelli, 1987; Rose et al, 1986). The time required to achieve spontaneous closure is reported to range from 4 to 7 weeks; 90% of enteric fistulas that close spontaneously will do so within 50 days (Allardyce, 1983; Berry and Fischer, 1996; Fischer, 1983; Rose et al, 1986; Kurtz, Heimann, and Aufses, 1981). Approximately 90% of simple type 1 fistulas close, whereas less than 10% of complex type 2 fistulas close spontaneously (Levy et al, 1989; Sitges-Serra, Jaurrieta, and Sitges-Creus, 1982).

Decision/Definitive Surgery. Several factors have been identified as impediments to spontaneous closure (Box 14-2). If these variables are present and closure of the fistula is the ultimate goal for the patient, a surgical approach is appropriate. Surgical procedures may also be indicated for palliation.

BOX 14-2 Factors that Delay Spontaneous Fistula Closure

- Complete disruption of bowel continuity
- Distal obstruction
- Foreign body in fistula tract
- Epithelium-lined tract contiguous with the skin
- Cancer in site
- Previous irradiation to site
- Crohn's disease
- Presence of large abscess

The exact timing for surgical intervention is variable, depending on the patient's status. Surgical intervention is emergent in the presence of bowel necrosis or abscess (Fazio et al, 1983). Otherwise, operative interventions to close the fistula tract should be delayed until the patient is in optimum condition (i.e., positive nitrogen balance and control of infection). Given that the patient is nutritionally and metabolically stable, definitive surgery for a simple or complex type 1 fistula is appropriate when a persistently draining fistula is in a sepsis-free environment for 6 to 8 weeks (Wong and Buie, 1993). It is important that definitive surgery be delayed until the abdominal wall is soft and supple; tissues should return to a normal soft pliable state, particularly in the presence of irradiated tissue (Rothenberger and Goldberg, 1983; Wong and Buie, 1993).

Complex type 2 fistulas invariably require definitive surgery; however, the timing of surgery is not well defined. Nutritional status, metabolic status, and immunocompetence should be normalized, and the obliterative peritonitis and the inflammation associated with chronic peritoneal contamination should be resolved (Wong and Buie, 1993). Judicious timing of surgery for complex type 2 fistulas is warranted. In one study, the time from fistula diagnosis to definitive operation ranged from 10 weeks to 13 months with a mean time of 4.2 months (Conter, Root, and Roslyn, 1988).

The surgical management of enterocutaneous fistulas usually involves either diversion or resection. Factors such as location, size, and cause of the fistula; the patient's overall status; and the presence of irradiated tissue will determine the approach selected (Smith et al, 1985).

Diversion techniques divert the fecal stream away from the fistula site; removal of the fistula is not accomplished. Resection of the fistula is not always appropriate or possible in the presence of extensive or recurrent malignancy or when there is inadequate tissue perfusion in the vicinity of the fistula (secondary to numerous surgical resections, scar formation, uncontrolled diabetes, or prior irradiation).

Diversion can be achieved by creation of a stoma proximal to the fistula or by the making of an anastomosis (end to end or side to side) of the two segments of bowel on both sides of the fistula (such as an ileotransverse anastomosis when the fistula communicates with the right colon). This latter procedure may be referred to as an *intestinal bypass* in which the segment of bowel containing the fistula is completely isolated and separated from the fecal stream.

When closure of the fistula is the goal, resection of the fistula will be necessary. The advantage of this technique is that the diseased tissue is removed. An end-to-end anastomosis of the intestine with resection of the fistula tract is performed. To protect the anastomosis, diversion of the fecal stream through a temporary stoma may be indicated. If the distal part of the rectum is not suitable for anastomosis or the anal sphincters are not competent, a permanent stoma with a Hartmann's pouch may be the safest procedure.

Enteric fistulas communicating with the urinary tract will always require diversion of the fecal stream proximal to the fistula site to prevent urinary tract infections and pyelonephritis.

NURSING MANAGEMENT

The occurrence of an enterocutaneous fistula is an unplanned event, a step backward in the recovery process (Phillips and Walton, 1992). Unlike the ostomy patient who has the benefit of a preoperative visit and ostomy site marking, the patient with a fistula is physically and psychologically unprepared for this outcome. The occurrence of a fistula lengthens recovery time whether closure is spontaneous or occurs with surgical repair. This section focuses on the technical management of the patient with a fistula. Principles are presented so that management can be tailored to achieve effective solutions. The care plan, however, must also include detailed attention to patient and family needs, involvement, education, and emotional support.

Technically, the fistula patient is the most challenging patient the wound care nurse may encounter. Critical thinking skills are necessary to synthesize assessment data, product knowledge (advantages, disadvantages, effectiveness, and guidelines for use), patient needs, and physiology into realistic goals. Principles of wound care and principles of ostomy management provide an im-

BOX 14-3 Nursing Goals for Fistula Management

- Perifistular skin protection
- Containment of effluent
- Odor control
- Patient comfort
- Accurate measurement of effluent
- Patient mobility
- Ease of care
- Cost containment

portant foundation (WOCN, 1998). Technique is important; the art of how to perform a procedure, what to use when, and how much all contribute to a successful outcome. There is no substitute for experience for complex fistulas; collaboration with an experienced colleague often proves rewarding.

Goals

Effective nursing management of the patient with a fistula strives to achieve eight goals as listed in Box 14-3. Optimally, all the goals are achieved simultaneously; however, that is not always possible and prioritizing is frequently necessary. For example, a pouching system may effectively contain output and odor as well as providing significant skin protection. However, complete mobility may not be possible or the pouching system may be expensive. Interventions to achieve the above goals begin as soon as the patient presents with a fistula; they are not contingent upon medical diagnosis.

Four rules of thumb are important when caring for a patient with a fistula (Rolstad and Wong, 1993):

1. Assess frequently and expect changes.
2. Build flexibility into the care plan.
3. Innovate using the easiest, most practical approach first.
4. Recognize that care of the patient is frequently provided by inexperienced caregivers.

Assessment

The method selected to manage a fistula is guided by the assessment of four key fistula characteristics as outlined in Box 14-4. Since fistulas change in shape and contours over time, repeat assessment and monitoring are necessary, Modifications to the initial containment system are invariably necessary (Scardillo and Folkedahl, 1998; Wiltshire, 1996; Zwanziger, 1999).

BOX 14-4 Fistula Assessment and Documentation Guide

1. Source (e.g., small bowel, bladder, esophagus)
2. Characteristics of effluent
   a. Volume
      (1) Low: <200 ml/24 hr
      (2) High: >200 ml/24 hr (pouching recommended)
   b. Odor? (If yes, describe)
   c. Consistency (e.g., liquid, semiformed, formed, gas)
   d. Composition
      (1) Color (e.g. clear, yellow, green, brown)
      (2) Active enzymes
      (3) Extremes in pH
3. Topography and size
   a. Number of sites
   b. Location(s)
   c. Length and width of each (include patterns)
   d. Openings (e.g., below skin level, at skin level, above skin level)
   e. Proximity to bony prominences, scars, abdominal creases, incision, drain(s), stoma
   f. Muscle tone surrounding opening (e.g., firm, soft, flaccid)
   g. Contours at the fistula opening (e.g., flat, shallow depth [<1/16 inch], moderate depth [1/16 to 1/4 inch], or deep [>1/4 inch])
4. Perifistular skin integrity at each location (e.g., intact, macerated, erythematous, denuded or eroded, ulcerated, infected)

Source. Initially, little information may be available regarding the origin of the fistula or the involved organs (if diagnostic studies have not yet been conducted). However, the nurse can determine probable origin of the fistula based on assessment of fistula output (volume, odor, consistency, and composition) (Table 14-3). This information provides insight into the patient's risk for altered skin integrity and provides decision points for selection of the management approach. For example, a fistula

TABLE 14-3 Characteristics of Gastrointestinal Secretions

					ELECTROLYTE CONCENTRATION			
SOURCE	SECRETIONS	pH	24-HOUR VOLUME	COLOR	Na	K	Cl	HCO_3
Saliva	Ptyalin, maltase	6.0-7.0	1000-1200	Clear	20-80	16-23	24-44	20-60
Gastric juice	Pepsin, rennin (chymosin) lipase, hydrochloric acid	1.0-3.5	2000-3000	Clear/green	20-100	4-12	52-124	0
Pancreatic juice	Amylase, trypsin, chymotrypsin, lipase, sodium bicarbonate	8.0-8.3	700-1200	Clear/milky	120-150	2-7	54-95	70-110
Bile	Bile salts, phospholipids	7.8	500-700	Golden brown–greenish yellow	120-200	3-12	80-120	30-50
Duodenum Jejunum Ileum	Peptidase, trypsin, lipase, maltase, sucrase, lactase	7.8-8.0	2000-3000	Gold–dark gold	80-130	11-21	48-116	20-30
Colon		7.5-8.9	50-200	Brown	4	9	2	—

Modified from Given BA, Simmons SJ: *Gastroenterology in clinical nursing,* ed 4, St Louis, 1984, Mosby; Rombeau J, Caldwell M: *Clinical nutrition: enteral and tube feeding,* ed 3, Philadelphia, 1997, W.B. Saunders.

producing semiformed, odorous effluent is likely communicating with the left transverse or descending colon. The effluent composition will be less damaging to the skin than effluent from the ileum, and containment of effluent and odor management would be the primary goals in management.

Characteristics of Effluent. Characteristics of effluent that must be considered in fistula management include volume, odor, consistency, and composition. In general, the fistula with volumes over 100 ml/24 hr requires a pouch or, in extreme situations, suction.

Odor is also a decision point when selecting a management method. The fistula patient with pungent malodorous output of 10 to 20 ml/24 hr is just as needy of a pouching system to contain odor as the patient with a high output fistula. Odor may originate from numerous sources, including exudate, necrotic or infected tissue, soiled dressings, dressing materials, and chemicals used in treatment.

Consistency of effluent is particularly important when using pouches becuase it affects the type of drainage spout needed and subsequently the type of pouch selected. It will also influence whether additional skin barriers are necessary. Liquid effluent is much more corrosive than thick effluent and results in premature erosion of the skin barrier.

The color of effluent also acts as an indicator of fistula source (see Table 14-3). In the presence of effluent with active enzymes or extremes in pH, the perifistular skin will require aggressive protection. However, all perifistular skin should be monitored and protected from moisture, even when effluent composition does not include active enzymes. Until radiographic studies are performed, the enzymatic and pH composition of the effluent can be implied from the volume and consistency of the drainage.

Cutaneous Opening. The size of the opening is determined by measuring the length and width in centimeters. A pattern is always useful since a fistula is usually an irregular shape and should be kept in the patient's room with supplies. The fistula opening may appear as a deep tunnel with the base not visible for assessment, or the base may be visible with the fistula exiting at a specific location. In some situations the fistula opening may exit above the skin level as mucosal or granulation tissue. Wound dressings may be warranted to pack the wound (e.g., alginates or foams) when the fistula is present in a deep wound base.

Abdominal Topography. Patient assessment is performed in a supine and semi-Fowler's position. The cutaneous fistula locations are identified and documented. The area is then assessed for the presence of irregular skin surfaces that are created by scars or creases (Plates 11 and 31). This assessment indicates how flexible the adhesive in contact with the skin must be and whether filling agents, such as skin barrier paste or strips, are needed to fill irregular surfaces (Plate 32). Additionally, the number of cutaneous fistula openings, the location of each, and the proximity to bony prominence or other obstacles (i.e., retention sutures or stoma) are assessed and documented. These characteristics will help to determine what size and shape of adhesive surface is needed to secure the sites, yet avoid impinging on the prominence or protrusion. If two cutaneous sites are too far apart to be pouched in one system, two pouches may be necessary.

Muscle tone in the area and skin contours are also assessed. Lack of exercise, weight gain, and aging result in decreased muscle tone. Aging affects subcutaneous tissue support. Muscle tone may be characterized as firm, soft, or flaccid.

It is also important to assess the level at which the fistula opening exits onto the skin. Contours of the skin surrounding the fistula opening may be classified as flat, shallow (<1/16 inch), moderate depth (1/16 to 1/4 inch), or deep (>1/4 inch) (Rolstad and Boarini, 1996). Fistulas emptying into deep open wounds require more pouch adaptations than fistulas emptying flush with intact skin.

Perifistular Skin Integrity. Perifistular skin condition should be assessed and documented at each dressing or pouch change. Constant exposure of the epidermis to moisture, active enzymes, extremes in pH of fluids, and mechanical trauma frequently lead to breaks in skin integrity. Denudation of perifistular skin is a common complication in fistula patients and is often present when the patient first presents with the fistula. Skin constantly bathed in fluid causes maceration, whereas effluent with enzymatic drainage or extremes in pH levels will create erythema and denuded or eroded perifistular skin. Although it is best to visually inspect the skin, data can also be obtained from the nursing staff and patient to aid assessment. For example, when frequent dressing changes (every 4 hours) are reported, skin will deteriorate quickly as a result of chemical and mechanical injury. Patient reports of burning or stinging sensations around the fistula or wound commonly indicate denudation of the epidermis.

Patients with fistulas may also develop an infection in the perifistular skin as a result of entrapment of moisture against the skin. The origin of the infection is most commonly fungal and is characterized by an erythematous, papular rash with satellite lesions (Plate 11). Although less common, herpes zoster skin lesions may also occur. At times it may be difficult to distinguish between the erythema caused by such an infection and the erythema caused by chemical irritation from contact with the effluent.

Planning and Implementation

Four key questions should be asked when planning the approach to technical management of a fistula:

1. Is the volume more than 100 ml/24 hr?
2. Is odor a problem?
3. Is the fistula opening less than 3 inches?
4. Is an access cap needed?

Figure 14-4 is an algorithm that incorporates these four questions to guide decision making for managing a fistula.

Fistulas can be managed with pouches, dressings, suction, or all three. When planning the specific fistula management approach, the nurse must consider the four key questions discussed previously and the goals that have been identified by the health care team and patient. In most situations, the priority goals are containment of effluent, odor control, and perifistular skin protection. Initially some goals may be compromised, such as ease of care, patient mobility, and cost containment because of the acuteness of the situation. This section presents nursing interventions that facilitate attainment of each goal for the nursing management of fistulas.

Goals

Perifistular skin protection. The potential for skin breakdown is always present when a fistula exists regardless of the management option selected. Preventive strategies should be implemented early with frequent monitoring. Protective strategies include atraumatic adhesive removal and protection of the skin from exposure to effluent. Dressings alone do not offer skin protection, thus the concurrent use of a skin barrier is often necessary. Skin barriers are available in various forms (Figure 14-5). Table 14-4 summarizes the characteristics and indications of each type.

If pouching is selected as the management approach, solid wafer skin barriers are usually integrated into the pouching system during manufacturing. However, additional skin-barrier products may be required to caulk edges, fill creases, and/or add convexity.

At times, skin-barrier wafers and pastes need to be applied over an intact incision as a part of the management system. This is done to secure the system and prevent leakage of effluent from the fistula onto the incision.

Skin-barrier powders are used to absorb moisture from denuded skin and to create a dry surface. Adhesives or ointments can then be applied to the dry surface. For severely denuded skin, it may be necessary to create an "artificial scab" with the skin-barrier powder by alternating layers of the skin-barrier powder and a skin sealant or skin cement. The pouching system may then be applied directly over the artificial scab. To enhance adherence, it may be desirable to apply either skin cement or spray adhesive to the artificial scab and pouch adhesive surface. Skin-barrier powders should not be confused with talc or cornstarch, which do not provide skin protection.

In non-pouching management approaches, petroleum-based or zinc-based ointments are used to provide skin protection. These products are particularly useful in low-volume, odorless fistulas and are usually inexpensive. They are applied to perifistular skin, particularly the edges, and covered with dressings. Ointments are not intended for use under adhesives. Frequency of application is indicated

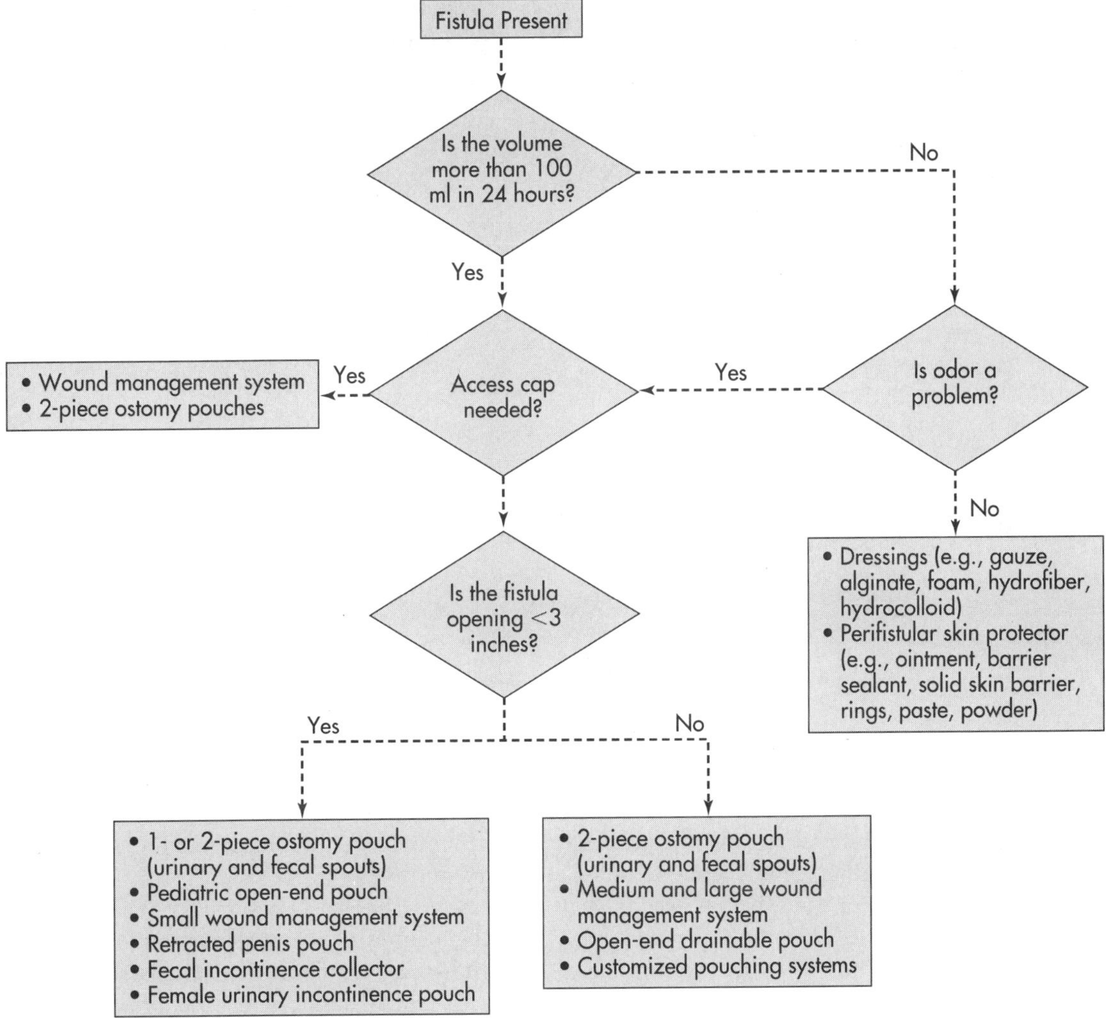

Figure 14-4 Selecting a fistula pouch: an algorithm. (Designed by B. Rolstad.)

on the product and may differ depending on the product formulation and use.

Containment of effluent. Containment of effluent is accomplished with nonpouching and pouching approaches. The volume of effluent, presence of odor, abdominal contours, and care setting influence which approach is most effective.

Nonpouching options. Nonpouching options are indicated when 1) fistula output is low (less than 100 ml/24 hr), 2) odor is not present, and 3) skin contours or the location of the fistula makes pouching impossible. Containment of effluent can be achieved with dressings intended for absorption, which include gauze (sponges or strip packing), alginates, foam, hydrofibers, hydrocolloids, and combinations of dressings (e.g., alginates covered with transparent film). When a cavity exists, semiocclusive products, such as

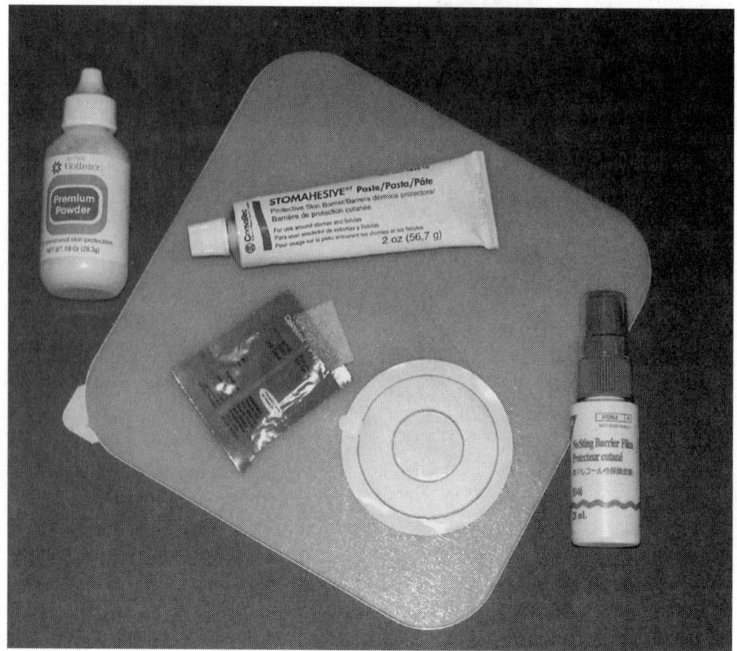

Figure 14-5 Examples of skin barriers: wafer, paste, ring, powder, sealant.

hydrocolloids, transparent films, and foams, are not recommended. Packing should only be done with dressing materials that may be retrieved from the wound. For example, a strip packing material may be gently packed into a low-volume drain site. A 2-inch tail of dressing material is left outside the wound and will be used to retrieve the packing at dressing changes.

When volume exceeds 100 ml/24 hr, dressings become less effective and more time intensive. The application of additional dressings will not increase the absorbency of the dressing or lengthen the time between dressing changes. Furthermore, entrapment of effluent against the skin may cause maceration and breakdown. A good rule is that when dressings have to be changed more often than every 4 hours, a pouching system should be used. Conversely, when a fistula site has low volume, a small pouching system may be used so that the patient does not have to change the pouch more than once in 7 days. This approach provides convenience and protects perifistular skin.

Suction catheters. Occasionally, a high-volume fistula requires a nonpouching option. Suction catheters attached to low, intermittent suction may be used when routine pouching is ineffective or overwhelmed by the volume of output (Beitz and Caldwell, 1998; Lange et al, 1989). Suction, however, does not provide complete containment of effluent; dressings and skin protection are still necessary. Effluent must be liquid if suction is to be effective; thick or particulate drainage will occlude the catheter. The wound is cleansed, and a layer of saline-moistened gauze is placed in the wound bed. The catheter is laid in the wound and directed toward the bottom of the setup. Another layer of moist gauze may be applied over the catheter, and a large transparent dressing may be applied as a secondary dressing (Hollis and Reyna, 1985; Jeter, Tintle, and Chariker, 1990). Skin-barrier paste is sometimes necessary to fill in irregular skin sur-

TABLE 14-4 Guide to the Use of Skin Barriers in Fistula Management

TYPE OF SKIN BARRIER	CHARACTERISTICS	INDICATIONS
Solid wafers (4″ × 4″ or 8″ × 8″)	• Pectin-based wafers with an adhesive surface • Available as wafers or rings • Have moist tack • Have varied flexibility • May be cut into wedges, rings, or strips • Have varied durability to effluent • Changed only when they loosen from the perifistular edges or once every 7 days	• Provide skin protection, referred to as *laying down a protective platform* • Level irregular skin surfaces • Protect perifistular skin from effluent when dressings are used or skin is exposed • Gauze dressings are applied over the skin-barrier wafer and taped to the wafer rather than the skin
Skin barrier rings	• Available in hydrocolloid and karaya formulations • Have moist tack • Have varied flexibility • Have varied durability to effluent • Hydrocolloid formulations • Recommended for fistula management	• Level irregular skin surfaces • Protect perifistular skin from effluent when dressings are used or skin is exposed
Paste (tube or strip forms)	• Commercial preparations contain alcohol, which can create burning sensation if skin is denuded • Extremely tacky; should be applied as a thin bead, smoothed into place with a damp gloved finger or tongue blade • Contains solvents; allow to dry briefly so that solvents can escape before other products are applied	• Level irregular skin surfaces • Protect exposed skin from effluent (i.e., with pouching) • Extend duration of solid wafer barrier when pouching
Powder	• Must be used lightly; may be used in combination with sealants to create an artificial scab • Residual powder alters adhesion	• Absorb moisture from superficial denudement before applying ointments or adhesives
Skin sealants	• Liquid, nonalcohol, and alcohol preparations • Nonalcohol skin sealants are indicated for use on denuded skin • Must be allowed to dry to permit solvents to dissipate • Available in various forms (wipes, gel, wands, roll-ons, and pump spray).	• May be used under adhesives to protect fragile skin during adhesive removal • Improve adherence of adhesives to skin (particularly oily skin) • Protect perifistular skin from effluent or maceration when dressings are used • Used in combination with skin barrier powders; creates an artificial scab

faces and to seal around the catheter as it exits from the transparent dressing. Suction tubing is then attached to the suction catheter and set at a low level of continuous suction. A hemovac can provide the suction for short periods of time to increase the patient's mobility. This dressing is usually changed every 1 to 2 days.

A catheter that is inserted into the fistula tract will act as a foreign body and may therefore interfere with healing and even increase fistula output (Welch,

1985). On the other hand, a catheter coiled in a defect above the orifice or in the open wound surrounding the fistula opening will not inhibit closure.

Because firm tubes can injure fragile tissue, only soft, flexible suction catheters should be used with fistulas (Welch, 1985). Suction catheters should be considered a short-term intervention because of the limitations placed on patient mobility and the time-intensive nature of the care

Vaginal fistula drain device. Vaginal fistulas occasionally develop secondary to pelvic irradiation and create a challenging situation where the patient is incontinent of feces through the vagina. The uncontrolled passage of fecal material vaginally results in severe perivaginal skin denudation and discomfort. Aggressive nursing care is essential to prevent these complications.

Skin protection can be achieved with ointments and pads. Frequent dressing changes are necessary to avoid entrapment of caustic drainage contents against the skin. Unfortunately, ointments and pads for vaginal fistulas are less than optimal because they are labor intensive, do not promote patient mobility, do not adequately contain the fecal contents, and fail to control odor. A female urinary incontinence pouch may be useful in these situations and may be connected to straight drainage. However, the difficult location and moist surface surrounding the vaginal orifice make application of an adhesive pouching system challenging.

A vaginal fistula drain device is another method of managing a vaginal fistula and does not require adhesives (Shield HealthCare). This type of system can also be constructed with a Davol breast shield, Evenflo nipple shield, or vaginal diaphragm and a large Malecot catheter (Figure 14-6) (O'Connor, 1983). A cruciate incision is made through the nipple shield or diaphragm through which the catheter is threaded. The shield or diaphragm serves to occlude the vagina so that the drainage is directed down the catheter.

The soft, cone-shaped device, shield, or diaphragm is inserted a short distance into the vagina. The discomfort that such manipulation of the labia and vagina can create for the patient can be minimized by lubrication of the device with a lidocaine (Xylocaine) lubricant. Tubing is attached to the device to channel the fistula contents into a straight drainage collection bag. The drainage tubing can be anchored to the patient's inner thigh.

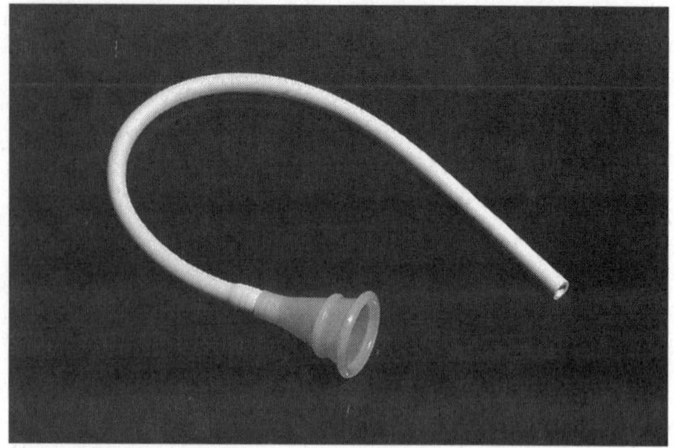

Figure 14-6 Vaginal drain device available commercially (Shield Health Care) or can be configured with Davol breast shield and large Malecot catheter.

A vaginal fistula drain device will remain in place effectively while the patient is reclining. As the patient becomes more ambulatory, the device may have a tendency to become dislodged; however, because the procedure is so easy, the patient can reinsert the vaginal drain as needed. Gentle irrigation of the tubing may be indicated if the tubing becomes occluded by fistula material. A vaginal fistula drain device may be a temporary or permanent management technique depending on the patient's status.

Pouching options. Volume and odor are the primary indications for pouching. Dressings are contraindicated when odor is problematic or the volume of effluent exceeds 100 ml/24 hr. However, patients with low volume, nonodorous output may elect to pouch for convenience. The pouch may be changed once a week and is less expensive than dressings.

Numerous techniques have been reported in the literature for managing fistulas (Boarini, Bryant, and Irrgang, 1986; Irrgang and Bryant, 1984; O'Brien, Landis-Erdman, and Erwin-Toth, 1998; Skingley, 1998; Smith, 1982, 1986). Ostomy pouches (fecal or urinary; adult or pediatric) can be used, as well as pouches specifically designed for managing complex wounds. Pouching offers a sense of control to the patient and nursing staff because effluent is contained and emptied at specific intervals. Pouch changing may be scheduled at convenient times. A routine pouch change procedure is

BOX 14-5 Sizable Pouch-Change Procedure: Fistula

1. Assemble equipment: pouch with attached skin-barrier, pattern, skin-barrier paste, scissors, paper tape, closure clip, water, gauze, or tissue.
2. Prepare pouch.
   a. Trace pattern onto skin-barrier surface of pouch.
   b. Cut skin-barrier pouch to size of pattern.
   c. Remove protective backing or backings from pouch.
3. Remove and apply pouch.
   a. Remove pouch, using one hand to gently push the skin away from the adhesive.
   b. Discard pouch and save closure clip.
   c. Control any discharge with gauze or tissue.
   d. Clean skin with water and dry thoroughly.
   e. Apply paste around fistula or stoma. Fill in any uneven skin surfaces with paste or skin barrier strips. Use a damp finger or tongue blade to apply paste.
   f. Apply new pouch, centering wound site in opening.
   g. Tape edges of adhesive surface in a picture-frame effect with paper tape.
   h. Close bottom of pouch with clip.

BOX 14-6 Features of a Fistula Pouch

Adhesive Surface
- Integrated skin barrier
- Size and shape of cutting surface
- Sizable versus presized adhesive surface
- Presence or absence of starter hole
- Degree of flexibility of skin-barrier wafer

Pouch Capacity
- Volume (3 to 4 hours' capacity preferred)

Pouch Material
- Odorproof or odor-resistant pouch film
- Transparent versus opaque film
- Fecal outlet spout
- Spout for liquids (urinary outlet)
- Wide drain for viscous material
- Wide tubular outlet can be converted to open-end drain

Wound Access
- Two-piece pouch
- Access window on wound-management system
- Wide tubular outlet can be converted to open-end drain

listed in Box 14-5. By preventing the embarrassment of odor and leaking dressings, the patient's dignity is also supported.

Historically, frequent modifications of skin barriers, adhesives, and/or pouches were required to effectively manage the complicated fistula. Few alternatives were available to manage the fistula with a large cutaneous opening, irregular contours of the skin, and other unique situations. Materials used for pouches included garbage bags, colostomy irrigation sleeves, and sandwich bags. Today, however, manufactured wound-management systems are designed for the difficult-to-manage site. Solid wafer skin barriers with new, durable formulations that provide longer wear time are integrated into most pouching systems. Cutting surfaces of the skin barriers are currently available to manage a broad range of fistula opening sizes, from the small opening of a starter hole to 9½ × 6 inches. However, it remains essential to fill irregular skin surfaces so that a flat, stable surface is attained for the pouching system.

Additionally, it may be necessary to select a pouching system that supports the perifistular tissue and stabilizes soft skin. In general, if the skin is soft or flaccid, a firm skin-barrier adhesive and possibly a belt may be indicated. In contrast, firm skin surrounding the fistula site will best be managed with a flexible, soft adhesive surface. Examples of soft, pliable materials include powder, skin-barrier paste, wafers, strips ,and rings, whereas methods to achieve firm support may include firm rings, convexity in ostomy pouching systems, or a belt.

Features of a pouching system. Knowledge of available features of products is essential for the nurse to make appropriate choices. Features include adhesive skin-barrier surface, pouch capacity, pouch film, pouch outlet, and wound access (Box 14-6 and Figure 14-7).

Adhesive skin-barrier surface. When the cutaneous opening is less than 3 inches, a one- or two-piece ostomy pouch may be used. For fistulas greater than 3 inches, commercially available wound-management systems or modifications of larger pouches are

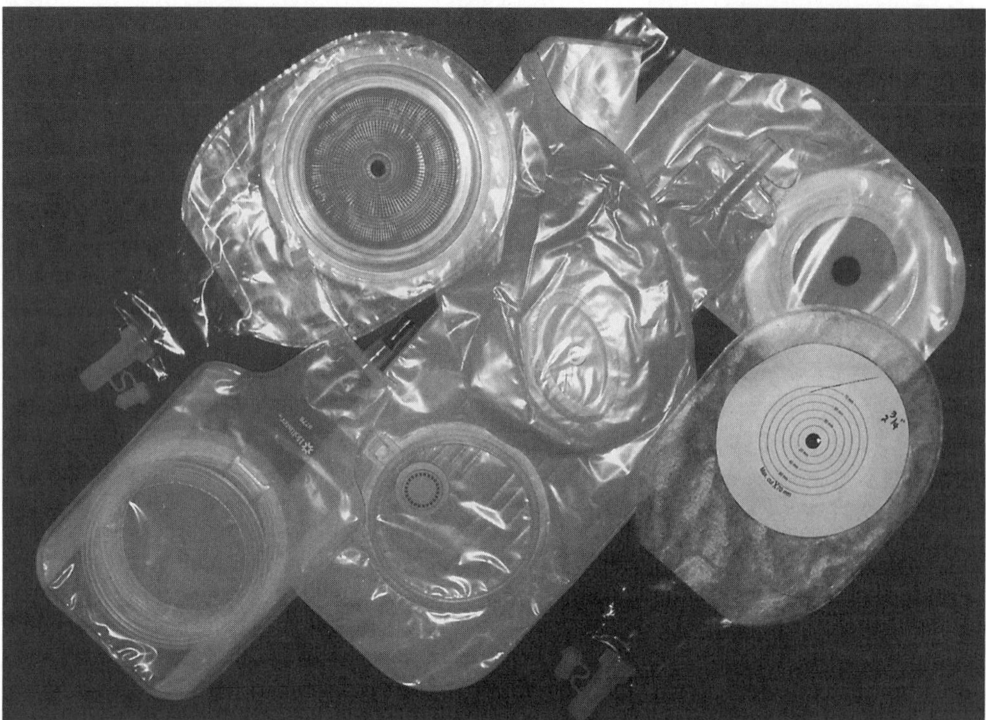

Figure 14-7 Examples of pouches. Notice the variety in sizes for the adhesive surface, the outlet spouts, and the access windows.

warranted. In either case, the adhesive skin-barrier surface must be large enough to accommodate the fistula opening and generally allow for 1 to 2 inches of adhesive contact around the fistula. The adhesive surface should be applied in such a fashion as to avoid obstacles in the perifistular skin area, such as a bony prominence or drain site. If this is not possible it may be necessary to find a pouch with a smaller adhesive surface. Conversely, a large amount of adhesive contact (over 4 to 5 inches) with the surrounding skin is generally not necessary and may be detrimental. Movement-induced skin changes under the adhesive surface will precipitate leakage and disruption of the pouch seal.

Pouching systems may have a starter hole for cutting the opening into irregular shapes or may be presized (e.g., for round, regular shapes). Although starter holes are convenient for cutting, they restrict the positioning of the opening in the adhesive, since the opening includes the starter hole. In some situations the opening may need to be covered with a skin barrier so that other locations on the adhesive may be cut to fit the size of the fistula.

A few pouches are available without an integrated skin-barrier wafer. In these situations, the fistula pattern must be used to cut a hole in the skin-barrier wafer and the pouch. The skin barrier is then attached to the pouch, and the system is applied directly to the skin.

Pouch volume capacity. The capacity of the pouch is predetermined by the size of the adhesive surface; typically pouches with larger adhesive surfaces have larger pouch capacities. Generally, a pouch with the capacity to contain 3 to 4 hours of effluent is recommended so that the risk of leakage is minimized. A smaller-capacity pouch may be used if the caregivers or patient is willing to empty the pouch more frequently or if the pouch can be connected to straight drainage. Small-volume closed-end pouches may also be indicated for the patient with minimal malodorous output. This pouch would be changed and discarded once or twice a week.

Pouch outlet spouts. Consistency and volume of the effluent dictate which outlet spout is best for management. Spouts are available with urinary (or liquid) outlets or fecal outlets (see Figure 14-7). The urinary outlet is indicated for liquid effluent and is convenient because it may be connected to straight drainage. Fecal outlets (or open-end drains) are appropriate for thick, mushy effluent. The two-piece ostomy system, fecal incontinence collectors, and wound-management systems offer the benefit of having a urinary outlet; however, this can be trimmed off to convert the outlet to a wide, drainable outlet while the seal remains intact.

Continuous drainage is still possible when particulate matter is present in the effluent by using a wider tubular outlet, by attaching a section of respiratory tubing or latex drainage tubing into the tail of an open-end drain, or by securing a urinary pouch adapter into a fecal pouch outlet (Box 14-7).

Wound access. At times, access to the fistula site may be desirable so that tubes can be advanced, the fistula can be assessed easily, or skin-barrier pastes can be reinforced. Access to the site without disruption of the pouch adhesive can be achieved with a two-piece pouch or with a pouch that has an attached "access window." When such access features are not available or have an inadequate adhesive surface size, wide open-end drains can be used. Limited access to the fistula site can be attained by cuffing the pouch film back.

Pouch film. Urinary drainage equipment and some fecal pouches may be more odor-resistent rather than odorproof. More frequent pouch changes may be necessary to control the odor from permeating the pouch film, or more aggressive odor-management techniques (e.g., oral deodorizers) may be required. Pouching systems marketed as wound-management systems are transparent to allow for visual inspection. Ostomy pouches adapted for fistula care provide choices in film color: transparent, opaque, or beige-tone.

Pouching system adaptations

Adhesives. Additional adhesive is available as cement, medical adhesive spray forms, and sheet form. Cements and sprays are applied according to the manufacturer's instructions; most require time to become tacky. They are used to enhance the tack of an existing adhesive and extend the adhesive surface on a pouch. Adhesives may also be warranted to improve the tack when several applications of skin-barrier powder are required in the presence of severe denudation. Occasionally, liquid adhesive may be used in combination with skin-barrier powders to protect exposed skin from caustic effluent. This procedure is similar to the "artificial scab" discussed previously.

Because fistulas vary in size and shape and abdominal contours can be dramatic, large and unusually shaped pouch apertures may be necessary. Sheets of adhesives (or double-faced adhesive disks) can be used to either create or increase the adhesive surface on a pouch. Box 14-8 describes the procedure for adding an adhesive sheet to a pouch.

Saddlebagging. Another method that can be used to acquire a large adhesive surface is to attach two open-end drainable pouches (Figure 14-8). Pouch features that facilitate saddlebagging include no attached solid-wafer skin barrier, no floating collar, and no starter hole. A large solid-wafer skin barrier is then attached to the new combined adhesive surface, and the pouch is prepared in the usual fashion. Box 14-9 describes the saddlebagging technique.

Bridging technique. The bridging technique is a procedure that can be used to isolate one area of a wound from another part of the wound. It has two primary indications for use:

1. Wounds may present with two distinct areas of "needs": one area of the wound has drainage and requires containment, whereas another area needs moist wound healing or packing.
2. Very large wounds may be more manageable if the wound is "divided." Solid-wafer skin barriers are cut into small pieces to fill the wound at the selected bridge location and layered into place (Figure 14-9). A routine pouch or more complicated pouching system can then be applied over the bridge that now exists in the wound.

Box 14-10 describes the steps involved in the bridging technique.

Catheter ports. When a catheter or tube is in place at a fistula site, leakage onto perifistular skin may occur. A pouching system with an attached catheter port may be used to collect the drainage. A catheter port is a nipple-shaped device that attaches to the external wall of a pouch. The catheter is disconnected, threaded through the

BOX 14-7 Addition of Continuous Drainage Tube to Fecal Outlet Pouch

Equipment

- Fecal pouch or open-end drain
- Connector to fit the tubing and bedside system
- 5 inches of wide lumen tubing or respiratory tubing
- Rubber band
- Bedside drainage system

Procedure

1. Cut the desired size for the fistula in the skin-barrier adhesive of a fecal pouch or open-end drain.
2. Insert the wide lumen tubing or respiratory tubing into the drain spout.
3. Working at the adhesive surface, reach inside the pouch and pull the drain spout and tubing through the opening cut in the skin-barrier adhesive.
4. Wrap a rubber band securely around the tubing to secure.
5. From the bottom of the pouch, pull the tubing through so that the outlet spout is in its normal location. The tail of the pouch is now cuffed around the tubing inside the pouch.
6. Attach to bedside drainage system.

NOTE: When the pouch is removed, the latex tubing and connector are discarded.

BOX 14-8 Procedure for Adding Adhesive Sheets to Enlarge Pouch Adhesive Surface

Equipment

- Pouch without floating collar
- Double-faced adhesive sheet or disk

Procedure

1. Remove protective paper from one side of adhesive sheet.
2. Attach this adhesive sheet adjacent to existing adhesive on pouch (edges may overlap slightly).
3. Trace desired opening size on protective paper, covering adhesive surface.
4. Cut to desired size.
5. Prepare solid skin-barrier wafer (usually 8 × 8 inches), attach to adhesive surface on pouch, and continue in usual fashion.

pouch opening on the adhesive surface, then threaded through the catheter port itself so that the catheter can be reconnected to drainage. The pouch is then secured to the skin in the usual fashion. Detailed instructions from the manufacturer accompany the catheter port. With this technique, drainage around the catheter is collected in the pouch while the catheter continues to drain by suction or gravity.

Silicone molding. A silicone molding technique has been reported using a dental mold material to fashion an impression of the fistula opening and perifistular area in an attempt to create a smooth surface to which a pouch can be applied (Laing, 1977). This procedure was reserved for the recessed fistula located in an open wound or the fistula surrounded by numerous irregular skin surfaces. However, the silicone mold procedure is less commonly used currently because of the advances in wound-management products.

Trough procedure. When fistulas are contained within the depressions of a wound such that a routine pouching system fails, this procedure may be useful. With the trough procedure, one or several strips of a transparent dressing are used to occlude the wound and trap effluent in the wound depression (Figure 14-10). A small opening is made in the transparent dressing at the most dependent aspect of the wound, and an ostomy pouch is applied over this opening; no pattern is required.

To enhance adherence of the transparent dressing to the skin peripheral to the fistula or wound (and to protect perifistular skin), strips of a solid-wafer skin barrier should be applied. Directions for the trough procedure are listed in Box 14-11.

Pouching technique. Technique is important to successful fistula management. The following are technique suggestions that will enhance the probability of a successful outcome:

- Schedule the procedure, if possible, to allow education and participation from nursing staff and other caregivers.

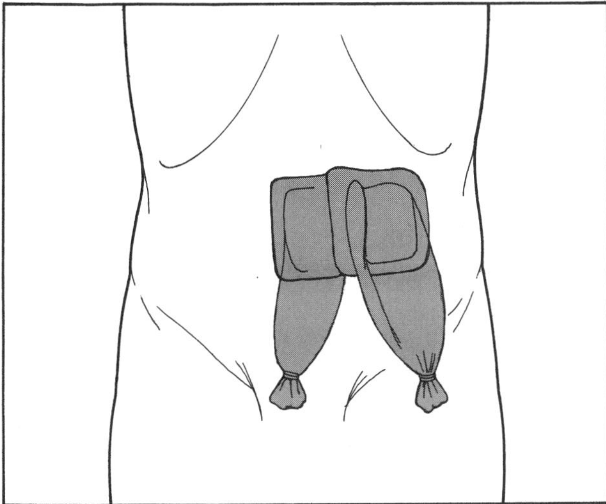

Figure 14-8 Sketch of saddlebagging technique where two open-ended drainable pouches are connected along the adhesive surface to create a large adhesive surface.

- Set up all equipment before starting the procedure; fistula function is unpredictable and may otherwise occur when adhesives are not completely set up.
- Cut the opening in the pouch adhesive approximately 1/8 inch larger than the fistula cutaneous opening. If periwound skin is exposed, a skin-barrier paste may be applied for protection. Apertures much larger than the actual fistula opening may be necessary with severe, deep depressions that create irregular skin surfaces. To prevent skin denudation, a skin-barrier paste is applied to the exposed skin (Plate 32).
- Follow universal precautions with clean technique during procedures. The care of fistulas or drain sites is seldom a sterile procedure. Sterile products are an unnecessary expense and are not shown to control infection.
- To remove adhesives from the skin, gently roll off adherent material with a dry gauze. Solvents may be used but must be cleansed thoroughly from the skin before adhesive application. Do not scrub or abrade the skin. It may be necessary to leave small amounts of residual paste or cement on the skin. This should not hinder pouch adhesion.

BOX 14-9 Saddlebagging Technique

Equipment

- Two open-end drains (without floating collar or attached skin barrier or starter hole)
- Solid-wafer skin barrier (8 × 8 inches)
- Skin-barrier paste

Procedure

1. Align pouches as final product is intended to appear on abdomen.
2. Peel protective backing away from adhesive along common edges of pouches approximately ½ to 1 inch.
3. Attach the two pouches along this ½- to 1-inch margin only.
4. Trace pattern of wound onto new adhesive surface (combined pouch adhesive surfaces).
5. Cut out pouch opening; do not cut into "seam" created by combining pouches.
6. Trace pattern onto solid-wafer skin barrier and cut out.
7. Remove protective paper backing from pouch adhesive surface and attach to solid-wafer skin barrier.
8. Prepare skin as indicated by wound contours and continue pouching procedure.

NOTE: Both pouches will fill with drainage and require emptying.

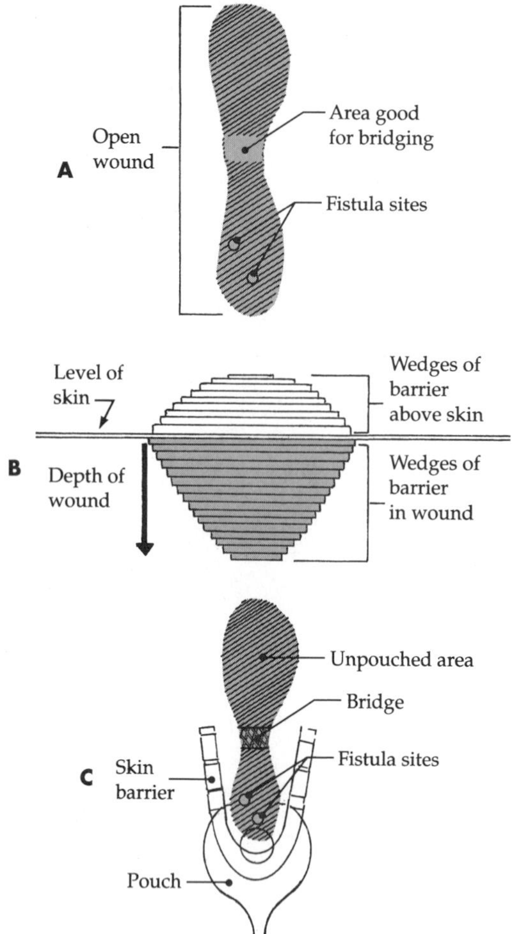

Figure 14-9 Bridging technique. A, Area of wound where fistula sites are located and identified can be separated from remainder of wound. B, Cross-section view of tapered skin-barrier wedges used to fill the wound defect and to extend slightly above the level of the skin. C, Demonstration of how a pouch is applied over a bridge and fistula, leaving the area of the wound that is not draining available for more appropriate wound care.

BOX 14-10 Bridging Technique

1. Assess wound and determine most appropriate location for "bridge." Be sure all sites from which drainage is produced are included in the side of wound to be pouched. For simplification of the bridging procedure, areas that are narrower or shallower should be selected.
2. Apply layered wedges of solid-wafer skin barrier and paste to create bridge. Wedges must be custom-cut to fit the dimensions of the wound at that level; usually the bottom wedge is narrowest because the deepest part of the wound is typically the narrowest area. Each successive wedge is a little wider until the skin-barrier wafer wedges reach skin level.
3. Continue to layer solid-wafer barrier wedges above skin level using progressively smaller and narrower wedges (to create a pressure-dressing effect).
4. Apply solid-wafer skin barrier to cover newly created bridge and extend onto intact skin. Paste may be needed to smooth "seams."
5. Continue with routine or complex pouching procedure as indicated.

NOTE: Skin barrier paste or adhesive spray or cement may be used between wedges but are not routinely necessary.

Control odor. In general, odor-control measures are indicated any time the patient and/or family perceive an odor to be objectionable, even if the odor seems almost imperceptible. The method of odor control depends on whether dressings or pouches are being used. Gauze dressings do not control odor; therefore charcoal-impregnated dressings may be needed over the gauze dressings. However, because charcoal becomes inactivated with moisture, these dressings should not come into contact with drainage materials. Charcoal dressings are most cost effective with low-output fistulas where the charcoal dressing remains intact for 24- to 48-hour periods. Pouches provide odor control. However, when the pouch is emptied, odor may be noticeable. Therefore, odor management must be a component of the care plan.

Odor is best controlled by use of a pouch to contain the effluent. A pouch may be the preferred management technique simply to contain the odor regardless of the volume of output. Although most pouches have an odorproof film, the quality of the film's ability to contain odor varies. For example, many urinary pouches and urinary drainable systems are not odorproof, and so may become saturated with odor quickly.

To control odor the nurse should 1) dispose of soiled linens and dressings from the room promptly,

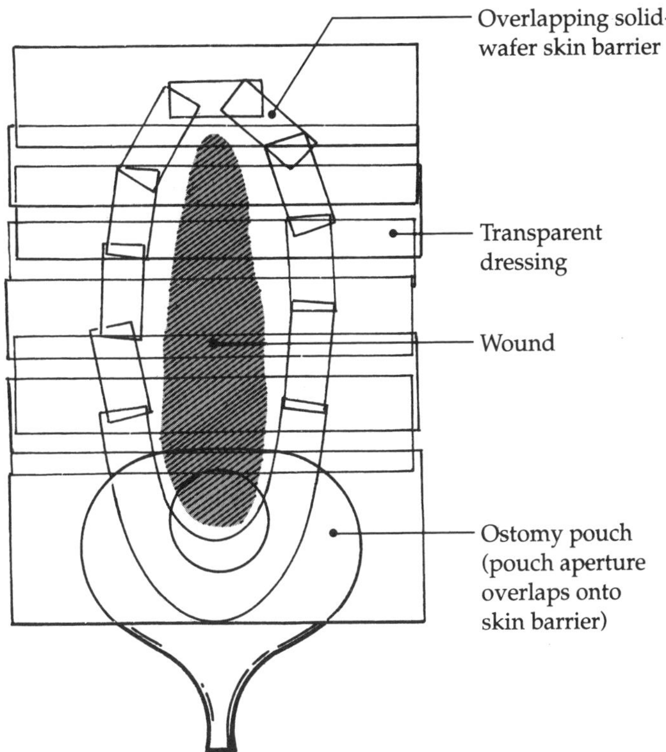

Figure 14-10 Sketch of trough procedure. Notice overlapping skin-barrier wafers and transparent dressing strips. Pouch opening must overlap onto the skin-barrier wafer at the inferior aspect of the wound.

2) use care in emptying pouches to prevent splashing effluent on the patient or on linens, 3) cleanse the tail of drainable fecal pouches after emptying, and 4) use deodorants appropriately.

Deodorants can be taken internally (orally) or used externally (in the pouch or as a room spray). Internal deodorants are in a tablet form but are generally discouraged in the presence of a pathologic condition such as a fistula. External deodorants are available in liquids, powders, and tablets and are placed in the pouch after each emptying. Room deodorants are particularly useful when the nurse is emptying the pouch, changing the pouch, or changing dressings. The room deodorant selected should be one that eliminates odor rather than masks odor. With the many types of deodorants now available, patients, families, and nurses should not have to tolerate the unfortunate odor that often accompanies fistulas.

Patient comfort. Areas to address in order to promote patient comfort include prevention and early treatment of perifistular skin irritation, pain control, and education to decrease anxiety. Leaking pouches, wet dressings on the skin, and odor in the patient's room all negatively affect morale. Medicating the patient before dressing changes may be indicated. Factors contributing to skin irritation include damp dressings, presence of caustic effluent in contact with the skin, and frequent tape application and removal. When selecting and evaluating a management technique, the nurse should consider interventions appropriate to prevent unnecessary patient discomfort.

Accurate measurement of effluent. Accurate measurement of effluent from a fistula or drain site is critical to the success of fluid and electrolyte resuscitation and nutritional support. As the patient becomes stabilized, accurate measurement of the

BOX 14-11 Trough Procedure

1. Prepare skin and fill irregular skin surface as usual.
2. Apply overlapping strips of solid-wafer barrier along wound edges.
3. Apply skin-barrier paste to smooth "seams" (between barrier edges and along skin edges). NOTE: Inferior aspect of wound should be bordered with a solid piece of barrier instead of overlapping strips to prevent leakage.
4. Cut strips of a transparent dressing so that they are wide enough to cover wound and skin-barrier strips. Calculate length of strips so that strips overlap intact skin with 1- to 2-inch margins.
5. Reserve one strip of transparent dressing to be applied to the most inferior aspect of the wound.
6. Attach a drainable pouch (can be urinary or fecal) to this one strip of transparent dressing.
7. Cut hole in pouch or transparent-dressing adhesive surface so that it is lower than the inferior wound margins (it should clear the wound edges to provide adequate drainage).
8. Beginning at top of wound, apply transparent dressing in overlapping strips.
9. Attach the final strip of the transparent dressing (with the attached pouch) so that the bottom of the pouch opening is secured onto the skin-barrier wafer.

effluent is less important. Seldom will the patient at home be required to monitor output volumes. Pouching offers the most objective method of monitoring output, and suction is accurate only if the effluent does not leak around the catheters. Dressings can provide an estimate of volume if the dressings are weighed; however, this method is time consuming, messy, and inconsistent from caregiver to caregiver.

Patient mobility. Consideration for optimizing the patient's activity should be of paramount importance when a fistula management method is being selected. Restrictions on physical activity predispose the patient to physical complications such as pneumonia, pressure ulcers, and thrombophlebitis as well as psychosocial complications such as depression and withdrawal. Because limitations on a patient's physical activity are sometimes necessary when suction or dressings are used to contain effluent, these interventions should be used only on a temporary basis. Pouches are less likely to restrict mobility.

Ease of use. Complex patient situations may necessitate unique pouching systems (initially, which are expensive and labor intensive). Unfortunately, these unique adaptations often increase the chance of error in application and care so that more caregiver education, reinforcement, and monitoring will be required. Seeking simplicity is important and is possible in most situations. Several conveniences are available and should be considered as long as effectiveness is not compromised:

1. Whenever possible, use a presized pouch rather than sizeable pouch.
2. Avoid suction when pouching is effective.
3. Fill skin defects with strip paste rather than tube paste in patients with manual dexterity problems.
4. Use pouching systems with convexity rather than creating convexity with layers of skin barriers.
5. Use one-piece rather than two-piece pouches.
6. Equipment should be selected that is easy to access in the community. Mail order of products is a convenience as long as orders are placed before the patient's supplies are depleted.

Cost containment. Accountable, appropriate fistula management also requires that the nurse select a treatment option that is cost effective. For example, a fistula pouch with a wound-access window that is changed every other day is more costly than a sizable ostomy pouch, which would probably yield the same wear time. However, if use of a pouch with an access window prolongs wear time by providing access for wound care and paste application, it may be the most cost-effective option. Cost containment implies attention not only to products and materials, but also to labor and time.

Evaluation

Accomplishment of Goals. The nurse should take time to reflect on the eight nursing management goals and evaluate how well these have been accomplished. Can steps be omitted? Is the skin intact? Is odor controlled? As the fistula stabilizes, the technical approach should be reevaluated and simplified as much as possible. One management system is seldom effective from the onset of the fistula until closure. For example, one fistula may be managed with a pouch, dressings, or suction, or all three. While in the hospital, suction may be a workable option; however, mobility is compromised and plans for home care are complicated. Therefore developing a pouching system that does not require suction would be an important simplification. Similarly, using products that are difficult to obtain is a complicating step and may be expensive. Planning to use an effective system that is easy and readily available is key to facilitating the delivery of care.

Making Changes. It is important to expect change in fistula care and modify interventions as needed. Seldom will the first pouch applied to a complex fistula be effective. Generally, modifications are necessary in the pouch pattern, size of adhesive surface, and use of skin-barrier pastes or wafer strips. It is best to make one change at a time so that the effect of these changes can be accurately assessed. The addition of a belt may be warranted to add security to the pouch system, particularly on obese patients, or when the perifistular skin is mobile.

Close monitoring by the nurse must be provided for the duration of the fistula regardless of the health care setting. An inquisitive, analytic approach will facilitate identifying steps to improve the duration of the pouching system. For example, if the pouch leaks, is it between the skin and barrier or the barrier and pouch? Is the pouch being emptied when it is one third to one half full to prevent overfilling?

SUMMARY

Patients with a fistula require complex, aggressive, and methodic care. Delivery of care necessitates mobility of the nurse across care settings and the use of multidisciplinary care teams. Successful nursing management of a patient with a fistula requires close monitoring and a plan for care that addresses the technical, educational, and emotional needs of these complex patients.

SELF-ASSESSMENT EXERCISE

1. List at least four factors that may contribute to fistula development after a surgical procedure.
2. Radiation-induced endarteritis may cause fistulas:
   a. Only in the first month after irradiation
   b. Between 1 and 3 years after irradiation
   c. From 3 to 5 years after irradiation
   d. At any time after irradiation
3. List three complications that contribute to death from fistulas.
4. Define the term *fistula.*
5. A high-output fistula is defined as one that produces more than:
   a. 75 ml/24 hr
   b. 150 ml/24 hr
   c. 200 ml/24 hr
   d. 600 ml/24 hr
6. Define the involved structures for the following fistulas:
   a. Enterocutaneous
   b. Colocutaneous
   c. Vesicovaginal
   d. Rectovaginal
   e. Colovesical
7. List the four phases of medical management for the patient with a fistula.
8. The major cause of death in the patient with a fistula is:
   a. Malnutrition
   b. Sepsis
   c. Operative complications
   d. Hypovolemia
9. List at least four factors known to delay spontaneous closure of fistulas.
10. List eight goals for nursing management of the patient with a fistula.
11. Which of the following is used to absorb moisture from irritated skin?
    a. Commercial skin-barrier pastes
    b. Adhesives
    c. Skin-barrier powders
    d. Skin sealants

12. Which of the following fistulas would be appropriately managed with gauze dressings?
    a. Volume of output 350 ml/24 hr
    b. Output noncorrosive and odorous
    c. Volume of output 50 ml/24 hr and noncorrosive
    d. Output with formed consistency and odorous
13. Explain when the bridging technique is indicated.
14. Identify options for odor control in wounds managed with dressings and wounds managed with pouches.
15. Skin-barrier paste is used with fistulas to achieve which of the following objectives?
    a. Absorb moisture from denuded skin
    b. Increase tack of pouch adhesives
    c. Level irregular skin surfaces
    d. Protect the skin from adhesives
16. The four most essential questions to ask when selecting a pouching system include:
    a. Volume, consistency, need for access, and ease of use
    b. Need for access, volume, odor, composition of effluent
    c. Opening size, odor, consistency, and ease of use
    d. Volume, opening size, odor, need for access

REFERENCES

Allardyce DB: Management of small bowel fistulas, *Am J Surg* 145:593, 1983.

Beitz JM, Caldwell D: Abdominal wound with enterocutaneous fistula: a case study, *J Wound Ostomy Continence Nurs* 25(2):102, 1998.

Berry SM, Fischer JE: Classification and pathophysiology of enterocutaneous fistulas, *Surg Clin North Am* 76(5):1009, 1996.

Boarini J, Bryant R, Irrgang S: Fistula management, *Semin Oncol Nurs* 2:287, 1986.

Chamberlain RS, Kaufman HL, Danforth DN: Enterocutaneous fistula in cancer patients: etiology, management, outcome and impact on further treatment, *Am Surg* 64(12):1204, 1998.

Conter RI, Root L, Roslyn JJ: Delayed reconstructive surgery for complex enterocutaneous fistulae, *Am Surgeon* 54:589, 1988.

Devereux DF, Sears HF, Ketcham AS: Intestinal fistula following pelvic exenterative surgery: predisposing causes and treatment, *J Surg Oncol* 14:227, 1980.

Edmunds LH Jr, Williams GM, Welch CE: External fistulas arising from the gastrointestinal tract, *Ann Surg* 152:445, 1960.

Eleftheriadis E et al: Early endoscopic fibrin sealing of high-output postoperative enterocutaneous fistulas, *Acta Chir Scand* 156:625, 1990.

Fazio VW, Coutsoftides T, Steiger E: Factors influencing the outcome of treatment of small bowel cutaneous fistula, *World J Surg* 7:481, 1983.

Fischer JE: Enterocutaneous fistulas. In Najarian JS, Delaney JP, editors: *Progress in gastrointestinal surgery,* St Louis, 1989, Mosby.

Fischer JE: The pathophysiology of enterocutaneous fistulas, *World J Surg* 7:446, 1983.

Hild P et al: Treatment of enterocutaneous fistulas and somatostatin, *Lancet* 2:626, 1986.

Hollender LF et al: Postoperative fistulas of the small intestine: therapeutic principles, *World J Surg* 7:474, 1983.

Hollis HW Jr, Reyna TM: A practical approach to wound care in patients with complex enterocutaneous fistulas, *Surg Gynecol Obstet* 161:179, 1985.

Hwang T-L, Chen M-F: Short note: randomized trial of fibrin tissue glue for low-output enterocutaneous fistula, *Br J Surg* 83(1):112, 1996.

Irrgang S, Bryant R: Management of the enterocutaneous fistula, *J Enterostom Ther* 11:211, 1984.

Jeter KF, Tintle TE, Chariker M: Managing draining wounds and fistulae: new and established methods. In Krasner D, editor: *Chronic wound care: a clinical source book for healthcare professionals,* King of Prussia, Penn, 1990, Health Management Publications.

Jones CR, Woodhouse CR, Hendry WF: Urological problems following treatment of carcinoma of the cervix, *Br J Urol* 56:509, 1984.

Kurtz R, Heimann T, Aufses A: The management of intestinal fistulas, *Am J Gastroenterol* 76:377, 1981.

Laing BJ: Making silicone casts for enterocutaneous fistulas, *ET J* Fall:11, 1977.

Lange MP et al: Management of multiple enterocutaneous fistulas, *Heart Lung* 18:386, 1989.

Lange V et al: Fistuloscopy. an adjuvant technique for sealing gastrointestinal fistuale, *Surg Endosc* 4:212, 1990.

Levy E et al: High-output external fistulae of the small bowel: management with continuous enteral nutrition, *Br J Surg* 76:676, 1989.

McIntyre PB et al: Management of enterocutaneous fistulas: a review of 132 cases, *Br J Surg* 71:293, 1984.

Moran JR, Greene HL: Digestion and absorption. In *Clinical nutrition: enteral and tube feeding,* ed 3, Philadelphia, 1997, W.B. Saunders.

Moser AJ, Roslyn JJ: Entereocutaneous fistula. In Cameron JS, editor: *Current surgical therapy,* ed 6, St Louis, 1998, Mosby.

Nubiola P et al: Treatment of 27 postoperative enterocutaneous fistulas with the long half-life somatostatin analogue SMS 201-995, *Ann Surg* 210:56, 1989.

O'Brien B, Landis-Erdman J, Erwin-Toth P: Nursing management of multiple enterocutaneous fistulae located in the center of a large open abdominal wound: a case study, *Ostomy Wound Manage* 44(1):20, 1998.

O'Connor E: Vaginal fistulas: adaptation of management method for patients with radiation damage, *J Enterostom Ther* 10(6):229, 1983.

Phillips J, Walton M: Caring for patients with enterocutaneous fistulae, *Br J Nurs* 1(10):496, 1992.

Reber HS, Austin J: Abdominal abscesses and gastrointestinal fistulas. In Sleisenger M, Fortran J, editors: *Gastrointestinal disease pathophysiology diagnosis management,* vol 1, ed 4, Philadelphia, 1989, W.B. Saunders.

Reber HA et al: Management of external gastrointestinal fistulas, *Ann Surg* 188:460, 1978.

Rolstad B, Boarini J: Principles and techniques in the use of convexity, *Ostomy Wound Manage* 42(1):24, 1996.

Rolstad B, Wong WD: Nursing considerations in intestinal fistulas. In MacKeigan JM, Cataldo PA, editors: *Intestinal stomas: principles, techniques and management,* St Louis, 1993, Quality Medical Publishing.

Rombeau J, Rolandelli R: Enteral and parenteral nutrition in patients with enteric fistulas and short bowel syndrome, *Surg Clin North Am* 67(3):551, 1987.

Rose D et al: One hundred and fourteen fistulas of the gastrointestinal tract treated with total parenteral nutrition, *Surg Gynecol Obstet* 163(4):345, 1986.

Rothenberger DA, Goldberg SM: The management of rectovaginal fistulae, *Surg Clin North Am* 63(1):61, 1983.

Sansoni B, Irving M: Small bowel fistulas, *World J Surg* 9:897, 1985.

Scardillo J, Folkedahl B: Management of a complex high-output fistula, *J Wound Ostomy Continence Nurs* 25:217, 1998.

Schein M, Decker GA: Postoperative external alimentary tract fistulas, *Am J Surg* 161(4):435, 1991.

Sitges-Serra A, Jaurrieta E, Sitges-Creus A: Management of postoperative enterocutaneous fistulas: the roles of parenteral nutrition and surgery, *Br J Surg* 69:147, 1982.

Skingley S. The management of a faecal fistula, *Nursing Times* 94(16):64, 1998.

Smith DB: Fistulas of the head and neck, *J Enterostom Ther* 9(5):20, 1982.

Smith DB: Multiple stomas, fistulas and draining wounds. In Smith DB, Johnson DR, editors: *Ostomy care and the cancer patient: surgical and clinical considerations,* New York, 1986, Grune & Stratton.

Smith DH, Pierce VK, Lewis JL Jr: Enteric fistulas encountered on a gynecologic oncology service from 1969-1980, *Surg Gynecol Obstet* 158:71, 1984.

Smith ST et al: Surgical management of irradiation-induced small bowel damage, *Obstet Gynecol* 65:563, 1985.

Soeters PB, Ebeid AM, Fischer JE: Review of 404 patients with gastrointestinal fistulas, *Ann Surg* 190:189, 1979.

Welch JP: Duodenal, gastric, and biliary fistulas. In Schwartz SI, Ellis H, editors: *Maingot's abdominal operations,* vol 1, ed 8, East Norwalk, Conn, 1985, Appleton-Century-Crofts.

Wiltshire BL: Challenging enterocutaneous fistula: a case presentation, *J Wound Ostomy Continence Nurs* 23(6):297, 1996.

Wong WD, Buie WD: Management of intestinal fistulas. In MacKeigan JM, Cataldo PA, editors: *Intestinal stomas: principles, techniques, and management,* St Louis, 1993, Quality Medical Publishing.

Wound Ostomy Continence Nursing Society: *Guidelines for management: caring for a patient with an ostomy,* Laguna Beach, Calif, 1998, WOCN.

Zwanziger PJ: Pouching a draining duodenal cutaneous fistula: a case study, *J Wound Ostomy Continence Nurs* 26(1):25, 1999.

CHAPTER 15

Management of Gastrointestinal Feeding Tubes

RUTH A. BRYANT

OBJECTIVES

1. Identify two primary reasons for use of gastrointestinal tubes.
2. Distinguish among the placement approaches for a gastostomy and jejunostomy, including indications and overview of technique.
3. Discuss guidelines for feeding tube site selection.
4. Explain why tube stabilization is a priority in management of the patient with percutaneous tubes.
5. Describe at least two options for stabilization of gastrostomy or jejunostomy tubes.
6. For each complication listed, identify a prevention and management approach: peritubular leakage, tube migration, candidiasis, and tube occlusion.
7. Describe routine site care for the patient with a gastrointestinal tube.

Within the gastrointestinal tract, tubes are placed through a variety of techniques for the purposes of feeding, decompression, or drainage. Although first described in the thirteenth century, the planned surgical gastrostomy as a procedure was first proposed in 1837 and performed in 1849, with the first reported survival of the procedure performed by S. Jones in 1875 (Gorman and Morris, 1997). Today the use of tubes is commonplace within the gastrointestinal tract as well as other organs and spaces on a temporary or a long-term basis. Malfunction of these tubes can result in skin erosion and irritation such that a referral to the wound care nurse becomes necessary. This chapter reviews the different types of gastrostomy and jejunostomy tubes, their purpose, procedures for placement, and nursing management. Potential complications are also presented.

Other percutaneous tubes may also come to the attention of the wound care nurse, such as empyema tubes, biliary drainage tubes, and nephrostomy tubes. Although the principles for use and method of placement are beyond the scope of this textbook, principles of care (in terms of tube stabilization to prevent migration, movement, and peritubular skin irritation) are similar to those that are discussed in this chapter.

Effective nursing management of the patient with tubes placed percutaneously requires an understanding of the anatomy and physiology of the affected body system, the pathology involved, the rationale for tube placement, the method of tube insertion, and the anticipated length of time that the tube will be necessary. Although specific care procedures vary depending on the body system involved and the purpose of tube placement, management should always include routine care designed to maintain tube function and prevent peritubular complications, patient/caregiver education, and routine surveillance for tube dysfunction or complications. Comprehensive care is best provided with a collaborative team approach involving but not limited to the interventional radiologist, gastroenterologist, surgeon or internist, and nurse.

GASTROSTOMY AND JEJUNOSTOMY DEVICES

A gastrostomy is an opening into the stomach, and a jejunostomy is an opening into the jejunum. Such

Thanks to Karen Huskey for her review of manuscript.

procedures may be used to provide decompression or enteral support for a patient unable to ingest adequate nutrients orally (Moran and Greene, 1997). Gastric enteral support is appropriate for long-term access (i.e., over 4 weeks) in the patient who is at low risk for aspiration (Gorman and Morris, 1997). When the risk of aspiration exists, postpyloric placement of a tube is preferred. The patient's history and physical examination, barium studies, fluroscopy, and manometry are useful when evaluating the patient's risk for aspiration. Consultation with the neurologist and speech pathologist is also beneficial. Box 15-1 provides a list of risk factors for aspiration.

BOX 15-1 Risk Factors for Aspiration

Altered mental status
Swallowing dysfuntion
History of aspiration
Severe gastroesophageal reflux
Gastric outlet obstruction
Gastroparesis

From Gorman RC, Nance ML, Morris JB: Enteral feeding techniques. In Torosian MH: *Nutrition for the hospitalized patient: basic science and principles of practice*, New York, 1995, Marcel Dekker.

Gastrostomy procedures were first performed successfully from 1875 to 1877 (Gorman and Morris, 1997). For over a century, gastrostomy placement required a surgical intervention involving anesthesia and the traditional preoperative preparation for abdominal surgery. Historically, a suture was placed around the base of the tube at skin level and then through the skin to immobilize the gastrostomy tube. Gastrostomy tubes were usually connected to suction for 12 to 24 hours to reduce tension on the suture line. Feedings were delayed until bowel sounds, tube patency, and proper placement of the tube was confirmed (McGee, 1987).

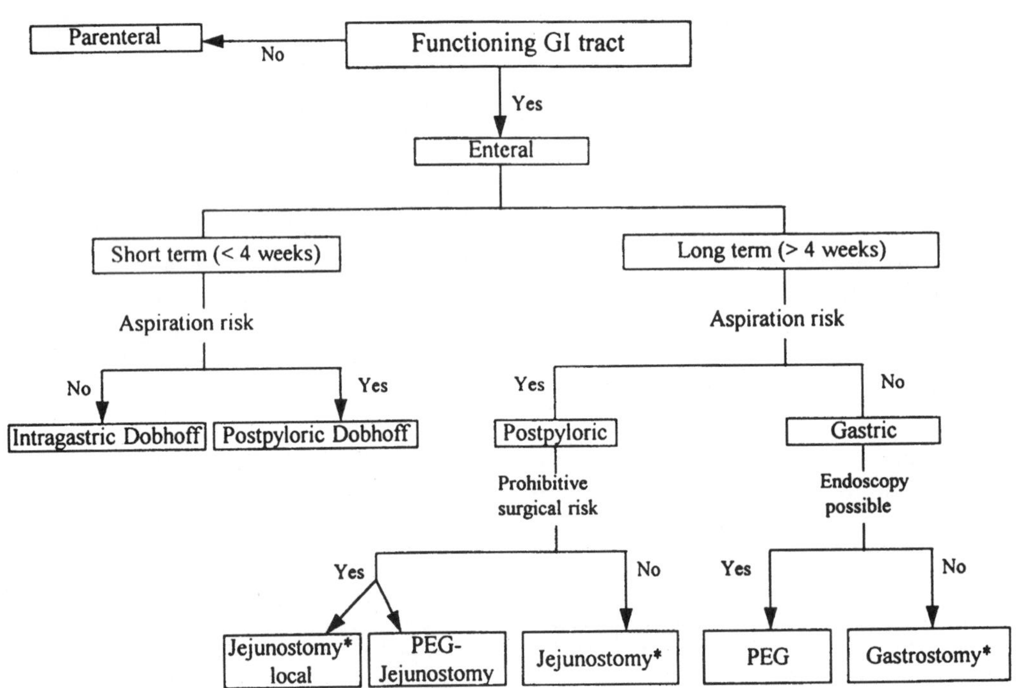

Figure 15-1 Enteral access algorithm for selecting the most appropriate technique for an individual patient. (From Gorman RC, Morris JB: Minimally invasive access to the gastrointestinal tract. In Rombeau JL, Rolandelli RH: *Clinical nutrition: enteral and tube feeding*, ed 3, Philadelphis, 1997, W.B. Saunders.)

Placement Approaches

Today, a gastrostomy or jejunostomy is created by one of three approaches: surgical, endoscopic, or radiologic intervention. When the purpose for accessing the gastrointestinal tract is for nutritional support, the most appropriate access technique must be selected. Figure 15-1 presents an algorithm for determining the most appropriate means of enteral access.

Surgical Approach. A surgically placed gastrostomy tube can be accomplished through an open surgical procedure or a laparoscopic procedure (Gauderer and Stellato, 1986). Surgical placement requires anesthesia and is usually reserved for the patient who is unable to undergo an endoscopic placement. An open surgical approach is considered when the patient is already undergoing a laparotomy. For the patient who is not undergoing a laparotomy, a laparoscopic approach is an option (Gauderer and Stellato, 1986).

Open surgical procedure. The most common open surgical procedures for gastrostomy tube placement are the Stamm, Witzel, and Janeway. The Stamm and Witzel are used when the need for feedings is temporary. Janeway is used when it is anticipated that a long-term or permanent access is necessary (Gincherman and Torosian, 1996).

Stamm gastrostomy. A Stamm gastrostomy is created when one makes a small incision in the left upper quadrant of the abdomen. Another small incision is made over and through the body of the stomach. A catheter (Foley, mushroom, Malicot, or gastrostomy replacement tube) is inserted through this incision, placed inside the stomach, and then directed toward the pylorus (Figure 15-2). Several purse-string sutures are used to invaginate the stomach around the tube. The stomach is then fixed to the abdominal wall at the catheter site, and traditionally a nonabsorbable suture is used to secure the catheter to the skin. Although the Stamm gastrostomy is the simplest surgical technique to perform and remove, it is frequently difficult to manage and is plagued with complications, such as peritubular leakage, wound infection, peritonitis, and tube dislodgement (Patterson, 1988).

Witzel gastrostomy. A Witzel gastrostomy is created similarly to the Stamm gastrostomy with the addition of a 4- to 6-cm seromuscular tunnel of the stomach wall through which the gastrostomy tube is placed (Figure 15-3). A decrease in peritubular

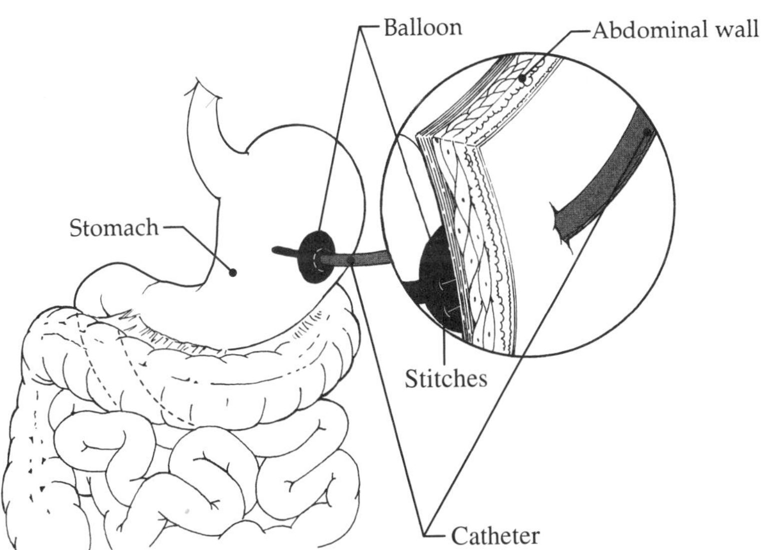

Figure 15-2 Stamm gastrostomy tube technique—oblique view. An incision is placed through the abdominal wall into the stomach, through which a catheter is passed.

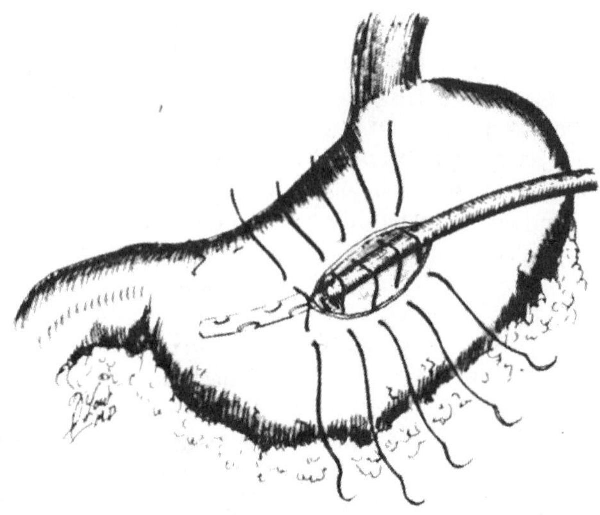

Figure 15-3 Witzel gastrostomy is similar to the Stamm gastrostomy with the addition of a 4 to 6 cm seromuscular tunnel of the stomach wall through which the gastrostomy tube is placed. (From Patterson RS: Enteral nutrition delivery systems, In Grant JA, Kennedy-Caldwell C, editors: *Nutritional support nursing*, Philadelpia, 1988, Grune & Stratton.)

leakage is anticipated by creating the tunnel; particularly when the stomach is distended or the tube is removed.

Janeway gastrostomy. A Janeway gastrostomy is a surgically constructed, mucosa-lined gastric passageway that is brought out the abdominal surface as a permanent mucocutaneous stoma. Figure 15-4 illustrates how the Janeway gastrostomy is constructed. Postoperatively, an inflated balloon-tip catheter is placed in the tract. Once the tract has matured (7 to 10 days), the tube is removed. A tube is inserted into the Janeway gastrostomy during each feeding and then removed. This type of permanent gastrostomy requires more operative time than the Stamm gastrostomy and results in many similar complications (Gorman, Nance, and Morris, 1995).

Witzel jejunostomy. The Witzel technique can also be used to create a jejunostomy either at the conclusion of a surgical procedure or as an isolated procedure. The usual site is the left upper quadrant. A loop of jejunum 15 to 20 cm from the ligament of Treitz is brought up to the wound, and a circular purse-string suture is placed in the antimesenteric border. An incision through the center of the purse-string suture is made, and a 14 French (Fr) feeding catheter is inserted into the jejunal lumen and advanced. A serosal tunnel is constructed at the exit site in the jejunal wall, extending approximately 5 to 6 cm proximally. The catheter is brought to the skin through a separate incision and secured, typically with sutures. The loop of intestine is anchored to the anterior abdominal wall (Bland, Karakousis, and Copeland, 1995).

Needle catheter jejunostomy. The needle jejunostomy is a simple procedure that is most often done at the conclusion of a surgical procedure when prolonged enteral support is anticipated. At approximately 30 to 40 cm distal to the ligament of Treitz, a 14- to 16-gauge needle is inserted into the jejunal wall. A feeding catheter is advanced through the needle 30 to 40 cm distally, and the needle is then withdrawn. A purse-string suture is then made around the tube to close the jejunal opening around the catheter. The loop of bowel is anchored to the anterior abdominal wall, and the catheter is secured to the skin (Figure 15-5) (Bland, Karakousis, and Copeland, 1995).

Laparoscopic surgical approach. The laparoscopic approach for insertion of the gastrostomy or jejunostomy is possible since the introduction of high-resolution video cameras and has the advantages of minimal invasion and few surgical side ef-

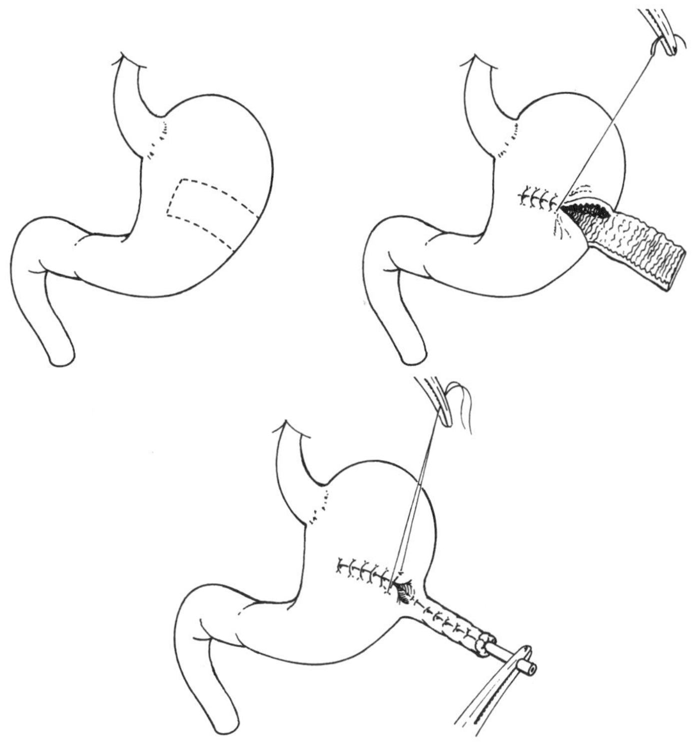

Figure 15-4 Janeway gastrostomy. A surgically constructed, mucosa-lined gastric passageway that is brought out the abdominal surface as a permanent mucocutanesous stoma.

fects (Georgeson, 1997). This approach also provides the opportunity to selectively determine the site of the tube within the stomach (i.e., lesser-curvature gastrostomy rather than the more commonly selected greater-curvature), which may be important in the patient who is at high risk for reflux or aspiration. A key advantage to a laparoscopic approach is that the abdomen can be examined under direct vision without the need for a large surgical incision so that biopsy specimens can be obtained if necessary or malignancy staging can be conducted (Coates and MacFadyan, 1996). This technique requires a smaller incision than the open surgical approach, and local or general anesthesia is still needed.

Laparascopic gastrostomy. The indication for a laparoscopic gastrostomy for feeding is when the percutaneous endoscopic gastrostomy cannot be performed, such as with an obese patient. A small supraumbilical incision is made through which the camera port is placed, and a 5 mm port is placed in the epigastrium. An atraumatic instrument is then used to grasp the stomach, and the site for the proposed gastrostomy is identified. An 18-gauge angiocatheter is passed through the anterior abdomen, at the site chosen for the gastrostomy, and into the stomach. The needle is then removed and a soft J-wire is passed into the stomach. Dilators (12 Fr and 14 Fr) are placed over this J-wire. A 16 Fr peel-away catheter is placed over the dilator, and a 16 Fr catheter is inserted through the sheath. The catheter is then positioned against the stomach wall by inflating the balloon or securing the internal bumper.

Laparoscopic jejunostomy. Several methods for laparoscopic jejunostomy are reported; however, the indications are just evolving. As a minimally invasive procedure, reduced postoperative pain and shortened recuperative time are desirable advantages; general anesthesia is required. The procedure

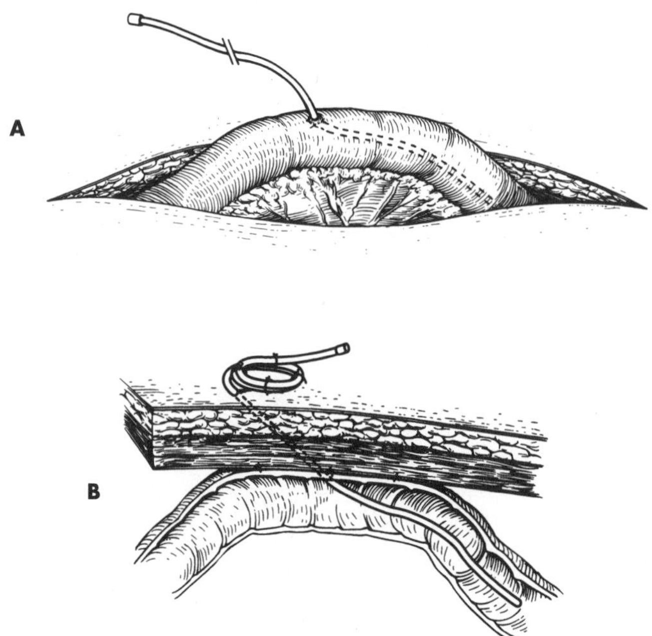

Figure 15-5 Needle catheter jejunostomy. Technique for placement of a needle catheter jejunostomy. **A,** The catheter is inserted into the lumen of the jejunum for a distance of 40 to 50 cm and secured into place with a purse-string suture. **B,** The jejunum is secured to the anterior abdominal wall. The feeding catheter is removed postoperatively when the patient is tolerating oral feedings. (Reprinted with permission from Bland KI, Karakousis CP, Copeland EM: *Atlas of surgical oncology*, Philadelphia, 1995, W.B. Saunders.)

remains more expensive than percutaneous or surgical placement. Two methods described in Gorman and Morris (1997) are briefly presented in this section.

The laparoscope is inserted through a small incision above the umbilicus. The proximal small bowel is identified, it is traced 25 cm distal to the ligament of Treitz, and the antimesenteric border is withdrawn into the umbilical wound. At this location in the small bowel, a Witzel tunnel is created or concentric purse-string sutures are placed and a #12 Fr catheter is inserted into the bowel. The bowel is secured to the fascia around the tube and returned to the abdominal cavity, and the fascia and skin are closed. The catheter is then tunneled subcutaneously to exit the skin at the site previously selected on the abdomen.

Another technique can be used in which T-fasteners are inserted through the skin into the bowel lumen to anchor and retract the bowel against the abdominal wall (Coates and MacFadyen, 1996). Once the bowel is anchored, a percutaneous jejunostomy tube can be placed directly through the abdominal wall (Figure 15-6).

Endoscopic Approach. The endoscopic approach to gastrostomy tube placement, known as the *percutaneous endoscopic gastrostomy* (PEG), was first described by Gauderer and colleagues in 1980 and has quickly become the procedure of choice. These devices can be placed under local anesthesia and conscious sedation outside the operating room, thus avoiding the complications associated with surgical procedures. The PEG can also be performed slightly faster than an open surgical technique at half the cost (Gorman and Morris, 1997).

Contraindications to the PEG include inability to perform upper endoscopy and inability to illuminate the abdominal wall. Because of the procedures involved for placement of a PEG, extreme caution is essential in the presence of massive ascites,

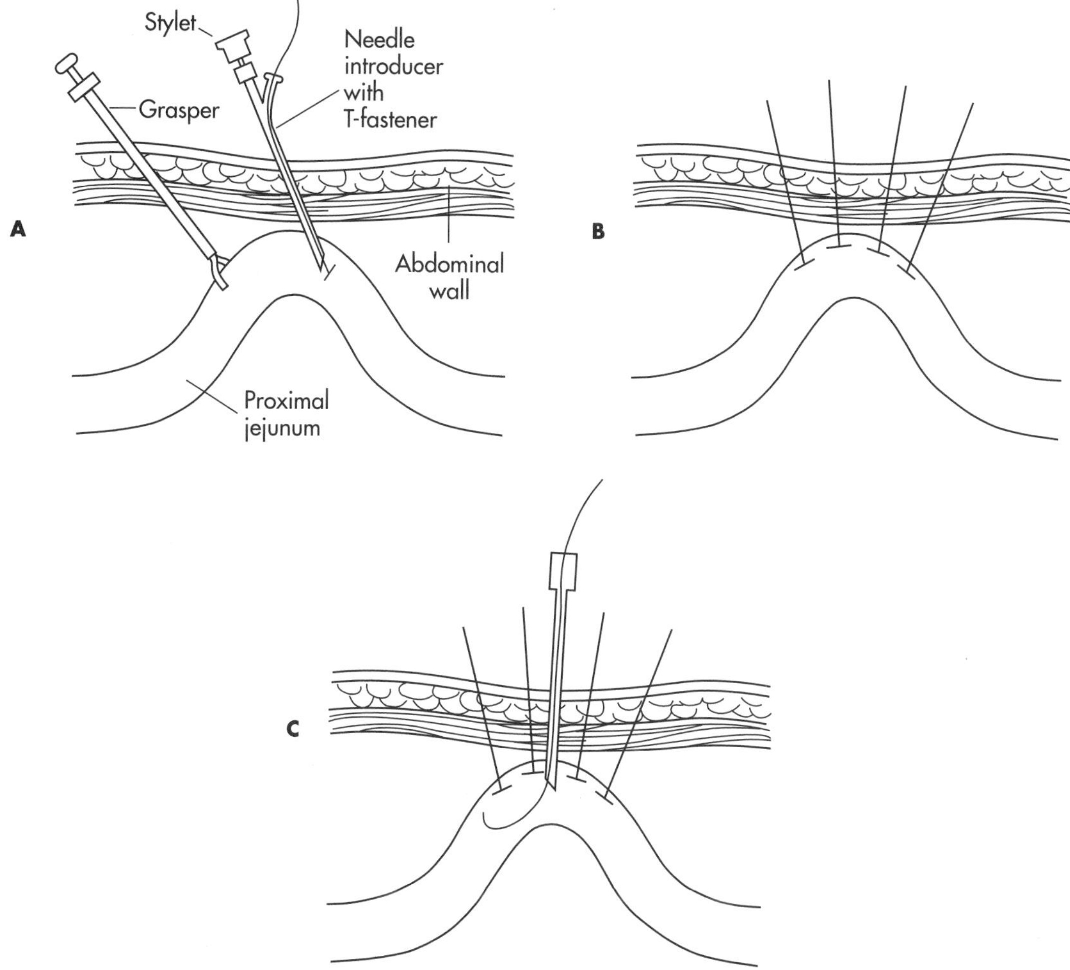

Figure 15-6 Laparoscopic jejunostomy with T-fasteners, which are inserted through the skin into the bowel lumen to anchor and retract the bowel against the abdominal wall, before inserting a percutaneous jejunostomy tube directly through the abdominal wall.

esophageal varices, intraabdominal sepsis, previous gastric resection, and coagulopathy (Gorman, Nance, and Morris, 1995).

Many variations to the original technique exists; however, the initial procedural steps remain similar (Mamel, 1989). The patient is NPO for 8 hours before the procedure. After application of a topical pharyngeal anesthetic and sedation, an endoscope is passed into the stomach. The stomach is distended with air, which distends the stomach against the anterior abdominal wall. The proposed gastrostomy site is then transilluminated. The endoscopy assistant indents the abdomen at the proposed gastrostomy site, which should be at least 2 cm below costal margin. At this point, several different techniques have been described to insert the PEG.

Pull (Gauderer-Ponsky) technique. A small incision is made over the illuminated site, and a large-gauge angiocatheter is inserted into the stomach. The needle is then withdrawn, and 60 inches of

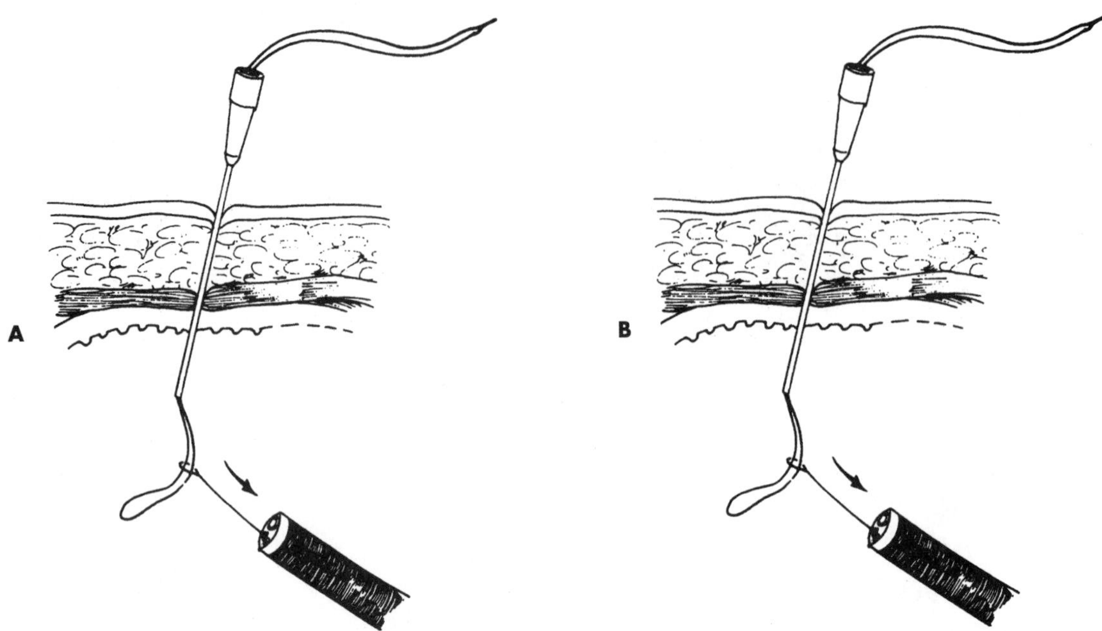

Figure 15-7 Gauderer-Ponsky PEG (pull) technique. **A,** After installation of local anesthesia, a 10 mm transverse incision is made, through which a tapered cannula needle is introduced under direct endoscopic vision. **B,** A looped heavy suture is directed through the catheter into the stomach, secured with a polypectomy snare, and withdrawn from the patient's mouth. **C,** The well-lubricated PEG catheter is now secured to the suture, and with steady traction directed down, the posterior pharynx into the esophagus. **D,** The endoscope is reintroduced, and under direct vision the catheter is pulled across the gastroesophageal junction and then approximated to the anterior gastric wall. It is imperative that the inner crossbar gently approximate the mucosa without excess tension to avoid ischemic necrosis. The stomach is decompressed by aspiration, and the gastroscope is withdrawn. **E,** The outer crossbar is gently approximated to the skin level and secured with two 0-0 Prolene sutures. (From Gorman RC, Morris JB: Minimally invasive access to the gastrointestinal tract. In Rombeau JL, Rolandelli RH: *Clinical nutrition: enteral and tube feeding*, ed 3, Philadelphis, 1997, W.B. Saunders.).

suture is passed through the catheter into the stomach. With a biopsy snare, the endoscopist grasps the suture and pulls so that the endoscope is removed with the suture attached (Figure 15-7). The gastrostomy tube is attached to the suture, and by pulling on the suture at the abdominal gastrostomy site, the tube is drawn through the esophagus into the stomach and positioned snugly against the anterior stomach wall. To verify proper position of the PEG, an endoscope is passed again. Once placement is confirmed, the endoscope is removed and the PEG is secured at the skin level.

Push (Sachs and Vine) technique. With this technique, a long flexible guidewire is inserted through the angiocatheter into the stomach. Again using the biopsy snare and endoscope, the wire is snared and pulled up through the esophagus, out the patient's mouth (Figure 15-8). The PEG tube is pushed over the guidewire and advanced through the esophagus to the stomach and positioned against the anterior stomach wall. As with the "pull" technique, PEG placement is checked with the endoscope, which is then removed, and the PEG is secured.

Modified techniques. Modifications to the push or pull technique of PEG insertion have been described in which the second passage of the endoscope is negated (Gorman, Nance, and Morris,

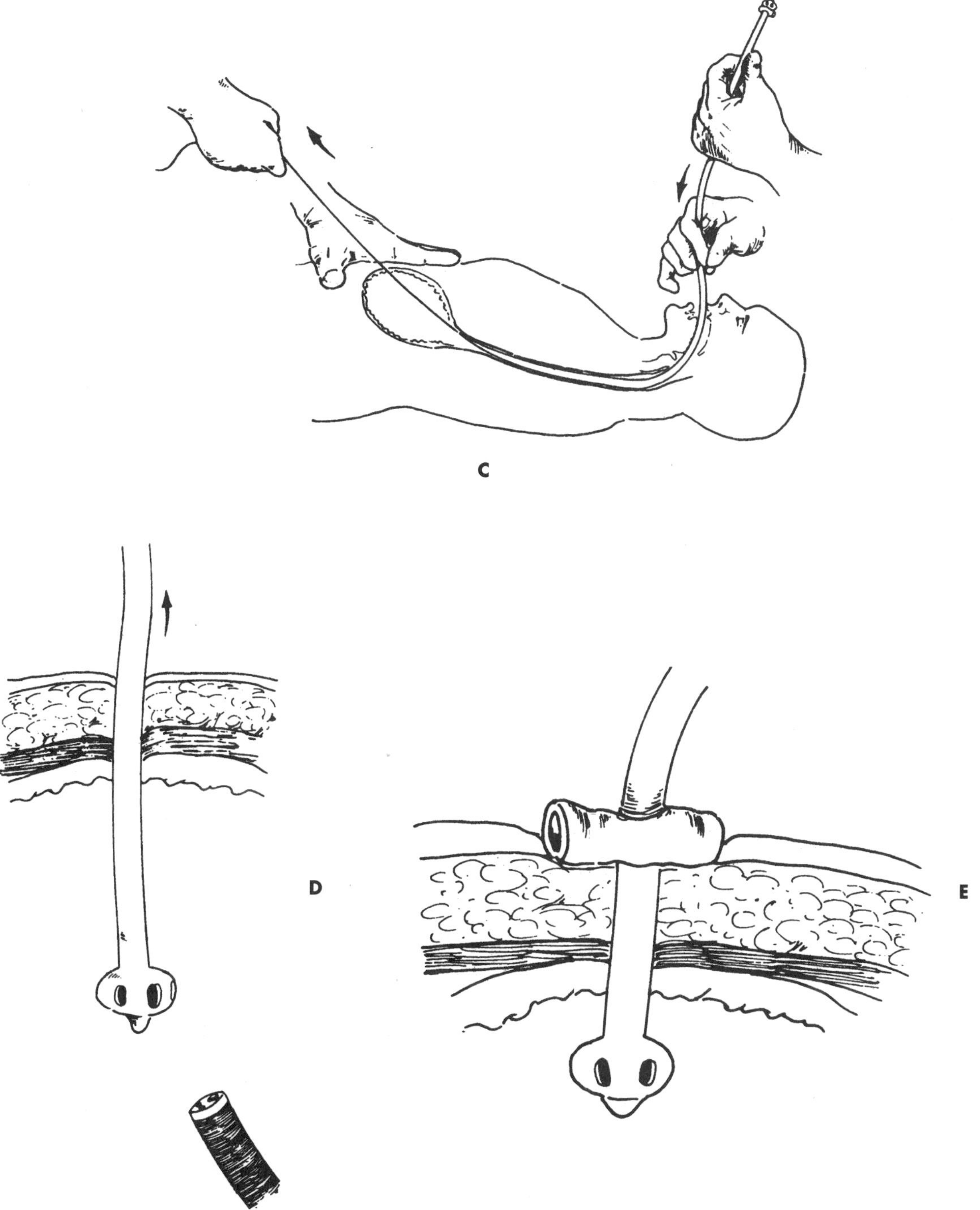

Figure 15-7, cont'd

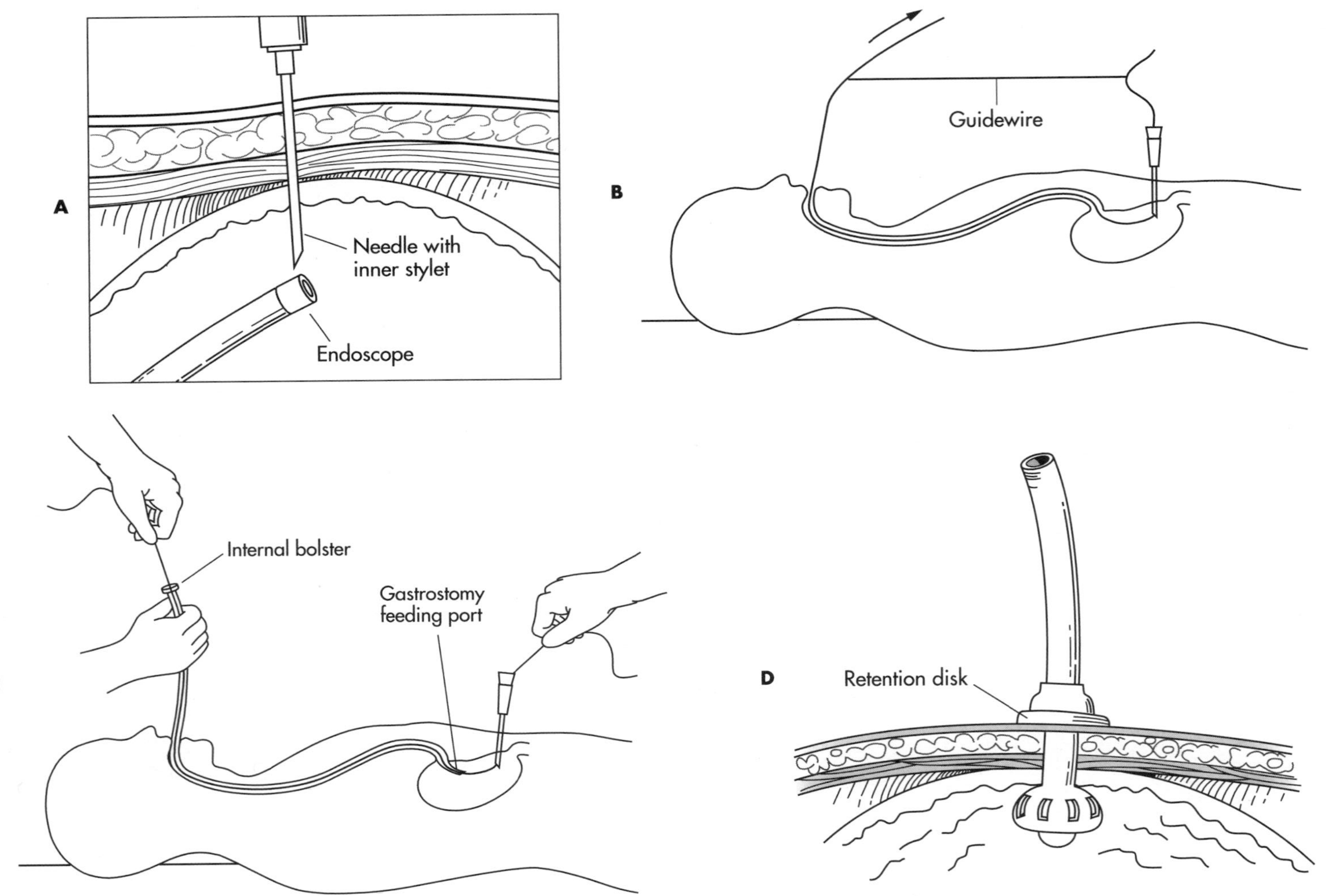

Figure 15-8 Sachs and Vine technique for PEG insertion. **A,** Needle inserted through abdomen into stomach under visualization by endoscopist. **B,** Endoscope is withdrawn, pulling guidewire up through the esophagus, out the patient's mouth. **C,** PEG tube is pushed over the guidewire and advanced through the esophagus to the stomach. **D,** PEG positioned against the anterior stomach wall.

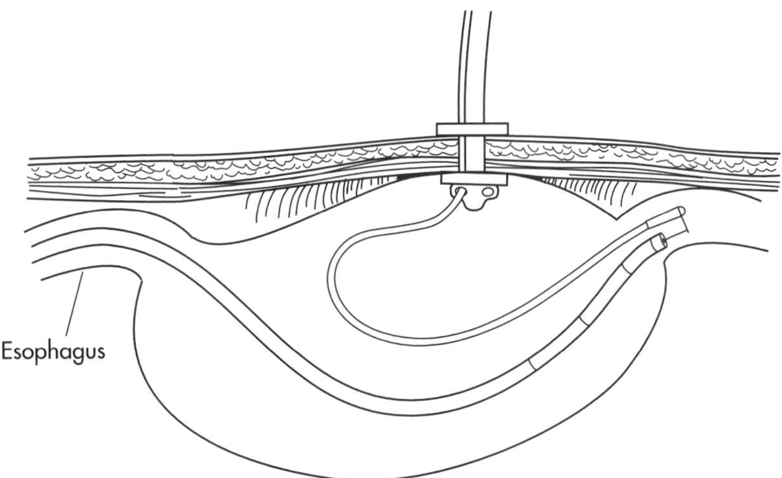

Figure 15-9 Transpyloric PEJ. Endoscopist guides the weighted tip of feeding tube into the duodenum.

1995). One technique involves using a PEG tube that has markings at 2-cm intervals so that proper positioning can be assessed by estimating the thickness of the abdominal wall. Another technique is a modification of the push technique and involves passing a dilator with a peel-away introducer over the guidewire. The position of the dilator is confirmed by the endoscopist, the dilator is removed, and a well-lubricated catheter is then placed through the introducer as the introducer is peeled away. The endoscopist verifies adequate placement of the catheter against the anterior stomach wall, and the endoscope is removed.

Percutaneous endoscopic jejunostomy (PEJ). Several innovative techniques have been described to obtain postpyloric enteral access through endoscopic placement of the percutaneous jejunostomy. The two basic approaches, transpyloric PEJ and direct PEJ, are briefly described.

Transpyloric PEJ. Through a previously established gastrostomy, a small feeding tube with a weighted tip and an attached heavy suture tie are passed. Under endoscopic visualization, the suture is grasped with a biopsy forceps and the suture and attached feeding tube are guided into the duodenum (Figure 15-9). The endoscope is withdrawn. An excess amount of tubing is left within the stomach to allow peristalsis to pull the weighted tip past the ligament of Treitz.

The transpyloric PEJ is associated with considerable long-term complications, including 1) separation of inner PEJ tube from outer gastrostomy tube, 2) clogging of the small diameter PEJ, and 3) kinking of the PEJ. Furthermore, the desired end point of reduced aspiration pneumonia has not been reported, which may be the result of retrograde migration of the tube back into the stomach or impaired pyloric sphincter function triggered by the presence of the tube (Gorman and Morris, 1997).

Directed PEJ. A PEJ can be placed directly through the abdominal wall into the jejunum using a modification of the Gauderer-Ponsky PEG procedure. In this approach the endoscope is advanced past the pylorus approximately 20 cm distal to the ligament of Treitz, and the abdominal wall is transilluminated. Using a small-gauge needle, the jejunum is cannulated through the abdominal wall, a heavy thread is inserted, a biopsy forceps is used to grasp the thread, and it is withdrawn through the mouth. The thread is tied to a feeding tube (typically mushroom tipped), which is then pulled into position under endoscopic observation.

Another direct PEJ technique involves a small incision in the upper quadrant. The endoscope is again inserted beyond the ligament of Treitz. The proximal end of the jejunum is clamped; in the small incision, a short segment of jejunum is eviscerated using the Witzel technique. The feeding tube is placed into the jejunum, the jejunum is returned to the abdominal cavity, and the proximal and distal ends of the jejunum are secured to the abdominal wall.

The direct PEJ seems to alleviate the problems associated with the transpyloric placement (tube migration, clogging, and aspiration). Evidence for the long-term benefits, efficacy, and use of this procedure is still inconclusive.

Interventional Radiologic Approach. Recent advances have led to the development of a radiographic approach to percutaneous gastrostomy tube placement. Although not the first choice for enteral access, percutaneous tubes placed radiologically become an alternative when surgical or endoscopic procedures are not feasible.

Percutaneous gastrostomy via radiologic intervention. In the radiographic approach the stomach is dilated with air and a needle is percutaneously inserted into the stomach. A J-wire is threaded into the stomach under fluoroscopic guidance, and the needle is then withdrawn. A 1-cm long incision is made into the skin at the exit site of the wire. When entry into the stomach has been determined, the tract is slowly dilated and the permanent catheter is inserted. These catheters usually have a balloon, which is inflated and positioned snugly against the gastric wall. Stabilization at the skin surface is achieved by use of a suture or a tube stabilization device.

Percutaneous jejunostomy via radiologic intervention. This technique first requires radiologic access to the stomach as described previously. A guidewire is then passed through the duodenum and into the jejunum. A balloon occluder catheter is inserted over the guidewire and placed in the jejunum. The balloon is inflated with air and water-soluble contrast so that the position can be checked by fluoroscopy. Still under fluoroscopic surveillance, an 18-gauge needle is inserted into the jejunum and the balloon is punctured. A guidewire is passed into the tract, and the tract is then dilated to approximately a 10 Fr size so that a feeding catheter can be inserted. The balloon occluder catheter is then removed, and the feeding catheter secured to the skin.

Conversion of gastrostomy to gastrostomy-jejunostomy tube (G-J tube). Repeat aspirations may make it necessary to convert an existing gastrostomy tube to a G-J tube. This can be done endoscopically or radiologically with a combined G-J tube or by inserting a smaller-diameter feeding tube through the gastrostomy tube. When a combined G-J tube is used, the gastrostomy tube is removed, and an angiocatheter and guidewire are inserted and advanced through the pylorus. The guidewire is further advanced distal to the ligament of Treitz at which point the angiocatheter is removed. A G-J tube is then inserted over the guidewire and advanced into the jejunum; the guidewire is then removed. The gastrostomy internal bumper or balloon is secured snugly against the stomach mucosa. An external securing device (bumper, flange, or commercial device) is used to secure the tube against the skin. Three ports will be apparent: gastric (proximal port), duodenal or jejunal (distal port), and balloon port (Figure 15-10).

When a combined G-J tube is not available, a jejunal tube can be placed and the external end of the jejunal tube can be threaded into a gastrostomy tube. The gastrostomy tube is then advanced over the jejunal tube, and the internal gastrostomy bumper is positioned against the anterior stomach wall. Again, external stabilization of the tube to the skin is necessary.

Summary of Placement Techniques

The type of patient who typically requires these tubes is a major reason for the high morbidity rate. Patients commonly have multiple medical problems and are malnourished. For these reasons, the surgical approach to tube placement is quickly being replaced by the endoscopic or radiographic approach.

Endoscopic techniques for enteral tube placement have a lower complication rate, are more cost effective than surgical methods, and can be performed on an outpatient basis. This technique requires the ability to insert an endoscope. Laparoscopic and radiologic techniques are less frequently used but are options when endoscopy is not anatomically feasible or when surgery is too risky.

A key consideration for type of tube placed is whether prepyloric or postpyloric delivery of enteral feedings is preferred (Welch, 1996). In the presence of significant gastroesophageal reflux, in-

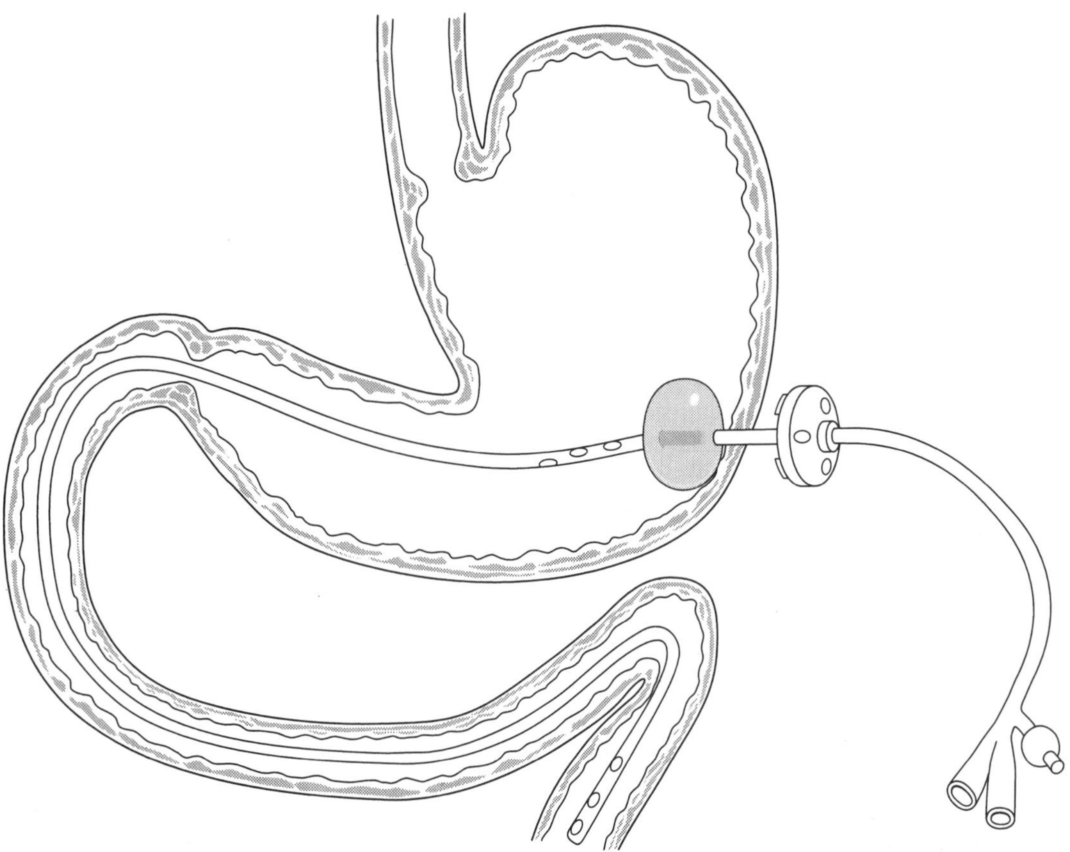

Figure 15-10 Transgastric jejunal tube. This dual lumen tube is placed surgically and allows for jejunal feedings while providing gastric decompression. (From Rombeau JL, Rolandelli RH: *Clinical nutrition: enteral and tube feeding,* ed 3, Philadelphia, 1997, WB Saunders.)

creased risk of aspiration, impaired gastric emptying, or primary disease of the stomach, a jejunostomy is preferred.

TUBE FEATURES

The type of tube used for a gastrostomy or jejunostomy depends in part on the anatomic site in which the tube is placed and the reason for its placement. The features of the tube to consider include material composition, tube size, and tip configuration.

Gastrostomy and jejunostomy tubes have traditionally been made of latex. Polyurethane and silicone have been used most frequently because these materials are associated with less soft-tissue reaction and longer wear time.

Tube size is generally the largest size tolerated by that anatomic site. For example, 24 to 30 Fr is an appropriate range of sizes for a gastrostomy tube in the adult. The best range for a jejunostomy is from 10 to 16 Fr (Apelgren, 1990). A PEG ranges from 20 to 24 Fr.

Several tip configurations are illustrated in Figure 15-11. Foley catheters are commonly used as gastrostomy tubes. However, they are not specifically designed for this purpose. Consequently, the balloon of the foley catheter is subject to decay from the gastric acid and requires periodic and regular replacement. In addition, Foley catheters do not have an external bumper and will migrate if an external tube stabilization device is not applied.

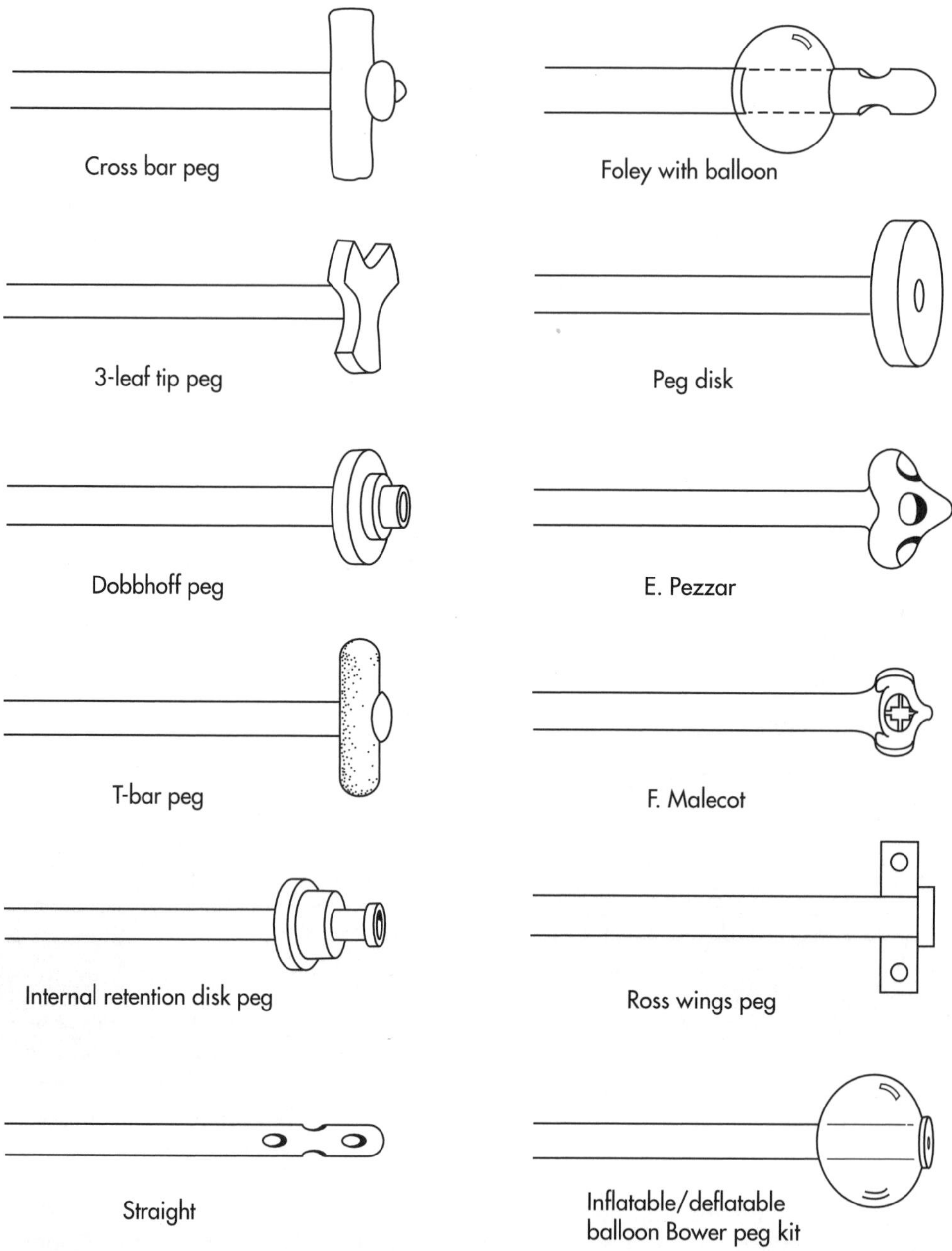

Figure 15-11 Tip configuration of enteral tubes.

Replacement gastrostomy tubes, which are silicone based, are preferable.

Another tip available and used to a great extent on the PEG is the disc. This tip cannot be removed by simple extraction through the skin and must be cut off. The tip is passed through the gastrointestinal tract or retrieved endoscopically. The PEG tip may also have a cross bar or bulb tip, which cannot be extracted through the skin.

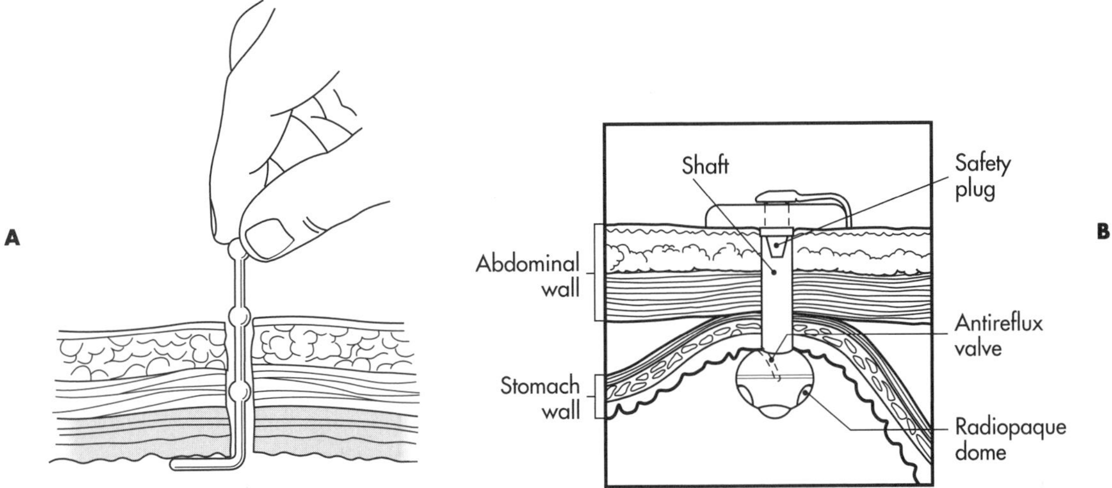

Figure 15-12 Gastrostomy button. **A,** Correct gastrostomy button size is determined by using a device to measure the width of the abdominal wall. **B,** Gastrotomy feeding button in place.

Tubes may also have a type of mushroom catheter known as a *pezzar tip*. These are rubber tubes with a stiff, round, pointed tip. The pezzar tip has minimal tiny holes present and unfortunately becomes easily plugged. This type of tip cannot be removed easily. The Malecot tube, also considered a mushroom catheter, has a bulbous tip with much larger openings. This type of tube can be more easily removed and is less inclined to become obstructed.

Multiple lumen tubes are also available. A triple-lumen tube may be used when patients require both proximal decompression and enteral feeding. This tube actually has four outlets or ports: a gastric lumen for gastric suction, a proximal duodenal lumen for duodenal suction, a distal duodenal lumen for feeding, and a gastric balloon. To maintain proper tube placement, the gastric balloon is inflated with sterile water or air (depending on the manufacturer's specific recommendation), and a retaining disk or tube stabilization device is applied at skin level. These tubes may be confusing to the staff because they are placed in the anticipated location for a gastrostomy tube but deliver feedings to the jejunum. Ports should be clearly labeled, and a diagram of the tube should be made available in the patient's care plan to provide clarity.

LOW-PROFILE GASTROSTOMY DEVICE (BUTTON)

A skin-level gastric conduit that is flush with the abdominal surface is known as a *gastrostomy button* (Foutch et al, 1989; Gauderer et al, 1988; Gauderer and Stellato, 1986). The button was first developed for use in children who require long-term gastrostomy feedings. It is a short silicone tube with a flip-top opening, a one-way antireflux valve (to prevent leakage of stomach contents around the tube), and a radiopaque dome that fits snugly against the stomach wall (Figure 15-12). Some devices have a special tubing that opens the reflux valve to permit decompression of the stomach.

To administer feedings, an adapter is passed through the one-way valve and connected to a feeding catheter. When the feeding is completed, the tube is flushed with water, the adapter is removed, and the flip-top opening is closed.

A button can be inserted in a clinic setting in an established gastrostomy tract and does not require anesthesia. It may also be placed as the initial device in a one-step procedure. The device is available in different shaft lengths and diameters. Correct shaft length is critical to ensure the proper position of the dome of the button against the anterior stomach wall, hence preventing gastric reflux around the button. By insertion of a special measuring device into the tract, the appropriate shaft length is determined. An obturator is then inserted into the button to straighten the dome of the button, making insertion of the button into the tract possible. The button should be lubricated to facilitate insertion. Once it is in place, the obturator is removed and the flip-top opening closed.

Disadvantages of the button include the potential for dysfunction of the antireflux valve with subsequent leakage and the need for replacement every 3 to 4 months. Studies and refinements of the device are ongoing; current reports demonstrate good success, few complications, and high user satisfaction.

NURSING MANAGEMENT OF ENTERIC TUBES

Optimal management for patients requiring long-term gastrostomy or jejunostomy tubes begins in the preplacement phase. Assessment of each patient should include the reason for the tube alternatives, risks and benefits associated with various treatment options, and the commitment of the patient or caregiver to long-term management. Preplacement information and instructions are critical to adequately prepare the patient and family for what they will be expected to do.

Nursing staff must also be prepared to care for the patient with an enteric tube. Much of the success of these tubes depends on proper care. Topics that must be addressed include preplacement site selection, site care, tube patency, tube stabilization, and management of complications. It is advisable to develop a competency checklist for the nursing staff who will care for a significant number of patients with feeding tubes.

Preplacement Site Selection

Tube exit sites should be selected preoperatively to reduce the potential for complications and to facilitate self-care. Site selection is commonly based on vague guidelines such as 3 to 5 cm below the costal margin and avoidance of the costal margin. However, in the person who has a protuberant hernia or is malnourished or wheelchair confined, this location may present a substantial problem such that it affects the integrity of their skin. Two techniques can be used to select a site preplacement, depending on whether the tube will be placed endoscopically or surgically (Hanlon, 1998).

Endoscopic Placement. When the tube is placed by the endoscopic approach, the location of the tube depends on transillumination. Therefore the specific site for the tube cannot actually be determined before the procedure. Nonetheless, by marking important abdominal landmarks (such as a skin crease, fold, or scar; the costal margin; belt line; prosthetic equipment; and hernia), the endoscopist can attempt to place the tube in a site that will avoid these landmarks. An indelible marker should be sufficient for these markings.

Surgical Placement. When the tube will be placed surgically, the technique used for preplacement site selection is the same as that used to mark a stoma site. The patient should be assessed standing, sitting, bending, and in the supine position. The objective is to find 1 inch of smooth skin surface that is free of creases, folds, and scars and avoids the beltline or bony structures. Again, a surgical marking pen can be used to place an X at the desired location. A transparent dressing may be applied over the marking when surgery is not scheduled for several days.

Site Care

Routine site care should include gentle cleansing with water; if desired a mild soap can be used but should also be rinsed off. To clean under an external bumper or disc, a cotton-tipped applicator may be necessary. Diluted hydrogen peroxide is only used to clean accumulated crusty drainage at the insertion site and when soap and water are ineffective. Routine and regular use of hydrogen peroxide should be avoided because hyperplasia at the tube site is associated with frequent use of hydrogen peroxide. Daily assessments should include the condition of the peritubular site and proper positioning of the stabilization device. The insertion site and surrounding tissue should be monitored for signs and symptoms of infection (i.e., erythema, induration, and pain). Soft tissue infections should be managed with culture-based antibiotics. Occlusive dressings for the tube site are generally unnecessary.

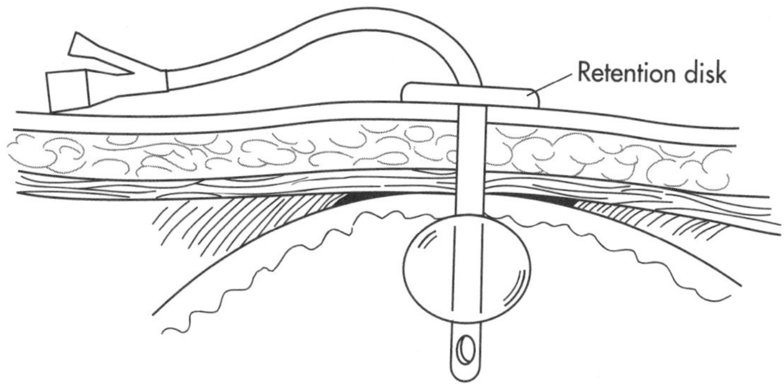

Figure 15-13 Proper stabilization of gastrostomy tube. Tube is secured between anterior wall of stomach and abdomen by a properly inflated internal balloon and externally with a tube stabilization device. Side-to-side mobility of the tube and tube migration are thus prevented.

Tube Stabilization

The most common complications related to gastrostomy or jejunostomy placement are 1) leakage of gastric or jejunal contents around the tube onto the skin and 2) tube dislodgment. These complications are frequently attributed to the failure to adequately stabilize the tube. Therefore postplacement nursing management must include measures to stabilize the tube (Powers et al, 1988).

Adequate tube stabilization is characterized by proper internal positioning and proper external (skin level) positioning. To achieve proper internal positioning, a tube is used that has a balloon, bumper, mushroom, or disc tip. These devices are snugly positioned against the anterior wall of the stomach (Figure 15-13). When a balloon tip is used, it must be inflated with an adequate volume of sterile water or air (in accordance with the manufacturer's guidelines) to work properly (Lord, 1997). Although saline may be readily available, it should not be used for balloon inflation because saline can crystalize and cause the balloon to rupture. Because water and air will diffuse through the walls of the balloon, adequacy of inflation should be checked weekly and any time that peritubular leakage is noted. Tubes with balloon tips should not be used as jejunal tubes; an inflated balloon within the jejunum is sufficient to obstruct the jejunum.

Adequate skin-level stabilization of the tube provides 1) minimal lateral movement in the tube at skin level and 2) avoidance of tube migration (in and out movements). Lateral movement of the tube contributes to leakage of gastric or intestinal contents onto the skin by eroding the tissue along the tract. Inflammation of the site can also develop from the presence of this chronic irritant. A stabilized tube should not allow lateral movement of the tube (Lord, 1997).

Migration of the tube in and out of the tract must be prevented. Nonstabilized tubes are subject to migration as a result of gastric and intestinal motility and abdominal wall motion. The tube can actually migrate and obstruct the gastric outlet (causing gastric distention, nausea, and vomiting) and compromise tube function.

Historically, sutures have been used to stabilize tubes. Unfortunately, sutures can cause tearing of the skin with subsequent inflammation and pain at the suture site. Additionally, although sutures prevent tube migration, they do not eliminate lateral tube movement.

Baby-bottle nipples have been used to secure gastrostomy tubes. Typically the nipple is cut along one edge, wrapped around the tube, and secured with tape as the tube exits from the nipple. Although popular and readily available, this technique in isolation is not completely effective at preventing lateral movement or tube migration. Effective tube stabilization can be accomplished only with a nipple when it is used with tape to secure the nipple to the

BOX 15-2 Methods of Tube Stabilization with Baby-Bottle Nipple

Use of Nipple with Skin-Barrier Wafer

1. Cut skin-barrier wafer to size of stomal opening at tube exit site.
2. Slit skin-barrier wafer along one edge so that wafer can be positioned around tube.
3. Remove protective paper backing and apply wafer to skin.
4. Slit nipple along one side and position around tube.
5. Secure nipple to wafer and tube with tape.

Use of Nipple with Skin-Barrier Flange and Convex Insert*

1. Cut opening in 1½-inch skin-barrier flange the size of stomal opening at tube exit site.
2. Peel off protective paper backing and apply barrier flange to skin.
3. Slit nipple along one side and position around tube so that the wide part of the nipple fits inside the flange.
4. Feeding the tube through the center of a convex insert (1¼-inch internal diameter), snap the convex insert into place inside the flange, securing the nipple. For ease of application, the convex insert can be applied so that the curve projects away from the patient's skin.
5. Tape nipple to tube. Note: A 1¼-inch skin-barrier flange can also be used. The wide end of the nipple will fit into the flange and is then secured with tape instead of a convex insert.

*Note: This procedure works best with Convatec SurFit flange and convex inserts.

abdomen or with a skin-barrier flange. Box 15-2 describes these two methods of tube stabilization.

Commercial external tube stabilization devices are also available (Figure 15-14). The commercial tube stabilization device is changed as needed; frequency is determined by the need to assess the tube site or provide site care. When frequent site care is required (as with newly placed tubes), a stabilization system that allows easy visualization of the site without removal of adhesives is desirable.

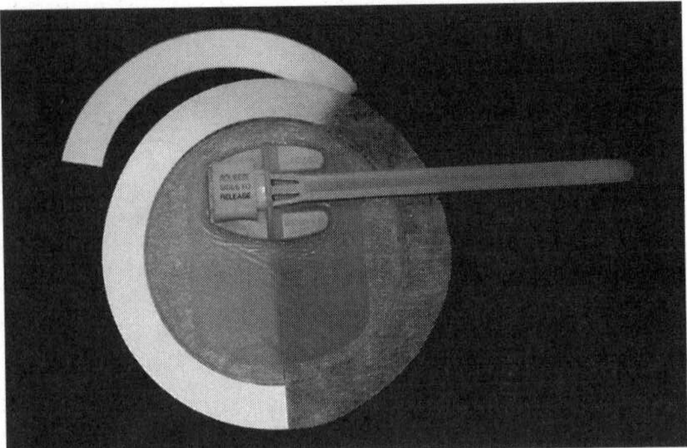

Figure 15-14 Commercial external tube stabilization device.

For selected patients the stabilization system may be discontinued once the tube site and tract are well healed. This usually occurs in 5 to 6 weeks after tube placement unless the patient is receiving corticosteroids, is immune compromised, or is malnourished. Before discontinuing stabilization measures, the nurse must assess the site to ensure that the tract is well granulated and that tube migration is no longer a potential complication.

Many tubes are being created specifically as gastrostomy tubes complete with stabilization features inherent in the design, thereby eliminating the need for commercial external stabilization devices. For example, the button has a dome, limited shaft length, and flip-top cap to ensure stabilization of the tube. PEG tubes are designed with an internal bolster and an external bolster. The internal bolster can be a bumper, disc, or balloon that when properly positioned lies up against the anterior stomach wall. Exteriorly, on the abdominal surface, the bolster is a bumper or disc that can be adjusted to lie snugly against the abdominal wall. This stabilization is critical to prevent dislodgment of the tube, mobility, obstruction, and peritubular leakage. A few Silastic catheter-feeding tubes (with a balloon to secure the tube against the anterior stomach wall) have an adjustable external flange (Figure 15-15). Once the Silastic catheter is in position and the balloon is inflated, the flange is slid down against the skin, stabilizing the catheter without the use of adhesives.

Regardless of the type of stabilization device or bolsters used, adequate stabilization is critical to

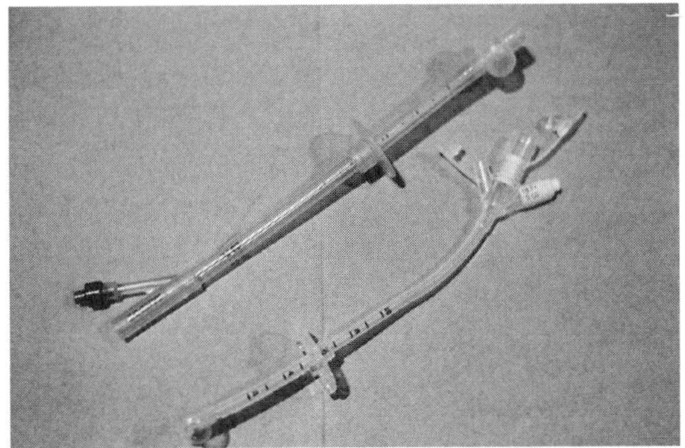

Figure 15-15 Sample replacement gastrostomy tubes.

the success of the tubes. They secure the tube against the abdominal wall and against the anterior stomach wall. The tension between the internal and external securing devices should allow slight leeway from the skin to prevent necrosis of the skin or gastric mucosa (Lord, 1997) This leeway should be monitored daily because changes in abdominal girth, such as with ascites, can develop, which then predisposes the patient to a pressure point under the external stabilization device. Modifications should be made as necessary.

Tube Patency

All enteral feeding tubes require routine flushing. This easy procedure is key to the prevention of tube clogging. In adults, the tube should be flushed with 20 to 30 ml of warm water every 4 hours during continuous feedings; with intermittent feedings the tube is flushed before and after the feeding. Tubes should always be flushed after medication administration.

COMPLICATIONS

Although the placement and care of gastric or jejunal tubes may appear to be relatively simple, they are associated with numerous significant complications. Complications may be related to the surgical technique or the tube. Examples include tube dislodgement, skin erosion at the exit site, skin-site wound infection, bleeding, peritonitis, and bowel obstruction. The first time the wound care nurse sees a patient with an intestinal tube may be when a skin complication develops. Although the skin problem must be addressed, it is also necessary to investigate and correct the underlying problem precipitating the skin irritation.

Skin Irritation

Skin irritation surrounding a tube is most commonly the result of chemical irritation (exposure to gastric or intestinal contents) or fungal infection. Leakage around the tube site warrants a thorough evaluation of the adequacy of tube stabilization, appropriate balloon placement, adequate inflation of the balloon, and tube patency. The balloon should be deflated and re-inflated with the amount of air or sterile water that is recommended by the manufacturer. Steps must be taken to correct any possible cause for the leakage. When all attempts to halt the leakage fail, the tube may need to be replaced.

If tube replacement is not an option and the leakage persists, methods to contain the drainage and protect the skin must be implemented. Hydrocolloids and absorbent dressings are not appropriate because they will trap drainage against the skin and cause chemical irritation.

To manage drainage around a tube site, an ostomy pouch and catheter port can be applied. By attaching a catheter port to the pouch, the tube can exit the wall of the pouch through the port, which allows for feeding, suction, or gravity drainage to continue. The ostomy pouch then contains peritubular drainage (Figure 15-16). Such a pouching system is cost effective and allows collection, identification, and measurement of the drainage as well as skin protection. Instructions for containing peritubular leakage are outlined in Box 15-3. Frequency of pouch change is determined by the duration of the pouch seal; on average the pouch is changed every 4 to 7 days. If a urinary pouch is selected, it may be necessary to "pop" the antireflux mechanism within the pouch, particularly when drainage is thick or contains particulate matter.

Fungal infections such as candidiasis can result when moisture is trapped at the insertion site. Corrective measures include protecting the skin from moisture with skin sealants or ointments or containing the moisture with appropriate dressings.

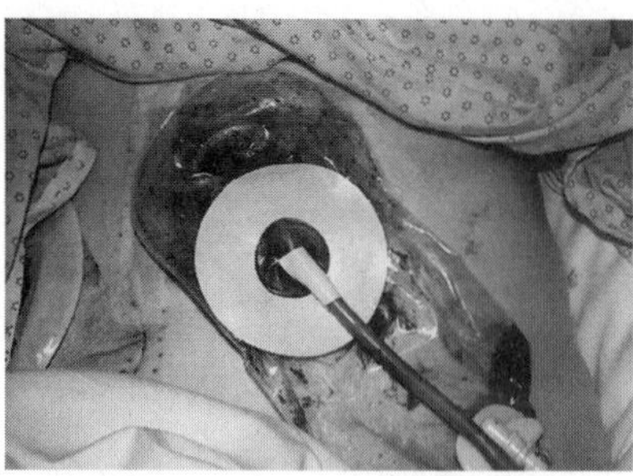
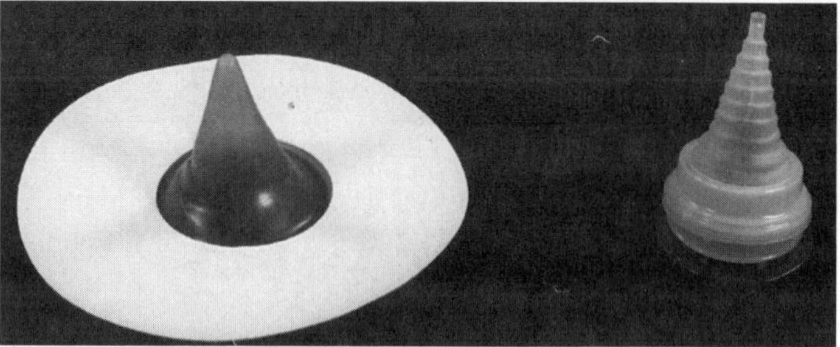

Figure 15-16 Catheter access port attached to drainable ostomy pouch *(left)*. Two examples of a catheter access port (NuHope and Hollister, Inc.).

BOX 15-3 Pouching Procedure for Leakage Around Tube

1. Assemble pouch and catheter access device.
   a. Cut opening in barrier and pouch to accommodate tube site.
   b. Make small slit in anterior surface of pouch.
   c. Attach an access device to the anterior surface of the pouch.
   d. Tear paper backing on pouch or wafer but leave in place.
2. Prepare skin.
   a. Clean and dry skin.
   b. Treat any denuded skin (skin-barrier powder to denuded area; water or skin sealant if needed to make powder tacky).
   c. Apply thin layer of skin-barrier paste to skin around insertion site, if needed.
3. Disconnect and plug tube.
4. Feed catheter through opening in pouch. Use water-soluble lubricant to pass tube, and use hemostat to pull tube through the pouch or barrier opening, anterior wall of the pouch, and the access device.
5. Reconnect tube.
6. Ensure dry skin; remove paper backing from wafer and secure pouch to skin.
7. Secure tube to stabilization device with tape.

Antifungal medications such as powders may be necessary when extensive candidiasis is present.

Peristomal Hyperplasia

An overgrowth of granulation tissue at the tube exit site can develop and is commonly referred to as *hyperplasia* or *granulation tissue.* This overgrowth of granulation tissue seems to be in response to chronic irritation or the tissue lining the tract. The source of the chronic irritation can be the type of tube material used (latex is more irritating that silastic material), tube mobility (particularly the in-and-out movement of the tube), and the chronic presence of excessive moisture. Hyperplasia may or may not be uncomfortable. However, when allowed to persist, seepage from the overgrowth will develop and compromise the integrity of the external stabilization and skin integrity. Treatment should address the underlying causative factor for the hyperplasia. Once this is corrected, the hyperplasia should resolve. Occasionally debridement and cautery with silver nitrate sticks may be warranted; however, this should be an infrequent procedure because it can be painful for the patient and should not be performed by an inexperienced care provider.

Tube Occlusion

The care plan should also incorporate measures to prevent or manage tube obstruction. Occlusion can result from inappropriate administration of medications in the feeding tube, viscous formulas, poor or inadequate flushing techniques, partially digested proteins, yeast, and aspiration of gastric or intestinal contents into the tube (Frankel et al, 1998). Water should be used initially to dislodge an occlusion. This process can also assist in distinguishing a kinked tube from a clogged tube; kinked tubes allow slow passage of water, whereas clogged tubes do not allow any passage of water (Frankel et al, 1998).

BOX 15-4 Sample Protocol for Enteral Tube Occlusion

Method A

1. Attach 5-ml luer-lok syringe and attempt to flush the tube with warm water and moderate pressure.
2. If irrigation is unsuccessful, attach an "Intro-Reducer" and attempt to irrigate with warm water using a 20- 60-mL syringe.
3. If unsuccessful, instill activated pancreatic enzyme mixture through "Intro-Reducer."

Method B

1. Attach a 30- 60-ml syringe to the end of the enteral tube and aspirate as much fluid as possible. Discard the fluid.
2. Fill the syringe with 5 ml of warm water and attach it to the end of the enteral device. Instill the water under manual pressure for 1 minute, using a back-and-forth motion with the plunger to loosen the clop.
3. Clamp the tube for 5 to 15 minutes.
4. Try to aspirate or flush the tube with warm water.
5. If the tube remains clogged, this procedure may be repeated with a pancrease and sodium bicarbonate solution (1 crushed Viokase tablet, or 1 teaspoon Viokase powder mixed with 1 nonenteric-coated sodium bicarbonate tablet, or 1/8 teaspoon baking soda dissolved in 5 ml warm water).

Adapted from Frankel EH et al: Methods of restoring patency to occluded feeding tubes, *Nutr Clin Pract* 13:129, 1998; Lord, LM: Enteral access devices, *Nurs Clin North Am* 32(4):685, 1997.

When irrigation with water fails, activated pancreatic enzymes should be instilled. The use of cranberry juice, chymotrypsin, carbonated drinks, and meat tenderizers is discouraged because they tend to precipitate in the feeding solution within the tube or cause adverse effects in patients with severe hepatic, renal, or coagulation abnormalities (Frankel et al, 1998; Metheny, Eisenberg, and McSweeney, 1988).

Declogging devices are also available. Some devices consist of a catheter that can be inserted into the feeding tube to which a syringe can be attached and a solution delivered to site of the occlusion. Some of these devices can be used to instill a mixture of pancreatic enzymes and sodium bicarbonate near the site of the clog. Devices that actually bore through the clog or brush the walls of the feeding tube are also available (Frankel et al, 1998). Box 15-4 provides a sample protocol for managing tube occlusion.

BOX 15-5 Instructions for Removal of Original PEG Tube

Equipment needed

Nonsterile gloves
Gauze, 4 × 4

Procedure

1. Obtain permission from physician.
2. Using dominant hand, grasp PEG tubing above bumper and rotate it 360 degrees. If it does not freely rotate, stop and call physician. If it rotates freely, wrap it around your hand to maintain a firm grip.
3. Use other hand to stabilize the patient's abdomen around the site.
4. Exerting moderate force, pull on PEG tube until inner bumper comes through skin opening. There may be slight bleeding. If resistance is too great, stop and call physician.
5. Cover opening with gauze until ready to insert replacement G-tube. This should be inserted immediately to prevent closure of the tract.

NOTE: Original PEG tube must be at least 2 weeks postinsertion before nurse should perform this procedure.
Courtesy Karen Huskey.

Tube Removal

Enteral tubes are removed when the patient is able to resume adequate nutrition orally and may need to be removed when hopelessly occluded, kinked, or malpositioned. The method of removal used will depend on the technique used to insert the tube and the type of tube tip used (Boxes 15-5 to 15-7). It is important to be familiar with the configuration of the tube in place and to have access to the manufacturer's information. Tube removal is a procedure

BOX 15-6 Instructions for Removal of Balloon Replacement G-Tube

Equipment

20 ml luer-lock syringe
4 × 4 gauze
Nonsterile gloves

Procedure

1. Connect 20 ml syringe to balloon port of tube and aspirate all water out of balloon. (NOTE: there may be less than 20 ml as a result of evaporation.)
2. Slowly withdraw the tube from abdominal site.
3. Cover opening with gauze until ready to reinsert replacement tube. The tube should be inserted immediately to prevent closure of the tract.

Courtesy Karen Huskey.

that should be reserved for nurses who have successfully completed a formal competency check.

PATIENT EDUCATION

Patient education is a key nursing responsibility and absolutely critical to the patient with a gastrostomy or jejunostomy tube. Since the hospitalization period after tube placement may be brief to nonexistent, detailed caregiver education is essential and outpatient follow-up care is imperative. In some situations, percutaneous tube placement may be performed strictly on an outpatient basis. In either case, home health care will be important to facilitate patient and caregiver independence in the process, safety with the procedure, and monitoring for complications. Key content areas to be included in a patient teaching plan are listed in Box 15-8.

SUMMARY

Percutaneous tubes are contributing both to quantity and quality of life for many patients. Nurses play a vital role in providing tube stabilization, maintaining tube patency, providing surveillance for complications, and teaching the patient self-care.

BOX 15-7 Instructions for Insertion of Balloon Replacement G-Tube

Equipment

Replacement G-tube of correct size
60 ml syringe with male tip
Lubricant (e.g., K-Y jelly)
Stethoscope
Nonsterile gloves
20 ml luer-lock syringe
20 ml sterile water

Procedure

1. Choose the replacement G-tube that is the same size as the previously used tube unless otherwise indicated.
2. Draw up 200 ml of sterile water into syringe. Do NOT use saline.
3. Insert syringe into the balloon port; fill balloon to assure proper inflation.
4. Withdraw water out of balloon and lubricate distal end of G-tube.
5. Gently insert G-tube into existing opening in abdomen. Tube should go in without resistance. If resistance is detected, pull back and attempt to insert again at a slightly different angle. If resistance is met again, stop and call physician.
6. Once G-tube is inserted into existing tract, gastric contents should return into the tube. To confirm proper placement, instill 30 ml of air into G-tube and auscultate for sound, which should be heard in the stomach (not the abdomen).
7. Once placement is confirmed, fill balloon with 20 ml water-filled syringe. (Check balloon port to determine the exact amount of water needed to fill balloon.)
8. After balloon is inflated, gently pull back on the tube until resistance is felt, then slide the external bumper or disc down until it rests lightly on the skin.
9. Rotate the catheter 360-degrees to confirm that tube has free rotation.
10. Cleanse skin around tube with soap and water; no dressing is necessary.

Courtesy Karen Huskey.

BOX 15-8 Key Content for Patient Education

1. Name of procedure
2. Purpose for tube insertion
3. Characteristics of normal tube function
4. Type of tube placed
5. Size of balloon (if present)
6. Tube stabilization (why it is important, how it is achieved)
7. Routine site care (daily)
8. Weekly balloon inflation checks (if present)
9. Signs and symptoms of complications, and appropriate response
10. Tube feeding schedule and procedure (when applicable)
11. Name of person to call with questions or problems
12. What to do if the tube falls out

SELF-ASSESSMENT EXERCISE

1. Identify two indications for the placement of a jejunostomy tube.
2. List the major content areas to be included in a teaching plan for the patient with a percutaneous enteral feeding tube.
3. Differentiate between:
   a. Janeway gastrostomy and Stamm gastrostomy
   b. PEG and gastrostomy button
   c. Foley catheter and a gastrostomy replacement catheter
4. Discuss the indications for a radiologic approach to gastrostomy tube placement as compared with an endoscopic approach.
5. Identify advantages and disadvantages of a gastrostomy button.
6. Describe the process of selecting a site for the placement of a PEG.
7. Describe the significance of stabilization as it applies to percutaneous enteral feeding tubes.
8. List three options for stabilization of gastrostomy or jejunostomy tubes.
9. In managing peritubular gastrostomy leakage, the initial goal should be:
   a. Determination of cause for leakage
   b. Initiation of skin-protection measures
   c. Establishment of an appropriate pouching system
   d. Cauterization of tract with silver nitrate
10. Which of the following interventions is key to preventing an obstructed feeding tube?
    a. Flushing the enteral tube with activated pancreatic enzymes once daily
    b. Flushing the enteral tube with 20 ml of cranberry juice every 4 hours
    c. Flushing the enteral tube with 20 ml of warm water every 4 hours
    d. Flushing the enteral tube with 20 ml of carbonated beverage every 4 hours
11. To cleanse the jejunostomy site, the nurse should:
    a. Use a skin cleanser three times daily
    b. Use a cotton-tipped applicator and warm water once daily
    c. Apply bacitracin ointment once daily
    d. Dab with diluted hydrogen peroxide once daily
12. The balloon on a PEG or replacement catheter is routinely filled with:
    a. Air
    b. Sterile water
    c. Normal saline
    d. Tap water

REFERENCES

Apelgren KN: Selection of tube type. In Apelgren KN, Dean RE, editors: *Enteral feeding in long-term care,* Chicago, 1990, Precept Press.

Bland KI, Karakousis CP, Copeland EM: *Atlas of surgical oncology,* Philadelphia, 1995, W.B. Saunders.

Coates NE, MacFadyen BV Jr: Laparoscopic placement of enteral feeding tubes. In Latifi R, Dudrick SJ, editors: *Medical Intelligence Unit: current surgical nutrition,* Austin, Tex, 1996, R.G. Landes.

Foutch PG et al: The gastrostomy button: a prospective assessment of safety, success and spectrum of use, *Gastrointest Endosc* 35(1):41, 1989.

Frankel EH et al: Methods of restoring patency to occluded feeding tubes, *Nutr Clin Pract* 13:129, 1998.

Gauderer MWL et al: Feeding gastrostomy button: experience and recommendations, *J Pediatr Surg* 23(1):24, 1988.

Gauderer MWL, Ponsky JL: Gastrostomy without laparotomy: a percutaneous technique, *J Pediatr Surg* 15:872, 1980.

Gauderer MWL, Stellato TA: Gastrostomies: evolution, techniques, indications and implications, *Curr Probl Surg* 23:657, 1986.

Georgeson KE: Laparoscopic versus open procedures for long-term enteral access, *Nutr Clin Pract* 12(1 suppl):S7, 1997.

Gincherman Y, Torosian M: Enteral nutrition: indications, methods of delivery and complications. In Latifi R, Dudrick SJ: *Current surgical nutrition,* New York, 1996, Chapman and Hall.

Gorman RC, Morris JB: Minimally invasive access to the gastrointestinal tract. In Rombeau JL, Rolandelli RH: *Clinical nutrition: enteral and tube feeding,* ed 3, Philadelphis, 1997, W.B. Saunders.

Gorman RC, Nance ML, Morris JB: Enteral feeding techniques. In Torosian MH editor: *Nutrition for the hospitalized patient: basic science and principles of practice,* New York, 1995, Marcel Dekker.

Hanlon MD: Preplacement marking for optional gastrointestinal and jejunostomy tube site locations to decrease complications and promote self-care. *Nutr Clin Pract* 13:167, 1998.

Lord LM: Enteral access devices, *Nurs Clin North Am* 32(4):685, 1997.

Mamel J: Percutaneous endoscopic gastrostomy, *Am J Gastroenterol* 84(7):703, 1989.

McGee L: Feeding gastrostomy, *J Enterostom Ther* 14(2):73, 1987.

Metheny N, Eisenberg P, McSweeney M: Effect of feeding tube properties and three irrigants on clogging rates, *Nurs Res* 37(3):165, 1988.

Moran JR, Greene HL: Digestion and absorption. In Rombeau JL, Caldwell MD, editors: *Clinical nutrition: enteral and tube feeding,* ed 3, Philadelphia, 1997, W.B. Saunders.

Patterson RS: Enteral nutrition delivery systems, In Grant JA, Kennedy-Caldwell C, editors: *Nutritional support nursing,* Philadelpia, 1988, Grune & Stratton.

Powers ML et al: A clinical report on the comparison of a drain/tube attachment device with conventional suture methods in securing percutaneous tubes and drains, *J Enterostom Ther* 15(5):206, 1988.

Rombeau JL et al: *Atlas of nutritional support techniques,* Boston, 1989, Little, Brown, and Company.

Welch SK: Certification of staff nurses to insert enteral feeding tubes using a research-based procedure, *Nutr Clin Pract* 11:21, 1996.

CHAPTER 16

Oncology-Related Skin Damage

MARGARET T. GOLDBERG & PEGGY McGINN-BYER

OBJECTIVES

1. Distinguish between extravasation and infiltration.
2. List at least five risk factors for extravasation.
3. Identify five cytotoxic and noncytotoxic agents that may cause tissue damage if extravasation occurs.
4. Discuss the parameters for assessment of potential extravasation.
5. Describe the roles of medical, nursing (including topical dressings and compresses), and pharmacologic interventions appropriate for extravasations resulting from at least three different medications.
6. Describe the etiology and clinical manifestations of a fungating wound.
7. List at least two goals for the management of a fungating wound, extravasation, and radiation-induced skin damage.
8. Describe at least four interventions used to achieve the goals associated with the care of the fungating wound.
9. Discuss the pathophysiologic basis for radiation-induced skin damage.
10. Differentiate between acute and late skin reactions to irradiation.
11. Define the Bruner and McGinn-Byer stages of skin reactions, including intervention options for each stage.
12. Identify key patient education information that will reduce the likelihood of acute radiation-induced skin reactions and prevent long-term complications in the irradiated field.

Thanks to Joseph G. Kusiak and Nancy L. Tomaselli for their review of this chapter.

Alterations in skin integrity may also develop as a consequence of medical therapy given for pathologic conditions such as cancer. This chapter presents three commonly encountered oncologic complications that involve the skin. These can develop during the course of cancer therapy or months to years later. The risk factors, assessment, prevention, and treatment for each condition are described.

EXTRAVASATION

The administration of intravenous fluids and or medications has the potential for tissue damage if these fluids or medications leak from the vein into the interstitial tissues surrounding the intravenous site. As defined by the Intravenous Nurses Society (*Intravenous Nursing,* 1998), *infiltration* is an inadvertent administration of nonvesicant solution or medication into surrounding tissue, whereas *extravasation* is an inadvertent administration of vesicant solution or medication into surrounding tissue. The incidence of extravasation varies in the literature but may occur at a frequency of 0.1% to 6.5% of all cytotoxic infusions (Murhammer, 1996). Later, Buck (1998) reported a review of the literature that describes a range from 10% to 30%. Boyle and Engelking (1995) suggests that actual extravasation injuries are both sporadic and underreported and that the incidence of extravasation from vascular access devices is unknown.

All intravenous medications and fluids can cause tissue injury after extravasation, but the severity of injury depends on the specific drug administered, its concentration, the amount of drug extravasated, the length of time that tissue is exposed to the drug, and the anatomic site of the extravasation (Ramu, 1996).

Prevention Of Extravasation

Recognizing patients at risk for extravasation, along with the risk profile of the medications, can signal the need for precautions that will decrease the occurrence of extravasation injuries.

Certain patients are more likely to have an extravasation injury. According to the *Standard of Care* (1998), such patients include those who are unable to communicate the presence of pain; confused; debilitated; elderly with impaired vascularity; and receiving vesicants over joints, tendons, nerves, or bony prominences. Patients with inadequate veins and preexisting venous or lymphatic impairment or obstruction in the involved extremity are at high risk for an extravasation injury. Buck (1998) concurs that age is the most significant risk factor, stating that infants and young children have more extravasations, possibly because of their need for smaller catheters and their inability to communicate pain at the IV site as an early warning sign. According to Buck (1998) additional risk factors include larger cannula gauge (therefore smaller internal diameter of the needle), use of steel needles, and infusion of substances known to cause direct cell damage. Individuals with darker complexions are also at risk because of the difficulty in assessing early warning signs such as erythema. Neonates and premature babies are particularly at risk of developing extravasation because of the small size of their vessels and the immature structure of their skin. Patients with prior radiation, decreased lymphatic drainage such as in those with a mastectomy, vascular ischemia, vascular obstruction, and small vessel diameter are deemed to be at risk by Lexi-Comp (1997).

Hyperosmolar solutions, vasopressor agents, and cytotoxic agents are the cause of the most frequently encountered wounds. Cytotoxic agents are classified as vesicants, irritants, and nonvesicants according to their potential to cause local toxicity. Not all cytotoxic agents cause local toxicity. Irritants can produce pain, burning, or inflammation without necrosis when extravasated. Nonvesicants do not usually cause a local reaction on administration. Vesicants can result in progressive and severe tissue destruction as well as significant pain. See Table 16-1 for a list of cytotoxic agents and their specific irritation and necrosis potential. Table 16-2 lists noncytotoxic agents that have the potential for significant local reactions.

Prevention of extravasation injuries includes a thorough assessment of the patient, the venous access, related risk factors, and knowledge of the vesicant potential of the drug. Vesicant agents should only be given through a newly established line. Infusions should be halted at the first sign of discomfort, altered infusion flow, or a local reaction (Murhammer, 1996).

The agents listed as vesicants can cause extensive necrosis. Doxorubicin, daunorubicin, epirubicin, and mitomycin bind to deoxyribonucleic acid (DNA), recycle locally, and may cause a progressive slough of tissue over several weeks, requiring excision and skin grafting (British Columbia Cancer Agency, 1997a). A recent article by Herrington and Figueroa (1997) suggests that paclitaxel, which is normally classified as an irritant, may actually be a vesicant, and cites a patient who experienced a delayed vesicant reaction to a paclitaxel extravasation that resulted in severe necrosis. No acute symptoms were reported at the time of extravasation. The site was erythematous and had areas of central necrosis requiring debridement and closure by a plastic surgeon. Boyle and Engelking (1995) note, however, that more than half of the available antineoplastic drugs have neither vesicant nor irritant potential.

Assessment

Extravasation is usually heralded by a burning pain and occasionally erythema at the injection site, often associated with a swelling or bleb formation. Flare involves development of an erythematous streak along the course of the vein with pruritus, patchy erythema, and/or urticaria. Flare occurs in about 3% of cytotoxic agent infusions, is transient in nature, disappears within 30 minutes, and does not have the serious sequelae of extravasations (Murhammer, 1996). Induration, or obvious ulcer formation, is not an immediate manifestation, and visual inspection cannot determine the potential for or extent of tissue impairment (Boyle and

TABLE 16-1 Irritation and Necrosis Potential of Cytotoxic Agents

	NONVESICANTS		
VESICANTS	IRRITANT	MINIMAL	RARE/NONE
Actinomycin D	Carmustine	Etoposide	Asparaginase
Amsacrine	Cisplatin	Methotrexate	BCG
Dactinomycin	Dacarbazine		Bleomycin
Daunorubicin	Fluorouracil		Carboplatin
Doxorubicin	Paclitaxel		Cyclophos-
phamide			
Epirubicin	Plicamycin		Cyproterone
Idarubicin	Teniposide		Cytarabine
Mechlorethamine			Octreotide
Mithramycin			Pentostatin
Mitomycin			Thiotepa
Mitoxantrone			
Vinblastine			
Vincristine			
Vindesine			
Vinorelbine			

Based on British Columbia Cancer Agency: *Drug manual,* 1997a. Available at www.bccancer.bc.ca/cdm/ appendices/extravasation-of-chemotherapy.shtml; Boyle DM, Engelking C: Vesicant extravasation: myths and realities, *Oncol Nurs Forum* 22(1):57, 1995; Buck ML: Treatment of intravenous extravasations, *Pediatr Pharmacother* 4(1):1998; Murhammer J: *Management of intravenous extravasations,* Pharmacy and Therapeutics Subcommittee, University Hospital Advisory Committee, and the Department of Pharmaceutical Care, The University of Iowa Hospitals and Clinics Virtual Hospital, 1996. Available at: www.vh.radiology.uiowa.edu/ providers/Publications/ PTNews/1996/12.96.PTN.html; National Institute of Health Clinical Center Nursing Department: *Guidelines for managing extravasation*

TABLE 16-2 Noncytotoxic Agents with Potential for Significant Local Reactions

ANTIBIOTICS	ELECTROLYTES	MISCELLANEOUS	VASOPRESSORS
Cephalothin	Calcium chloride	Acyclovir	Dopamine
Chloramephenicol	Calcium gluconate	Aminophylline	Epinephrine
Gentamicin	Potassium chloride	Dextrose .10%	Metaramenol
Nafcillin	Sodium bicarbonate	Diazepam	Norepinephrine
Oxacillin		Dobutamine	
Vancomycin		Mannitol	
		Phenytoin	
		Radiocontrast media	
		Total parenteral nutrition solutions (not IV lipids)	

Based on Chen JL, Oshea M: Extravasation injury associated with low-dose dopamine, *Ann Pharmacother* 32(5):545, 1998; Boyle DM, Engelking C: Vesicant extravasation: myths and realities, *Oncol Nurs Forum* 22(1):57, 1995; Murhammer J: *Management of intravenous extravasations*, Pharmacy and Therapeutics Subcommittee, University Hospital Advisory Committee, and the Department of Pharmaceutical Care, The University of Iowa Hospitals and Clinics Virtual Hospital, 1996. Available at: www.vh.radiology.uiowa.edu/providers/ Publications/PTNews/1996/12.96.PTN.html; National Institute of Health Clinical Center Nursing Department: *Guidelines for managing extravasation with vesicant and irritant drugs*, 1996. Available at www.cc.nih.gov/nursing/APNDXA.htm.
NOTE: Always check individual drug information and institutional policies for the irritation and necrosis potential for every intravenously administered drug. Most institutions have guidelines for managing extravasation of vesicant and irritant drugs.

TABLE 16-3 Assessment of Intravenous Sites

	EXTRAVASATIONS			
PARAMETER	IMMEDIATE	DELAYED	FLARE REACTION	SPASM/IRRITATION OF THE VEIN
Discomfort	Pain or burning could be stinging or other discomfort at IV site	Within 48 hr	Pain or burning uncommon; itching predominates	Aching and tightness along vein
Erythema	May or may not be blotchy redness around the needle site	Occurs later	Diffuse, irregular blotches or streaks along the vein; may subside within 30 min	Redness or darkening along the full length of the vein
Ulceration	Develops insidiously; may occur 48 to 96 hr later	Occurs later	Not usually	Not usually
Swelling	Severe swelling usually occurs immediately	Up to 48 hr	Not likely; wheals may appear along the vein line	Not likely
Blood return	Absent or sluggish	Possible blood return during administration	Usually; not always	Usually; not always
Other	Changes in rate or quality of infusion	Local tingling and sensory deficits	Urticaria	Possibly resistance felt on injection

Based on British Columbia Cancer Agency: *Drug manual*, 1997a. Available at www.bccancer.bc.ca/cdm/ appendices/extravasation-of-chemotherapy.shtml; Boyle DM, Engelking C: Vesicant extravasation: myths and realities, *Oncol Nurs Forum* 22(1):57, 1995; National Institute of Health Clinical Center Nursing Department: *Guidelines for managing extravasation with vesicant and irritant drugs*, 1996. Available at www.cc.nih.gov/nursing/APNDXA.htm.

Engelking, 1996). Although extravasation can occur without symptoms, the injection site should be observed for swelling, stinging, burning, bleb formation, pain, or redness. Lack of blood return may suggest extravasation, but alone it is not always indicative of such (*Standard of Care,* 1998). Table 16-3 lists the parameters that should be included when conducting an intravenous site skin assessment for possible extravasation or infiltration.

As noted previously, infiltration and extravasation are separate processes. An infiltration scale is available in Table 16-4. The infiltration of any amount of blood product, irritant, or vesicant is classified as a grade 4 infiltration because of the potential for patient harm.

Interventions

Early intervention after extravasation can lessen the severity of tissue injury. There is very little agreement on treatment measures in the literature. Modalities include thermal devices to alter the temperature of superficial skin, manipulation of the pH of exposed tissue, and injection of antidotes into the affected area to reverse the action of the infiltrated agent or to otherwise interfere with the process of cell destruction.

Once infiltration is noted, infusion should be discontinued with thorough examination of the site. If the catheter appears to be lodged in the tissues, an attempt to aspirate any fluid remaining in the catheter can be made to decrease the amount of drug at the site (Buck, 1998). Lexi-Comp (1997) recommends leaving the needle in place, aspirating any residual drug and blood in the IV tubing, needle, and suspected extravasation site. Furthermore, for all drugs *except* mechlorethamine (nitrogen mustard) and vinca alkaloid (vinblastine, vinorelbine, vincristine) where highly effective

TABLE 16-4 Infiltration Scale

GRADE 0	GRADE 1	GRADE 2	GRADE 3	GRADE 4
No symptoms	• Skin blanched • Edema <1 inch • Cool to touch with or without pain	• Skin blanched • Edema 1 to 6 inches • Cool to touch with or without pain	• Skin blanched, translucent • Gross edema >6 inches • Mild to moderate pain • Possible numbness	• Skin blanched, translucent • Skin tight, leaking • Skin discolored, bruised, swollen • Gross edema >6 inches • Deep pitting tissue edema • Circulatory impairment • Moderate to severe pain • Infiltration of any amount of blood product, irritant, vesicant

From Intravenous nursing: standards of practice: Intravenous Nurses Society, *J Intraven Nurs* 21(1 suppl):S36, 1998.

antidotes are well known, the needle should be removed.

Pressure is always contraindicated because even slight pressure on an extravasated area could spread the vesicant agent over a much broader area. Elevation of the affected limb is recommended to decrease swelling and increase net blood flow away from the area.

There is much debate in the literature about the application of warm or cold compresses. A small study found no benefit from warm or cold compresses on healthy volunteers given intentional extravasation of normal or hypertonic saline (Hastings-Tolsma et al, 1993). However, in another very small study, Yucha, Hastings-Tolsma, and Szevereny (1994) found that elevation had no effect on pain, surface area of induration, or volume of infiltrate remaining. Although elevation and compresses may not reduce the amount of drug penetration, those therapies may significantly improve patient comfort (Buck, 1998). In most cases the choice of treatment should be tailored to the individual patient. Moist heat, however, should be avoided because it can lead to maceration and necrosis.

The appropriate type of compress (cold versus hot) for specific medications when they extravasate are listed in Table 16-5. Cold will actually increase the toxicity of vinca alkaloid extravasations and should be avoided (Murhammer, 1996). Doxorubicin toxicity is significantly reduced by cold and increased by heat. Cold is preferred for all extravasations by cytotoxic agents except for vincristine, vinblastine, vonorelbine, and etoposide. Intermittent cold as a compress is preferred because continuous application of ice to the area may cause an increase in tissue necrosis. Since the optimal frequency and duration for the application of warm or cold compresses is not known, each intermittent application should be for as long as the patient can comfortably tolerate it (NIH, 1996).

Pharmacologic Interventions

Sodium Thiosulfate. Sodium thiosulfate has been found to be an effective antidote for mechlorethamine extravasation. Mechlorethamine extravasation can produce severe prolonged skin ulcers along with immediate pain and swelling as a result of rapid fixation to all tissues by alkylation of protein and DNA. Prompt use of sodium thiosulfate after mechlorethamine extravasation is vital for maximal efficacy because of the drug's rapid local effects. This means that whenever mechlorethamine is administered, the antidote should be readily available (Murhammer, 1996).

Hyaluronidase. Hyaluronidase has been shown to reduce the extent of tissue damage after extravasation of parenteral nutrition solutions, electrolyte infusions, antibiotics, aminophylline mannitol, and

TABLE 16-5 Thermal Application Guide

HOT PACK	COLD PACK
Dopamine	Amsacrine
Etopside	Daunorubicin
Navelbine	Doxorubicin
Paclitaxel	Mechlorethamine
Teniposide	Paclitaxel
Vinblastine	
Vincristine	
Vindesine	
Vinorelbine	

Based on British Columbia Cancer Agency: Extravasation of chemotherapy, *Cancer management manual*, 1997b. Available at www.bccancer.bc.ca/cmm/19-10.html; Lexi-Comp: *Extravasation treatment of drugs*. Available at www.lexi.com/HTMLSample/appendix/section/ extreat.htm; Murhammer J: *Management of intravenous extravasations*, Pharmacy and Therapeutics Subcommittee, University Hospital Advisory Committee, and the Department of Pharmaceutical Care, The University of Iowa Hospitals and Clinics Virtual Hospital, 1996. Available at www.vh.radiology.uiowa.edu/providers/Publications/PTNews/1996/ 12.96.PTN.html; National Institute of Health Clinical Center Nursing Department: *Guidelines for managing extravasation with vesicant and irritant drugs*, 1996. Available at www.cc.nih.gov/ nursing/APNDXA.htm. Always follow institutional policies for care of vesicant or irritant extravasations.

chemotherapeutic agents, including the vinca alkaloids (Buck, 1998). Disa and colleagues (1998) describes hyaluronidase's ability to temporarily decrease the viscosity of the hyaluronic acid component of the ground substance, thus allowing greater diffusion of doxorubicin into surrounding tissues and therefore decreasing its local concentration. Timely administration is a key factor in achieving positive results with hyaluronidase. Treatment should occur within 2 hours after infiltration to be most effective (Buck, 1998). In a small study, Bertelli and colleagues (1994) used this enzyme as a local treatment after extravasation of vinca alkaloids. No patient suffered subsequent skin necrosis.

Phentolamine. Norepinephrine and dopamine are vasopressors that, when extravasated, cause circulation to the area to become impaired through their strong vasoconstrictive action. If not corrected, tissue damage may be severe enough to cause peripheral ischemia and gangrene, necessitating skin grafting and occasional extremity amputation. The extravasation site will appear cold, hard, and pale. Phentolamine is an alpha-adenergic blocking agent that causes vasodilatation, thereby decreasing the local vasoconstriction and ischemia and subsequently restoring circulation. It should be administered within 6 to 12 hours of the extravasation (Murhammer, 1996).

Dimethyl Sulfoxide. Dimethyl sulfoxide (DMSO) is a solvent that can penetrate tissues when applied topically to the skin. It has been evaluated for the management of extravasations because of its potent free-radical scavenging properties and possibly its ability to speed up the removal of extravasated drugs from the tissues. According to St. Germain, Houlihan, and D'Amata (1994) the application of DMSO topically with cooling has been shown effective at reducing skin ulcerations caused by doxorubicin. Bertelli and colleagues (1995) reports a 3-year experience with extravasations of varied etiologies (doxorubicin, epirubicin, mitomycin, mitoxantrone) in which all patients tolerated the treatments well with only one ulceration. Strum (1993) noted a stinging or burning sensation during the initial application as the only toxicity associated with DMSO.

Corticosteroids. It has been theorized that the antiinflammatory effects of corticosteroids can ameliorate the effects of vesicant extravasations. However, histologic studies have shown that inflammation is not prominent in the etiology of tissue necrosis. In fact, when high doses or multiple injections of hydrocortisone were given, they significantly increased doxorubicin and vincristine skin ulcers in experimental settings (Murhammer, 1996). Lexi-Comp (1997) reports that an injection of hydrocortisone is of doubtful benefit for amsacrine, daunorubicin, doxorubicin, epirubacin, and idarubicin and is contraindicated with etopside, teniposide, navelbine, vinblastine, vincristine, and vindesine.

Sodium Bicarbonate. Sodium bicarbonate has been proposed as an antidote, primarily for doxorubicin extravasation. Manipulation of local pH at the extravasation site may decrease the cellular uptake of doxorubicin and increase its removal from the area. Animal studies have described no antidotal effects and, mice studies indicate that sodium bicarbonate may increase doxorubicin skin toxicity (Murhammer, 1996).

Since most small extravasations do not result in serious problems even when antidotes are not used, injection of specific antidotes should likely be restricted to larger extravasations (>1 to 2 ml) (British Columbia Cancer Agency, 1997a; Kusiak, 1999).

Topical Skin Care

There are few recommendations in the literature for topical skin treatments of extravasations. Thomas and colleagues (1997) describe a topical method of treatment specifically for treating extravasation injuries in the hands or feet of small infants, but it can easily be adapted for treating similar injuries in patients of all ages. The technique involves the use of a sterile amorphous hydrogel applied to the affected area in a sterile polythene bag forming a "glove" or "boot." The treatment may be started as soon as extravasation is detected or suspected but should not preclude the use of other more immediate or specific measures, such as removal of the extravasated drug by needle aspiration if there are more obvious signs of fluid swelling. If tissue damage is apparent, treatment should be started immediately. Gel is applied liberally to the injury, and the affected limb is placed inside the plastic bag. If required, additional gel may be delivered into the bag with a syringe in sufficient amounts to ensure that the wound remains covered at all times and that the bag does not come into contact with the wound surface. The neck of the bag is closed using surgical tape, ensuring that the tape does not come into contact with the patient's skin. If necessary a splint may be applied to the affected limb to support the weight of the gel. Because both the gel and the bag are transparent, the wound may be examined without disturbing the dressing, which can usually be left in place for 2 to 3 days. If the wound shows any clinical evidence of infection, the dressing should be replaced daily and appropriate antibiotic therapy should be initiated. Dressing changes are accomplished by gently sliding the bag off the limb and irrigating the wound with sterile isotonic saline. During this treatment it should not be necessary to touch the surface of the wound, which does not need to be dried before the dressing is replaced. The limb is redressed as described every 3 days.

Amorphous hydrogels are used extensively for the treatment of sloughy or necrotic lesions where they are believed to facilitate autodebridement of the wound by rehydrating slough and enabling autolysis to take place at an enhanced rate. In the current application, the gel also prevents dehydration of damaged tissue and limits further devitalization of exposed dermis.

Silvadene (silver sulfadiazine) may also be used with open or closed bullae (Kusiak, 1999). The cream should be applied once to twice daily to a thickness of approximately 1/16 inch. Whenever necessary, the cream should be reapplied to any areas from which it has been removed by patient activity.

Surgery

In the presence of painful necrosis, early surgical intervention is recommended. Areas of extensive blistering or ulceration, progressive induration, and erythema or persistent severe pain are indications for surgical assessment and possible excision of the injured tissue (British Columbia Cancer Agency, 1997b). Induration and erythema may also herald the onset of infection, especially in the leukopenic patient; therefore antibiotics should also be considered in this type of patient (Kusiak, 1999). Skin sloughing has been known to occur in extravasations involving doxorubicin and epirubicin. Early debridement with delayed closure has been shown to be effective in some of these cases (Heitmann, Durmus, and Infianni, 1998). However, since as few as one third of all vesicant extravasations will ulcerate, the routine use of excision is not warranted (Murhammer, 1996).

Summary

Murhammer (1996) proposes a systematic approach to the treatment of extravasation that includes the elements of early detection to halt further drug delivery, conservative treatment, use of proven antidotes, and when necessary, surgical excision. Patient and family education are critical, especially if the patient will be receiving ambulatory continuous infusion of a vesicant agent. The patient must be instructed that although the risk for extravasation can be minimized, it cannot be entirely eliminated. The patient should be taught to examine the needle site every 4 to 8 hours and to report any possible symptom of an extravasation immediately. Ambulatory infusion pumps with occlusion alarms should be used, and the patient should be provided with written instructions of whom to call 24 hours a day if extravasation is suspected (Wickham, Purl, and Welker, 1992).

FUNGATING WOUNDS

Fungating tumors or wounds are a devastating complication resulting from complicated underlying pathology such as metastasis. The incidence of fungating wounds has not been established. Although they appear to be a rare yet troublesome occurrence, Lookingbill, Spangler, and Helm (1993) reports a 10% incidence among a series of patients with metastatic disease. Fungating wounds present a physical and emotional challenge to patients, families, and caregivers.

Definition

The fungating wound is an ulcerating malignant skin lesion and is defined by the British Columbia Cancer Agency (1997c) as "a cancerous lesion involving the skin which is open and may be draining." The wound may be a result of a primary cancer, a metastasis to the skin from a local tumor, or a tumor at a distant site. The lesion can present as a rapidly growing fungus or with a cauliflower-like appearance that also may ulcerate and form shallow craters. Associated sinus or fistula formation can create malodorous fungating wounds (Collier, 1997).

Etiology

Fungating wounds are most commonly associated with breast cancer but may also originate from cancers of the head, neck, kidney, lung, ovary, colon, and penis (Young, 1997). Lymphoma, leukemia, and melanoma can also produce fungating skin lesions. Collier (1997) notes the infiltration of the skin involves the spread of malignant cells along pathways that offer minimal resistance, such as tissue planes and blood and lymph capillaries, and through the perineural spaces. These wounds often become infected with aerobic and anaerobic organisms that produce volatile fatty acids and other molecules with a pungent odor that can be a source of great embarrassment and distress to the patient, family, and caregivers (Thomas, 1992). There are few published studies regarding the management of these wounds; Moody and Grocott (1993) maintain that current practice relies more upon an exploratory approach rather than research-based evidence.

Assessment

The management of fungating wounds is based on achieving the objectives of symptom control and patient comfort rather than wound healing. As with all wound care, objectives of therapy must derive from a thorough and indepth wound assessment. See Table 16-6 for a list of wound-assessment parameters pertinent to the fungating wound (Goldberg, 1997).

In addition, the patient, family, and caregivers should be involved in setting the principal aim of the treatment. It is useful to begin the assessment by asking the patient what aspect of this wound is the most disturbing. It may be surprising to learn that the dressing changes two to three times daily do not upset the patient as much as the odor from the wound or the constant drainage. Toward this end, care is targeted to the areas of most concern to the patient and family while maximizing the effects of the intervention.

The patient's psychologic assessment should include their coping skills, feelings, and reactions to their wound as well as their reaction to their disease. Potential isolation and social ostracism are possible if the lesions are visible and/or odor is apparent (NCI, 1997b).

Nursing Interventions

Treatment options for the fungating wound are aimed at the underlying pathology and include radiotherapy, chemotherapy, hormone therapy, surgery, cryotherapy, or laser therapy (NCI, 1997b). Wound and local treatment must be congruent with the goals and objectives that were identified through the process of psychosocial and physical assessment. These interventions may or may not support wound

TABLE 16-6 Assessment of Fungating Wounds

ASSESSMENT PARAMETER	DESCRIPTION
Appearance	Necrosis, slough, bleeding, ulceration
Odor	Sweet, foul (offensive)
Drainage/exudate	Clear, thick, thin; low, moderate, copious amount
Presence of infection	Increased drainage; fever, leukocytosis
Periwound skin	Erythemia, maceration, edema, tenderness, maculopapular rash
Size and shape of site	Interference with dressing application

Based on British Columbia Cancer Agency: Guidelines for the care of chronic ulcerating malignant skin lesions, *Cancer management manual,* 1997c. Available at www.bccancer.bc.ca/cmm/ulcerating-lesions/01.shtml; Moody M, Grocott P: Let us extend our knowledge base: assessment and managment of fungating malignant wounds, *Prof Nurse* 8(9):586, 1993.

healing since wound healing, seldom a realistic expectation, is unlikely to be the primary objective.

Dressing selection for the fungating wound includes considerations other than efficacy; issues such as costs, reimbursement, local availability, number of applications required, complexity of the procedure, additional patient care needs, anticipated care provider, and extent of education necessary for appropriate dressing use must also be considered. As Doughty (1992) notes, there is no one correct dressing for each wound; a variety of dressings are available so that care can be tailored to the patient's specific needs. There is no ideal dressing for malignant fungating wounds. Individual situations should be assessed and dealt with according to the wound presentation at that time (Young, 1997). The nurse or caregiver should use dressings that will accomplish the goal of treatment within the realm of those dressings available to them.

Management of fungating wounds typically addresses three key objectives: 1) wound pain management, 2) odor control, and 3) control of exudate (Collier, 1997; Williams, 1997; Young, 1997). Table 16-7 lists appropriate intervention options for each of these treatment objectives. The following section further describes treatment options for these key objectives. Table 16-8 contains a partial list of specific examples of dressings by generic dressing category.

Pain Management. The fungating wound is characteristically painful, but a key source of pain is the trauma associated with dressing changes. Consequently, to control or minimize pain requires attention to the reduction or elimination of mechanical trauma. Two primary interventions are 1) minimization of trauma associated with dressing changes and 2) infrequent dressing changes. The fungating wound site also has an increased tendency to bleed when disturbed, which may aggravate the presence of pain. Infrequent dressing changes also reduce the potential for bleeding. When bleeding is a concern, appropriate dressings must be selected to reduce the potential for a bleeding episode. The skin surrounding the malignant fungating wound is often delicate and friable and requires diligent attention to maintain integrity and control pain (Collier, 1997).

Nontraumatic dressing changes. Dressings whose interface will not adhere to the wound but will remain absorbent are used to encourage nontraumatic dressing removal. Dressing selection options include a contact-layer dressing, nonadherent gauze, impregnated gauze such as a hydrogel- or Vaseline-impregnated gauze, and semipermeable foam dressings. To eliminate unnecessary dressing changes, dressings should have a long wearing time, such as every other day. Protective barrier films, particularly those without alcohol applied to the surrounding skin, will also decrease trauma to periwound skin. Nontraumatic tapes and mesh netting can be used to affix dressings, thereby avoiding trauma to the surrounding skin upon removal.

Control of bleeding. Erosion of blood capillaries can lead to significant spontaneous bleeding. Many different types of dressings are available that assist in the control of bleeding. A comprehensive wound assessment should direct which dressing is most appropriate. Absorbable

TABLE 16-7 Interventions for the Fungating Wound

PAIN MANAGEMENT	ODOR MANAGEMENT	EXUDATE CONTROL
Nontraumatic dressing changes • Contact layer • Gauzes, nonadherent or coated • Foam • Protective barrier films • Nontraumatic tapes **Control of bleeding** • Hemostatic dressings • Nonadherent gauze • Alginates • Sliver nitrate sticks **Periwound skin management** • Nontraumatic tapes • Skin sealants (alcohol free) • Barrier ointment/cream • Hydrocolloid wafer	**Wound cleansing** • Ionic cleansers • Sodium-impregnated gauze • Antimicrobials • Polysaccharide beads **Deodorizers** • Charcoal dressings • Chloromycetin solution **Debridement** • Dry, hard, necrotic tissue (hydrogel, enzymatic debriders) • Wet sloughy tissue (polysaccharide beads, starch, copolymer dressing) **Reduction of bacterial burden** • Irrigation with ionic cleansers • Antimicrobial dressings and creams • Absorptive dressings • Sodium-impregnated gauze • Oral antimicrobials	**Exudate collection and containment** • Foam, alginates, hydrofiber dressings, hydrofibers, absorptive powders • Wound drainage pouch **Dressings changes at appropriate time interval** • When pooling on intact skin occurs • When strikethrough occurs

hemostatic dressings and silver nitrate cautery sticks can be used to specifically control the bleeding on an individual basis. Alginates have also been demonstrated to exhibit hemostatic effects and are also useful in the wound that is heavily exudative. Nonadherent gauze is an option and will absorb exudate without adhering to the wound bed. Significant bleeding events may also require oral antifibrinolytics, radiotherapy, and embolization. Although vasoconstrictive effects can result in ischemia and consequently necrosis, topical adrenaline 1:1000 may be applied for emergent situations (Grocott, 1999).

Periwound skin management. The skin surrounding the fungating wound is particularly fragile and therefore vulnerable to epidermal stripping, maceration, and infection. Routine skin assessments should be obtained to monitor for signs and symptoms of a bacterial infection (induration, localized erythema, heat, or pain) and fungal infection (erythematous, papular rash). Using nontraumatic, microporous tapes, skin sealants, and creams or ointment barriers can provide additional skin protection. When applied to the periwound skin, hydrocolloid dressings provide protection from exudate and also act as an anchor for tape.

Collier (1997) reports that excessive exudate production that is allowed to remain on intact skin will result in tissue maceration. Toxins contained in the wound exudate are particularly caustic and will exert a detrimental effect. Maceration and the resulting contact dermatitis may be decreased by use of skin barriers. Skin sealants can be used under adhesive or nonadhesive dressings to protect the skin from the wound drainage and prevent epidermal stripping associated with adhesive removal. Creams or ointment barriers may be applied under nonadhesive dressings and provide slightly more aggressive protection from wound exudate. Hydrocolloid wafers can be applied to the skin surrounding the wound to protect the skin from exudate and to act as an anchor for tape.

Odor Management. Odor can be caused by necrotic tissue, infection, or saturated dressings. It

TABLE 16-8 Dressing Examples

DRESSING CATEGORY	EXAMPLE (MANUFACTURER)
Alginates	Kaltostat (ConvaTec), Sorbsan (Dow Hickman Pharmaceuticals, Inc.)
Antifungal	Triple Care (T.J. Smith & Nephew, Ltd.)
Antimicrobial	Topical metronidazole, silver sulfadiazine
Barrier cream	Critic Aid (Coloplast Corp.), BAZA (Coloplast Corp.)
Charcoal odor-absorbent dressings	Carbonet, Lyofoam C (ConvaTec)
Coated gauze (gel)	Carragauze (Carrington Laboratories, Inc.)
Coated gauze (petrolatum)	Adaptic
Contact-layer dressing	N-Terface (Winfield Labs)
Enzymes	Elase, Santyl (Knoll Pharmaceuticals), Papain (Healthpoint)
Hemostatic dressings	Gelfoam (Healthpoint)
Hydrofiber dressing	Aquacell (ConvaTec)
Hydrogel	Amorphous: Intrasite (T.J. Smith & Nephew, Ltd.), Hypergel (Mölnycke Health Care) Wafer: Aquasorb (DeRoyal), Vigilon (C.R. Bard, Inc.)
Maltodextrin powder	Multidex (DeRoyal Wound Care)
Nonadherent gauze	Telfa, Exudry (T.J. Smith and Nephew, Ltd.)
Nontraumatic tape	Medipore (3M Health Care), Mefix (Mölnycke Health Care)
Nontraumatic wound cleansers	Shur clens (ConvaTec), Puri Clens (Coloplast Corp.)
Polysaccharide beads	Iodosorb (Healthpoint)
Protective barrier film	NoSting (3M Health Care), Skin Prep (T.J. Smith & Nephew, Ltd.)
Semipermeable foam	Allevyn (T.J. Smith & Nephew, Ltd.), Lyofoam (ConvaTec)
Sodium-impregnated gauze	Mesalt (Mölnycke Health Care)
Starch copolymer	Bard Absorption Dressing (C.R. Bard, Inc.)
Wound drainage pouches	Wound Manager (Hollister, Inc.), Wound drainage collector (ConvaTec)

Courtesy Margaret Goldberg and Margaret McGinn-Byer.

is difficult to objectively assess the presence of odor, but subjective reporting by the patient should guide interventions (Collier, 1997). Interventions appropriate for control of odor include wound cleansing, use of wound deodorizers, debridement, and treatment of infection. Many of these interventions can be used simultaneously to aggressively attack the problem of odor. For example, the topical application of the antimicrobial metronidazole has also been reported effective in the reduction of odor from fungating wounds (Finlay et al, 1996).

Wound cleansing. Gentle removal of exudate and debris from the wound base can aid in odor management. Ionic irrigants may help with mechanical removal of odorous necrotic tissue. Absorbent dressings, polysaccharide beads, sodium-impregnated gauze, and alginates absorb fluid from the wound surface and further assist in containing odors.

Deodorizers. Although not appropriate when the objective is to heal the wound, Chloromycetin solution is an effective wound deodorant. Gauze is moistened with the Chloromycetin solution and applied to the wound surface; it is generally changed twice daily so that the dressing will remain moist. Skin protection should be implemented to keep the solution from contacting the surrounding skin because Chloromycetin will cause an irritant reaction to intact skin. Puri-Clens (Coloplast Corp.) has also been applied to wounds to control odor.

As an outer covering, charcoal-impregnated dressings can be used either as a primary dressing (when the wound is not exudative) or as a secondary dressing (over a primary absorptive dressing) to suppress odor. These dressings are changed when they become moist (moisture inactivates the charcoal) and when the charcoal is saturated so that it is no longer effective. Charcoal dressings may require changes ranging from daily to every 2 or 3 days depending on the extent of the odor.

Debridement. Necrotic tissue can be extremely pungent and malodorous. Conservative debridement such as with autolysis or enzymes is a fundamental measure to control odor. Hydrogel dressings are a gentle method of debridement because they soften the necrotic tissue to facilitate its separation from the wound bed (Young, 1997). These dressings have the additional benefit of providing a soothing effect and providing pain control. The amorphous hydrogel should be used with crater wounds, whereas the wafer hydrogel is most appropriate for shallow wounds.

When the fungating wound is wet with slough-like necrosis, polysaccharide beads or starch copolymer beads can be used. Surgical debridement is less commonly used with odorous fungating wounds. Mechanical debridement is not recommended because of the tendency for fungating wounds to bleed and because of the pain that is triggered by wet-to-dry dressings (Young, 1997).

Reduction of bacterial burden. The presence of infectious materials in the wound can render a wound odorous. Actisorb Plus (Johnson & Johnson Medical) (odor-absorbent charcoal dressing with antibacterial activity), antimicrobial creams, and sodium-impregnated gauze all may assist in reducing bacterial numbers. Anecdotally, gauze dressings soaked in crushed 250-mg metronidazole tablets and mixed with 250 ml of normal saline serve to decrease bacterial load at the wound site. Dressings are placed on the wound and changed daily. Although effective suppression of odor has been reported, this is not an approved use for metronidazole.

Exudate Control. The surrounding tissue of a fungating wound is often edematous, and even a small ulcer or nodule can produce prolific amounts of exudate. Interventions that aid in exudate control include 1) collection and containment of exudate and 2) changing dressings at an appropriate interval.

Collection and containment of exudate. Moderately or highly exudative wounds require dressings that are capable of absorbing high volumes of exudate. Moderate to large amounts of exudate can be contained with semipermeable foam dressings and alginates. Very heavily exudative wounds may require a superabsorbent pad in conjunction with an alginate dressing, a hydrofiber dressing, or maltodextrin powder. A contact-layer dressing can be used to line the wound so that absorbent dressings can be applied and removed without traumatizing the wound bed. Two-layer permeable vented dressings may also be used. With these dressings, the perforated nonadherent layer protects the sound surface and permits passage of exudate to an absorbent and permeable layer (Grocott, 1999).

Wound drainage pouches are available from most ostomy manufacturers. These are indicated when the volume of exudate produced exceeds the capabilities of the dressings. Pouching should be considered when dressings must be changed more often than two to three times daily, when the skin begins to show early signs of damage, when the patient's ability to ambulate is hampered, or when odor is uncontrolled. These products have various desirable features such as attached skin barriers, flexible adhesive surfaces, and an access window over the wound site. Many wound pouches also have an attached tubular drain spout that facilitates connecting the pouch to a drainage container so that the fluid does not pool over the wound site.

Changing dressings at an appropriate time interval. As with other wounds, dressings for fungating wounds should be changed when exudate is pooling over intact skin or when "strikethrough" occurs. This time interval appears to be a function of the volume of exudate produced, volume of necrotic tissue present, and the patient's hydration status and activity level.

Evaluation

Patient reaction to many dressings is varied and difficult to predict. It is therefore important to elicit the patients' reaction to the selected dressing. The health care team, including the patient and family, must review the initial goals often. If, for example, debridement was an original objective, once necrotic tissue has been removed, a new goal or objective is decided upon by the team. In this way, the changing needs of the dynamic wound are met.

Assessment and management of the metabolic effects of the fluid losses from these open wounds should be ongoing. The management of fungating wounds is predominantly palliative with the aim of controlling symptoms at the wound site and reducing the physical and psychologic effects of the wound on the patient's daily life (Grocott, 1997). In most situations, the quality of care given to patients with malignant fungating wounds is the most important factor in determining their quality of life (Williams, 1997).

IRRADIATION TISSUE DAMAGE

Definition

Radiation therapy is an established, common treatment for cancer. Although the techniques and technologies for radiotherapy have been improved, skin reactions and complications still occur and continue to be a problem for patients (Lopez et al, 1998). The use of combined modality treatments such as chemotherapy with radiation increases the cytotoxic effect of radiation on the skin (Margolin et al, 1990). Unfortunately the effects of radiation therapy are not restricted to malignant cells. When the skin receives a significant dose of radiation, a reaction will develop that progresses through erythema to dry desquamation and then moist desquamation (British Columbia Cancer Agency, 1998). In addition, radiation recall, whereby a tissue reaction is produced by a chemotherapeutic agent in a previously irradiated field (Schweitzer et al, 1995), is not uncommon.

Historically, the management of these skin reactions has been inconsistent, and at present there are few reports of clinical trials regarding specific treatment modalities. Research about the most practical, comfortable, and cost-effective method of managing these problems is needed.

Etiology/Pathology

Ionizing radiation generates free radicals and reactive oxygen intermediates that damage cellular components, including DNA. Rapidly proliferating tissues such as intestinal mucosa, bone marrow, and skin are more susceptible to radiation. In skin, the rapidly dividing cells (keratinocytes, hair follicles, and sebaceous glands) are more sensitive to radiation (Hall and Cox, 1989). Skin is particularly vulnerable to the effects of radiation since it is in a continuous state of cellular renewal. At risk for highest stages of reaction are those body areas within the treatment field that include skin folds and bony prominences (Strohl, 1989). Patients receiving combination therapy are also at risk because the concomitant use of chemotherapy may sensitize the basal cells to radiation (Thomas et al, 1997).

Acute reactions are an expected adverse effect of radiation and may occur 2 to 3 weeks after beginning therapy or when completing therapy (Strunk and Maher, 1993). Acute radiation therapy reactions are a function of the dose delivered, multiplied by the volume treated over time exposed to radiation, rather than the total applied dose. Since acute radiation effects are cumulative, the greatest reactions occur toward the end of therapy. However, side effects are usually self-limiting, and most subside 1 to 3 months after therapy has ended (Bruner and McGinn-Byer, 1993).

Late radiation therapy reactions are a function of the total dose and volume of the area irradiated. Late effects usually occur within 6 to 18 months after the completion of radiation therapy (Bruner and McGinn-Byer, 1993).

Landthaler, Hagspiel, and Braun (1995) conducted a 10 year retrospective study and found that irradiation-induced ulcers appeared after a mean latency period of 8 years and 7 months. The frequency increased with total dose of irradiation and decreased with the increasing age of the patient. When ulceration and necrosis occur years after radiation therapy, according to Dunne-Daly (1995) they usually occur after trauma or infection. These lesions can become very painful and difficult to manage.

Assessment

Clinically, irradiated skin looks dry because of sweat and sebaceous gland destruction. There is loss of elasticity because of atrophy and fibrosis, and telangiectasia and discoloration occur with loss of hair. Other skin complications include ulceration, necrosis, shedding or deformity of the nails,

TABLE 16-9 Radiation Skin Reaction: Stages and Treatment Goals

STAGE	DEFINITION	TREATMENT GOALS
Stage I	Inflammation and slight edema	Protection and prevention of trauma
Stage II	Dry desquamation	Protection and prevention of trauma Rehydration of dry areas
Stage III	Wet desquamation and blistering	Protection and prevention of trauma Absorption of moisture
Stage IV	Epilation and suppression of sweat glands	Protection and prevention of trauma

Adapted from Bruner DW, McGinn-Byer M: Ostomy care considerations for patients before and after radiation therapy, *Progressions* 5(3):18, 1993.

malignant tumors, and lymphedema caused by fibrosis of the lymph glands (Lopez, 1998). The effects experienced by the normal tissues can be categorized as early or late. Acute effects occur during radiotherapy and in the immediate weeks and months after treatment. Late effects of radiation therapy develop gradually over several months or years. In those few individuals with serious late effects (less than 5% of patients who have received high-dose irradiation), the results are often disastrous and treatment is extremely difficult (British Columbia Cancer Agency, 1998).

Stages of Skin Reactions. Bruner and McGinn-Byer (1993) have described four stages of skin reactions to radiation therapy (Table 16-9). Early skin manifestations can range from erythema to moist desquamation and blistering. Late skin changes include epilation and suppression of sweat glands.

Erythema is a red, macular rash, on warm-appearing skin that may feel sensitive and tight. It is an inflammatory response thought to be caused by dilation of the capillaries and increased vascular permeability. Edema may accompany erythema. Dunne-Daly (1995) reports that this reaction appears about 3 weeks into treatment, usually confined to the treatment area.

Dry desquamation is red- or tanned-appearing skin that is dry, itchy, and peeling. This reaction is a result of the decreased ability of the basal cells of the epidermis to replace the surface-layer cells and the decreased ability of the sweat and sebaceous gland to produce sweat. This reaction could appear as early as 2 weeks into treatment (Dunne-Daly, 1995).

If the desquamation process continues, the dermis is eventually exposed and moist desquamation results. This reaction increases the risk of infection, discomfort, and pain, possibly requiring interruption of the treatment plan to allow for healing (NCI, 1999). This reaction could occur by the fourth week of treatment.

Prevention

Patients treated with identical radiotherapy schedules show a substantial variation in the degree of acute and late normal tissue reactions (Turesson et al, 1996). This makes it difficult to identify those at risk for severe radiation-induced skin reactions. Treatment schedule and total dosage in radiation therapy are based on the tumoricidal doses and the tolerance dose of the perifocal normal tissue. Fernando and colleagues (1996) conclude that there are both treatment and patient related factors that will increase the acute skin reaction after breast irradiation. According to Nachtrab and colleagues (1998), since large scale variations occur between patients concerning side effects, one of the major goals of radiation research recently has been the development of a predictive in vitro assay. In a very small study, Nachtrab and colleagues (1998) found a radiation dose-dependent increase in micronucleus frequency. They concluded that the micronucleus test seemed to be a very promising tool in the evaluation of radiation sensitivity before therapy. However, larger studies are needed to confirm these findings and to optimize the methodology. Dubray, Delanian, and Lefaix (1997) attempted to develop biologic assays, which would potentially be able to predict the probability of increased normal tissue injury after irradiation in individual patients. Such a test would allow the adaptation of the treatment modalities to the radiobiologic behavior of normal tissues. To date, these expectations have not been met. The quality of the irradiation and its modalities, including total dose, fractionation, and interfractional interval, remain the main ways to achieve an optimal functional and cosmetic outcome.

Some other researchers have attempted to find a form of protection for the skin during radiation treatments. Goebel and colleagues (1997) tested a liquid adhesive, which when applied to the skin, polymerizes rapidly to form a clear, tough, flexible, and waterproof skin sealant. Prophylactic use of the skin sealant on a small number of patients was well tolerated and appeared to be effective in minimizing radiation-induced desquamation.

Fernando and colleagues (1996), in a small study (n = 197), investigated the delivery method of the radiotherapy. It was found that the semisupine positioning technique during treatment may have enhanced the skin reaction in patients who received breast irradiation.

Campbell and Farrell (1998) emphasize that the nurse should prepare the patient for potential toxicities, thereby enabling proactive management in relation to diet and skin care.

Intervention

Radiation therapy treatment centers differ greatly on the most effective way to manage radiation-induced skin problems. Thomas and colleagues (1997) reports that many cancer treatment centers require the treatment area to be left open to the air, encouraging drying or crusting, in direct opposition to moist wound-healing principles. Furthermore, he reports that other treatment centers recommend covering the affected area with a cream or nonadherent dressing, neither of which ease the discomfort experienced by some patients (Thomas et al, 1997).

As noted previously, there are few evidence-based recommendations for the care of irradiated skin. More research is needed to support the use of many nursing measures used in skin care and wound management in radiation oncology. Nursing care during and after radiation is aimed at minimizing patient discomfort, promoting healing, and reducing the physiologic effects of radiation (Dunne-Daly, 1995). Patients and caregivers are included in planning care and selection of goals and objectives. These goals form the basis for evaluation of outcomes of nursing care and are reviewed and evaluated regularly. At every stage, patient comfort should be promoted.

Patient education concerning skin care is critical when preparing for radiation and during the course of the therapy (Figure 16-1). The primary focus of skin care is more on trauma prevention (Table 16-10). During the course of treatment, the focus becomes rehydration and moisturization. If skin damage occurs, the focus of skin care becomes absorption. Intervention options that support these three needs are listed in Table 16-10.

Many anecdotal reports are available for a variety of topical products used to prevent and manage skin damage associated with radiation. The following discussion is representative of a recent literature review.

A hypotonic oil-in-water emulsion (Biafine RE [Kinetic Concepts, Inc.]) is advertised for use as prophylaxis and for management of both wet and dry desquamation in radiotherapy patients. For prophylaxis, erythema, and dry desquamation, a small amount of Biafine RE is recommended to be gently massaged on and around the irradiated area three times per day, 7 days per week. For moist desquamation, the recommendation is a thick layer (¼ to ½ inch of Biafine RE) on and around the affected area, covered with a moist or petroleum gauze, and secured with tape as necessary. The dressing should be renewed every 24 hours. However, there are no clinical studies that show the efficacy of this regimen; there are merely advertisements and statements by the distributor after 20 years of use in France in the management of radiodermatitis.

Topical steroid creams (Cortaid, Topicort, hydrocortisone cream 1%) are sometimes used for the itching in erythematous and dry desquamation areas. Caution should be used with these preparations because steroids reduce itching by vasoconstriction, reducing blood flow to the skin. In addition, they can cause atrophy of dermal collagen, which can result in thinning of the skin and increased susceptibility to infection (Dunne-Daly, 1995). Steroid applications can also reduce wound healing.

PATIENT INFORMATION -- IRRADIATED SKIN

HOW TO HELP PREVENT SKIN IRRITATION TO TREATMENT AREAS

*Use mild soaps.

*Pat dry with soft towel (avoid rubbing).

*Do not use perfumes, deodorants, or makeup.

*Do not wear tight-fitting clothes or girdles.

*Avoid using heating pads and/or ice packs.

*Check with your nurse or physician about creams or lotions that are safe to put on your skin.

*Avoid sun exposure. Use cover-ups, hats, umbrella, etc. Ask your nurse or physician about sunblocks.

WOUND CARE (circle or highlight)

Mild to moderate discharge (leakage)   Moderate to excessive discharge (leakage)

Your treatment

Creams/lotions you *can* use:	How often:
____________________	____________
____________________	____________
____________________	____________

Type of dressing

____

____

____

Dressing change schedule

____

____

If you have questions call ____________________ **at** ______________
(Contact person) (Phone number)

Figure 16-1 Patient information regarding irradiated skin.

TABLE 16-10 Care of Irradiated Skin

OBJECTIVES	INTERVENTIONS
I. Prevent trauma to irradiated tissue	1. Use mild soaps. 2. Pat dry with towel (do not rub). 3. Avoid bathing or soaking in hot water, especially with bubble bath or detergent soaps. 4. No perfumes, deodorants, or makeup is allowed in treatment area. 5. Avoid tight-fitting clothes or girdles if in treatment field. 6. Avoid use of heating pad or ice packs to area. 7. Avoid sun exposure to irradiated area; use sunblocks, hats, coverups, T-shirts, umbrella, etc. 8. Use microporous adhesives only in treatment area. 9. Apply skin sealants as necessary under adhesives. 10. Avoid scratching of skin in treatment area.
II. Rehydrate and moisturize skin in treatment area	Apply only lotions or moisturizers to treatment area that are approved by radiation therapy physician. Commonly used products include Aquaphor (Beiersdorf) and Biafine (Kinetic Concepts, Inc.).
III. Care for radiation damaged skin appropriately	1. Apply hydrogel wafer or sheet to reddened or inflamed area as needed for comfort. 2. Use only nonadhesive dressings in irradiated skin field. 3. If irradiated skin is "weepy," consult with wound- and skin-care nurse for most appropriate type of dressings to contain drainage (such as foam, alginate, impregnated gauze, etc.) 4. Notify radiation therapy physician of skin condition.

Compiled from National Cancer Institute: *Pruritus (PDQ)*, June 1997a. Available at cancernet.nci.nih.gov/clinpdq/supportive/Pruritus_Physician.html 1997; Dunne-Daly CF: Skin and wound care in radiation oncology, *Cancer Nurs* 18(2):144, 1995; Metz J: *OncoTip: skin care and radiation therapy*, 1999, University of Pennsylvania Cancer Center. Available at oncolink.upenn.edu/support/tips/tip39.html.

A moisture vapor permeable (MVP) film dressing resulted in faster wound healing and greater patient comfort than a gauze dressing coated in lanolin in a small study by Shell, Stanutz, and Grimm (1986), who also reported that the film dressing did not have to be removed for radiation therapy treatments.

A hydrogel dressing (Vigilon [C.R. Bard, Inc.]) was used successfully by Strunk and Maher (1993) on a patient with moist desquamation. An advantage of this type of dressing is that they are nonadhesive and can be removed for radiation therapy treatments and replaced afterwards without causing trauma to the area. In addition, hydrogel dressings are cool, and patients report a soothing sensation on erythematous areas.

A hydrocolloid dressing was used on moist skin desquamation in a small study (n = 18) whereby all patients' skin reactions healed (Margolin et al, 1990). In addition, there were no wound infections evident.

Lopez and colleagues (1998) report that in the presence of ulceration after radiation, a biopsy should be performed to rule out any residual or recurrent malignancy. The treatment of these ulcers involves local wound care and surgical debridement with removal of all poor-quality tissue and timely reconstruction with well-vascularized soft tissue flaps.

Williams and colleagues (1992) reported a study of radiation-induced necrotic wounds that failed to heal after 3 months of conservative therapy. These were successfully treated with hyperbaric oxygen (HBO). Neovius, Lind, and Lind (1997) studied 15 patients consecutively who had soft tissue wounds without signs of healing, whereby the healing processes seemed to be initiated and accelerated by HBO. It is believed that HBO raises oxygen levels in hypoxic tissue, stimulates angiogenesis and fibroplasia, and has antibacterial effects.

Recent modalities for treatment using growth factors and biologic skin substitutes may be useful in this patient population, but according to Lopez and colleagues (1998) these have not yet been studied in controlled clinical trials.

Evaluation

Ongoing and consistent review of the goals of interventions are necessary to readjust treatments tailored to the reactions of the skin. Systemic measures are as important as local skin care. Optimal nutrition and hydration, wherever possible, are crucial to wound healing and should be included in the overall treatment plan.

It is imperative that patients are advised about the potential effects of treatment (Holmes, 1997). Patients also need to be aware of the possibility that skin reactions can be magnified by chemotherapy, as in radiation recall. Campbell and Farrell (1998) cautions that patients should be educated to avoid the use of any product within the treatment field and to put nothing on the skin that has not had the prior approval of the health care team. Potential irritants must be avoided for the remainder of the patient's life. Patients must be instructed that any area of the body that has received radiation treatment should be treated tenderly for the rest of their life.

SUMMARY

Although the wound care nurse is not expected to be proficient in the day-to-day care of the oncology patient, the potential skin complications associated with cancer are amenable to the application of wound-healing principles. As with other chronic wounds, the goals for these types of wounds range from healing to palliation and symptom management. The wound care nurse should collaborate closely with the oncology nurse, chemotherapy nurse, and radiation oncology personnel to establish guidelines for the prevention, early detection, and care of oncologic complications, such as extravasation, fungating lesions, and radiation skin damage.

SELF ASSESSMENT EXERCISE

1. The key distinction between extravasation and infiltration is:
   - a. Extravasation occurs only with chemotherapeutic agents
   - b. Extravasation occurs only with vesicant solutions or agents
   - c. Infiltration involves less tissue than an extravasation
   - d. Infiltration can occur with any intravenous solution or agent
2. Which of the following agents is known to precipitate significant local tissue reactions?
   - a. Thiotepa
   - b. Vinblastine
   - c. Cyclophosphamide
   - d. Bleoycin
3. Which of the following interventions is generally appropriate when an extravasation occurs?
   - a. Apply a warm compress
   - b. Remove the intravenous needle immediately
   - c. Apply pressure to the extravasation site
   - d. Aspirate any remaining fluid in the catheter
4. All of the following objectives are appropriate for the management of fungating wounds EXCEPT:
   - a. Odor control
   - b. Wound healing
   - c. Exudate management
   - d. Pain management
5. The primary objective of wound cleansing or debridement in the fungating wound is to:
   - a. Reduce exudate production
   - b. Promote a healing wound environment
   - c. Control odor
   - d. Provide pain relief
6. A stage III radiation skin reaction is characterized by:
   - a. Dry desquamation
   - b. Slight edema
   - c. Epilation
   - d. Blistering
7. Which of the following products should be avoided to minimize trauma to irradiated skin?
   - a. Deodorants
   - b. Emollients
   - c. Hydrogels
   - d. Skin sealants

REFERENCES

Bertelli G et al: Hyaluronidase as an antidote to extravasation of Vinca alkaloids: clinical results, *J Cancer Res Clin Oncol* 120(8):505, 1994.

Bertelli G et al: Topical dimethylsulfoxide for the prevention of soft tissue injury after extravasation of vesicant cytotoxic drugs: a prospective clinical study, *J Clin Oncol* 13(11):2851, 1995.

Boyle DM, Engelking C: Vesicant extravasation: myths and realities, *Oncol Nurs Forum* 22(1):57, 1995.

British Columbia Cancer Agency: *Drug manual*, 1997a. Available at www.bccancer.bc.ca/cdm/appendices/extravasation-of-chemotherapy.shtml.

British Columbia Cancer Agency: Extravasation of chemotherapy, *Cancer management manual*, 1997b. Available at www.bccancer.bc.ca/cmm/19-10.html.

British Columbia Cancer Agency: Guidelines for radiation therapy, *Cancer management manual*, 1998. Available at www.bccancer.bc.ca/cid/22.html.

British Columbia Cancer Agency: Guidelines for the care of chronic ulcerating malignant skin lesions, *Cancer management manual*, 1997c. Available at www.bccancer.bc.ca/cmm/ulcerating-lesions/01.shtml.

Bruner DW, McGinn-Byer M: Ostomy care considerations for patients before and after radiation therapy, *Progressions* 5(3):18, 1993.

Buck ML: Treatment of intravenous extravasations, *Pediatr Pharmacother* 4(1):1998.

Campbell T, Farrell W: Palliative radiotherapy for advanced cancer symptoms, *Int J Palliative Nurs* 4(6), 1998.

Chen JL, Oshea M: Extravasation injury associated with low-dose dopamine, *Ann Pharmacother* 32(5):545, 1998.

Collier M: The assessment of patients with malignant fungating wounds: a holistic approach. Part 1, *Nurs Times* 93(44):suppl 1, 1997.

Disa JJ et al: Prevention of adriamycin-induced full thickness skin loss using hyaluronidase infiltration, *Plast Reconstr Surg* 101(2):370, 1998.

Doughty D: Principles of wound healing and wound management. In Bryant R, editor: *Acute and chronic wounds: nursing management*, St Louis, 1992, Mosby.

Dubray B, Delanian S, Lefaix JL: Late effect of mammary radiotherapy on skin and subcutaneous tissues, *Cancer Radiother* 1(6):744, 1997.

Dunne-Daly CF: Skin and wound care in radiation oncology, *Cancer Nurs* 18(2):144, 1995.

Fernando IN et al: Factors affecting acute skin toxicity in patients having breast irradiation after conservative surgery, *Clin Oncol* 8(4)226, 1996.

Finlay IG et al: The effect of topical 0.75% Metronidazole gel on malodorous cutaneous ulcers, *J Pain Symptom Manage* 11(3):158, 1996.

Goebel RH et al: *A new approach to the prevention of radiation-induced skin desquamation using a polymer adhesive skin sealant: final results of a prospective study.* Poster Presentation Cancer Therapy and Research Center's Annual Breast Cancer Symposium, San Antonio, Tex, 1997.

Goldberg MT: Management of wound and pressure sores. In Berger A et al, editors: *Principles and practices of supportive oncology*, Philadelphia, 1997, J.B. Lippincott

Grocott P: Evaluation of a tool used to assess the management of fungating wounds, *J Wound Care* 6(9):421, 1997.

Grocott P: The management of fungating wounds, *J Wound Care* 8(5):232, 1999.

Hall E, Cox J: Physical and biological basis of radiation therapy. In Moss W, Cox J, editors: *Rationale, technique, results*, ed 6, St Louis, 1989, Mosby.

Hastings-Tolsma MT et al: Effect of warm and cold applications on the resolution of IV infiltrations, *Res Nurs Health* 16:171, 1993.

Heitmann C, Durmus C, Infianni G: Surgical management after doxorubicin and eiprubicin extravasation, *J Hand Surg [Br]* 23(5):666, 1998.

Herrington JD, Figueroa JA: Severe necrosis due to paclitaxel extravasation, *Pharmacotherapy* 17(1):163, 1997.

Holmes S: The maintenance of health during radiotherapy: a nursing perspective, *J R Soc Health* 117(6)393, 1997.

Intravenous nursing: standards of practice: Intravenous Nurses Society, *J Intraven Nurs* 21(1 suppl):S36, 1998.

Kusiak JF: Personal communication, Philadelphia, Penn, May, 1999.

Landthaler M, Hagspiel HJ, Braun F: Late irradiation damage to skin caused by soft x-ray radiation therapy of cutaneous tumors, *Arch Dermatol* 131:182, 1995.

Lexi-Comp: *Extravasation treatment of drugs.* Available at www.lexi.com/HTMLSample/ appendix/section/extreat.htm.

Lookingbill DP, Spangler N, Helm KF: Cutaneous metastases in patients with metastatic carcinoma: a retrospective study of 4020 patients, *J Am Acad Dermatol* 29(2 Part 1):228, 1993.

Lopez AP et al: What is your diagnosis? *Wounds* 10(4):132, 1998.

Margolin SG et al: Management of radiation-induced moist skin desquamation using hydrocolloid dressing, *Cancer Nurs* 13(2):71, 1990.

Metz J: *OncoTip: skin care and radiation therapy.* University of Pennsylvania Cancer Center, 1999. Available at oncolink.upenn.edu/support/tips/tip39.html.

Moody M, Grocott P: Let us extend our knowledge base: assessment and managment of fungating malignant wounds, *Prof Nurse* 8(9):586, 1993.

Murhammer J: *Management of intravenous extravasations*, Pharmacy and Therapeutics Subcommittee, University Hospital Advisory Committee, and the Department of Pharmaceutical Care, The University of Iowa Hospitals and Clinics Virtual Hospital, 1996. Available at www.vh.radiology.uiowa.edu/providers/Publications/PTNews/1996/12.96.PTN.html.

Nachtrab U et al: Radiation-induced micronucleus formation in human skin fibroblasts of patients showing severe and normal tissue damage after radiotherapy, *Int J Radiat Biol* 73(3):279, 1998.

National Cancer Institute: *External radiation therapy: what to expect*, 1999. Available at rex.nci.nih.gov/ NCI_Pub_Interface/Radiation/radexther.html.

National Cancer Institute: *Pruritis (PDQ),* June 1997a. Available at cancernet.nci.nih.gov/ clinpdq/supportive/Pruritus _Physician.html.

National Cancer Institute: *Skin integrity changes secondary to cutaneous metastases (PDQ),* June 1997b. Available at cancernet.nci.nih.gov/Skin_intergrity_changes_secondary_ to_cutaneous_metastases.

National Institute of Health Clinical Center Nursing Department: *Guidelines for managing extravasation with vesicant and irritant drugs,* 1996. Available at www.cc.nih.gov/ nursing/APNDXA.htm.

Neovius EB, Lind MG, Lind FG: Hyperbaric oxygen therapy for wound complications after surgery in the radiated head and neck: a review of the literature and a report of 15 consecutive patients, *Head Neck* 19:315, 1997.

Ramu A: *Compounds and methods that reduce the risk of extravasation injury associated with the use of vesicant antineoplastic agents,* Houston, Tex, 1996, Baylor College of Medicine, BCM Technologies, Inc. Available at www. bcm.tmc.edu/bvmt/techs/tech-96-30.html.

Schweitzer VG et al: Radiation recall dermatitis and pneumonitis in a patient treated with paclitaxel, *Cancer* 1576(6):1069, 1995.

Shell JA, Stanutz F, Grimm J: Comparison of moisture vapour permeable (MVP) dressings to conventional dressings for management of radiation skin reactions, *Onc Nurs Forum* 13:11, 1986.

St. Germain B, Houlihan N, D'Amata S: Dimethyl sulfoxide therapy in the treatment of vesicant extravasation: two case presentations, *J Intraven Nurs* 17(5):261, 1994.

Standard of care: medical guide for the legal profession, Chemotherapy extravasation issue, 4(2), 1998. Available at info@standardofcare.com.

Strohl RA: Radiation skin reactions, *Progressions* 1(3):3, 1989.

Strunk B, Maher K: Collaborative nurse management of multi-factorial moist desquamation in a patient undergoing radiotherapy, *J ET Nurs* 20(4):152, 1993.

Strum SB: Treating extravasation injury, *Contemp Oncol* 10:9, 1993.

Thomas S: *Current practices in the management of fungating lesions and radiation damaged skin,* Surgical Materials Testing Laboratory, Brigend General Hospital, Mid Glamorgan, 1992. Available at www.smtl.co.uk./WMPR/ Fungating-Wounds/fung.html.

Thomas S et al: *The management of extravasation injury in neonates,* Mid Glamorgan, Wales, 1997, World Wide Wounds, Surgical Materials Testing Laboratory, Brigend General Hospital. Available at www.smtl.co.uk/World-Wide-Wounds/1997/October/Neonates/Neonate Paper. html#ID6.

Turesson I et al: Prognostic factors for acute and late skin reactions in radiotherapy patients, *Int J Radiat Oncol Biol Phys* 36(5):1065, 1996.

Wickham R, Purl S, Welker D: Long-term central venous catheters: issues for care, *Semin Oncol Nurs* 8(2):133, 1992.

Williams C: Management of fungating wounds, *Br J Community Nurs* 2(9):423, 1997.

Williams JA et al: The treatment of pelvic soft tissue radiation necrosis with hyperbaric oxygen, *Am J Obstet Gynecol* 167:412, 1992.

Young T: The challenge of managing fungating wounds, *Community Nurse* 3(9):41, 1997.

Yucha CB, Hastings-Tolsma M, Szevereny NM: Effect of elevation on intravenous extravasations, *J Intraven Nurs* 17(5):231, 1994.

CHAPTER 17

Managing Wound Pain

DIANE KRASNER

OBJECTIVES

1. Briefly discuss research efforts related to wound pain.
2. Discuss the AHCPR recommendations related to pressure ulcer pain.
3. Describe the different types of pain experienced by patients with wounds.
4. Identify two ways to assess wound pain.
5. Define the Chronic Wound Pain Experience Model.
6. Discuss four assumptions about wound pain that are taken for granted.
7. State three strategies for managing procedural wound pain.
8. State three strategies for managing nonprocedural wound pain.
9. Discuss the effects of wound pain on quality of life.
10. Explain why an interdisciplinary approach to wound pain is optimal.

For people with painful acute and chronic wounds, coping with the wound pain can be as challenging as coping with the wound itself. For health providers and caregivers, the psychosocial aspects of pain management are very real issues. Although the wound-pain problem is significant, little attention has been paid to this phenomenon until relatively recently.

This chapter reviews the current literature on wound pain and the assessment of pain. The Chronic Wound Pain Experience Model and recent research on chronic wound pain are discussed in detail. Pragmatic suggestions for addressing procedural and nonprocedural pain are then presented.

In the current climate of outcome-focused healthcare, nurses should consider the use of "no-pain" or "reduced-pain" outcome measures. These can be highly measurable target goals, or they can serve as intermediate goals on the way to healing outcomes. Furthermore, in the case of palliative care where healing may not be a realistic outcome measure, reduction in pain may be an appropriate long-term goal. From a suffering patient's perspective, wound pain can be a significant problem, affecting quality of life and general well-being. The following words of an ancient Greek epigrapher should be kept in mind while reading this chapter: To cure—occasionally. To relieve—often. To comfort—always.

BRIEF REVIEW OF THE LITERATURE

Pain is defined as "the sensation which one feels when hurt (in body or mind); suffering, distress" (Oxford English Dictionary, 1933). Historically, research on pain has focused on such illnesses as low back pain (Cavanaugh and Weinstein, 1994; Frymoyer and Gordon, 1989; Mayer, Mooney, and Gatchell, 1991), headache pain (Olesen, Tfelt-Hansen, and Welch, 1993; Schoenen and Maertens de Noordhout, 1994), and arthritis pain (Grennan and Jayson, 1994; McCarthy, Cushnaghan, and Dieppe, 1994). The research that has been published on wound pain has generally involved acute wounds or burns (Choiniere, 1994; Cousins, 1994).

Over the past decade there has been an explosion of interest in pain as evidenced by the proliferation of algologic literature. There has also been a growing interest in the issue of wound pain (Dallam et al,

1995; Field and Kerstein, 1994; Franks et al, 1994; Hamer, Cullum, and Roe, 1992; Hollinworth, 1995; Krasner, 1995a, 1995b; Krasner, 1997; Krasner, 1998a, 1998b, 1998c; Pieper, Rossi, and Templin, 1998; Rice, 1994; van Rijswijk, 1999). In December of 1994 the Agency for Health Care Policy and Research (AHCPR; currently known as the Agency for Healthcare Research and Quality [AHRQ]) published Clinical Practice Guideline #15, *Treatment of Pressure Ulcers* (Bergstrom et al, 1994). This guideline addressed pressure ulcer pain, particularly as it relates to wound dressings and debridement, and stimulated interest in the subject (Appendix C). The panel noted that although there is only cursory mention of pressure-ulcer pain in the literature, clinicians report anecdotally that pressure-ulcer–related pain is experienced by patients. Clinicians were urged to assess for pain (not to assume that pain does not exist in nonverbal or nonresponsive patients) and to undertake the clinical research that is needed for evidence-based practice in this area. The panel recommended three specific guidelines related to pressure ulcer pain:

- Assess all patients for pain related to the pressure ulcer or its treatment.
- Manage pain by eliminating or controlling the source of pain (e.g., covering wounds, adjusting support surfaces, repositioning). Provide analgesia as needed and appropriate.
- Prevent or manage pain associated with debridement as needed.

Treatment of Pressure Ulcers further details these guideline recommendations. The reader may also wish to refer to the other AHCPR Clinical Practice Guidelines related to pain, which are discussed in the next section of this chapter: Guideline 1, *Acute Pain Management: Operative or Medical Procedures and Trauma* (Acute Pain Management Guideline Panel, 1992) and Guideline 9, *Chronic Malignant Pain* (Jacox et al, 1994).

In 1999, van Rijswijk and Braden revisited the AHCPR Pressure Ulcer Treatment Guideline recommendations as part of a special supplement to *Ostomy/Wound Management* entitled "Moving Beyond the AHCPR Guidelines: Wound Care Evolution Over the Last Five Years." The authors point out that research subsequent to the guideline release, although not extensive, confirms the panel's first recommendation on pain as quoted previously. Leg ulcer research has demonstrated that although sharp debridement can be painful, the use of topical anesthetics can significantly reduce debridement pain (Holm, Andren, and Grafford, 1990). The authors' cite numerous studies demonstrating that moisture-retentive dressings reduce wound pain. They suggest that "at this time, the most effective pain management technique is unknown, but data suggest that a combination of techniques designed to eliminate or control the source of pain (i.e., pressure, movement, exposure, or manipulation of the wound) may help. In addition, analgesia to treat chronic wound pain and/or procedure-related pain, should be provided" (p. 63S). Therefore the authors propose revising the second and third AHCPR recommendations to read as follows:

> Manage pain by eliminating or controlling the source of pain (i.e., covering wounds, adjusting support surfaces, and repositioning) and provide analgesia as needed to treat procedure-related, as well as chronic, wound pain (p. 63S).

Three nursing studies on wound pain deserve closer scrutiny. Using a qualitative case-study approach, Hollinworth (1995) found that nurses' assessment, management, and documentation of pain at wound dressing changes was most often inadequate and uninformed. She observed nurses' failure to assess pain verbally or to use pain assessment tools. Instead, there was reliance on nursing experience or nonverbal patient indicators to assess pain. Hollinworth found inadequate pain management and poor accountability. Pain assessment and management efforts were not documented, leading the researcher to conclude that "the future management of patients' pain at dressing changes may be compromised owing to impaired communication between healthcare professionals" (Hollinworth, 1995, p. 83).

In a cross-sectional quantitative study of 132 patients with pressure ulcer pain, Dallam and colleagues (1995) found that 59% reported having pain of some type; however, only 2% were given analgesics for the pain (within 4 hours of interview). The researchers recommend the following: "... the domain of pain must be added to the assessment of pressure ulcers. Further investigation should be completed to identify and quantify pain associated with pressure ulcers. Additional research is also needed to identify which combinations of strategies will most effectively relieve the pain associated with pressure ulcers. Educational programs should be developed to sensitize healthcare providers to the association of pain with pressure ulcers and to increase timely and appropriate assessment and treatment" (p. 216).

In 1996, Pieper published a retrospective analysis of venous ulcer healing in current and former users of injected drugs. More recently, Pieper, Rossi, and Templin (1998) explored the pain experienced by injected drug users with venous ulcers. Thirty-two patients answered questionnaires and had their wounds traced for this study. The researchers found that three variables were significantly related to larger wound area: greater current pain, worse pain in 24 hours, and higher levels of pain relief from medications. The strategies that ranked highest in alleviating pain were ibuprofen, compression dressings, Unna's boot, and heroin. The activities that caused the most pain were working, walking outside, standing, and stairclimbing. About 41% of the patients who completed the questionnaires said that they did not like to bother others about their pain. The researchers conclude that "providers need to listen to patient concerns about pain medication, and with the patient, determine the best medication protocol. Patients who have used injected drugs should not be denied pain therapy based upon their history (pp. 64-65)."

ASSESSMENT OF PAIN

McCaffery's widely accepted definition says that pain "is whatever the experiencing person says it is and exists whenever he says it does" (1972, p. 8). Because of the subjective nature of pain and in light of this definition, most of the pain assessment tools developed over the last 35 years have been based on or have incorporated patient self-report. The AHCPR Acute Pain Management Guideline Panel endorses, in the strongest terms, this approach to pain assessment, stating the following: "The single most reliable indicator of the existence and intensity of acute pain—and any resultant affective discomfort or distress—is the patient's self-report" (1992, p. 11).

The pain assessment tools in general use today range from simple visual analog scales to complex multidimensional, multipage instruments. All have their purpose and place. For example, visual analog scales measure only one dimension of the pain phenomenon at a time (e.g. intensity, from "no pain" to "worst possible pain"), using words, numbers, faces or other culturally congruent objects (e.g., coins, poker chips). Examples of several pain assessment scales are provided in Figures 17-1 to 17-3. Visual analog scales are particularly useful in clinical practice for patients who are actively in pain and do not have the capacity to complete a long, arduous questionnaire. Visual analog scales may also be used to measure pain distress and have been shown to be highly reliable instruments, even with the elderly (Herr and Mobily, 1993). More complex pain assessment tools, such as the McGill Pain Questionnaire (Melzack, 1975; Wall and Melzack, 1994) and its modifications like the Dartmouth Pain Questionnaire (Corson and Schneider, 1984) are used primarily in specialized pain centers and for clinical research.

Many pain history-taking tools have also been developed, and the reader is referred to the AHCPR Clinical Practice Guidelines #1 (Acute Pain Management Guideline Panel, 1991) and #9 (Jacox et al, 1994) for further specifics on pain history-taking and examples. Nurses should include relevant North American Nursing Diagnosis Association (NANDA) nursing diagnoses in their assessments, such as "Alteration in Comfort: Pain" and "Alteration in Comfort: Chronic Pain." There is no question that the assessment and management of pain in patients with severe wounds, in the elderly, or in nonverbal or nonresponsive patients presents very special challenges (Herr and Mobily, 1991; McCaffery and Beebe, 1989; Watt-Watson and Donovan, 1992) and that more research in this area is needed.

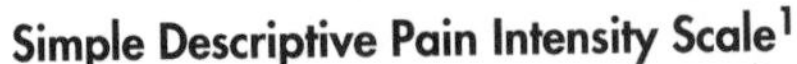

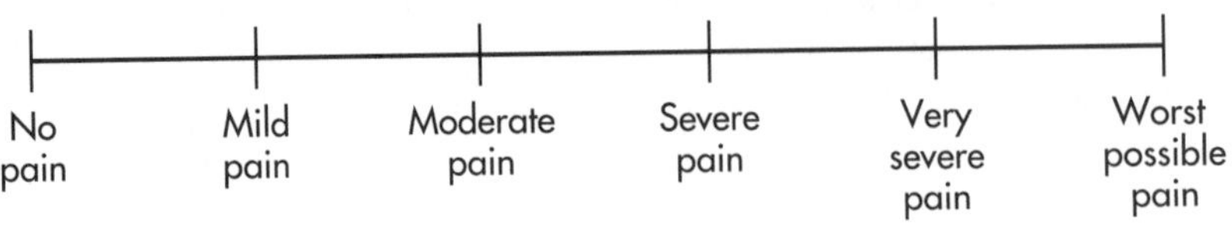

0-10 Numeric Pain Intensity Scale[1]

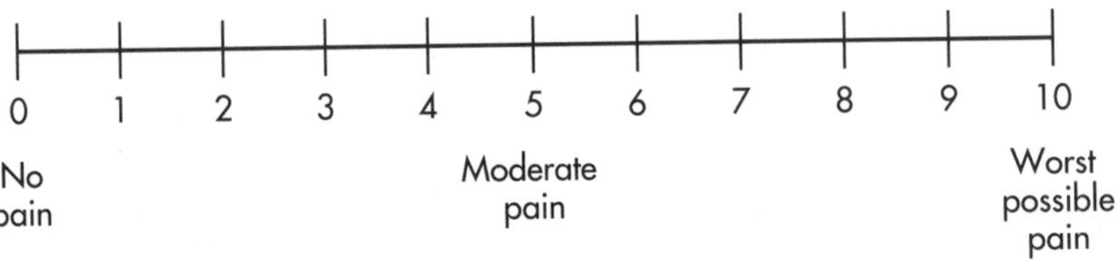

Visual Analog Scale (VAS)[2]

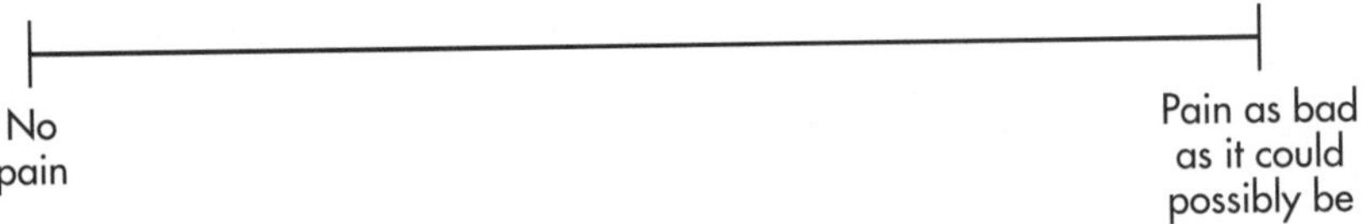

[1] If used as a graphic rating scale, a 10 cm baseline is recommended.

[2] A 10 cm baseline is recommended for VAS scales.

Figure 17-1 Three examples of pain intensity scales as published by the AHCPR. (Bergstrom N et al: *Treatment of pressure ulcers*, Clinical Practice Guideline #15, Rockville, Md, 1994, USDHHS, PHS, AHCPR Pub. No. 95-0622.)

CHRONIC WOUND PAIN EXPERIENCE MODEL

Scientists and researchers have traditionally classified pain as acute (often defined as pain lasting for less than 6 months) or chronic (often defined as pain lasting for greater than 6 months). At the 1986 National Institutes of Health (NIH) Consensus Development Conference on pain, a different pain classification with three pain categories was proposed: acute, chronic malignant, and chronic nonmalignant (NIH, 1986). Neither classification system adequately reflected the complex pain experience of most patients with chronic wound pain because the chronic wound pain experience does not fit neatly into any one of these proposed categories. Furthermore, the cutoff point of 6 months seemed arbitrary and inconsistent with definitions of chronic wounds.

Wong-Baker FACES Pain Rating Scale

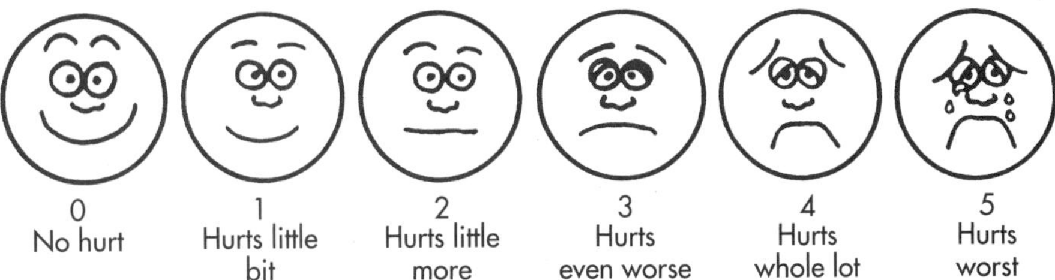
0
No hurt
1
Hurts little bit
2
Hurts little more
3
Hurts even worse
4
Hurts whole lot
5
Hurts worst

Figure 17-2 Wong-Baker FACES Pain Rating Scale. Directions for use: Explain to the person that each face is for a person who feels happy because he or she has no pain (hurt) or feels sad because he or she has some or a lot of pain. *Face 0* is very happy because he or she does not hurt at all. *Face 1* hurts just a little bit. *Face 2* hurts a little more. *Face 3* hurts even more. *Face 4* hurts a whole lot. *Face 5* hurts as much as you can imagine, although you do not have to be crying to feel this bad. Ask the person to choose the face that best describes how he or she is feeling. Recommended for persons 3 years of age to older. (From Wong DL et al: *Whaley and Wong's nursing care of infants and children,* ed 6, St Louis, 1999, Mosby, p. 1153. Copyrighted by Mosby, Inc. Reprinted with permission.)

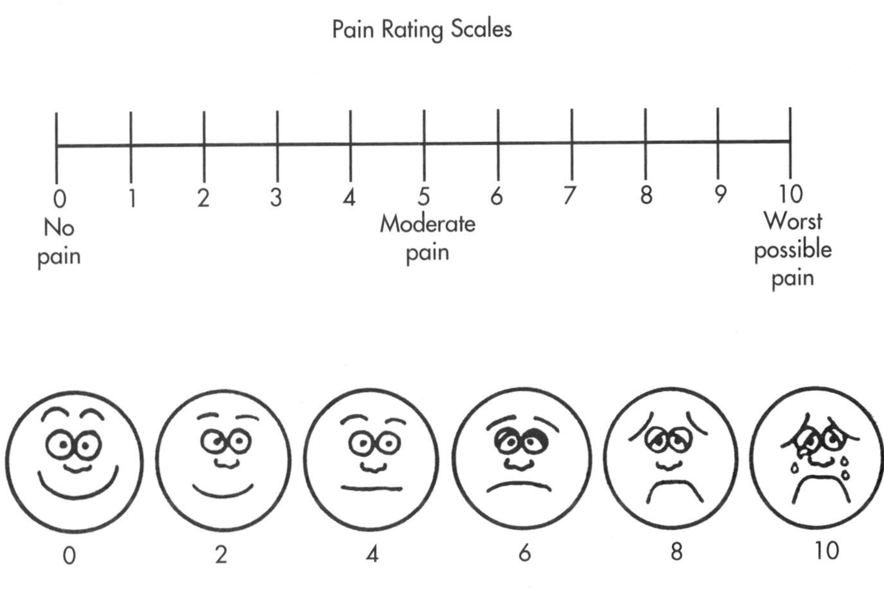

Point to each face using the words to describe the pain intensity. Ask the person to choose the face that best describes their own pain and record the appropriate number. Rating scale is recommended for persons age 3 years and older.

Figure 17-3 Example of how a numerical pain rating scale with word anchors and the Wong-Baker FACES scale can be combined onto one piece of paper so that the patient has a choice of pain rating scales. In this example, the numbers beneath the faces have been changed from a scale of 0 to 5 to a scale of 0 to 10 so that the recording of pain intensity is consistently on a 0 to 10 scale. (From Wong DL et al: *Whaley and Wong's nursing care of infants and children,* ed 6, St Louis, 1999, Mosby, p. 1153. Copyrighted by Mosby, Inc. Reprinted with permission.)

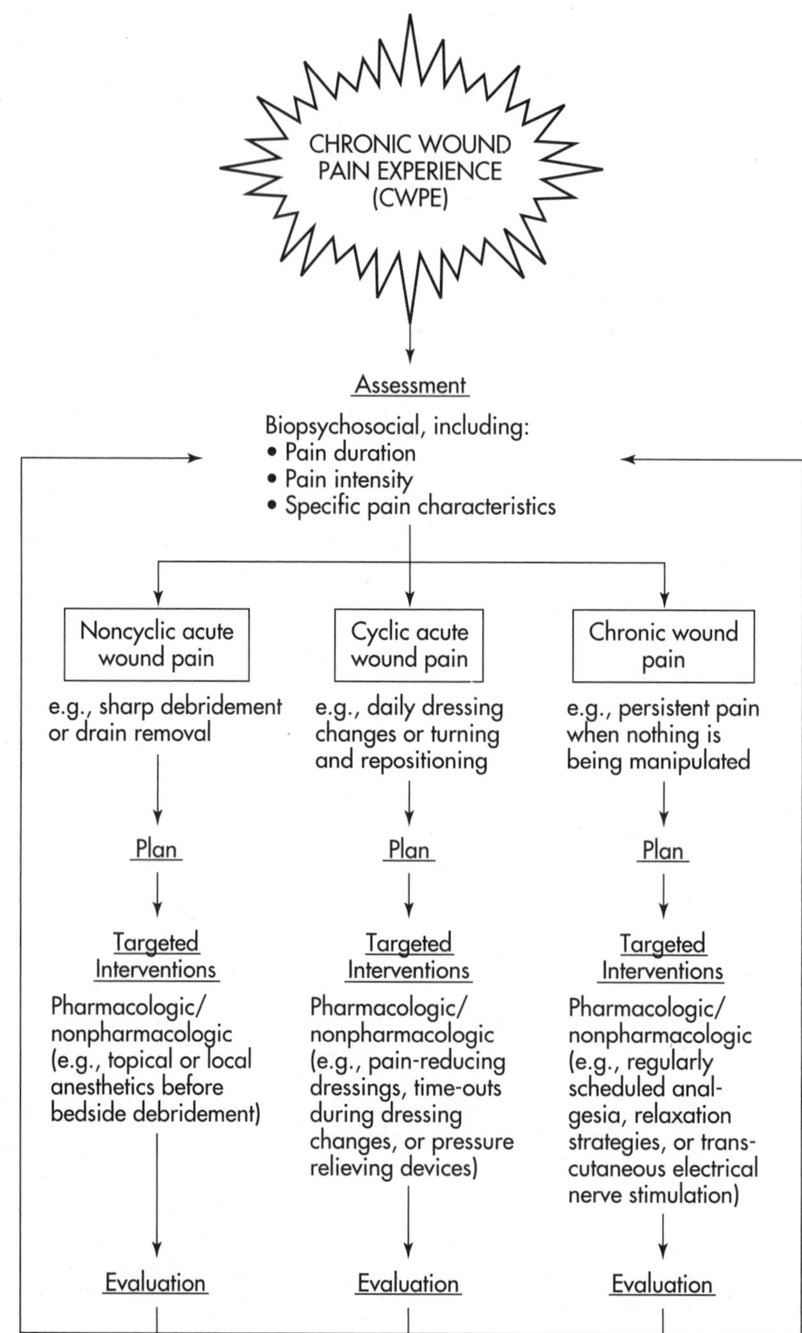

Figure 17-4 Chronic Wound Pain Experience (CWPE) Model. (Used with permission. Copyright ©1995, Diane Krasner.)

In 1991, 1993, and 1995, the author underwent surgeries for endometriosis, first experiencing an open wound, then an infected wound, and finally hypertrophic scarring. These experiences (Krasner, 1992; Ponder and Krasner, 1993), plus previous experiences caring for patients with chronic wounds for over 10 years, were the stimulus for considering a different conceptual model with definitions that would be more congruent with the lived experience of patients with chronic wound pain. In 1995, the Chronic Wound Pain Experience (CWPE) Model (Figure 17-4) (Krasner, 1995a) with theoretical definitions (Box 17-1) was proposed. The model was empirically and inductively derived. It relates the CWPE to the nursing process and to NANDA nursing diagnoses.

The model divides the CWPE into three distinct pain categories: noncyclic acute wound pain, cyclic acute wound pain, and chronic wound pain. An assumption is that *most* chronic wound patients will experience all three types of pain at some time, although not necessarily simultaneously. It is also recognized that some patients may not experience or be able to indicate pain at all. Others may not experience one of the pain types because of the particular course of their treatment or disease (e.g., the patient who has never had sharp debridement may never experience noncyclic acute wound pain). Another assumption is that many assumptions about wound pain may lack validity (e.g., diabetics do not experience wound pain resulting from neuropathy).

The CWPE Model can be used to guide wound pain assessment, plan strategies related to prevention and relief of wound pain, evaluate the efficacy of targeted strategies, or guide research in this area. It is proposed that specific plans and targeted strategies (both pharmacologic and nonpharmacologic) be initiated based on the type of wound pain that is being experienced. Future research is necessary to confirm which strategies or groups of strategies optimize pain relief for which type of pain. So, for example, applying a topical anesthetic compress before sharp debridement might be more effective for this type of acute noncyclic pain than taking an oral pain medication. Around-the-clock medications might be most effective for continuous chronic wound pain. Applying pain-reducing dressings or selecting pressure-reducing devices may prove to reduce acute cyclic pressure ulcer pain more effectively than pharmacologic measures. Would dressing-related wound pain be reduced if able patients were allowed to change their own dressings or to call "time-outs" during dressing changes?

Modeling of the CWPE presents a conceptual road map that can guide the way for future descriptive, intervention, and outcome research for patients with chronic wound pain. The need for conceptual clarity derives from the complexity of health care concepts as Vincent and Coler articulated: "Classification in nursing is complex because the phenom-

BOX 17-1 Chronic Wound Pain Experience (CWPE): Theoretic Definitions

Concept

The chronic wound pain experience (CWPE) is the complex, subjective phenomenon of extreme discomfort experienced by a person in response to skin and/or tissue injury. Chronic wounds include, but are not limited to, lower leg ulcers, diabetic ulcers, pressure ulcers, and open surgical wounds. Biopsychosocial assessment of the CWPE should address pain duration (e.g., periodic, intermittent, persistent), pain intensity (e.g., mild, severe) and other specific descriptive characteristics (e.g., "throbbing," "burning"; effect on ADLs and functional status).

Subconcepts

- *Noncyclic acute wound pain* is single-episode acute wound pain (e.g., the pain of sharp debridement or of drain removal).
- *Cyclic acute wound pain* is periodic acute wound pain that recurs as a result of repeated treatments or interventions (e.g., daily dressing changes or turning and repositioning).
- *Chronic wound pain* is the persistent pain that occurs without manipulation (e.g., throbbing of an abdominal wound when a patient is lying in bed).

ena within the discipline are multifaceted and evolving. Given the uniqueness and complexity of human behavior, the categories in an empirical science such as nursing overlap and intertwine, unlike the traditional classification systems of mathematics in which classes are mutually exclusive" (1990). Waltz, Strickland, and Lenz state the following: "Because key nursing concepts tend to be complex and relatively abstract, they must be defined and operationalized carefully, if they are to be useful in building and applying knowledge" (1991). It is hoped that the CWPE Model will help to clarify concepts, inspire clinicians and researchers to explore the chronic wound pain experience more closely, and ultimately lead to a comprehensive approach to chronic wound pain management that will optimize outcomes for patients who experience chronic wound pain.

"USING A GENTLER HAND"

In a qualitative study conducted by the author (Krasner, 1996), nurse generalists and advanced practice nurses who care for patients with pressure ulcers who experience pain were asked to reflect and write a story about the phenomenon. Stories from 42 participants were analyzed for the meanings derived from the nurse caregiver's reflections. A Heideggerian hermeneutical approach (Allen, Benner, and Diekelmann, 1986; Benner, 1994; Diekelmann, 1991; Diekelmann and Allen, 1989; Heidegger, 1962; van Manen, 1990) was used for analysis. Text analysis included the identification of themes, common meanings, and constitutive patterns that were shared and discussed with two separate qualitative research teams. Comments and insights from both groups informed and stimulated the thinking of this researcher.

Three constitutive patterns and eight themes emerged from the text (Box 17-2). For "nursing expertly" the themes that emerged were "reading the pain," "attending to the pain," and "acknowledging and empathizing." These were the skills that nurses identified as making a difference for patients with pressure ulcer pain. The following paradigm story portrays how one expert nurse described these skills (Krasner, 1996):

BOX 17-2 Reflections on Patients with Pressure Ulcers Who Experience Pain: Constitutive Patterns and Related Themes

1. Nursing expertly
   a. Reading the pain
   b. Attending to the pain
   c. Acknowledging and empathizing
2. Denying the pain
   a. Assuming it does not exist
   b. Not hearing the cries
   c. Avoiding failure
3. Confronting the challenge of pain
   a. Coping with the frustrations
   b. BEING WITH the patient

> My experiences with patients with pressure ulcers always involve pain, fear, and anxiety . . . My experiences have taught me this: if I can guarantee that a patient will not suffer pain with pressure ulcer care (during debridement, dressing changes, etc.), I see an immediate response of decreased anxiety and fear, but if I have inflicted pain with care, when I return to repeat that care, patients have cried and asked, "Please don't hurt me," or have exhibited signs of increased anxiety (such as sweating, bulging eyes, increased respirations, and exaggerated movement in bed). Patients who cannot verbalize their pain show me these signs of pain, which oftentimes go overlooked by caregivers. My response now is *a gentler hand,* a slower pace, speaking with patients and explaining every step of care, letting them know that a procedure may be uncomfortable, and offering pain medications prior to painful procedures.

For "denying the pain," the themes that were reflected in the nurses' stories were "assuming it doesn't hurt," "not hearing the cries," and "avoiding failure." Although these may be effective coping strategies for healthcare providers, they leave the patient in a vulnerable position (Krasner, 1996):

> I've observed failure of medical and nursing staff to recognize or treat [pressure ulcer] pain. It's almost [as if there's the assumption that when] there's an absence of tissue or skin, there must be an absence of sensation in the same location. I've experienced surgeons performing

debridement of nonviable tissue, which apparently is not painful, but then continue into viable tissue without anesthesia or analgesia. They soon realize this hurts as evidenced by the patient's response but persist as if this is acceptable or expected and should not be resisted. Nurses tend not to regularly medicate pressure ulcer patients for pain as they would for other types of surgical wounds. Maybe they perceive pressure ulcers as being the patient's fault or disgusting or not a "solid" reason for pain.

For "confronting the challenge of pain," two themes emerged from the text: "coping with the frustrations" and "BEING WITH the patient." Clearly, when it comes to pressure ulcer pain, there can be a great deal of anger, helplessness, hopelessness, and even pain experienced by healthcare professionals and by lay caregivers as well by patients themselves. An effective strategy for confronting the pain problem that the participants identified is BEING WITH the patient. Those participants who could just BE WITH the patient in pain felt that they had been able to answer the call to care. Some were even able by BEING WITH the patient to gain insight into the meaning that the pain experience held for the patient. For example, for one patient with a stage 3 pressure ulcer, the pain was a marker that she was still alive (Krasner, 1996):

> She came to us on the telemetry unit, we did dressing changes, and then sent her off to surgery for skin grafts when she was strong enough. The entire time caring for this woman amazed me because she was not angry to have these wounds (which I felt were the nurses fault). She instead felt that this was just a side effect of being ill and she was happy to be alive. She was so positive and so helpful when I was changing her dressings, and after surgery she still remained so pleasant. I don't think I could have been as gracious as she was.

Taken together these stories form a tapestry of practical insight gained through experience about patients with pressure ulcers who experience pain. Healthcare professionals possess a vast body of experiential knowledge (Benner, 1983, 1984; Benner and Tanner, 1987; Heidegger, 1962, 1971, 1972) related to wound pain, even though they may not always articulate or share that knowledge with others. Becoming more sensitive to this phenomenon and focusing on the experiences of the patients in pain (rather than just the wound) can transform care. As Heidegger (1972) stated, we must confront the challenge of pain and suffering when patients cry out to us: "The point is not to listen to a series of propositions, but rather to follow the movement of showing."

VENOUS ULCER PAIN

Hofman and colleagues (1997), in a study of venous ulcer pain, found that for 69% of the patients in the study, pain was "the worst thing about having an ulcer," disrupting sleep and negatively affecting quality of life. Similar findings were identified by Phillips and colleagues (1994) and Walshe (1995).

Krasner's dissertation study of the experience of patients with venous ulcer pain used Heideggerian hermeneutic phenomology to identify themes and patterns related to this experience (Krasner 1997, 1998a, 1998b, 1998c). The pattern that emerged from the study was "Carrying On Despite the Pain." Eight themes were identified:

- Expecting pain with the ulcer
- Swelling = pain
- Not standing
- Starting the cycle of pain all over again: painful debridement
- Feeling frustrated
- Interferring with the job
- Making significant life changes
- Finding satisfaction in new activities

For many of the patients in this study, their venous ulcer pain seemed to be a combination of nociceptive and neuropathic pain, a finding that has important ramifications for medicating for pain with polypharmacy. Another ironic finding was that patients expected their wounds to be painful and therefore often did not request pain medication, whereas healthcare professionals often assume and have frequently been taught that arterial ulcers, not venous ulcers, are painful; therefore healthcare professionals often do not even assess for venous ulcer pain. Undertreatment of chronic wound pain patients is far too common.

PRAGMATIC SUGGESTIONS FOR MANAGING PROCEDURAL AND NONPROCEDURAL WOUND PAIN

Despite the lack of research and information to guide practice related to procedural and nonprocedural wound pain, nurses who care for patients with wound pain must do their best to address these problems. It is no longer acceptable to use expressions like "bite the bullet" or "you have to hurt to heal." The ethical principle of nonmaleficence admonishes healthcare providers to "do no harm." With that in mind, various strategies for dealing with procedural and nonprocedural wound pain are provided for the reader's consideration (Krasner, 1998; Rook, 1996; van Rijswijk, 1999). These strategies reflect best practices. In the future, evidence-based science is needed to support these best practices.

1. Eliminate Cause of Pain

Often the procedures chosen to *treat* a wound, such as irrigation, adherent dressings, or debridement, cause nociceptive wound pain. The AHCPR *Treatment of Pressure Ulcers,* Clinical Practice Guideline #15 states the following: "Manage pain by eliminating or controlling the source of pain (e.g., covering wounds, adjusting support surfaces, repositioning). Provide analgesia as needed and appropriate" (Bergstrom et al, 1994, p. 31). Wound pain can be controlled or eliminated by carefully choosing dressings that cover the wound bed and exposed nerve endings, that adhere as little as possible to the wound bed, and that leave minimal residue behind (Thomas, 1989). Avoiding cytotoxic topical agents (such as antiseptics and antimicrobials), harsh chemicals, or highly concentrated agents for wound cleansing can significantly reduce wound pain. In general, the use of these agents should be avoided unless the wound warrants such intervention (e.g., a traumatic wound) and has been adequately anesthetized (van Rijswijk, 1999). Allowing the patients to perform their own dressing changes if they are able or to call "time-outs" can reduce the pain experienced by some patients. Whenever possible, timing the dressing change at a time of day when the person is most "psyched" for it can be extremely beneficial. Give an analgesic and then schedule the dressing change when its peak effect occurs.

Wound cleansing can be used as a strategy to reduce wound pain. The build-up of exudate in a wound bed can cause pressure and pain. Removal of the exudate by gentle flushing, low-pressure irrigation, or by the cautious use of whirlpool in selected patients can bring pain relief.

Positioning patients for comfort and off their wounds can reduce pain at the wound site. If this is not possible, the judicious use of support surfaces can offer pain relief to bedbound or chairbound patients. Medicating patients before turning, repositioning, sitting, or ambulation is logical but requires planning and coordination and therefore is too often omitted. Using lift sheets (to lift and move) instead of draw sheets (that drag) to move patients in bed prevents friction and shear that can cause painful injuries to the skin and deeper tissues. For many patients, splinting or immobilizing the wounded area (e.g., the use of an abdominal binder for a midline incision or wound) can offer significant comfort.

2. Protect Wound Margins

Eroded or denuded wound margins can contribute significantly to the pain experienced by wound patients. The use of skin sealants on skin that is still intact can prevent painful denuding of skin or skin stripping. The use of ointments or skin barriers on open areas can prevent and/or minimize the pain secondary to damaged wound margins.

3. Select Among Debridement Options Carefully

Although many factors enter into the decision about which method to select for debriding a wound containing necrotic tissue, pain is a frequently neglected consideration. The AHCPR *Treatment of Pressure Ulcers,* Clinical Practice Guideline #15, states, "Regardless of the method [of debridement] selected, the need to assess and control pain should be considered" (1994, p. 6). Many effective topical anesthetic agents are available for use before sharp debridement, including 2% to 4% xylocaine compresses (for 10 to 15 minutes with caution about reactions) and eutectic mixture of local anesthetics (EMLA) for use on intact skin, not eroded, open, or mucosal surfaces (Holm, Andren, and Grafford, 1990). Using autolysis for debridement, when feasible and appropriate, can significantly reduce the pain associated with debridement.

4. Control Inflammation and Edema

Inflammation and edema contribute to wound pain, so any measures that reduce inflammation and edema will likely also provide pain relief. This includes thoughtful positioning (e.g., elevation of swollen legs as much as possible), appropriate selection of dressings and devices to reduce edema (e.g., compression bandaging, sequential compression pumps), and the use of systemic medications to reduce edema and inflammation.

5. Stabilize the Wound

The use of binders, splints, body positioners, and other devices that stabilize a wound can significantly reduce pain, especially pain related to mobilization. Care must be taken to fit these devices properly so that the wound dressing is appropriately accomodated and increased pressure on the wound does not result.

6. Address the Ache and Anguish

For many patients, the suffering that accompanies the wound pain experience can exacerbate the pain that the person feels if it is not addressed. Whether it is holding the person's hand during care, a pat on the back, a hug, or in selected cases referral to a counselor or psychologist, acknowledging the suffering and BEING WITH the person can make a tremendous difference in the outcome. The following case is instructive (Krasner, 1996):

> A woman in her thirties developed breakdown of her wound after a radical mastectomy. The sight of the wound and the torture three times a day of wet-to-dry dressing changes compounded her suffering. In consulting on the case, I sought to select a dressing that would hide the wound from sight, that would not need to be changed so often, that would be less traumatic to the granulating tissue in the wound bed, and that might be bulky enough to parallel her remaining breast so that she would be more "in balance" until the wound healed enough for a prosthetic device. The solution was a nonadherent impregnated gauze dressing, covered by an ABD with Montgomery straps changed daily. The dressing was effective because it not only addressed moist wound healing but more importantly acknowledged this patient's ache and anguish.

SUMMARY

"When wounds are painful, they are trying to communicate that something is wrong. All we have to do is listen." – Lia van Rijswijk

"The real voyage of discovery consists not in seeking new landscapes but in having NEW EYES." – Marcel Proust

Opening our ears and eyes to the issue of wound pain is an important first step in managing this problem, which is significant for many people with acute and chronic wounds. Acknowledging the subjective, multidimensional nature of wound pain challenges us to work together as a healthcare team, giving respect to the person's own expression of the wound pain experience. Although the wound care community has tended to minimize or even ignore the problem of wound pain over the years, it is now time to become sensitized to the issue. We must listen, look, assess, and then try pragmatic approaches for managing procedural and nonprocedural wound pain. It is important that we share our best practices for wound pain with our colleagues and that we undertake the research to support evidenced-based practices for managing wound pain.

SELF-ASSESSMENT EXERCISE

1. Wound pain can affect which of the following dimensions?
   - a. Productivity
   - b. Quality of life
   - c. Sleep
   - d. All of the above
2. The AHCPR Pressure Ulcer Treatment Guideline recognizes the importance of:
   - a. Routinely assessing for and treating pressure ulcer pain
   - b. The routine use of the Faces Pain Rating Scale
   - c. The provider determining the patient's pain score
   - d. Using a topical anesthetic cream before debridement

3. List at least 5 suggestions for managing procedural and nonprocedural wound pain.
4. Which of the following dimensions of the Chronic Wound Pain Experience Model best describes the pain of conservative sharp debridement?
   a. Noncyclic acute wound pain
   b. Cyclic acute wound pain
   c. Chronic wound pain
   d. All of the above
5. True or False: According to the Chronic Wound Pain Experience Model, patients with wound pain may experience noncyclic acute wound pain, cyclic acute wound pain, and chronic wound pain at the same time.
6. Procedural (nociceptive) wound pain is frequently caused by:
   a. Adhesive dressings
   b. Wet-to-moist gauze
   c. Debridement
   d. All of the above
7. Best practices for managing wound pain include:
   a. Assuming that the pain is bearable
   b. Medicating for pain after the procedure
   c. Using a combination of strategies
   d. Addressing nonprocedural pain before procedural pain
8. The most likely cause of leg ulcer pain is:
   a. Nociceptive
   b. Neuropathic
   c. Nociceptive and neuropathic
   d. Psychologic
9. True or False: Decreasing swelling by compression in patients with venous ulcers has been shown in several recent studies to reduce venous ulcer pain.
10. Describe two methods that can be used to assess a patient's wound pain.

REFERENCES

Acute Pain Management Guideline Panel: *Acute pain management: operative or medical procedures and trauma,* Clinical Practice Guideline #1, Rockville, Md, 1991, USDHHS, PHS, AHCPR Pub. No. 92-0032.

Allen D, Benner P, Diekelmann N: Three paradigms for nursing research: methodological implications. In Chinn P, editor: *Nursing research methodology: issues and implementation,* Rockville, Md, 1986, Aspen.

Benner P: *From novice to expert: excellence and power in clinical nursing practice,* Menlo Park, Calif, 1984, Addison Wesley.

Benner P: Uncovering the knowledge embedded in clinical practice, *Image* 15(2):36, 1983.

Benner P, editor: *Interpretive phenomenology: embodiment, caring and ethics in health and illness,* Thousand Oaks, Calif, 1994, Sage.

Benner P, Tanner C: How expert nurses use intuition, *Am J Nurs* 87(1):23, 1987.

Bergstrom N et al: *Treatment of pressure ulcers,* Clinical Practice Guideline #15, Rockville, Md, 1994, USDHHS, PHS, AHCPR Pub. No. 95-0622.

Cavanaugh J, Weinstein J: Low back pain: epidemiology, anatomy and neurophysiology. In Wall P, Melzack R, editors: *Textbook of pain,* Edinburgh, 1994, Churchill Livingstone.

Choiniere M: Pain of burns. In Wall P, Melzack R, editors: *Textbook of pain,* Edinburgh, 1994, Churchill Livingstone.

Corson J, Schneider M: The Dartmouth pain questionnaire: an adjunct to the McGill pain questionnaire, *Pain* 19:59, 1984.

Cousins M: Acute and postoperative pain. In Wall P, Melzack R, editors: *Textbook of pain,* Edinburgh, 1994, Churchill Livingstone.

Dallam L et al: Pressure ulcer pain: assessment and quantification, *J Wound Ostomy Continence Nurse* 22(5):211, 1995.

Diekelmann N: The emancipatory power of the narrative. In *Curriculum revolution: community building and activism,* New York, 1991, NLN.

Diekelmann N, Allen D: A hermeneutic analysis of the NLN criteria for the appraisal of baccalaureate programs. In Diekelmann D, Allen D, Tanner C: *The NLN criteria for appraisal of baccalaureate programs: a critical hermeneutic analysis,* New York, 1989, NLN.

Field C, Kerstein M: Overview of wound healing in a moist environment, *Am J Surg* 167(1A):2S, 1994.

Franks P et al: Community leg ulcer clinics: effect on quality of life, *Phlebology* 9:83, 1994.

Frymoyer J, Gordon S, editors: *New perspectives on low back pain,* Park Ridge, Ill, 1989, American Academy of Orthopaedic Surgeons.

Grennan D, Jayson M: Rheumatoid arthritis. In Wall P, Melzack P, editors: *Textbook of pain,* Edinburgh, 1994, Churchill Livingstone.

Hamer C, Cullum N, Roe B: Patients' perceptions of chronic leg ulceration. In *Proceedings of the 2nd European Conference on Advances in Wound Management,* London, 1992, Macmillan Magazines.

Heidegger M: *Being and time,* New York, 1962, Harper & Row.

Heidegger M: *On time and being,* New York, 1972, Harper & Row.

Heidegger M: *Poetry, language and thought,* New York, 1971, Harper & Row.

Herr K, Mobily P: Comparison of selected pain assessment tools for use with the elderly, *Appl Nurs Res* 6(1):39, 1993.

Herr K, Mobily P: Pain assessment in the elderly: clinical considerations, *J Gerontol Nurs* 17(4):12, 1991.

Hofman D et al: Pain in venous leg ulcer, *J Wound Care* 6(5):222, 1997.

Hollinworth H: Nurses' assessment and management of pain at wound dressing changes, *J Wound Care* 4(2):77, 1995.

Holm J, Andren B, Grafford K: Pain control in the surgical debridement of leg ulcers by the use of a topical Lidocaine-Prilocaine cream, EMLA, *Acta Derm Venereol* Suppl (Stockh) 70:132, 1990.

Jacox A et al: *Management of cancer pain,* Clinical Practice Guideline #9, Rockville, Md, 1994, USDHHS, PHS, AHCPR Publication No. 94-0592.

Krasner D: *Carrying on despite the pain: living with painful venous ulcers: a Heideggerian hermeneutic analysis* (doctoral dissertation), Ann Arbor, Mich, 1997, UMI.

Krasner D: Chronic wound pain. In Krasner D, Kane D: *Chronic wound care: a clinical source book for healthcare professionals,* Wayne, Penn, 1998a, Health Management Publications.

Krasner D: Managing pain from pressure ulcers. In Pasaro C: Pain control, *Am J Nurs* 6:22, 1995b.

Krasner D: Painful venous ulcers: themes and stories about living with the pain and suffering, *J Wound Ostomy Continence Nurs* 25(3):158, 1998b.

Krasner D: Painful venous ulcers: themes and stories about their impact on quality of life, *Ostomy Wound Manage* 44(9):38, 1998c.

Krasner D: The chronic wound pain experience: a conceptual model, *Ostomy Wound Manage* 41(3):20, 1995a.

Krasner D: Using a gentler hand: reflections on patients with pressure ulcers who experience pain, *Ostomy Wound Manage* 42(3):20, 1996.

Krasner D: Using a hydrogel, foam and dressing retention sheet, *Ostomy Wound Manage* 38(3):28, 1992.

McCaffery M: *Nursing management of the patient with pain,* Philadelphia, 1972, J.B. Lippincott.

McCaffery M, Beebe A: *Pain: clinical manual for nursing practice,* St Louis, 1989, Mosby.

McCarthy C, Cushnaghan J, Dieppe P: Osteoarthritis. In Wall P, Melzack R, editors: *Textbook of pain,* Edinburgh, 1994, Churchill Livingstone.

Mayer T, Mooney V, Gatchell R, editors: *Contemporary conservative care for painful spinal disorders,* Philadelphia, 1991, Lea & Febriger.

Melzack R: The McGill pain questionnaire: major properties and scoring methods, *Pain* 1:277, 1975.

National Institutes of Health: *The integrated approach to the management of pain,* Consensus Development Conference Statement, Bethesda, Md, 1986, NIH.

Olesen J, Tfelt-Hansen P, Welch K editors: *The headaches,* New York, 1990, Raven Press.

Oxford English Dictionary, vol 7, Oxford, England, 1933, Oxford at the Claredon Press.

Phillips T et al: A study of the impact of leg ulcers on quality of life: financial, social and psychologic implications, *J Am Acad Dermatol* 31(1):49, 1994.

Pieper B: A retrospective analysis of venous ulcer healing in current and former drug users of injected drugs, *J Wound Ostomy Continence Nurs* 23(6):291, 1996.

Pieper B, Rossi R, Templin T: Pain associated with venous ulcers in injecting drug users, *Ostomy Wound Manage* 44(11):54, 1998.

Ponder R, Krasner D: Gauzes and related dressings, *Ostomy Wound Manage* 39(5):48, 1993.

Rice A: Pain, inflammation and wound healing, *J Wound Care* 3(5):246, 1994.

Rook J: Wound care pain management, *Adv Wound Care* 9(6):24, 1996.

Schoenen J, Maertens de Noordhout A: Headache. In Wall P, Melzack R, editors: *Textbook of pain,* Edinburgh, 1994, Churchill Livingstone.

Thomas S: Pain and wound management, *Community Outlook,* July 11, 1989.

van Manen M: *Researching lived experience: human science for an action sensitive pedagogy,* New York, 1990, State University of New York.

van Rijswijk L: Wound pain. In McCaffery M, Pasero C: *Pain clinical manual,* ed 2, St Louis, 1999, Mosby.

van Rijswijk L, Braden B: Pressure ulcer patient and wound assessment: an AHCPR clinical practice update, *Ostomy Wound Manage* 45(1A):56S, 1999.

Vincent K, Coler M: A unified nursing diagnostic model, *Image* 22(2):93, 1990.

Wall P, Melzack R: *Textbook of pain,* ed 2, Edinburgh, 1994, Churchill Livingstone.

Walsche C: Living with a venous leg ulcer: a descriptive study of patients' experiences, *J Adv Nurs* 22:1092, 1995.

Waltz C, Strickland O, Lenz E: *Measurement in nursing research,* ed 2, Philadelphia, 1991, W.B. Saunders.

Watt-Watson J, Donovan M: *Pain management: nursing perspective,* St Louis, 1992, Mosby.

CHAPTER

18 Surgical Approaches to Wound Closure

DONALD J. MORRIS

OBJECTIVES

1. Describe the role of subcutaneous tissue and muscle in preventing pressure ulcers.
2. Identify four factors that cause pressure ulcer formation.
3. Describe one situation when surgical intervention for a pressure ulcer is preferred and one situation when surgical intervention is not preferred.
4. Identify the major principles underlying all surgical procedures.
5. Distinguish between fasciocutaneous flap and myocutaneous flap.
6. Describe the nursing implications in the care of a patient after a myocutaneous flap with regard to wound drainage, positioning, and activity level.

Superficial pressure ulcers (limited to the epidermis) heal by regeneration, whereas deeper pressure ulcers (dermis and below) heal by scar formation. Although the wound that heals by scar formation is resurfaced, the durability of the wound is decreased, leaving it vulnerable to mechanical stresses. In addition, allowing a full-thickness pressure ulcer to heal by scar formation requires time and restricted mobility, which delays an individual's ability to resume day-to-day activities or to return to work. For these reasons, surgical closure of the full-thickness pressure ulcer is often desirable.

Before any planned surgical treatment for pressure ulcers, the general condition of the patient must be optimized. A team approach, including an internist, rehabilitation specialist, nursing staff, surgeon, wound care nurse, nutritionist, orthopedist, and physical therapist, must be used to obtain good results.

OPTIMIZE PATIENT

Along with fine tuning of the basic functional processes, there are specific requirements before operative intervention. All spasticity must be controlled, either pharmacologically or surgically. Infection at the site of the ulcer or elsewhere must be overcome by intravenously administered antibiotics and appropriate debridement. The cause of the ulcer must be identified (whether secondary to repeated shear forces, immobility, or trauma) and corrected. Most importantly, the patient must be nutritionally sound because protein malnutrition is a leading cause of flap failure. Serum albumin is a readily available test that can act as a rough guide to the patient's condition. With rare exception, flap closure of a pressure ulcer should not be done with a serum albumin level of less than 3.0 g/dl.

EVALUATE TISSUE DAMAGE

Coincident with optimization of the patient's general condition, the ulcer itself should be evaluated and staged (see Chapter 4). Surgical therapy is based on ulcer staging (Linder and Morris, 1990).

Stage I

Stage 1 lesions should be considered as a warning. They heal spontaneously, without operative intervention, provided that the cause of the lesion is understood and measures are taken to correct the patient's poor positioning, hygiene, or susceptibility to shear forces.

Stage 2

Stage 2 lesions appear similar to partial-thickness burns with loss of epidermis and exposed, injured dermis. Careful evaluation of the wound is needed because these lesions may herald a larger, deeper stage 3 lesion. The true stage 2 lesion, with only partial-thickness skin loss, should also heal with local therapy if one assumes that there is correction of the cause. These lesions heal by reepithelialization from remaining epidermal structures (hair follicles, sweat glands, and so forth). In the true stage 2 lesion there is little or no role for surgical intervention because viable dermis still exists.

Stage 3

Stage 3 lesions show full-thickness skin loss with injury to underlying tissue layers. On presentation, many often contain a large amount of necrotic material and show significant associated cellulitis. Systemic toxicity is not uncommon. Necrotic tissue must be removed, and infection must be controlled. Such steps are usually best accomplished by intravenous antibiotics and immediate surgical debridement. Debridement may be done at the bedside; however, a more thorough job can be done in the operating room.

Most of these patients show clear physical and biochemical signs of protein malnutrition. Intervention in this regard is at least as crucial as operative intervention. Because of the significant protein loss from the wound, these patients require an unusually high caloric intake with protein supplementation. If the patient is unable to maintain adequate protein intake, then nasogastric tube feedings or parenteral hyperalimentation, or both, are warranted.

Once debridement of any grossly necrotic tissue is complete, appropriate topical therapy is begun. Standard gauze dressings moistened with saline solution are frequently used and are an appropriate choice to support wound debridement. The gauze should be loosely placed into the depths of the wound and not packed because vigorous packing prevents the naturally helpful process of wound contraction from occurring. With adequate nutritional support and proper positioning, the wound will clean up rapidly. Healthy, red granulation tissue at the wound base and new epithelialization at the wound margin are sure signs that the wound is ready for surgical closure. If there is a lack of granulation tissue present or if no new epidermis is present at the wound edge, surgical closure should be delayed. The patient should be further evaluated for the presence of factors affecting wound healing (such as nutritional status, uncorrected causes, infection), which may need to be corrected before surgical closure.

Most stage 3 ulcers will heal on their own; however, spontaneous closure may take months and may result in an unstable scar that is predisposed to recurrence. For this reason, it is frequently preferable to manage these lesions with surgical excision and closure, barring contraindications.

Stage 4

Stage 4 lesions are handled in a fashion similar to the stage 3 lesion. Debridement is often more radical because there is bony involvement. Localized osteomyelitis is the rule. Deeper extension into the pelvis and fistulas (such as urethroperineal) must be ruled out.

SURGICAL OPTIONS

There is a variety of surgical procedures that may be used to close chronic wounds. The most common are skin grafts and tissue flaps (Black and Black, 1987).

Skin Grafts

Skin grafts may be either split thickness (the most common) or full thickness. These grafts involve transfer of the epidermis and a measured portion of the dermis from a donor site to a shallow, well-vascularized wound (Stueber and Goldberg, 1985). Skin grafts provide superficial coverage but do not replace deeper tissue layers, such as subcutaneous tissue and muscle; thus they are unable to provide the padding needed to protect bony prominences from recurrent breakdown (Black and Black, 1987). They are rarely, if ever, used in the surgical management of pressure ulcers. They may, however, be used to close donor sites after layer flap procedures (Stueber and Goldberg, 1985).

Survival of skin grafts depends on revascularization of the grafted skin. This is accomplished by ingrowth of capillaries from the vascularized surface into the graft. The two factors most commonly associated with graft failure are 1) failure to adequately immobilize the graft, which is critical to revascularization, and 2) infection (Stueber and Goldberg, 1985). The donor site for the skin graft is a partial-thickness wound, which heals by reepithelialization.

Tissue Flaps

Tissue flaps are the procedures most commonly used for surgical management of pressure ulcers (Black and Black, 1987). They involve the transfer of skin and underlying structures (such as subcutaneous tissue, fascia, and muscle) to fill a defect. Tissue flaps may be further classified according to tissue layers involved and surgical method used to transfer the tissue into the defect. All flaps involve partial detachment of the tissue from its original site. The base remains attached and provides circulatory support to the flap (Stueber and Goldberg, 1985).

Flaps may be classified as fasciocutaneous (also sometimes called *skin flaps*) and myocutaneous. Fasciocutaneous flaps involve elevation and rotation of the epidermis, dermis, and subcutaneous tissue and provide padding and superficial coverage. These flaps may be further divided into "random" flaps and "axial" flaps. Random flaps depend on the dermal and subdermal vessels for their blood supply. Since these vessels are rather small, the blood supply to these flaps is somewhat tenuous (Black and Black, 1987). Axial flaps are designed to include a major cutaneous artery, which increases vascularity and the chances for flap survival (Stueber and Goldberg, 1985).

Myocutaneous flaps involve rotation of all tissue layers (i.e., skin, subcutaneous tissue, fascia, and muscle). These flaps provide optional coverage for a bony prominence and are therefore frequently used in surgical reconstruction of pressure ulcers. Myocutaneous flaps are well-vascularized flaps containing major vessels that originate from the base of the flap. These vessels nourish the flap until new capillary systems are established between the flap and the wound bed (Stueber and Goldberg, 1985).

Flaps can also be classified according to surgical technique. Common flaps include the advancement flap, the rotation flap, and the transposition flap (Stueber and Goldberg, 1985).

Advancement flaps involve elevation of the tissue to be transferred, undermining of the wound edges, and advancement of the tissue into the defect. Advancement flaps are useful in areas where there is significant stretch of the skin (Stueber and Goldberg, 1985).

Rotation flaps are used to fill defects adjacent to the donor tissue. A flap is outlined on three sides, the tissue is elevated, and the flap is "rotated" into the defect. The donor site may be closed surgically or may require a split-thickness skin graft in closure. Skin-graft closure is adequate since the tissue is rotated from a site adjacent to but not overlying a bony prominence (Stueber and Goldberg, 1985).

Transposition flaps are rotation flaps that are moved across normal skin to fill a defect (as opposed to being directly adjacent to the defect).

The *free flap* is performed less commonly because it requires microvascular surgery techniques. In this approach, the donor tissue is completely removed from the donor site and transferred to the graft site. The vessels are anastomosed by microvascular techniques to vessels in the wound bed (Stueber and Goldberg, 1985).

Tissue Expansion

An additional surgical option for pressure ulcer closure is tissue expansion. This option may be used when there is not enough tissue adjacent to an ulcer to provide flap coverage. Silastic "expanders," or hollow pouches, are placed surgically into the subcutaneous or submuscular tissue layer in an area adjacent to the defect. Sterile fluid is injected into the expander at routine intervals until the pouch is fully expanded. This process induces expansion of the overlying tissue layers. When there is sufficient tissue to provide coverage of the defect, the expander is removed and the ulcer is closed (Stueber and Goldberg, 1985).

PRESSURE ULCER CLOSURE

Principles

Although many different techniques and flaps have been described, all follow basic principles:

1. The patient is positioned in the operating room to mimic the position of maximal

tension on the flap. This prevents postoperative wound dehiscence secondary to tension upon patient positioning.

2. Perioperative prophylactic antibiotic therapy specific to wound culture is in order. Forty eight hours of intravenous therapy is required. Although some authors have found quantitative cultures helpful, most have not found them necessary. Even in patients with a radiologic diagnosis of osteomyelitis, additional antibiotic therapy is not needed because all involved bone should be excised at the time of closure.
3. Ostectomy of bony prominence is necessary to increase the surface area upon which the patient rests. Total ischiectomy is no longer favored because the weight redistribution results in ulcers on the opposite side or on the perineum.
4. The entire ulcer is excised in "pseudotumor" fashion, leaving only healthy, unscarred tissue. This also removes the contaminated granulation tissue, thereby decreasing postoperative infection rates.
5. Incisions are planned to allow for possible recurrences in the same or a different location. Since recurrences are common, the surgeon must be sure that planned incisions do not violate potential future flaps.
6. Incisions are planned to avoid suture lines over bony prominences. Scar tissue directly over a bony prominence predisposes the patient to future pressure ulceration.
7. The defect resulting from excision is filled with healthy, unscarred, well-vascularized tissue. This filling in prevents seroma formation and allows for rapid wound healing.
8. A closed drainage system is used to prevent seroma formation. Drainage can be significant in the early postoperative period. Drainage systems can be discontinued when drainage is minimal (usually 5 to 7 days).
9. Postoperatively the patient is placed in a prone position or on a specialty bed, which provides pressure relief and eliminates shear (such as an air-fluidized bed) (Parish and Witkowski, 1980). Three weeks prone or in a specialty bed is a minimum requirement.
10. Mobility is gradually increased, beginning 3 weeks after the procedure, with careful monitoring of skin and suture lines.
11. Skin grafts are not used to close pressure ulcers because they are usually lack long-term durability.

Adherence to these basic principles will decrease overall perioperative complications regardless of the site of the ulcer. The ischial ulcer is the most common in the chair-bound patient with a spinal cord injury, whereas sacral and trochanteric sores are more common in patients confined to bed.

Ischial Ulcer

Ischial ulcers occur secondary to prolonged sitting without change in position. There is rarely a large skin defect present. The underlying cavity however is frequently very large (Figure 18-1). The ischial tuberosity is the pressure point and is always involved. As part of the ulcer excision, ischial ostectomy should be carried out to create a smooth, broad surface, theoretically to distribute weight over a greater surface area (Figure 18-2).

The gluteus maximus muscle flap offers a large amount of well-vascularized tissue with which to fill the defect (McCraw and Arnold, 1986). Even in the patient with a spinal cord injury, significant muscle exists. Skin closure of the donor site can be obtained by linear closure in some cases or by a separate, inferiorly based fasciocutaneous rotation flap.

The hamstring V-Y myocutaneous flap may be used for patients with recurrent ulcerations in extremely large defects or when the gluteus is nonusable (Figures 18-3 and 18-4). This flap is particularly valuable for layer defects because thorough dissection yields 10 to 12 cm of advancement. It is called a "V-Y flap" because the flap is raised with V-shaped incisions and then closed as a Y (Tobin et al, 1981). This flap is well vascularized by segmental perforators from the hamstrings originating from the profunda femoris artery (Tobin et al, 1981). Because the origins and insertions of the muscles are severed, however, this flap cannot be used in an ambulatory patient.

Additional myocutaneous flaps for ischial ulcer closure include the tensor fasciae latae flap, the rectus abdominis flap, and the gracilis flap.

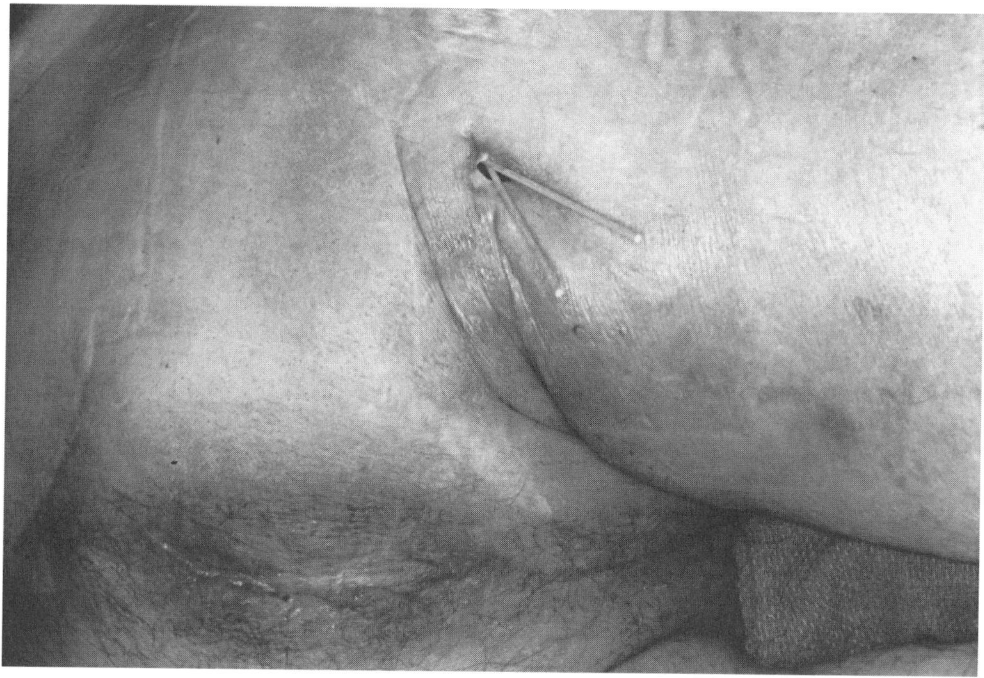

Figure 18-1 Typical ischial ulcer with small skin defect and large cavity.

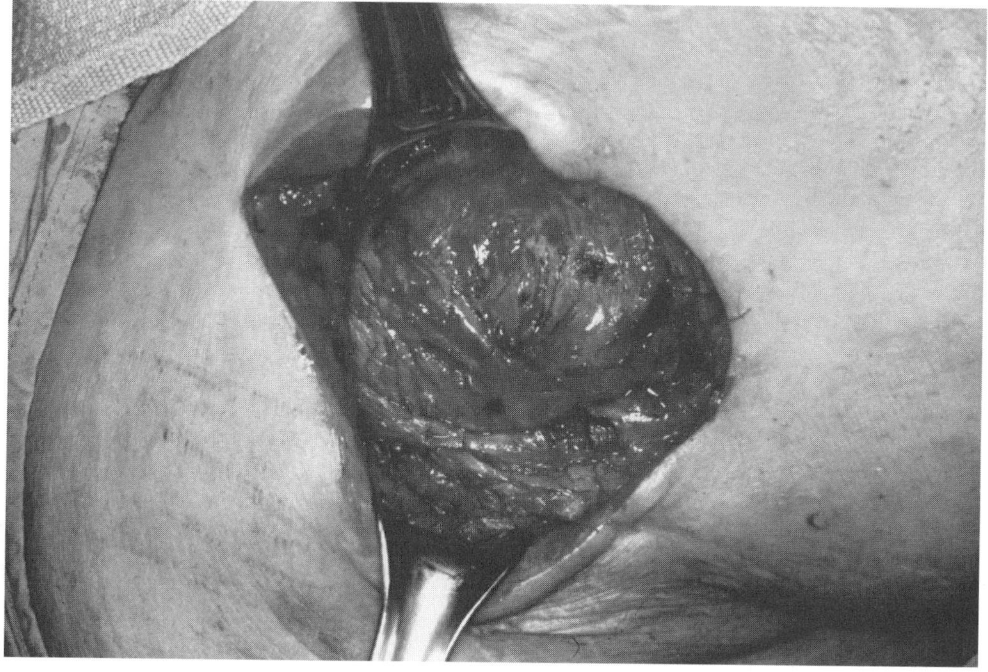

Figure 18-2 Resultant large defect after excision and ostectomy.

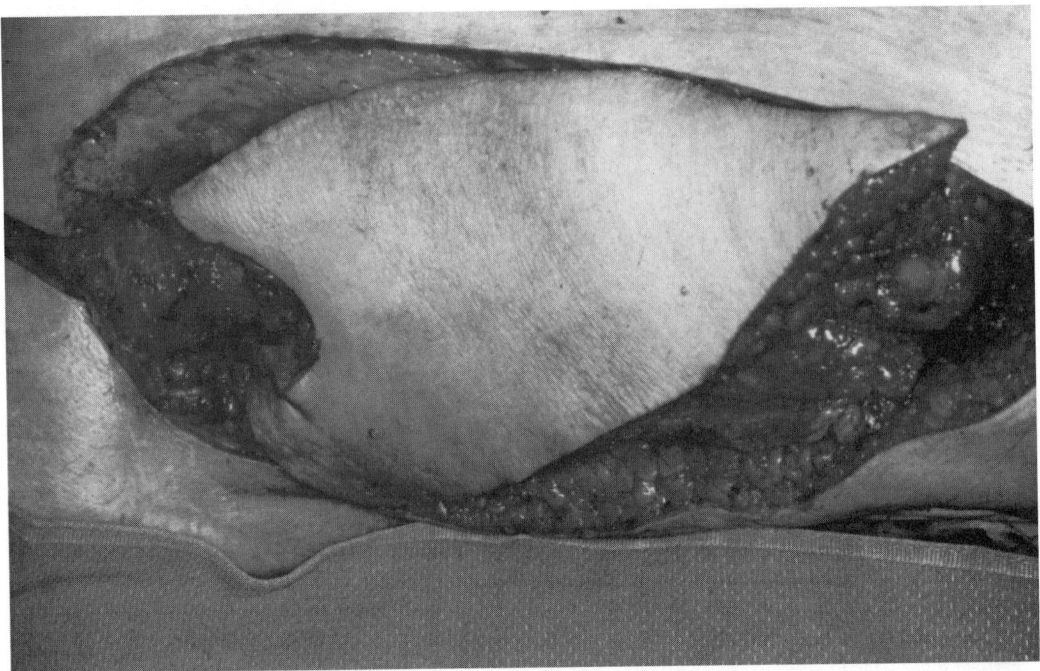

Figure 18-3 Mobilized hamstring V-Y flap.

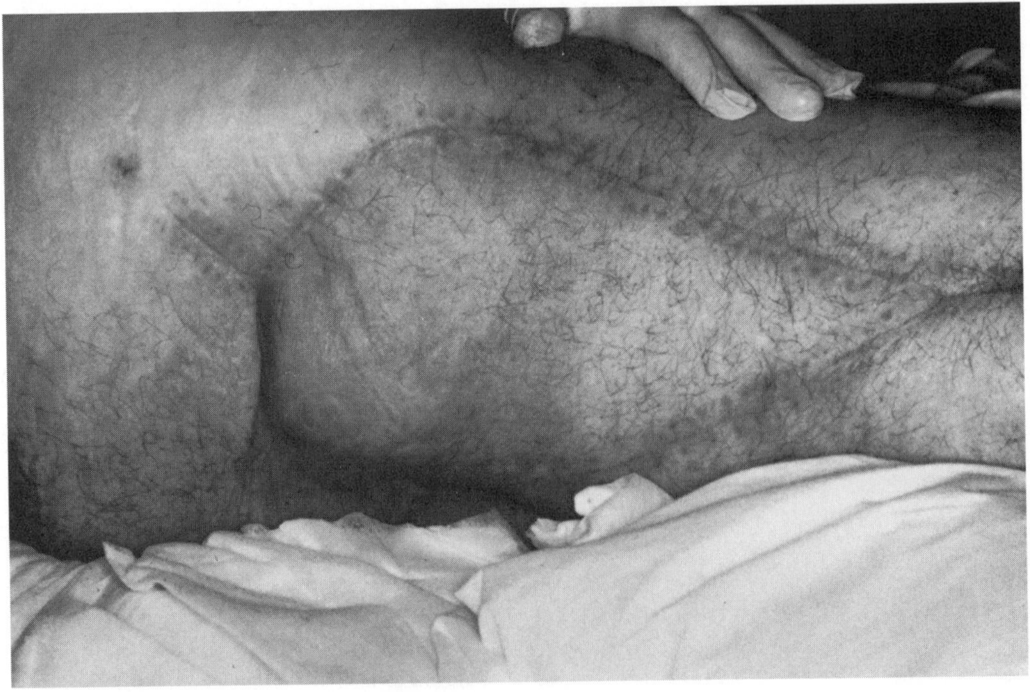

Figure 18-4 Well-healed flap.

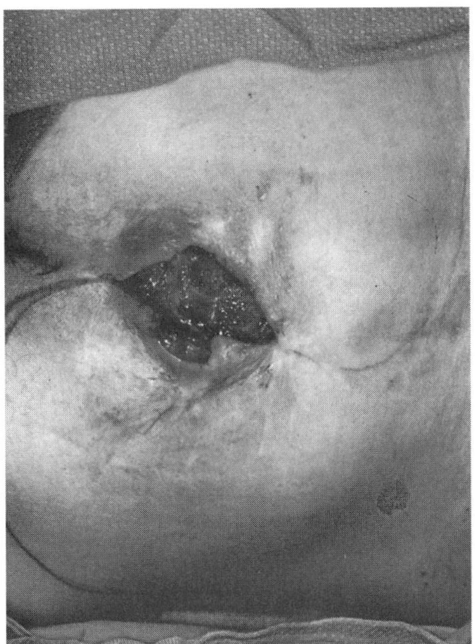

Figure 18-5 Recurrent sacral ulcer. Notice scar from prior inferiorly based rotation flap.

Sacral Ulcer

Unlike ischial ulcers, large skin defects in the sacral area are not uncommon and can be associated with even larger areas of undermining. Fortunately, these ulcers are rarely deep. Ostectomy of the sacral prominence is still mandatory. Coverage is most commonly obtained with a large fasciocutaneous buttock rotation flap (Figures 18-5 and 18-6). Other useful flaps include the rhomboid (a diamond-shaped flap) and a simple Z-plasty (a double transposition flap designed to lengthen in one direction and shorten in the other) (Stueber and Goldberg, 1985) (Figures 18-7 and 18-8). Gluteus maximus musculocutaneous V-Y flaps have been advocated but are extensive procedures that are usually more than is needed for these ulcers (McCraw and Arnold, 1986).

Greater Trochanteric Ulcers

The tensor fasciae latae (TFL) myocutaneous flap is the workhorse of this region (Nahai, 1980). It is most commonly designed as a transposition flap with a large resultant dog-ear (Figures 18-9 to 18-11). V-Y advancement and rotation of the TFL flap

Text continued on p. 451

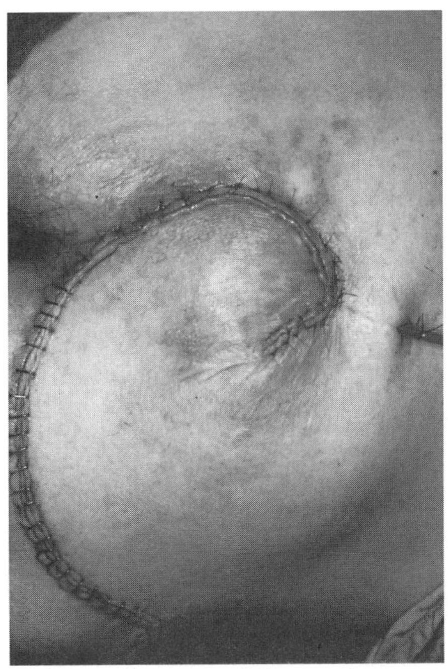

Figure 18-6 Closure with superiorly based buttock rotation flap.

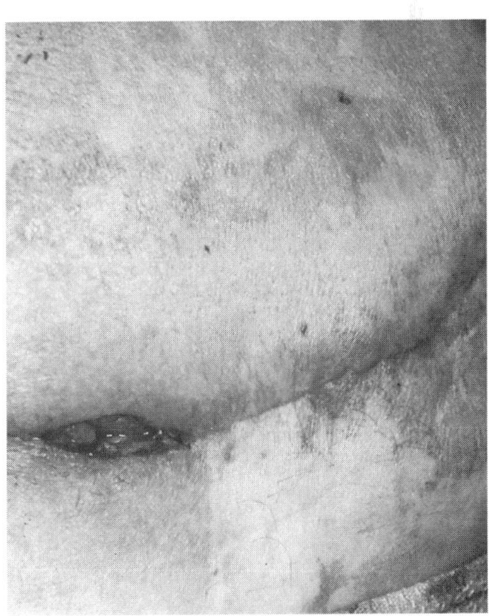

Figure 18-7 Recurrent sacrococcygeal ulcer at distal end of prior buttock rotation flap.

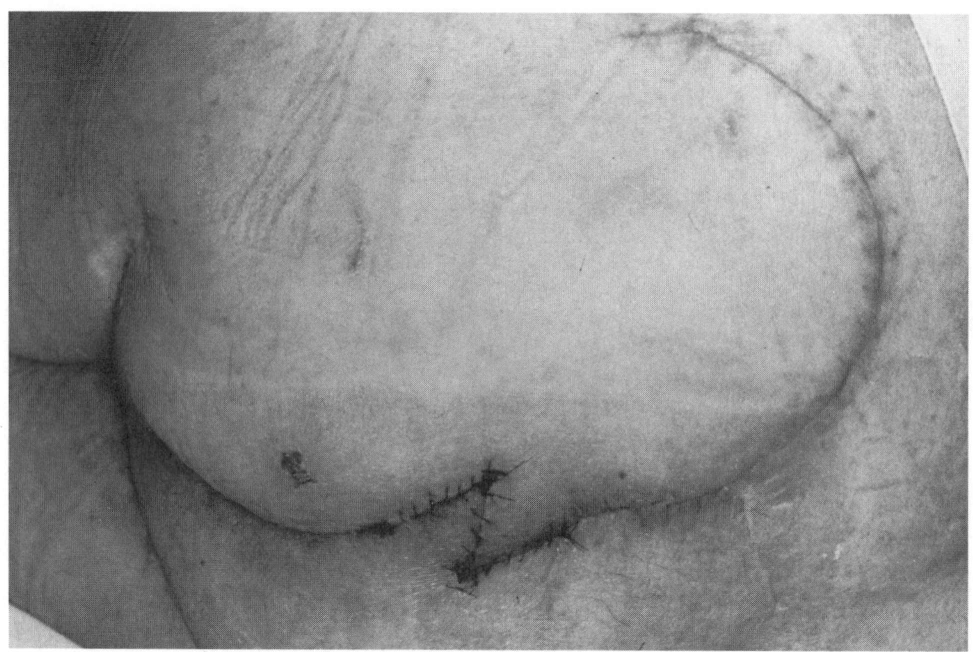

Figure 18-8 Closure with simple Z-plasty.

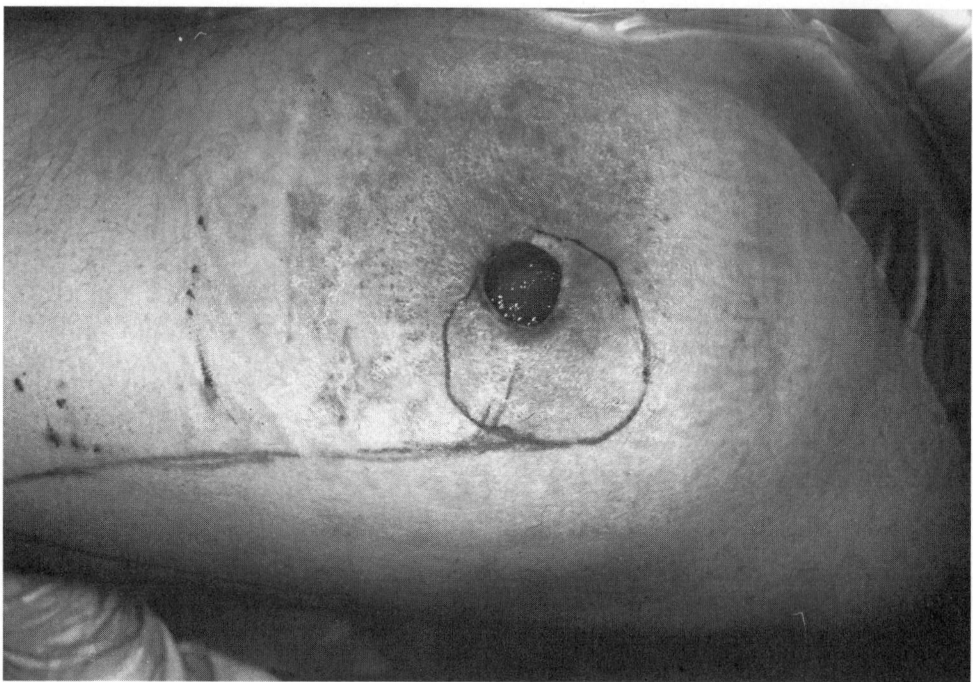

Figure 18-9 Greater tochanteric ulcer. Markings demonstrate large area of undermining and tensor fasciae latae (TFL) flap design.

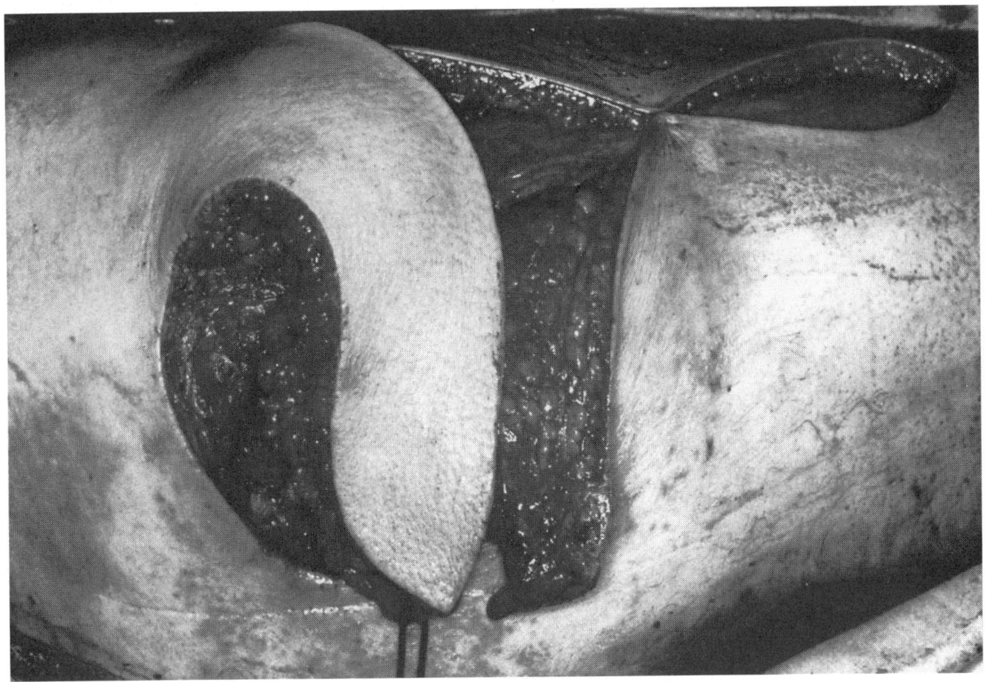

Figure 18-10 Flap transposed.

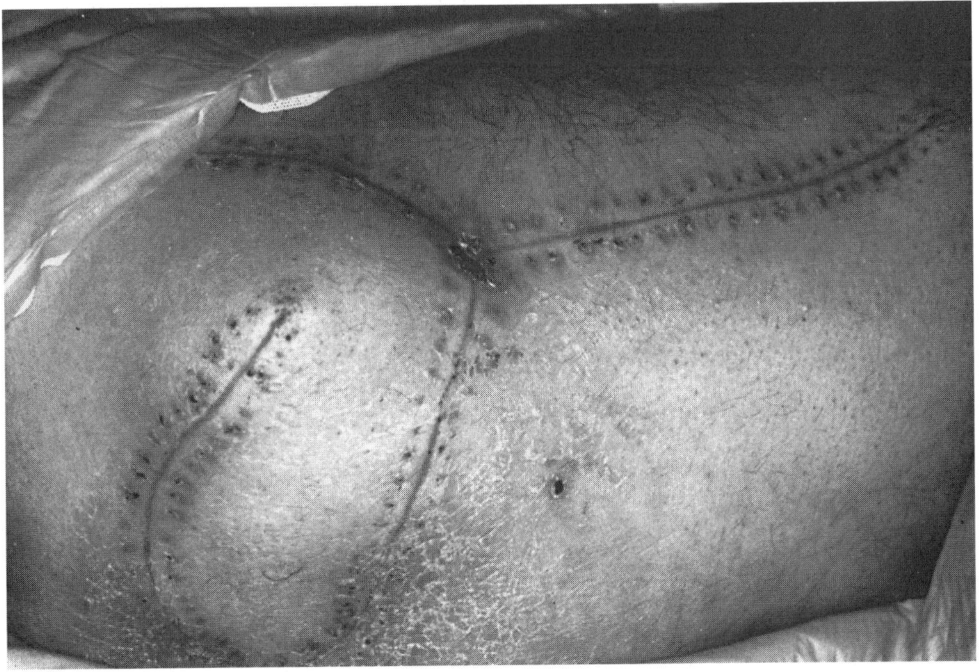

Figure 18-11 Well healed with large dog-ear.

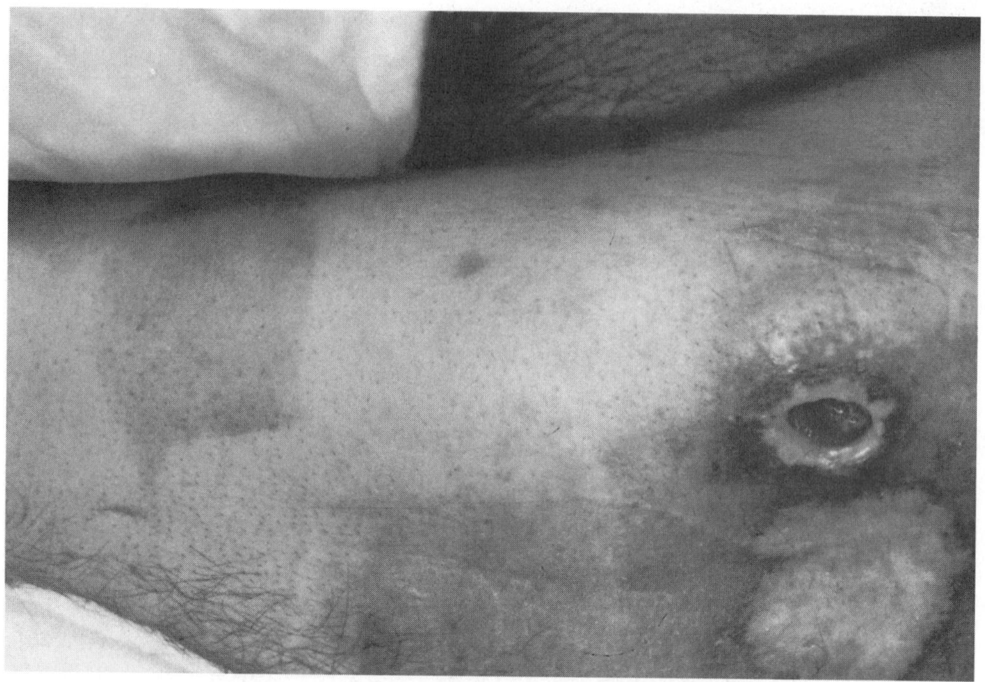

Figure 18-12 Recurrent greater trochanteric ulcer.

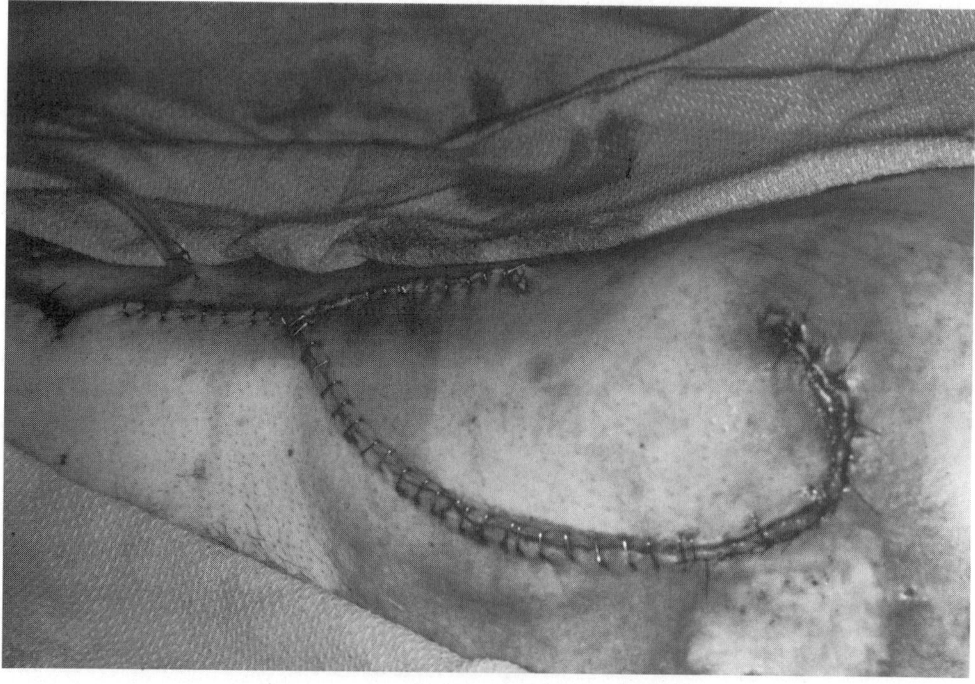

Figure 18-13 Completed tensor fasciae latae flap. V-Y rotation-advancement flap closure.

often give an excellent functional and better esthetic result (Figures 18-12 and 18-13).

Other flaps include the rectus femoris myocutaneous flap and random bipedicle or unipedicle fasciocutaneous flaps.

Other Sites

The olecranon, malleolar, and heel areas are particularly susceptible to pressure injury. Repair of these ulcers follows the same principles outlined previously; local and regional fasciocutaneous flaps are most commonly employed.

SUMMARY

Surgical closure of a pressure ulcer is indicated in select situations. The result is a more durable, functional skin covering over a bony prominence that will resist mechanical stresses better than a wound healed by secondary intention (i.e., scar formation).

Successful surgical treatment of pressure ulcers is based on optimizing the patient's physiologic needs, a team approach, accurate staging, and fundamental surgical principles. Preventive strategies must then be employed to avoid a recurrence of these problem ulcers. The nurse must be familiar with the types of surgical options available for pressure ulcer management and their indications and contraindications to effectively care for these patients.

SELF-ASSESSMENT EXERCISE

1. What is the role of muscle in preventing pressure ulcers?
   - **a.** Muscle redistributes pressure load
   - **b.** Muscle provides the blood supply to the skin
   - **c.** Muscle enables blood vessels to resist shear injury
   - **d.** Muscle concentrates pressure over the bony prominence
2. Describe four conditions that must be controlled before surgical intervention for the patient with pressure ulceration.
3. Briefly describe 11 principles underlying successful surgical management for the patient with pressure ulcers.
4. Myocutaneous flaps such as the gluteus maximus flap are frequently the procedure of choice in pressure ulcer closure because:
   - **a.** They provide well-vascularized tissue to fill the defect
   - **b.** They are almost always successful, even in the malnourished patient
   - **c.** Postoperative healing time is half that required for fasciocutaneous flaps and skin grafts
   - **d.** They are 25% more resistant to repeat breakdown than normal tissue
5. Which of the following flaps should not be used in an ambulatory patient?
   - **a.** Gluteus maximus myocutaneous flap
   - **b.** Tensor fasciae latae (TFL) flap
   - **c.** Large fasciocutaneous flap
   - **d.** Hamstring V-Y flap
6. Patients undergoing flap closure of pressure ulcers are best managed postoperatively on:
   - **a.** An alternating air mattress with frequent position changes
   - **b.** A kinetic therapy device with air-support surface
   - **c.** A water-flotation device
   - **d.** An air-flotation device with nonshear surface
7. Which of the following patients should be referred to plastic surgery?
   - **a.** A 32-year-old male patient with a spinal cord injury with multiple partial-thickness lesions secondary to friction
   - **b.** A 90-year-old woman with late-stage Alzheimer's disease and stage 4 sacral pressure ulcer
   - **c.** A 45-year-old woman with a full-thickness venous hypertension ulcer that is granulating
   - **d.** A 26-year-old paraplegic with a stage 4 ischial pressure ulcer

REFERENCES

Black J, Black S: Surgical management of pressure ulcers, *Nurs Clin North Am* 22(2):4291, 1987.

Linder RM, Morris DM: The surgical management of pressure ulcers: a systematic approach based on staging, *Decubitus* 3(2):32, 1990.

McCraw J, Arnold P: Gluteus maximus. In McCraw J, Arnold P, editors: *Atlas of muscle and musculocutaneous flaps*, Norfolk, Va, 1986, Houston Press.

Nahai F: The tensor fasciae latae flap, *Clin Plast Surg* 7:51, 1980.

Parish LC, Witkowski JA: Clinitron therapy and the decubitus ulcer: preliminary dermatologic studies, *Dermatology* 19:517, 1980.

Stueber K, Goldberg N: Wound coverage: grafts and flaps. In Dagher FJ, editor: *Cutaneous wounds*, Mt Kisco, New York, 1985, Futura Publishing Co.

Tobin GR et al: The biceps femoris myocutaneous advancement flap: a useful modification for ischial pressure ulcer reconstruction, *Ann Plast Surg* 6(5):396, 1981.

CHAPTER 19

Molecular Regulation of Wound Healing

GREGORY S. SCHULTZ

OBJECTIVES

1. Describe the importance of adhesion and migration of leukocytes in inflammation.
2. Identify important processes in wound healing that are regulated by growth factors, cytokines, protease, or hormones.
3. Describe the molecular environment that growth factors need to promote wound healing.
4. For each of the five families of growth factors, list at least one member, a key target cell, and one main action.

Wound healing in the skin has been studied extensively in animal models and in humans, and much has been learned about the cells and the molecules that regulate this complex process. At the cellular level, healing of skin wounds involves platelets, leukocytes, epidermal cells, fibroblasts, and vascular endothelial cells. At the molecular level, results of cell culture studies, animal wound models, and human clinical trials have demonstrated that many growth factors, cytokines, proteases, and hormones regulate most of the key actions of cells during wound healing.

These actions include the directed movement of the cells into a wound (chemotactic migration), replacement of damaged epidermal and dermal cells (mitosis), growth of new blood vessels (neovascularization), formation of scar tissue (synthesis of extracellular matrix proteins), and remodeling of scar tissue (proteolytic turnover of extracellular matrix proteins) (Bennett and Schultz, 1993a, 1993b). Any condition that disrupts the normal actions of these molecular regulators in wounds will directly impair healing and promote the establishment and maintenance of chronic wounds (Mast and Schultz, 1996; Tarnuzzer and Schultz, 1996). If these two concepts are correct, then it should be possible to identify abnormalities in the actions of these molecules in chronic wounds and design therapies that reestablish an environment in chronic wounds that permits these molecular regulators to function normally and lead to healing of chronic wounds.

BIOLOGIC ROLES OF CYTOKINES AND GROWTH FACTORS IN WOUND HEALING

General Phases of Wound Healing

The processes that occur during healing of skin wounds can be grouped into four general phases: hemostasis, inflammation, proliferation and repair, and remodeling. There is considerable temporal overlap of these phases of healing, and the entire process lasts for several months. Immediately after injury the process of blood clotting in initiated by activation of a proteolytic cascade, which ultimately converts fibrinogen into fibrin. As the fibrin molecules self-associate into a web-like net, red blood cells (RBCs) and platelets become entrapped. The aggregate of fibrin, RBCs, and platelets quickly grows large enough to form a tampon that blocks an injured capillary and stops the flow of blood.

The process of blood clotting also induces platelet degranulation, which releases a burst of preformed growth factors stored in platelet granules. These include platelet-derived growth factor (PDGF), transforming growth factor-beta (TGF-β), epidermal growth factor (EGF), and insulin-like growth factor-I

(IGF-I). These growth factors initiate two major processes: inflammation and initiation of tissue repair. The growth factors released from platelets quickly diffuse from the wound into the surrounding tissues and attract leukocytes into the injured area (Bennett and Schultz, 1993a, 1993b).

Adhesion Molecules and Adhesion Receptors in Inflammation

Chemotactic attraction of leukocytes to a wound and their movement from the blood into wounded tissue (extravasation) involves expression and activation of adhesion molecules and adhesion receptors on leukocytes, platelets, and vascular endothelial cells. Cytokines and growth factors play key roles in these processes (Arai et al, 1990; Frenette and Wagner, 1996a, 1996b; Springer, 1990). Among the many types of adhesion molecules and receptors on the cell surface, four major families of transmembrane proteins stand out in the process of inflammation: integrins, selectins, cell adhesion molecules, and cadherins (Figure 19-1).

1. *Integrins* are glycoproteins composed of two different types of subunits, designated α and β. In simple terms, integrins are cellular receptors for extracellular matrix proteins, as shown with $\alpha_5\beta_1$, which is a receptor for fibronectin. A short amino acid sequence, such as arginine-glycine-aspartate (RGD), is often the site of recognition by the integrin receptor. Integrins are important because they are capable of generating signals inside cells when the integrin receptor binds to a specific extracellular matrix protein in much the same way as the insulin receptor generates intracellular signals, which regulates glucose transport into a cell when insulin binds to its cellular receptor. Expression of $\beta2$ integrins is limited to leukocytes, whereas

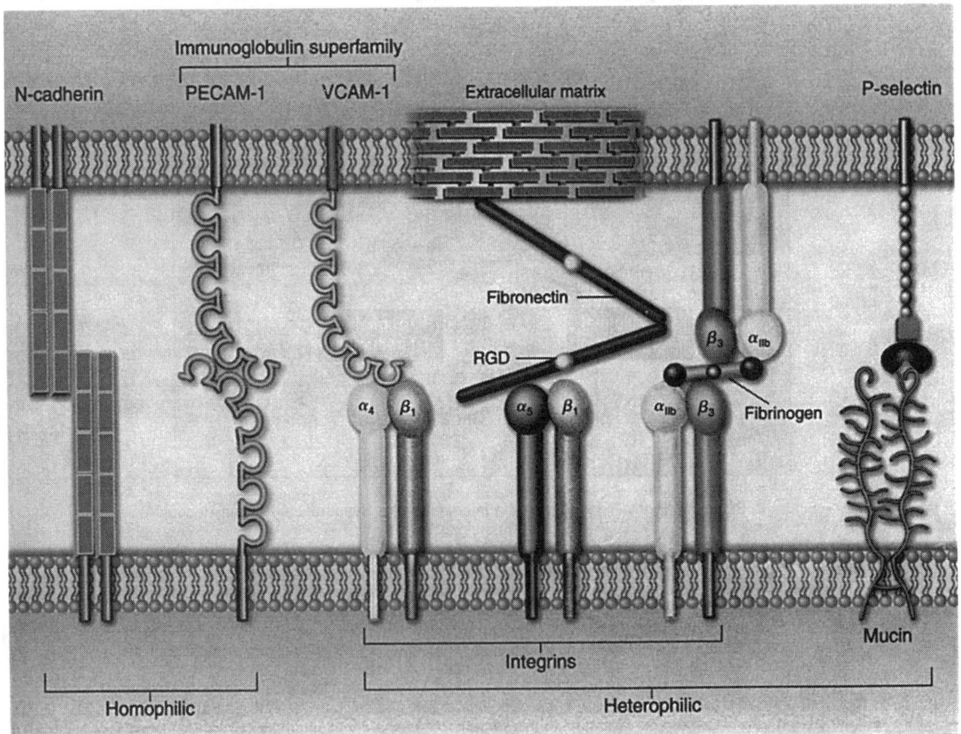

Figure 19-1 Four major classes of adhesion proteins and adhesion receptors embedded in a theoretic plasma membrane (integrins, selectins, cell adhesion molecules [PECAM-1 and VCAM-1], and cadherins). (From Frenette PS, Wagner DD: Adhesion molecules. Part 1, *N Engl J Med* 334:1526, 1996. Massachusetts Medical Society. All rights reserved.)

$\beta1$ integrins are expressed on most cell types. $\beta1$ integrins primarily bind to extracellular matrix components such as fibronectin, laminin, and collagens.

2. *Selectins* are proteins that have a unique structure called a *lectin domain* at the distal end, which can bind specific carbohydrate groups of glycoproteins or mucins on adjacent cells. So unlike other adhesion proteins, which recognize specific protein structures, selectins recognize and bind to carbohydrate ligands on leukocytes and vascular endothelial cells. E-selectin appears on endothelial cells after they have been activated by inflammatory cytokines, and P-selectin is stored in α-granules of platelets and the storage granules of endothelial cells (Weible-Palade bodies).
3. *Cell adhesion molecules* (CAMs) are members of the immunoglobulin superfamily of proteins, and CAMs can bind to other CAMs or to integrins on cells. CAMs that are important in inflammation include the platelet-endothelial-cell adhesion molecule (PECAM), vascular-cell adhesion molecule (VCAM), and intercellular adhesion molecule-1 (ICAM-1).
4. *Cadherins* are important in establishing molecular links between adjacent cells, especially during embryonic development. They form zipper-like structures of dimers at specialized regions of contact between neighboring cells called *adherens junctions.* Cadherins are linked to the cytoskeleton through molecules called *catenins,* which associate with actin microfilaments.

During the process of extravasation of inflammatory cells into a wound, important interactions occur between blood vessels and blood cells (Arai et al, 1990; Frenette and Wagner, 1996a, 1996b; Springer, 1990). Initially, circulating leukocytes begin rolling on endothelial cells through the binding of glycoproteins expressed on their cell surface to selectins, transiently expressed by activated endothelial cells of venules (Figure 19-2). The binding affinity of selectins is relatively low, but it is enough to serve as a biologic brake, making leukocytes quickly

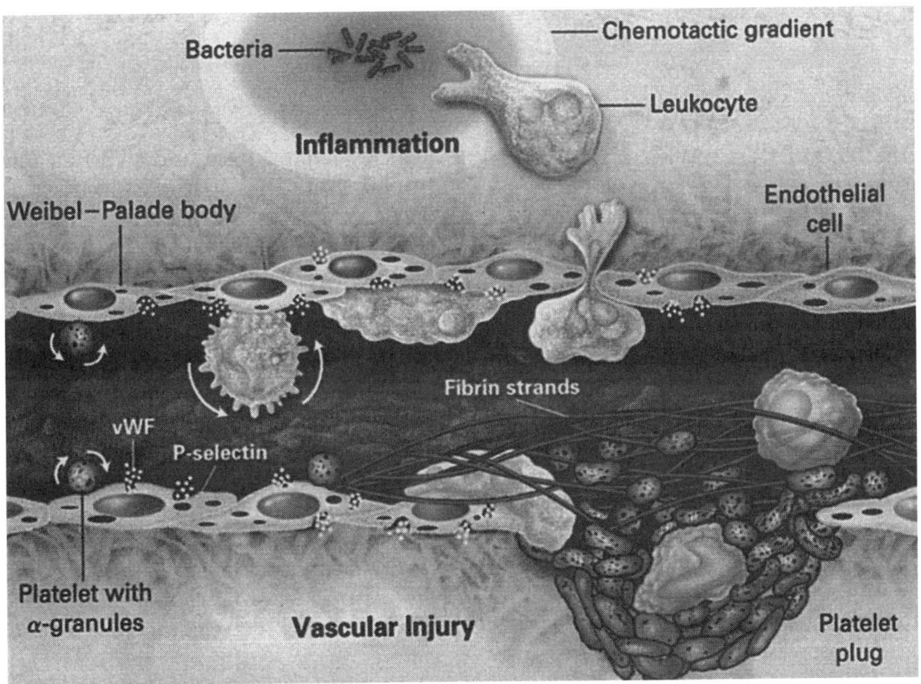

Figure 19-2 Interactions between blood cells and a stimulated or injured venule. (From Frenette PS, Wagner DD: Adhesion molecules. Part II: Blood vessels and blood cells, *N Engl J Med* 335:43, 1996. Massachusetts Medical Society. All rights reserved.)

decelerate by rolling on endothelial cells. While rolling, leukocytes can become activated by chemoattractants (cytokines, growth factors, or bacterial products). After activation, leukocytes firmly adhere to endothelial cells as a result of the binding between their $\beta 2$ class of integrins and ligands, such as VCAM and ICAM expressed on activated endothelial cells. Chemotactic signals present outside the venule induce leukocytes to squeeze between endothelial cells of the venule and migrate into the inflammatory center by using their $\beta 1$ class of integrins to recognize and bind to extracellular matrix components.

Adhesion and degranulation of platelets at sites of vascular injury also use a system of adhesion molecules and adhesion receptor proteins. Vascular injury immediately induces endothelial cells to release the contents of their storage granules (Weible-Palade bodies), including the proteins P-selectin and von Willebrand factor. P-selectin promptly moves to the plasma membrane of endothelial cells where it induces rolling of platelets on endothelial cells, and von Willebrand factor is quickly deposited on the exposed extracellular matrix, where it plays a crucial role in the adhesion of platelets to the damaged site.

Inflammatory Cell Proteases

When the inflammatory cascade is activated, neutrophils enter the wound initially followed by macrophages. Neutrophils and macrophages become activated and engulf and destroy bacteria through their production of reactive oxygen species (super oxide anion, oxygen free radicals, or hydrogen peroxide). Activated neutrophils and macrophages also release several proteases, including neutrophil elastase (a serine-type protease), neutrophil collagenase (a matrix metalloproteinase-type protease designated as MMP-8) and macrophage metalloelastase (MMP-12). These proteases play important beneficial roles in initiating normal wound healing by removing (proteolytically degrading) damaged extracellular matrix components, which must be replaced by new, intact extracellular matrix molecules for wound healing to proceed. These proteases also are important for enabling inflammatory cells to move through the basement membrane that surrounds capillaries.

Inflammatory Cell Cytokines and Growth Factors in Proliferation and Repair

The growth factors released by platelets diffuse away from a wound within a few hours, but they are replaced by growth factors and cytokines that are produced by neutrophils, macrophages, activated fibroblasts, vascular endothelial cells, and epidermal cells that are drawn into the wound area. For example, activated macrophages secrete several important cytokines, including tumor necrosis factor alpha (TNFα) and interleukin 1 beta (IL-1β), which have a variety of actions on different cells. TNFα and IL-1β are potent inflammatory cytokines, which further stimulate inflammation. TNFα also induces macrophages to produce IL-1β, which is mitogenic for fibroblasts and upregulates expression of MMPs. Both TNFα and IL-1β directly influence deposition of collagen in the wound by inducing synthesis of collagen by fibroblasts and by upregulating expression of MMPs. Additionally, these cytokines downregulate expression of the tissue inhibitors of metalloproteinases (TIMPs), which are the natural inhibitors of MMPs. Interferon gamma (IFN-γ), produced by lymphocytes attracted into the wound, inhibits fibroblast migration and downregulates collagen synthesis.

Inflammatory cells secrete other growth factors, including TGF-β, transforming growth factor alpha (TGF-α), heparin-binding epidermal growth factor (HB-EGF) and basic fibroblast growth factor (bFGF). The growth factors secreted by macrophages continue to stimulate migration of fibroblasts, epithelial cells, and vascular endothelial cells into the wound. As the fibroblasts, epithelial cells, and vascular endothelial cells migrate into the site of injury, they begin to proliferate, and the cellularity of the wound increases. This begins the proliferative and repair phase, which often lasts several weeks. If the wound is not infected, the number of inflammatory cells in a wound begins to decrease after a few days. Other types of cells drawn into the wound, such as fibroblasts, endothelial cells, and keratinocytes, begin to synthesize growth factors.

Fibroblasts secrete IGF-1, bFGF, TGF-β, PDGF, and keratinocyte growth factor (KGF). Endothelial cells produce vascular endothelial cell growth factor (VEGF), bFGF, and PDGF. Keratinocytes synthesize TGF-β, TGF-α, and IL-1β. These growth factors continue to stimulate cell proliferation and synthesis of extracellular matrix proteins and to promote formation of new capillaries.

Remodeling Phase

After the initial scar forms, proliferation and neovascularization cease and the wound enters the remodeling phase, which can last for many months. During this last phase, a new balance is reached between the synthesis of extracellular matrix components in the scar and their degradation by metalloproteinases such as collagenase, gelatinase, and stromelysin. Fibroblasts synthesize a majority of the collagen, elastin, and proteoglycans that comprise the dermal scar matrix. Fibroblasts also are a major source of the MMPs that degrade the scar matrix as well as their inhibitors, the TIMPs. They also secrete lysyl oxidase, which is an enzyme that covalently cross links components of the extracellular matrix such as collagen and elastin molecules, producing a stable extracellular matrix. Keratinocytes secrete much of the type 4 collagen that reforms the basement membrane, which separates the epidermal and dermal layers and forms the surface on which keratinocytes prefer to migrate. Angiogenesis ceases and the density of capillaries decreases in the wound site as a result of programmed cell death of the vascular endothelial cells (apoptosis). Eventually remodeling of the scar tissue reaches equilibrium, although the mature scar is never as strong as uninjured skin.

GENERAL PROPERTIES OF GROWTH FACTORS AND THEIR RECEPTORS

Discovery, Purification, and Cloning of Growth Factors

Protein growth factors initially were discovered because of their ability to stimulate multiple cycles of cell growth (mitosis) when added to cultures of normal, quiescent cells. This distinguishes growth factors from essential nutrients such as vitamins, cofactors, and trace minerals (such as selenium), which are required for metabolic processes but are not sufficient to initiate cell division by themselves. Both nutrients and growth factors are necessary for mitosis, but only growth factors can initiate mitosis of quiescent cells.

Based on the ability of growth factors to stimulate continuous mitosis of cells in culture, it is not surprising that many growth factors initially were isolated from medium conditioned by tumor cells. Other sources of growth factors included platelets,

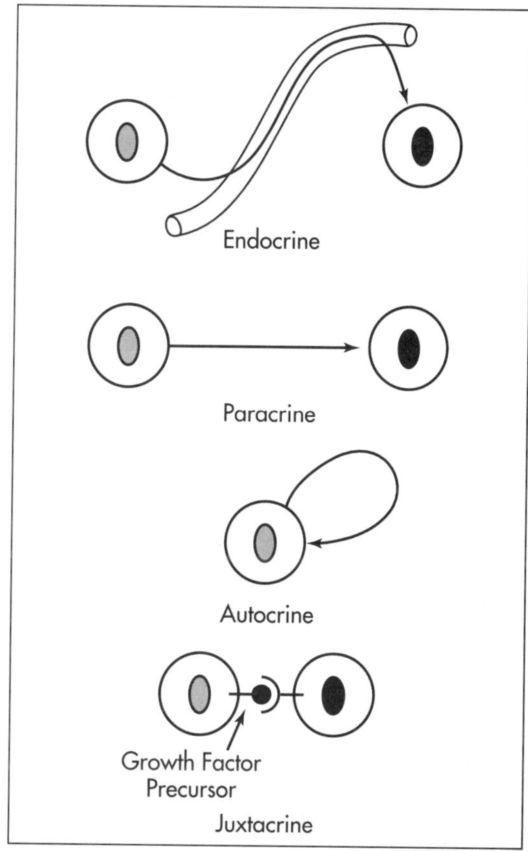

Figure 19-3 Growth factor action. Secreted growth factors act predominately by autocrine (self-stimulation) or by paracrine (adjacent cells) pathways and not usually by classical endocrine pathways. Membrane-bound growth factors may also interact with adjacent cells by juxtacrine stimulation. (From Bennett NT, Schultz GS: Growth factors and wound healing: biochemical properties of growth factors and their receptors, *Am J Surg* 165:728, 1993. With permission, Excerpta Medica Inc.)

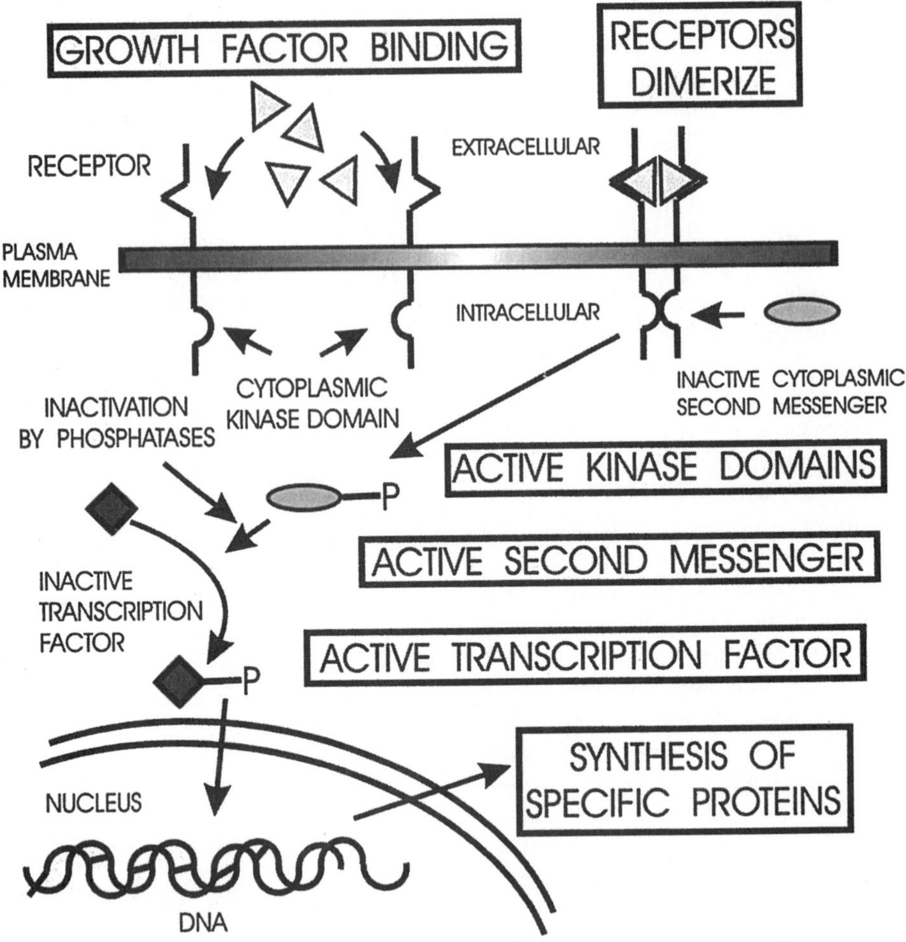

Figure 19-4 Growth factor receptor signal generation. Growth factors typically affect cells by binding to specific, high-affinity receptor proteins located in the plasma membrane of target cells, which then dimerize and activate tyrosine or serine/threonine kinase domains located in the cytoplasmic region of the receptor. The activated receptor then phosphorylates second messenger proteins, which also are frequently kinases that participate in a cascade of phosphorylation/activation steps that ultimately activate an RNA transcription factor, which selectively initiates synthesis of proteins that alters the behavior of the target cell. The second messenger system is turned off by enzymes called *phosphatases* that remove phosphate groups from proteins.

macrophages, and normal tissues that can proliferate rapidly, such as ovarian follicles or placenta. Although growth factors were present in minute quantities from these natural sources, tiny amounts eventually were purified using traditional biochemical methods of column chromatography, ion-exchange chromatography, high-pressure liquid chromatography (HPLC), ultracentrifugation, and gel electrophoresis. The amino acid sequences of the proteins were determined, which permitted the growth factor genes to be cloned and sequenced. With the development of recombinant DNA technology, large amounts of synthetic human growth factors were produced from cultures of bacteria, yeast, or human cells that carried the gene for the growth factor. The availability of large amounts of the synthetic growth factors enabled research to be performed that led to a better understanding of the biologic roles of growth factors in wound healing and other physiologic processes, such as fetal development, aging, and cancer. Ultimately, this lead to experiments that evaluated the effects of the synthetic growth factors in animal wound healing models and eventually to clinical trials in patients.

Autocrine and Paracrine Action of Growth Factors

Growth factors are synthesized and secreted by many types of cells involved in wound healing, including platelets, inflammatory cells, fibroblasts, epithelial cells, and vascular endothelial cells. Moreover, growth factors usually act either on the producer cell (autocrine stimulation) or on adjacent cells (paracrine stimulation). In contrast to classical endocrine hormones, growth factors generally do not enter the blood stream and act on cells at a great distance (Figure 19-3).

Receptors for Growth Factors

All peptide growth factors initiate their effects on target cells by binding to specific, high-affinity receptor proteins located in the plasma membrane of target cells (Fantl, Johnson, and Williams, 1993). Only cells that express the specific receptor protein can respond to the growth factor. Binding of the growth factor to its receptor usually initiates dimerization of two receptor proteins, which activates a region of receptor protein called a *kinase domain* that is located inside the cell (Figure 19-4). Kinase domains have the enzymatic ability to covalently transfer a phosphate group from the high-energy molecule (ATP) to an amino acid, such as tyrosine, serine, or threonine, in a protein. The activated receptor protein is the "first messenger" in the response system of a cell to a growth factor.

The activated receptor kinase domain then phosphorylates amino acids on a small number of specific cytoplasmic proteins. These cytoplasmic proteins become activated when phosphorylated and are the first in a series of second messenger proteins that eventually generate a response in the cell to the growth factor. Second messenger proteins also typically contain kinase domains that are activated when the proteins are phosphorylated. The activated cytoplasmic kinase proteins in turn phosphorylate other cytoplasmic proteins in a sequential cascade of phosphorylations and activations that eventually leads to the activation of special proteins called *RNA transcription factors*. Activated RNA transcription factors bind with selected regions of the DNA to help initiate transcription of genes into messenger RNAs (mRNAs), which are translated into proteins that ultimately alter the functions of the target cell.

Another system of cytoplasmic proteins acts to turn off the transcription of genes that are turned on by growth factors. These proteins are called *phosphatases*, and they remove the phosphate groups that were added to the amino acids of the second messenger kinase proteins and to the RNA transcription factors. Removal of the phosphate groups inactivates the second messenger proteins and the transcription factors. Thus the effects of growth factors on target cells require an integrated balance between receptor proteins, second messenger kinase proteins, RNA transcription factors, and phosphatases.

MAJOR FAMILIES OF GROWTH FACTORS

The first attempt to use growth factors to promote healing of human wounds was based on the concept that platelets contained numerous growth factors that were released at the time of injury. Furthermore, substantial amounts of activated platelet supernatant could be obtained either from individual patients with chronic skin ulcers or from apheresis donors. This would permit patients to be treated with their own activated platelet supernatant or from carefully screened platelet donors. To test this concept, an FDA-approved, randomized, controlled, multicenter, dose-response trial of topically applied activated platelet supernatant in chronic, nonhealing, diabetic wounds was conducted (David et al, 1992; Holloway et al, 1993).

A total of 97 patients from four sites were randomized to receive either placebo or one of three dilutions of activated platelet supernatant (CT-102). The study population consisted of patients who had diabetes mellitus with at least one chronic, nonhealing, diabetic ulcer of at least 8 weeks' duration with no signs of systemic wound infection and a

TABLE 19-1 Growth Factors Involved in Skin Wound Healing

GROWTH FACTOR FAMILY	MEMBERS	GENERAL ACTIONS
Epidermal growth factor	EGF, TGF-α, HB-EGF	Strongly stimulate migration and mitosis of epidermal cells; weakly angiogenic; small increase in scar formation
Platelet-derived growth factor	PDGF-AA, PDGF-BB, VEGF, CTGF	PDGF: simulates migration and mitosis of fibroblasts CTGF: large increase in scar formation VEGF: very angiogenic
Fibroblast growth factor	aFGF, bFGF, KGF	aFGF and bFGF: stimulate migration and mitosis of fibroblasts and epidermal cells; angiogenic; moderate increase in scar formation KGF: only stimulates epidermal cells
Insulin-like growth factor	IGF-I, IGF-II, insulin	Functions with growth hormone; moderate increase in mitosis of fibroblasts and epidermal cells; moderate increase in scar formation
Transforming growth factor-beta	TGF-β1, TGF-β2, TGF-β3	TGF-β1, TGF-β2: large increase in scar formation; promote bone formation

supine periwound transcutaneous oxygen tension of at least 30 mm Hg. Before topical application of double-blind therapy, the wounds were debrided of all necrotic and infected soft and bony tissues. Wounds were treated daily until they healed or until a total of 20 weeks of treatment was achieved. The use of placebo treatment, combined with good basic wound care, reduced wound area 77% and reduced wound volume 83% from baseline to final visit, although only 29% of the placebo group healed completely. However, all healing parameters were significantly improved in patients treated with all doses of platelet releasate. For example, 63% of the patients treated with platelet releasate achieved complete healing ($p = 0.01$), with a 93% mean area reduction ($p = 0.002$) and a 95% mean volume reduction at the final visit ($p = 0.005$). The adverse experience profile of patients receiving platelet releasate was similar to that of patients receiving placebo. These results demonstrated the benefit of treatment of chronic diabetic wounds with a mixture of growth factors and proteins released from platelets.

Table 19-1 presents an overview of the five major families of growth factors and includes those growth factors that have been shown to play roles in wound healing in animals or humans (not all known growth factors are included).

Epidermal Growth Factor Family

EGF was the first growth factor to be purified and biochemically characterized (Carpenter and Cohen, 1990). Other members of the EGF family that influence wound healing are TGF-α (Massague, 1990) and HB-EGF (Shigeki et al, 1992). Members of the EGF family are small (about 6000 molecular weight) single-chain proteins that contain a characteristic triple loop structure, which is required for biologic activity. They bind to a common receptor protein (EGF-receptor) that has tyrosine kinase activity and is expressed on almost all types of cells. Members of the EGF family have similar, but not identical, biologic effects on target cells. They are chemoattractants and mitogens for epidermal cells, fibroblasts, and vascular endothelial cells but are most effective for epidermal cells.

EGF or TGF-α are synthesized as membrane-bound precursors that are released by proteolysis in a wide range of cells, including cells of the lacrimal gland and salivary gland. EGF and TGF-α are present in saliva and tears, and data from many different types of experiments strongly suggest that EGF and TGF-α play important roles in both the normal turnover of epithelial cells of the gut and cornea and in the healing of wounds in these tissues. Specifically, in the skin, epidermal cells synthesize large amounts of TGF-α, and mice that lack TGF-α or EGF receptor have abnormal hair and skin architecture. Levels of EGF-receptor are elevated in the leading edge of epidermal cells in burn wounds (Nanney et al, 1996). Specific inhibition of the EGF receptor delays healing of partial-thickness skin injuries in animals. HB-EGF is produced by macrophages and presumably is retained in a wound for longer periods of time than EGF or TGF-α because of reversible binding to heparin.

Current models of skin wound healing propose that TGF-α is the growth factor that is primarily responsible for the normal maintenance and turnover of epidermal cells of the skin. When a skin injury occurs, epidermal cell proliferation and migration is stimulated by TGF-α produced by epidermal cells; EGF produced by epithelial cells lining the hair follicles, sweat glands, and sebaceous glands; and HB-EGF produced by macrophages that enter the wound. In addition, fibroblasts surrounding the wound secrete KGF, a member of the fibroblast growth factor system, which exclusively promotes migration and mitosis of keratinocytes.

Therapeutic Uses. EGF has been evaluated in burn care and venous ulcers. Early studies in normal animals showed accelerated healing of partial-thickness burns or excisional wounds when treated with EGF, TGF-α, or HB-EGF (Brown et al, 1986). In a prospective, double-blind, paired study of 12 patients with split-thickness skin donor sites, EGF treatment significantly decreased the average length of time to 25% healing and 50% healing by approximately 1 day and decreased healing times to 75% healing and 100% healing by approximately 1.5 days ($p < 0.02$) as compared with silver sulfadiazine cream (Brown et al, 1989). These results demonstrated that recombinant human growth factors could accelerate healing of acute skin wounds in patients and prompted the evaluation of EGF in chronic skin ulcers.

Because epidermal regeneration is an important component of healing venous ulcers, a prospective, randomized, double-blind, placebo-controlled study was conducted evaluating topical use of recombinant human EGF for treatment of chronic venous ulcers (Falanga et al, 1992). Thirty-five patients with venous ulcers were randomly assigned to either a placebo group or treatment with an aqueous solution of EGF (10 μg/ml). All patients applied a nonadherent dressing pad saturated with the EGF or placebo solutions to the ulcer twice daily; a gauze bandage and a compression roll were also applied. At the end of the 10-week study, 6 of 17 ulcers treated with EGF had completely epithelialized compared with 2 of 18 ulcers treated with saline ($p = 0.01$). The mean (and median) percent reduction and ulcer size at the end of the study was 48% (73%) for EGF compared with 13% (33%) for placebo ($p = 0.32$). Although topical application of EGF in the dose and manner used in this study did not significantly enhance epithelialization of venous ulcers, a greater reduction in ulcer size and a larger number of healed ulcers occurred with the use of the EGF. Further investigations with EGF in venous ulcers seem warranted.

Platelet-Derived Growth Factor Family

The PDGF family comprises two major proteins, PDGF and VEGF, that influence wound healing (Heldin and Westermark, 1996). PDGF and VEGF share about 25% amino acid sequence homology, and both are composed of two subunits that are covalently linked by disulfide bonds. PDGF has two different subunits (designated A and B types). Human platelets contain high levels of PDGF, and many types of human cells important in skin wound healing can secrete PDGF, including fibroblasts, vascular smooth muscle cells, and vascular endothelial cells.

Macrophages secrete a growth factor named *connective tissue growth factor* (CTGF), which binds to the PDGF receptors but has minimal sequence homology to PDGF (Bradham et al, 1991; Frazier et al, 1996). PDGF and VEGF bind to different receptor proteins (both are tyrosine kinases) and stimulate different biologic actions. Two distinct PDGF receptors have been characterized. The PDGF-α receptor recognizes both A- and B-subunits of PDGF, whereas the PDGF-β receptor only recognizes the B-subunit of PDGF.

PDGF is a chemoattractant and mitogen primarily for fibroblasts, whereas VEGF is a chemoattractant and mitogen primarily for vascular endothelial cells. VEGF is one of the most effective angiogenic factors yet discovered, and synthesis of VEGF by vascular endothelial cells is increased by hypoxia.

Therapeutic Uses. PDGF, effective at stimulating formation of extracellular matrix and granulation tissue, has been evaluated clinically in pressure ulcers and diabetic ulcers. The PDGF-BB isoform was chosen for evaluation in clinical studies because it is able to bind to both PDGF-α and PDGF-β receptors.

Robson and colleagues (1992a) first studied PDGF-BB in 20 patients with pressure ulcers. Topical synthetic human PDGF-BB was applied daily to chronic pressure ulcers for 28 days. In this prospective, randomized, double-blind, placebo-controlled phase I/II trial, dosing solutions containing 1, 10, or 100 μg/ml of PDGF-BB was evaluated. Patients treated with 100 μg/ml of PDGF-BB had pronounced healing responses compared with patients treated with placebo, 1 μg/ml, or 10 μg/ml PDGF-BB. Although the results of this initial, small study did not achieve statistical significance at the 95% confidence level for both reduction of ulcer depth and reduction of ulcer volume, it strongly suggested that PDGF-BB improved healing of chronic pressure ulcers.

In a second major clinical study, PDGF-BB was evaluated for the treatment of noninfected, lower-extremity diabetic ulcers. All ulcers had a transcutaneous partial pressure of oxygen of 30 mm Hg or greater on the dorsum of the foot or at the ulcer margin (Steed and the Diabetic Ulcer Study Group, 1995). A total of 118 patients with chronic, full-thickness, lower-extremity diabetic ulcers were enrolled in this prospective, double-blind, placebo-controlled, multisite clinical trial. PDGF-BB was formulated at 30 μg/g in a gel. Ulcers were treated once a day at a dose equivalent to approximately 2.2 μg PDGF-BB/cm^2 ulcer area for 20 weeks or until complete wound healing was achieved. The gel was spread evenly over the entire ulcer surface, a nonadherent saline-soaked gauze dressing was placed directly over the ulcer, and the foot was wrapped circumferentially with roll gauze. Patients were assessed weekly for the first month and thereafter every 2 weeks until completion of the study. The wound area was measured, and complete healing was defined as the achievement of 100% wound closure with no drainage present and no dressing required.

About 48% of the 61 patients randomized to the PDGF-BB treatment group achieved complete wound healing during the study compared with only 25% of 57 patients randomized to the placebo group ($p = 0.01$). The median reduction from initial wound area for the PDGF-BB group was 99% compared with 82% reduction for the placebo group ($p = 0.09$). These results demonstrated that once-daily topical application of PDGF-BB is safe and effective in stimulating the healing of chronic, full-thickness, lower-extremity diabetic neurotrophic ulcers. This study was the basis for approval of PDGF-BB (Regranex) by the U.S. Food and Drug Administration (FDA) for treatment of diabetic foot ulcers.

Another important result that emerged from the study of PDGF-BB–treated diabetic foot ulcers was the contribution of debridement (Steed et al, 1996). A lower rate of healing was observed in centers that performed less frequent debridement. Furthermore, the improved response rate associated with more frequent debridement occurred in both the PDGF-BB–treated group and the placebo group. These data indicate that wound debridement is a vital adjunct in the care of diabetic foot wounds.

Transforming Growth Factor-Beta Family

The TGF-β family of proteins is the newest family to be discovered (Roberts and Sporn, 1996). Three distinct TGF-βs have been identified in humans: TGF-β1, TGF-β2, and TGF-β3. All three TGF-β isoforms are homodimers with covalently linked subunits of 12,500 molecular weight. They are synthesized as inactive proteins that must be activated by proteolytic removal of a segment of the proteins. The TGF-βs are synthesized by a variety of cell types, including platelets, macrophages, lymphocytes, fibroblasts, bone cells, and keratinocytes, and nearly all nucleated cells have TGF-β receptors. Thus TGF-βs are probably the most broadly acting of all the families of growth factors.

Three different TGF-β receptor proteins have been identified and are designated type I, type II, and type III receptors. Although all three TGF-β iosforms bind to all three types of TGF-β receptors, they do not appear to have the same biologic effects on target cells. This may be due to differences in the ways the TGF-β isoforms interact with the three TGF-β receptor proteins. Two of the most important actions of TGF-βs in the context of skin wound healing are their ability to stimulate chemotaxis of inflammatory cells and to stimulate synthesis of extracellular matrix. Elevated, chronic production of TGF-β has been strongly implicated in nearly all fibrotic diseases, including hepatic cirrhosis, pulmonary fibrosis, kidney glomerulonephritis, and pelvic adhesions (Border and Noble, 1994). This has stimulated research into methods to inhibit the action of TGF-β in vivo. For example, neutralizing antibodies to TGF-βs have been reported to reduce scar formation in rat skin incisions (Kurt et al, 1992; Shah, Foreman, and Ferguson, 1992, 1994). Excessive scar formation is an important area for future research.

Recently, TGF-βs were shown to induce synthesis of another important protein, CTGF (Frazier et al, 1996; Steed and Diabetic Ulcer Study Group, 1995). CTGF is a potent inducer of extracellular matrix synthesis, and much of the increase in extracellular matrix that occurs in the skin after treatment with TGF-β may be due to the action of CTGF. TGF-βs and related proteins have potent activity in formation of bone.

Therapeutic Uses. Although TGF-β has been reported to stimulate healing in a large number of animal models, it has been evaluated in only one clinical trial in patients with chronic skin ulcers (Robson et al, 1995). In a three-arm, prospective, randomized, observer-blinded, placebo-controlled study, 36 patients were randomly assigned to one of three treatment groups consisting of 12 patients each: conventional dressing only, placebo collagen vehicle group, and TGF-β group. Ulcers were located at or proximal to the malleolus and distal to the tibial tuberosity, had an ankle-brachial index (ABI) greater than 0.5, had no clinical signs of infection, and had a bacterial count less than 10^5 bacteria/g tissue. During the 6-week treatment period, the mean ulcer area expressed as a percentage of initial ulcer area decreased more rapidly for ulcers treated with TGF-β_2 than for ulcers treated with placebo or conventional dressings. Three ulcers in the TGF-β group, three in the placebo group, and two in the standard dressing group healed completely during the treatment period. Overall, these differences favored treatment with TGF-β_2 but were not statistically significant.

Fibroblast Growth Factor Family

Three proteins of the FGF family are thought to be important regulators of wound healing: acidic FGF (aFGF or FGF-1), basic FGF (bFGF or FGF-2), and keratinocyte growth factor (KGF or FGF-7) (Abraham and Klagsbrun, 1996). Over 30 synonyms have appeared in the literature to describe proteins that eventually were shown to be either aFGF or bFGF. As their names imply, aFGF and bFGF are potent mitogens for fibroblasts that share many similar biochemical and biologic properties. Both aFGF and bFGF are single-chain proteins that are proteolytically derived from precursor molecules to generate biologically active proteins of about 15,000 molecular weight. Their names reflect their different isoelectric points of pH 5.6 and 9.6. Neither aFGF nor bFGF have a conventional secretory peptide sequence at their amino-terminus that usually is necessary for secretion of proteins, and the mechanism of release for aFGF and bFGF from cells is not clear.

An important characteristic of FGFs is the ability to bind the glycosoaminoglycans heparin and its protein-bound counterpart, the proteoglycan, heparan sulfate. Immunohistochemical analysis of tissues for bFGF often reveals bFGF in association with the extracellular matrix and in basement membranes attached to heparan sulfate. The binding of bFGF to extracellular matrix constituents may serve several functions. Heparan sulfate protects bFGF from proteolytic degradation, and binding of aFGF to heparin or to heparan sulfate proteoglycans in the membranes of cells increases the affinity of FGF binding to its receptor, which results in a substantial increase in cell division. Release of matrix-degrading enzymes such as heparinase, cathepsin D, or collagenase after an injury to the skin may liberate bound FGF. These data imply that binding of FGFs by heparin-containing components of the extracellular matrix may regulate the activity of FGF by acting as a potential storage and release site and by potentiating its effects on receptors of target cells.

FGFs appear to play major roles in wound healing. FGFs stimulate proliferation of the major cell types involved in wound healing, including fibroblasts, keratinocytes, and endothelial cells. FGFs and VEGF probably are the major angiogenic factors in wound healing. Many of the cells that respond to FGF also synthesize the peptide, including fibroblasts, endothelial cells, and smooth muscle cells.

KGF has 37% sequence homology to bFGF and shares the ability to bind to heparin. KGF is a single-chain polypeptide of 28,000 molecular weight that is proteolytically derived from a larger precursor. In contrast to aFGF and bFGF, synthesis of KGF is restricted to fibroblasts, and KGF expression is rapidly upregulated in fibroblasts after an injury (Werner et al, 1992). More importantly, KGF only stimulates mitosis of keratinocytes and not fibroblasts since the receptor for KGF in not expressed by fibroblasts. This has lead to the concept that KGF is a paracrine effector of epithelial cell growth.

Four FGF receptors have been identified (FGFR1, FGFR2, FGFR3, and FGFR4), and they share about 60% sequence homology. All four of the FGF receptors can bind aFGF, but the receptors and their multiple splice variants (different mRNAs generated from a single gene) differ in their ability to bind bFGF and KGF. Expression of different FGF receptor variants by cells may provide another method to regulate the response of cells to FGFs.

Therapeutic Uses. FGF has been studied in both pressure ulcers and burns. A prospective, randomized, blinded, placebo-controlled trial was performed on 50 patients with grade 3 and 4 pressure ulcers using three different concentrations of bFGF (Robson et al, 1992b). More patients treated with bFGF achieved >70% wound closure compared with patients treated with vehicle ($p = 0.05$). Histologically, bFGF treatment produced a marked increase in fibroblasts and capillaries compared with ulcers treated with vehicle. These data demonstrated that bFGF was an effective adjuvant treatment for chronic pressure ulcers.

A synthetic bovine bFGF has also been evaluated for treatment of second-degree burns (Fu et al, 1998). Compared with placebo treatment, bFGF treatment significantly reduced the time for complete healing of superficial second-degree burns from 12.4 ± 2.7 days to 9.9 ± 2.5 days ($p = 0.0008$) and reduced healing of deep second-degree burns from 21.2 ± 4.9 days to 17.4 ± 4.6 days ($p = 0.0003$). Histologic evaluation of granulation tissue in biopsies of burns after 7 days of treatment also showed more capillaries sprouts or tubes in bFGF-treated wounds than in placebo-treated wounds. After more than 1½ years of follow-up since treatment has stopped, neoplasia at the burn site has not been observed.

Insulin-Like Growth Factor Family

IGF-I and IGF-II have substantial amino acid sequence homology to proinsulin, and both are synthesized as precursor molecules that are proteolytically cleaved to generate active monomeric proteins of about 7000 molecular weight. IGF-II is synthesized more prominently during fetal development, whereas IGF-I synthesis persists at high levels in many adult tissues, especially the liver in response to stimulation by pituitary-derived growth hormone. Many of the biologic actions originally attributed to growth hormone such as cartilage and bone growth are mediated in part by IGF-I. However, combinations of growth hormone and IGF-I are more effective than either hormone alone.

Unlike other growth factors, plasma contains substantial levels of IGF-I, which primarily reflects hepatic synthesis. Almost all the IGF-I in plasma is reversibly bound by high-affinity IGF-binding proteins. Because the IGFs are inactive while bound to their binding proteins, the dynamic balance between free and bound IGFs has a substantial influence on the effects of IGF-I in wound healing. IGF-I also is found in high levels in platelets and is released during platelet degranulation. IGF-I is a potent chemotactic agent for vascular endothelial cells, and IGF-I released from platelets or produced by fibroblasts may promote migration of vascular endothelial cells into the wound area, resulting in increased neovascularization. IGF-I also stimulates mitosis of fibroblasts and may act synergistically with PDGF to enhance epidermal and dermal regeneration.

IGF-I and IGF-II each have distinct receptor proteins. The IGF-I receptor is similar in structure to the insulin receptor, and consists of two α subunits that contain the IGF-I binding site linked by disulfide bonds to the two β subunits that contain the transmembrane and cytoplasmic regions with the tyrosine kinase domain. The IGF-I receptor binds IGF-I with high affinity, binds IGF-II with lower affinity, and binds insulin weakly. The IGF-II receptor is a monomeric protein that has no kinase activity but binds proteins that contain the sugar mannose-6-phosphate. The IGF-II receptor binds IGF-II with high affinity, binds IGF-I with low affinity, and does not bind insulin.

Therapeutic Uses. There are no published reports of clinical studies evaluating IGF-I treatment of wounds. However, IGF-I and growth hormone may act synergistically to promote wound healing. Topical growth hormone treatment of chronic leg ulcers was reported to improve healing (Rasmussen et al, 1991). In a prospective, double-blind, placebo-controlled trial, 37 patients with chronic leg ulceration were randomized to receive either topical synthetic human growth hormone or placebo in addition to a standard treatment of compression and hydrocolloid dressing. Patients receiving growth hormone treatment had a significantly faster rate of ulcer healing than the placebo group, and more patients treated with growth hormone achieved 50% reduction in initial ulcer size.

A prospective, randomized, double-blind, placebo-controlled study was conducted to test the efficacy of systemic administration of synthetic human growth hormone on healing times of split-thickness skin graft donor sites in pediatric patients with severe burns. The total body surface area (TBSA) of burns was greater than 40%, and the TBSA of full-thickness burns was greater than 20% (Gilpin et al, 1994). Donor sites in patients receiving growth hormone healed at approximately 6½ days, whereas donor sites in patients receiving placebo healed at 8½ days ($p < 0.01$). These studies suggest that topical application of growth hormone to leg ulcers or systemic dosing of growth hormone to severely burned patients may enhance healing.

Cytokines

Proliferation and differentiation of nonimmune system cells is regulated primarily by the proteins described in the five major families of growth factors. Although the term *cytokine* can be used broadly to include the classical growth factors, it frequently is used in a more restricted definition to describe molecules that primarily regulate the interactions between cells that participate in the immune response (Frenette and Wagner, 1996a, 1996b; Springer, 1990). These molecules could be further classified as lymphokines or monokines depending on their major target cells. They are produced extensively by activated T cells and macrophages, although nonimmune system cells such as keratinocytes and vascular endothelial cells also produce some cytokines. Studies have revealed that cytokines generally induce multiple biologic activities (pleiotropic) and that a single cytokine can act both as a positive signal and a negative signal, depending on the type of the target cell. Cytokines such as IL-1, IL-2, IL-3, IL-4, IL-5, IL-6, IL-10, granulocyte-monocyte colony-stimulating factor (GM-CSF), granulocyte colony-stimulating factor (G-CSF), IFN-γ and TNF-α are key mediators of immune and inflammatory responses. Two cytokines in particular, TNF-α and IL-1β, have activities that substantially influence skin wound healing through their ability to increase production of MMPs and suppress production of tissue inhibitors of metalloproteinases.

Therapeutic Uses. Cytokines have not been investigated extensively in human wound healing studies. IL-1β was evaluated in a prospective, randomized, double-blind, placebo-controlled trial performed on 26 patients with pressure ulcers of grade 3 and 4 (Robson et al, 1994). Measurements of the pressure ulcer area and volume determined with alginate mold were made at weekly intervals. No statistically significant differences were seen in the percentage decreases of wound volumes between the treatment groups over the 4-week treatment evaluation.

POTENTIAL LIMITATIONS OF GROWTH FACTOR TECHNOLOGY

From practical and theoretic standpoints, growth factor therapy has certain limitations. One major limitation is the concept of "barren soil." If a growth factor or a mixture of growth factors is applied to a wound, the cells in or adjacent to the wound must be properly prepared so they can respond. This means the cells must have adequate levels of oxygen, nutrients, and intact extracellular matrix components to be able to support cell mitosis, migration, and attachment. The underlying condition that caused the wound to become chronic must be corrected.

Because the molecular environment of chronic wounds is different from that of acute wounds (Figure 19-5), the imbalances in cytokines and proteases in chronic wounds also need to be corrected

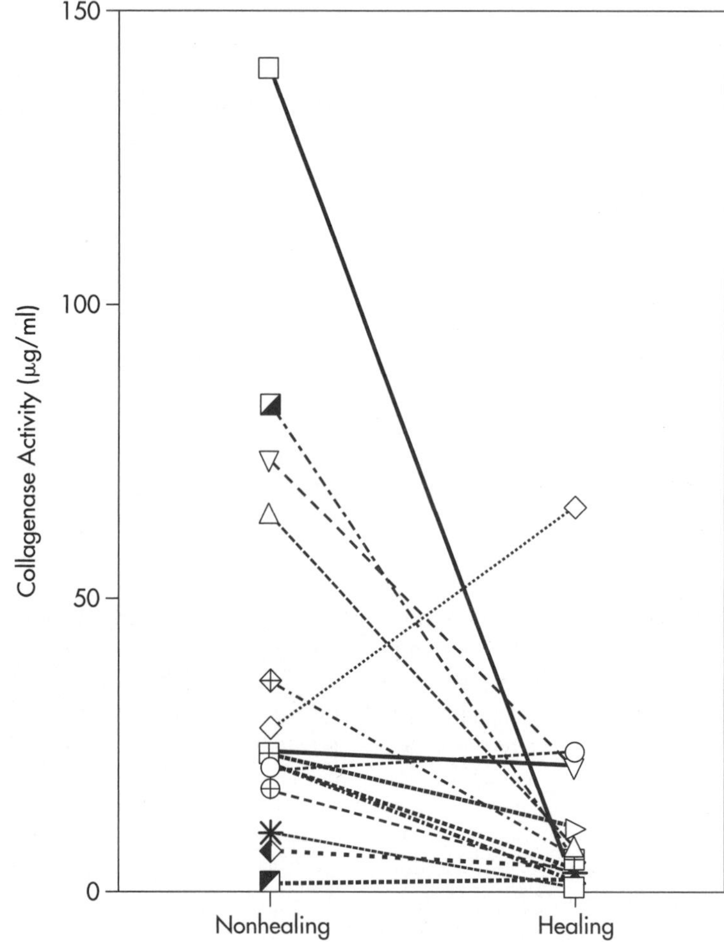

Figure 19-5 Protease levels in fluids from chronic venous ulcers before and after initiating healing. Protease activity was measured in fluids collected from chronic venous leg ulcers of 15 patients at the start of hospitalization (*nonhealing*) and 2 weeks later, after the ulcers had clinical evidence of healing (*healing*). Lines connecting the protease levels measured in the two samples from each patient (*nonhealing and healing*) indicate that protease activity tends to decrease as ulcers begin to heal. (From Schultz GS, Mast BA: Molecular analysis of the environment of healing and chronic wounds: cytokines, proteases and growth factors, *Wounds* 10:1F, 1998. Health Management Publications, Inc., Wayne, Penn.)

as much as possible before exogenous growth factors are added. Three key differences in the molecular environment of chronic wounds have been identified:

1. Chronic wound fluid does not consistently stimulate growth (mitosis) of skin fibroblasts (Alper, Tibbetts, and Sarazen, 1985; Bucalo, Eaglstein, and Falanga, 1993; Katz et al, 1991).
2. Ratios of proinflammatroy cytokines (TNF-α and IL-1β) and natural receptors are significantly increased (Harris et al, 1995; Mast and Schultz, 1996).
3. Protease activity in chronic wounds is significantly elevated (Bullen et al, 1995; Harris et al, 1995; Mast and Schultz, 1996; Nwomeh et al, 1998; Rogers et al, 1995; Tarnuzzer and Schultz, 1996; Yager et al, 1996, 1997).

Protease activity and levels may be one of the most important factors preventing chronic wounds from healing because proteases can degrade proteins that are essential for healing, such as growth factors, their receptors, and extracellular matrix proteins. Experiments have shown that growth factors added to chronic wound fluids are quickly degraded by the proteases (MMPs and serine proteases such as neutrophil elastase) present in the fluid. Fortunately, levels of protease activity decrease in chronic wounds as they begin to heal (Figure 19-6). Frequent sharp debridement may be instrumental in converting the detrimental chronic wound environment into a pseudo-acute wound molecular environment in which growth factors can function more effectively.

Another major limitation of growth factor therapy of chronic wounds may be the status of the wound cells themselves. Addition of exogenous growth factors may have little effect on cells in long-established chronic wounds if the cells are approaching senescence and unable to respond (Agren, 1998). Healing would depend on repopulation of chronic wounds with healthy cells that migrate either from areas adjacent to the chronic wound or from artificial skin substitutes, such as

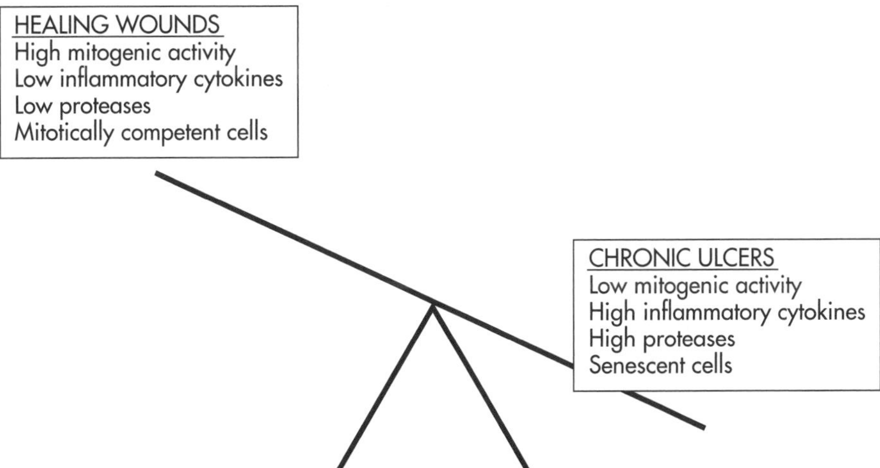

Figure 19-6 Imbalanced activities in acute and chronic wounds. Healing wounds generally have high levels of mitogenic activity, low levels of inflammatory cytokines, low levels of proteases, high levels of growth factors, and mitotically competent fibroblasts. In contrast, chronic skin wounds tend to have low levels of mitotic activity, high levels of inflammatory cytokines, high levels of proteases, low levels of growth factors, and nearly senescent fibroblasts. (From Schultz GS, Mast BA: Molecular analysis of the environment of healing and chronic wounds: cytokines, proteases and growth factors, *Wounds* 10:1F, 1998. Health Management Publications, Inc., Wayne, Penn.)

Dermagraft-TC (Advanced Tissue Sciences, Inc.) and Apligraf (Organogenesis, Inc. and Novartis Pharmaceuticals Corp.), applied to the chronic wound.

A third consideration relates to the cost-effectiveness of growth factor therapy. For this high-priced technology to find broad application, it must ultimately be shown to have a significant positive effect (e.g., decreased duration of confinement, reduced cost of supplemental therapies, reduced amputations rate). The promise of growth factor therapy remains enormous but will require additional clinical investigations that are carefully conducted and properly designed.

SUMMARY

The clinical management of skin wounds is entering a new phase because of the increased understanding of the roles that growth factors, adhesion molecules, extracellular matrix molecules, cytokines, and proteases play in healing of acute wounds and how these key molecules are altered in chronic wounds. New products, including recombinant growth factors (PDGF) and biologically active engineered artificial skin substitutes, are a direct result of this increased understanding of the molecular regulation of wound healing. However, these new products only function optimally when properly applied to wounds that are able to respond to them. Thus the wound care nurse must stay abreast of new discoveries in these areas of basic wound research to be able to effectively integrate these new advances into clinical practice.

SELF-ASSESSMENT EXERCISE

1. Name three types of adhesion molecules or adhesion receptors that participate in inflammation.
2. True or false: Growth factors are proteases
3. All of the following growth factors have shown significant benefit in healing acute or chronic wounds in clinical trials EXCEPT?
   a. Fibroblast growth factor
   b. Epidermal growth factor
   c. Transforming growth factor-beta
   d. Insulin-like growth factor

REFERENCES

Abraham J, Klagsbrun M: Modulation of wound repair by members of the fibroblast growth factor family. In Clark RAF, editor: *The molecular and cellular biology of wound repair*, New York, 1996, Plenum Press.

Agren M: Fibroblast growth in acute and chronic wounds, *European Tissue Repair Society Annual Meeting Abstract*, abstract #33, 1998.

Alper JC, Tibbetts LL, Sarazen AAJ: The in vitro response of fibroblasts to the fluid that accumulates under a vapor-permeable membrane, *J Invest Derm* 84:513, 1985.

Arai K et al: Cytokines: coordinators of immune and inflammatory responses, *Annu Rev Biochem* 59:783, 1990.

Bennett NT, Schultz GS: Growth factors and wound healing: biochemical properties of growth factors and their receptors, *Am J Surg* 165:728, 1993a.

Bennett NT, Schultz GS: Growth factors and wound healing. Part II. Role in normal and chronic wound healing, *Am J Surg* 166:74, 1993b.

Border WA, Noble NA: Transforming growth factor-β in tissue fibrosis, *N Engl J Med* 10:1286, 1994.

Bradham DM et al: Connective tissue growth factor: a cysteine-rich mitogen secreted by human vascular endothelial cells is related to the SRC-induced immediate early gene product CEF-10, *J Cell Biol* 114(6):1285, 1991.

Brown GB et al: Enhancement of epidermal regeneration by biosynthetic epidermal growth factor, *J Exp Med* 163:1319, 1986.

Brown GL et al: Enhancement of wound healing by topical treatment with epidermal growth factor, *N Eng J Med* 321:76, 1989.

Bucalo B, Eaglstein WH, Falanga V: Inhibition of cell proliferation by chronic wound fluid, *Wound Rep Reg* 1:181, 1993.

Bullen EC et al: Tissue inhibitor of metalloproteinases-1 is decreased and activated gelatinases are increased in chronic wounds, *J Invest Dermatol* 104:236, 1995.

Carpenter G, Cohen S: Epidermal growth factor, *J Biol Chem* 265:7709, 1990.

David LS et al: Randomized prospective double-blind trial in healing chronic diabetic foot ulcers, *Diabetes Care* 11:1598, 1992.

Falanga V et al: Topical use of human recombinant epidermal growth factor (h-EGF) in venous ulcers, *Phlebology* 18:604, 1992.

Fantl WJ, Johnson DE, Williams LT: Signaling by receptor tyrosine kinases, *Annu Rev Biochem* 62:453, 1993.

Frazier K et al: Stimulation of fibroblast cell growth, matrix production, and granulation tissue formation by connective tissue growth factor, *J Invest Dermatol* 107:404, 1996.

Frenette PS, Wagner DD: Adhesion molecules, blood vessels and blood cells, *N Engl J Med* 335:43, 1996a.

Frenette PS, Wagner DD: Molecular medicine, adhesion molecules, *N Engl J Med* 334:1526, 1996b.

Fu X et al: Randomised placebo-controlled trial of use of topical recombinant bovine basic fibroblast growth factor for second-degree burns, *Lancet* 352:1661, 1998.

Gilpin DA et al: Recombinant human growth hormone accelerates wound healing in children with large cutaneous burns, *Ann Surg* 220:19, 1994.

Harris IR et al: Cytokine and protease levels in healing and non-healing chronic venous leg ulcers, *Exp Dermatol* 4:342, 1995.

Heldin C, Westermark B: Role of platelet derived growth factor in vivo. In Clark RAF, editor: *The molecular and cellular biology of wound repair*, New York, 1996, Plenum Press.

Holloway GA et al: A randomized, controlled, multicenter, dose response trial of activated platelet supernatant, topical CT-102 in chronic, nonhealing, diabetic wounds, *Wounds* 5:198, 1993.

Katz MH et al: Human wound fluid from acute wounds stimulates fibroblast and endothelial cell growth, *J Am Acad Dermatol* 25:1054, 1991.

Kurt S et al: Transforming growth factor-β acts as an autocrine growth factor in ovarian carcinoma cell lines, *Cancer Res* 52:341, 1992.

Massague J: Transforming growth factor-α, *J Biol Chem* 265:21393, 1990.

Mast BA, Schultz GS: Interactions of cytokines, growth factors, and proteases in acute and chronic wounds, *Wound Rep Regen* 4:411, 1996.

Nanney LB, King LE: Epidermal growth factor and transforming growth factor-α. In Clark RAF, editor: *The molecular and cellular biology of wound repair*, New York, 1996, Plenum Press.

Nwomeh BC et al: Dynamics of the matrix metalloproteinases MMP-1 and MMP-8 in acute open human dermal wounds, *Wound Rep Regen* 6:127, 1998.

Rasmussen LH et al: Topical human growth hormone treatment of chronic leg ulcers, *Phlebology* 6:23, 1991.

Roberts AB, Sporn MB: Transforming growth factor-β. In Clark RAF, editor: *The molecular and cellular biology of wound repair*, New York, 1996, Plenum Press.

Robson MC et al: Recombinant human platelet-derived growth factor-BB for the treatment of chronic pressure ulcers, *Ann Plast Surg* 29:193, 1992a.

Robson MC et al: Safety and effect of topical recombinant human interleukin-1β in the management of pressure sores, *Wound Rep Regen* 2:177, 1994.

Robson MC et al: Safety and effect of transforming growth factor-B2 for treatment of venous stasis ulcers, *Wound Rep Regen* 3:157, 1995.

Robson MC et al: The safety and effect of topically applied recombinant basic fibroblast growth factor on the healing of chronic pressure sores, *Ann Surg* 216:401, 1992b.

Rogers AA et al: Involvement of proteolytic enzymes—plasminogen activators and matrix metalloproteinases—in the pathophysiology of pressure ulcers, *Wound Rep Regen* 3:273, 1995.

Shah M, Foreman DM, Ferguson MWJ: Control of scarring in adult wounds by neutralising antibody to transforming growth factor beta, *Lancet* 339:213, 1992.

Shah M, Foreman DM, Ferguson MWJ: Neutralising antibody to TGF-β1,2 reduces cutaneous scarring in adult rodents, *J Cell Sci* 107:1137, 1994.

Shigeki H et al: Structure of heparin-binding EGF-like growth factor, *J Biol Chem* 267:6205, 1992.

Springer TA: Adhesion receptors of the immune system, *Nature* 346:425, 1990.

Steed DL, Diabetic Ulcer Study Group: Clinical evaluation of recombinant human platelet-derived growth factor for the treatment of lower extremity diabetic ulcers, *J Vasc Surg* 21:71, 1995.

Steed DL et al: Effect of extensive debridement and treatment on the healing of diabetic foot ulcers, *J Am Coll Surg* 183:61, 1996.

Tarnuzzer RW, Schultz GS: Biochemical analysis of acute and chronic wound environments, *Wound Rep Regen* 4:321, 1996.

Werner S et al: Large induction of keratinocyte growth factor expression in the dermis during wound healing, *Proc Natl Acad Sci* 89:6896, 1992.

Yager DR et al: Ability of chronic wound fluids to degrade peptide growth factors is associated with increased levels of elastase activity and diminished levels of proteinase inhibitors, *Wound Rep Regen* 5:23, 1997.

Yager DR et al: Wound fluids from human pressure ulcers contain elevated matrix metalloproteinase levels and activity compared to surgical wound fluid, *J Invest Dermatol* 107:743, 1996.

CHAPTER

20

Adjuvant Wound Therapies

CRAIG L. BROUSSARD, SUSAN MENDEZ-EASTMAN, & RITA FRANTZ

OBJECTIVES

1. Define *hyperbaric oxygenation.*
2. Describe the steps necessary to prepare a patient for hyperbaric treatment.
3. List at least five indications and three contraindications for hyperbaric oxygenation as identified by the Undersea and Hyperbaric Medical Society (UHMS).
4. Explain how to reduce the risk of developing three complications associated with hyperbaric oxygen treatment.
5. Describe the biologic basis for and effects of hyperbaric oxygenation and electrical stimulation.
6. Describe the waveforms that characterize low-voltage continuous direct current (LVCDC), high-voltage pulsed current (HVPC), and low-voltage pulsed current (LVPC).
7. Define *galvanotaxic effects.*
8. For each type of current (LVCDC, HVPC, LVPC), describe the most common placement for the cathode and anode.
9. Describe a typical protocol for applying HVPC or LVPC, including parameters such as amps, pulse duration, interpulse interval, frequency of treatment, and duration of treatment.
10. Describe the scientific basis of negative pressure wound therapy.
11. Define the indications and contraindications for negative pressure wound therapy.
12. Discuss nursing interventions related to negative pressure wound therapy.

Adjuvant wound therapies are treatment modalities that are applied in conjunction with conventional topical wound management. This chapter discusses hyperbaric oxygenation, negative pressure wound therapy, and electrical stimulation. These adjuvant treatments are most commonly used when the wound response has been marginal to conventional therapies. Although it is unusual to use these techniques in isolation for acute or chronic wounds, there are situations when hyperbaric oxygenation is considered the primary intervention (e.g., necrotizing soft tissue infections, compromised skin grafts and/or flaps, and clostridial myonecrosis).

The use of these adjuvant therapies varies geographically and by professional preparation. For example, electrical stimulation is more familiar to, and therefore more commonly employed by, physical therapists. Hyperbaric oxygenation is most often available in large academic or government medical centers and is coordinated by physicians.

The level of evidence in terms of efficacy and effectiveness for most adjuvant therapies is limited. Furthermore, the few clinical studies that exist have numerous design inadequacies. For example, treatment allocation may not be randomized, the standard treatment or control arm is incomplete or poorly controlled, outcome measures are inconsistent or obtained in a potentially biased fashion, and sample size is commonly too small to detect a difference. There are many clinical trials in the literature involving electrical stimulation; however, designs vary greatly with inconsistent outcome measures, making it difficult to draw any clear conclusions.

Despite these limitations, the wound care nurse must be cognizant of these techniques so that he or she understands the biologic basis and plausibility for the modality. The nurse should also be aware of the indications, contraindications, and side effects of these treatments. Although the wound care nurse may or may not actually perform the adjuvant therapy, he or she should understand the method used to apply these interventions.

HYPERBARIC OXYGENATION

Hyperbaric oxygenation is the systemic, intermittent administration of oxygen delivered under pressure. A hyperbaric environment exists when atmospheric pressure is greater than 1 atmosphere absolute (ATA) (Hammarlund, 1995). A medically significant hyperbaric exposure is occurs when atmospheric pressure is increased to greater than 1.4 ATA or 10.2 pounds per square inch gauge pressure (psig) (UHMS, 1996). The typical hyperbaric oxygen treatment takes place at a pressure of 2.0 to 2.4 ATA or 14.7 to 17.6 psig. For hyperbaric oxygenation to occur, the patient must breathe 100% oxygen while physically exposed to the hyperbaric environment (Shilling and Faiman, 1984). Topical application of oxygen is *not* hyperbaric oxygenation and has shown no significant benefit to wound healing. Oxygen under pressure functions as a pharmacologic agent in that it has a therapeutic dose, a toxic dose, side effects, contraindications, interactions with other drugs, and incompatibilities with other drugs (Heimbach, 1998).

The effects of hyperbaric oxygen are twofold:

1. *Mechanical effect.* The mechanical effect follows the physical law described by Boyle, which states that as barometric pressure increases, volume decreases. Therefore in the case of decompression sickness or air/gas embolism, hyperbaric treatment can be used to decrease the size of the embolism.
2. *Increased oxygenation of tissue.* This physiologic effect follows the physical law described by Henry Law, which states that the amount of gas dissolved in a liquid is directly proportional to the partial pressure of the dissolved gas (Hammarlund, 1995; Sheffield, 1998b). The result is that oxygen tensions can be raised 10 to 13 times higher that breathing oxygen at ambient pressure (Hammarlund, 1995).

Hyperbaric Treatment in History

Much of what is know about the physical effects of hyperbaric treatment came from observations and studies of caisson workers and divers. The first description of a pressurization vessel dates to 1662 when Henshaw used bellows to increase and decrease pressures to treat respiratory problems. The nineteenth century saw the advent of caisson workers for bridge construction and the subsequent description of caisson's disease (or decompression sickness), bubble theory, and oxygen toxicity by Paul Bert in 1878. Eleven years later, Moir used recompression to treat decompression sickness in caisson workers building the Hudson River tunnel. The twentieth century also brought about extensive research and application of hyperbaric therapy for decompression sickness by the military.

Modern use of hyperbaric oxygenation began in 1955 to potentiate the effects of radiation on cancer patients (Kindwall, 1995a; Sheffield, 1998a). The National Academy of Science—National Research Council appointed a committee to review the physiologic basis for hyperbaric oxygenation in 1962 (UHMS, 1996). In 1966, this group published *Fundamentals of Hyperbaric Medicine*, which describes the physical and physiologic effects of hyperbaric oxygen; however, it does not address clinical conditions that were currently being given hyperbaric treatment (UHMS, 1996). The Undersea Medical Society (UMS) was founded in 1967 and was primarily devoted to diving and undersea medicine. The UMS became the Undersea Hyperbaric Medical Society (UHMS) in 1986. The UHMS is the primary, worldwide source of information on hyperbaric and diving medicine. The purpose of the UHMS is to ". . . improve the scientific basis of hyperbaric oxygen therapy, [and] promote sound treatment protocols and standards of practice . . ." (UHMS, 1999).

Indications for Hyperbaric Oxygenation

The UHMS is the primary source of investigative information related to hyperbaric medicine and diving medicine worldwide. The UHMS sets forth treatment protocols and practice standards. The UHMS, as the global source of hyperbaric information, has designated the conditions or disease

BOX 20-1 Indications for Hyperbaric Therapy

Air/gas embolism
Decompression sickness
Carbon monoxide poisoning
Crush injury, compartment syndrome, acute traumatic ischemia
Exceptional blood loss
Clostridial myonecrosis
Necrotizing soft tissue infections
Chronic refractory osteomyelitis
Thermal burns
Radiation tissue damage
Compromised skin grafts and/or flaps
Select problem wounds
Intracranial abscess adjunctive treatment

processes listed in Box 20-1 as an indication for hyperbaric therapy (Abramovich et al, 1997; Cianci and Sato, 1994; Elliot, 1995; Goad et al, 1984; Hirn, 1993; Hsu and Wang, 1996; Kindwall, 1995c, 1999; Lee et al, 1989; Ludwig, 1989; Mader, Ortiz, and Calhoun, 1996; Marx, 1995; Siriwanij, Vattanavongs, and Sitprija, 1997; Stegmen, 1998; Stephens, 1996; Tai et al, 1992; UHMS, 1999; Zonis et al, 1995). Hyperbaric oxygenation is the primary therapy for arterial gas embolism, carbon monoxide poisoning, and decompression sickness. When used for any other indication, hyperbaric therapy must be integrated with the appropriate clinical and surgical treatments.

Hyperbaric oxygenation has been and is being used for other disease processes and conditions (Box 20-2). Although the UHMS does not currently recognize the use of hyperbaric treatment in these instances, research continues and is providing support (Carl et al, 1998; Gottlieb and Neubauer, 1988; Hughes, Schwarer, and Miller, 1998; Kindwall, 1999; Laden, 1998; Neubauer, 1998; Nighoghossian and Trouillas, 1997; Pascual, 1995; Reillo and Altieri, 1996; Sparacia, Sparacia, and Sansone, 1999; Wallace et al, 1995).

Hyperbaric Oxygen and Wound Healing

Disease states, such as diabetes, peripheral vascular disease, compromised skin flaps or grafts; irradiation, and crush injury, contribute to the development of chronic, problematic wounds. It is well documented in the literature that a relative state of hypoxia is needed for wound healing to occur; however, oxygen is essential for wound healing. The role of oxygen is multifaceted in wound healing. Oxygen is required for energy metabolism, collagen synthesis, neovascularization, polymorphonuclear cell function, and antibacterial activity. Cellular function and integrity cannot be maintained, nor can cellular repair occur, without oxygen.

BOX 20-2 Situations for Hyperbaric Therapy Under Investigation

Acute myocardial infarction
Acute cerebral vascular accident
Closed head injury
Spinal cord injury
Sickle cell crisis
Rheumatic diseases
Migraine/cluster headache
Multiple sclerosis
Radiation cystitis/proctitis
HIV/AIDS
Cerebral palsy

Hyperbaric oxygenation increases the capacity of blood to carry and deliver oxygen to tissues. This hyperoxygenation occurs because oxygen is administered under pressure to the patient. Consequently hyperbaric treatment significantly enhances oxygen delivery to compromised tissues, increase oxygenation to the tissues, and may restore perfusion to compromised areas. The increased capacity of blood to carry oxygen assists in the restoration of cellular function. The volumetric levels of diffusion achieved with hyperbaric oxygenation are 2 to 3 times those obtained under normobaric conditions. Increased oxygen at the wound site thus promotes neovascularization and healing. The effect of hyperbaric oxygenation is instantaneous in blood with a subsequent plateau in soft tissues approximately 1 hour after exposure. The effect of hyperbaric oxygen declines steadily over 2 to 4 hours after exposure.

Another effect of hyperbaric oxygenation is vasoconstriction. Oxygen is a powerful vasoconstrictor and can be helpful in managing edema related to traumatic wounding or crush injuries. Although hyperbaric oxygen may seem injurious by decreasing blood supply to an injured area, the increase in diffusion of oxygen overcomes the decrease in circulation associated with vasoconstriction (Hammarlund, 1995; Sheffield, 1998b; Shilling and Faiman, 1984; Swanson, 1998).

Patient Selection

Rigorous assessment of the patient must be completed to rule out contraindications to hyperbaric therapy. According to Boyle's law, any air-filled cavity must be assessed. Ears and sinus cavities must be assessed for the patient's ability to equalize pressure. A chest x-ray examination will rule out trapping of air in the lungs. Patients with a history of seizure activity should be assessed for seizure control. Hyperbaric treatment is absolutely contraindicated for patients who have a history of receiving bleomycin because this increases the risk for oxygen toxicity. Hyperbaric treatment is also contraindicated for patients receiving Cis-Platinum, Sulfamylon, and disulfiram. Another absolute contraindication is untreated pneumothorax. Relative contraindications to hyperbaric treatment include pregnancy, known malignancy, emphysema, pneumonia, bronchitis, and hyperthermia (Heimbach, 1998; Foster, 1992).

Treatment Protocol

Hyperbaric treatment protocols depend upon the specific disease process. Acceptable protocols for hyperbaric exposure have been outlined by the UHMS. This does not, however, preclude physician preference and individualization to meet the patients needs. Typically, a patient will receive a daily hyperbaric exposure five to seven times per week. The treatment will last for 90 minutes at 2.0 to 2.4 ATA. The patient generally receives 40 to 60 treatments. Continuous assessment of the patient's progress assists the physician in determining when the maximum benefit from hyperbaric oxygen therapy has been reached (UHMS, 1996).

Patient Preparation and Safety. Two factors dictate that rigorous procedures be followed for patient preparation and patient safety. The first factor is the nature of hyperbarics (e.g., atmospheric pressure changes). Patient instruction should include air equalization techniques to prevent aural or sinus barotrauma. The patient should also be instructed not to hold his or her breath during ascent to prevent pneumothorax. The caregiver responsible for assessing the patient before treatment should assess breath sounds to prevent exposing a patient with compromised pulmonary status to the hyperbaric environment. A random blood sugar measurement before the treatment should be obtained on all patients with diabetes because hyperbaric oxygenation can significantly lower blood sugar levels. Vital signs are obtained to assess for hypertension and hyperthermia. Hyperbaric oxygenation is a potent vasoconstrictor and can predispose the patient to a hypertensive crisis. An oral temperature of greater that 102° F predisposes the patient to an oxygen toxicity seizure.

The second factor affecting patient preparation and safety is the pressurized high oxygen environment. This is significant in any hyperbaric environment and is of extreme importance when the patient is pressurized in a 100% oxygen environment. Patients should be instructed not to use products that have a petroleum or alcohol base before going into the chamber. Cosmetic products such as hair spray, hair creams, lotions, Vaseline, deodorants, and perfumes must be removed before the treatment. Only cotton linens and clothing are allowed into the chamber to decrease spark potential. Prosthetics should be removed, including hearing aides. Glasses, contacts lenses, and dentures are not absolutely contraindicated in the hyperbaric environment but should be removed if the patient is at risk for seizure activity or if the patient has an altered mental condition (Hart, 1995; Kindwall, 1995b, 1995e; UHMS, 1994; Weaver and Straas, 1991).

Hyperbaric Procedure. To achieve a hyperbaric state, the patient is placed into either a monoplace chamber or a multiplace chamber. The monoplace chamber has rapidly become the predominant chamber seen in outpatient settings. A monoplace chamber is typically compressed with oxygen. These chambers have a maximum pressurization of 44 psi, or 3 ATA. The major advantages of using a monoplace chamber are that they are relatively inexpensive. The chamber may be placed anywhere that an adequate gas supply is available and can be housed in most areas without significant construction costs. Another advantage is that the monoplace chamber may be staffed with either a technician or nurse and a physician. Current reimbursement guidelines dictate that a physician must be present for the duration of a hyperbaric treatment. Disadvantages of the monoplace chamber include lack of direct patient contact and difficulty monitoring the patient other than visually. Methods are available to monitor electrocardiogram (ECG), arterial blood pressure, pulmonary artery pressure, wedge pressure, central venous pressure, cuff blood pressure, temperature, and transcutaneous oxygen monitoring ($TcPO_2$). It is also possible to ventilate a patient in the monoplace chamber (Hart, 1995; Weaver and Straas, 1991).

The multiplace chamber allows a caregiver to enter the chamber with the patient. The caregiver, or tender, may be a technician, nurse, or physician. The multiplace chamber can accommodate multiple patients. The number of patient's that can be treated simultaneously depends on the size of the chamber and whether the patient is ambulatory or chair- or bed-bound. The multiplace chamber can easily be equipped to handle the critically ill. The critically ill patient can be monitored the same as in the monoplace chamber. To breathe oxygen, the patient wears either a mask or a hood. The major disadvantages of the multiplace chamber include cost and housing of the chamber. The National Fire Protection Association (NFPA, 1993) sets forth structural requirements for a multiplace chamber. Another disadvantage of the multiplace chamber is that if a patient is unable to equalize pressure during pressurization, a multioccupant dive must be aborted. A final consideration of the multiplace chamber is staffing. The multiplace chamber requires a greater expenditure of staff than the monoplace chamber. The multiplace chamber is staffed with a chamber operator, tender, nurse, and physician (Kindwall, 1995e; NFPA, 1993; UHMS, 1994).

Side Effects

The most common side effect or complication of hyperbaric oxygenation is claustrophobia. Patients who experience claustrophobia should be reassured, and a tender should be present and in contact with the patient at all times. In the multiplace chamber the tender can offer direct physical comfort. In the monoplace chamber, the tender should maintain both visual and verbal contact with the patient. Benzodiazapenes offer relief of claustrophobia in most cases. Occasionally, a treatment is aborted and subsequent hyperbaric therapy is discontinued as a result of claustrophobia (Kindwall, 1995d).

Aural barotrauma, referred to as an "ear squeeze," will present as ear pain and may result in a hematoma to the tympanic membrane, hemorrhage in the middle ear, or tympanic rupture. If a patient experiences an ear squeeze, a myringotomy or placement of pressure equalization (PE) tubes may be necessary. Sinus barotrauma, or sinus squeeze, results in extreme sinus pain and may lead to hemorrhage of the sinus. The patient who presents for a hyperbaric treatment with a congested nasal passage may benefit from nasal decongestant sprays before the treatment. Oral decongestants may be indicated for a more long-term approach (Capes and Tomaszewski, 1996; Kidder, 1995; Vrabec, Clements, and Mader, 1998).

Visual acuity changes are not rare during hyperbaric therapy. Myopia may worsen after twenty or more hyperbaric exposures. Frequently, a patient who uses glasses to correct presbyopia will find that he or she is able to read without corrective lenses. The exact mechanism behind these visual changes is not known. The patient who experiences a visual change should be instructed not to change prescription eye wear for 2 to 3 months after hyperbaric treatment because the visual change is usually temporary (Maki, 1996).

A physiologic anomaly, breath holding, or cessation of respiration can cause air to be trapped in the lungs. This trapped air can lead to a tension pneumothorax. Should this occur in a multiplace chamber, the patient can be recompressed and the pneumothorax can be corrected within the chamber before decompression of the chamber. In a monoplace environment, the patient should be recompressed to treatment depth until supplies, equipment, and personnel are available. Once the team and supplies are assembled, the patient should be decompressed and treated immediately upon removal from the chamber.

Seizure activity from oxygen toxicity, although ominous in appearance, is self-limiting and benign. The patient in the monoplace environment should be maintained at pressure until seizure activity has stopped. If the patient is breathing oxygen by mask or hood, the oxygen should be stopped and the patient placed in air. Once the seizure has stopped, the patient can be removed from the chamber. Generally, no further precautions or anticonvulsant medications are necessary for subsequent treatments. Patients with a known history of seizure or who are predisposed to seizure activity would benefit from periodic, scheduled discontinuation of oxygen breathing (air breaks) during the treatment (Clark, 1995).

Summary

Hyperbaric oxygenation should be considered an adjunct to wound treatment practices. Not all wounds benefit from hyperbaric treatment, nor are all wounds a candidate. Under no circumstance should patients be treated with hyperbaric oxygenation "just to see if it works." Patient selection should focus on the hypoxic nature of wounds. Wound hypoxia should be demonstrated with $TcPO_2$. The origin of the wound must be considered. A pressure ulcer is best treated with pressure reduction, and a hypoxic wound is best treated by maximization of oxygen to the wound.

Frequently, caregivers question the efficacy of hyperbaric oxygenation for wounds. Many wound care providers complain that hyperbaric treatment does not work and is extremely expensive. A response to these statements would be that hyperbaric oxygenation is often the "last ditch effort" for problem wounds. These wounds may have responded extremely well had hyperbaric treatment been instituted earlier. Although it is understood that not all wounds heal, consideration for hyperbaric treatment should be given for those patients with lower-extremity wounds when it is known that these wounds may not heal. Hyperbaric treatment could mean the difference between a below- or above-the-knee amputation with appropriate circulatory assessment and preamputation preparation with hyperbaric oxygenation.

Just as wound care is not a subspecialty of hyperbaric oxygenation, neither is hyperbaric oxygenation a subspecialty of wound care. Hyperbaric treatment is indicated for conditions that are not wound related (e.g., carbon monoxide poisoning, osteomyelitis, decompression sickness). Nurses may obtain national certification in hyperbaric nursing through the Baromedical Nurses Association (BNA), an association that promotes the status and standards of baromedical nursing practice.

NEGATIVE PRESSURE WOUND THERAPY

Introduction

Negative pressure wound therapy (NPWT) is a mechanical wound care treatment that uses controlled negative pressure to assist and accelerate wound healing. Also known as *vacuum-assisted closure* (VAC®) (KCI, San Antonio, Texas), NPWT is used to provide evacuation of wound fluid, stimulation of granulation tissue formation, and reduction of bacterial colonization counts. This therapy is achieved by placing an open-cell foam sponge into the wound bed, sealing it with an adhesive drape, and applying subatmospheric pressure via an evacuation tube by a computerized pump. The pump is adjustable and can be programmed to deliver the appropriate amount of negative pressure based on the individual characteristics of the wound.

NPWT is thought to benefit wound healing by assisting the body's capacity to heal itself (Figure 20-1). Increased local, functional blood perfusion, increased nutrient delivery to wounded tissue, acceleration of the rate of granulation tissue formation, and decreased wound bacterial counts are among the benefits of NPWT (Argenta, Morykwas, and Rouchard, 1993). Mullner and colleagues (1997) noted granulation tissue formation over previously exposed bone or implants in 14 soft tissue defects with the use of negative pressure. Studies have reported reduced recovery time for patients with chronic problem wounds and earlier grafting of wounds (Morykwas et al, 1997; Mullner et al, 1997).

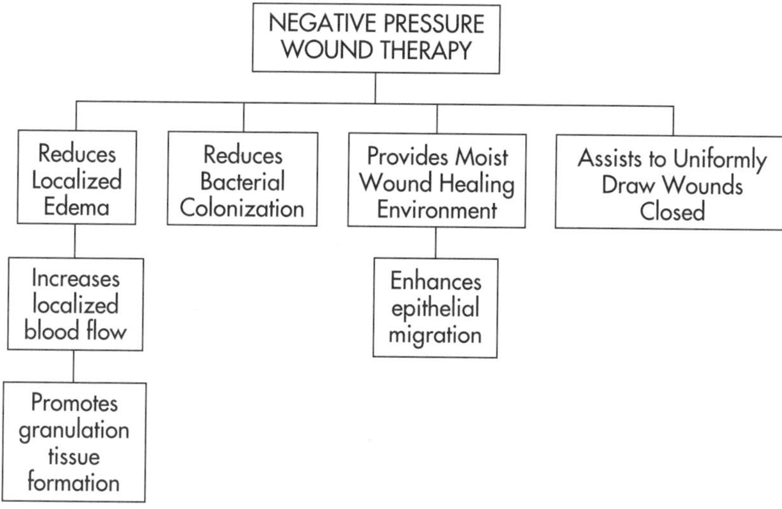

Figure 20-1 Science behind negative pressure wound therapy.

Wounds refractory to more traditional topical therapy have demon-strated a healing response to NPWT (Hartnett, 1998) (Figure 20-2).

Physiologic Basis

The cellular and molecular processes that occur in delayed wound healing often include the trapping of third-space fluid around the wound bed. Localized edema can compress the circulatory supply surrounding a wound. Application of NPWT assists in the reduction and evacuation of third-space fluids and edema via negative pressure. Morykwas and colleagues (1997), the initial founders of negative pressure wound therapy, found that the use of intermittent negative pressure at 125 mm Hg provided a peak blood flow four times that of non–NPWT-treated wounds. Observations from this research also indicate that intermittent negative pressure results in a repetitive release of biochemical messengers that assists in the wound healing process. Increased blood flow stimulated by NPWT provides the wound with a more nutrient-rich environment in which to heal. Increased blood supply around a wound also assists with the formation of granulation tissue, which is an essential ingredient for wound healing.

Granulation tissue relies on the development of new capillary growth to develop a collagen matrix. Capillaries are a major component of the support structure that intermingles with delicate collagen fibers to develop healthy granulation tissue. The mechanical stretch experienced by cells in the environment of negative pressure undergoes an increased rate of cellular proliferation (Ryan and Barnhill, 1983). This stretch also encourages neo-angiogenisis, uniform wound size reduction, and eventually epithelialization.

Wound fluid is an excellent medium for bacterial growth. By removing stagnant wound fluid, the amount of bacterial colonization within a wound is decreased. This, along with increased circulation that results in higher nutrient and oxygen levels available to the wound, enhances resistance to infection. This process is beneficial to the process of wound healing because infection delays any phase of the wound-healing trajectory. A transparent dressing secures the NPWT to the wound and protects the wound from possible environmental bacterial assaults. Bacterial counts obtained from wound fluid in wounds with and without NPWT suggest a significant reduction in bacterial colonization in those receiving NPWT (Argenta, Morykwas, and Rouchard, 1993).

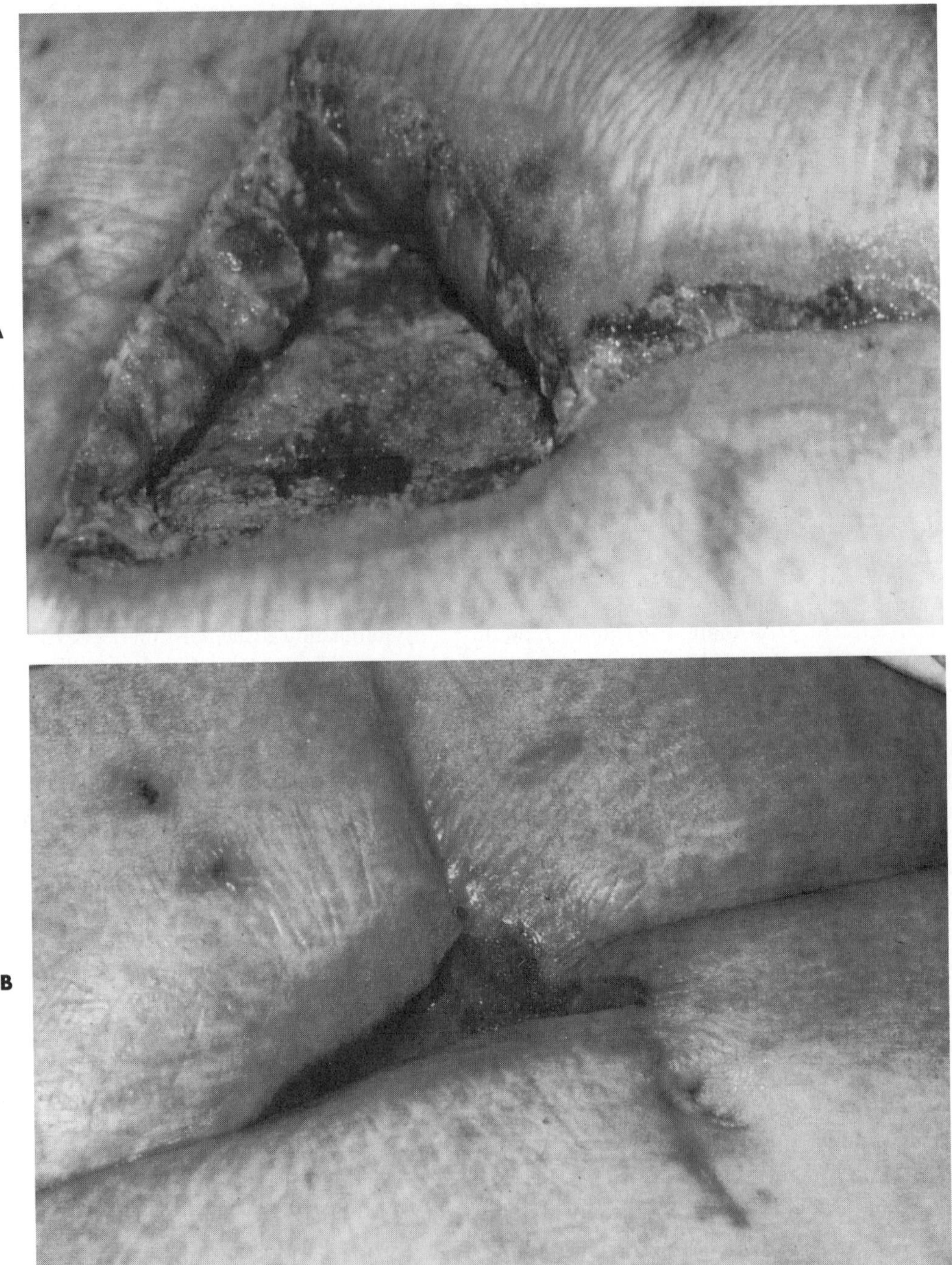

Figure 20-2 A, Dehisced abdominal wound after 1 week of NPWT. Note the clean, moist, well-granulated wound bed. **B,** Same wound after 14 days of NPWT. Note the reduction in size and depth and the continued clean moist wound bed.

The design of NPWT provides an occlusive, moist wound-bed environment. The continual influx of third-space fluid encourages a moist, clean wound, which is important for granulation tissue formation, epithelialization, and sustained viability of growth factors and cytokines.

Indications and Contraindications

NPWT evolved from a desire to develop a treatment for chronic, debilitating wounds. As successful treatment of chronic, unsalvageable wounds with NPWT mounted, the treatment expanded to use with subacute and acute wounds. Chronic wounds, such as stage 3 and 4 pressure ulcers, vascular wounds, and neuropathic ulcers, have all proven to be appropriate for NPWT. Dehisced incisions, split-thickness mesh skin grafts, and muscle flaps also benefit from the properties provided by negative pressure. Because the NPWT uses the body's own healing qualities to assist and accelerate wound healing; a patient must have an overall physiologic capacity to heal in order to be an appropriate candidate. Contraindications for NPWT include nonviable tissue within the wound bed, untreated osteomyelitis, and malignancy in the wound margins.

Before the application of NPWT, a wound must be free of all necrotic or dead tissue. Granulation tissue is difficult to form in the presence of necrotic tissue, and therefore all nonviable tissue must be removed before initiation of NPWT. The type of debridement used to clear the wound should be based on a thorough assessment of the patient and the wound and must result in a clean wound bed free of any nonviable tissue.

A wound complicated with osteomyelitis must be treated with antibiotics and/or debridement of infected bone for appropriate use of NPWT as an adjunct treatment. Negative pressure alone cannot treat an infection of the bone and is not appropriate for untreated osteomyelitis. Response of tissue to mechanical forces is characterized by increased proliferation of cells. These forces are not discriminatory and therefore will stimulate rapid reproduction of normal and malignant cells in an environment of negative pressure and the resulting mechanical stretch. Therefore wounds with malignancy in or surrounding a wound are considered inappropriate for NPWT.

Any treatment must be evaluated for appropriateness via a thorough assessment of the patient and that patient's wound. Precautions include unstable hemostasis. Active bleeding or use of anticoagulants does not deem a patient inappropriate for negative pressure wound therapy, but continued frequent assessment must be maintained and considered throughout the therapy. When vital organs are exposed, precautions such as the placement of mesh products over the organs should be deliberated. The VAC has been successfully placed directly over the heart, lung, liver, and spleen (Morykwas et al, 1997).

Wound Management

Once a patient has been deemed appropriate for NPWT and the device is applied, dressing changes are performed every 48 hours for most wounds. The reticulated polyurethane dressing is made of open cell foam to ensure equal distribution of the applied nega-tive pressure force to every surface of the wound communicating with the foam. The foam is trimmed to fit the entire surface of the wound. Once the foam is placed, evacuation tubing is laid on top of the foam. This tubing has slits cut into the proximal end, which will evacuate the wound fluid into a collection chamber located on the computerized vacuum pump. The pump is approximately 14 inches long, 12 inches high, and 8 inches wide and weighs approximately 9 pounds (Figure 20-3). This unit can be powered by either an AC outlet or a battery. A smaller, portable unit that is about 4 inches by 2 inches and weighs approximately 2 pounds is also available and can be hooked to the patient's belt and runs on a rechargeable battery (Figure 20-4). A clear, adhesive dressing is placed over the foam and tubing to secure the unit to the wound site. The distal end of the evacuation tubing is attached to a collection canister, and the controlled negative pressure is applied. The target pressures for negative pressure wound therapy vary from 75 mm Hg to 125 mm Hg, depending

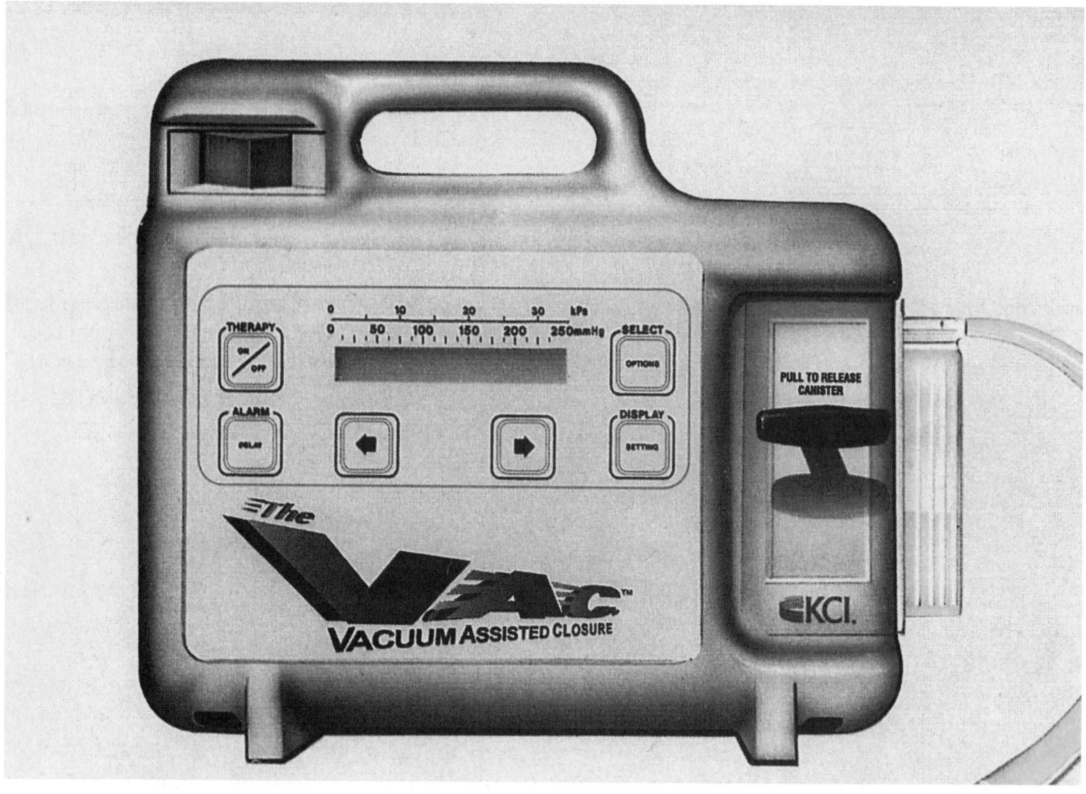

Figure 20-3 The VAC® pump. (Courtesy Kinetic Concepts, Inc. San Antonio, Texas.)

on the characteristics of the individual wound. The cycle of therapy, continuous or intermittent, is also based on predetermined guidelines (Table 20-1). Continuous therapy maximizes removal of wound fluid and surrounding edema. Intermittent therapy usually runs on a preset cycle of 5 minutes of negative pressure followed by 2 minutes of no pressure. The intermittent cycle capitalizes on the effects of mechanical stretch and repetitive release of biochemical messengers to the wound by alternating pressure and nonpressure. The parameters for negative pressure can be changed if necessary to accommodate excessive drainage or infection in the wound.

The patient is attached to the negative pressure pump throughout the treatment. The evacuation tubing is long enough to allow limited movement around the pump. The tubing can also be clamped and disconnected for short periods of time (no more than 2 hours at a time for a maximum of 6 hours per day). This mobility allows the patient to move freely and encourages increased activity as wound healing continues. If the negative pressure must be off for an extended amount of time, the sponge should be removed and replaced with a moisture-retentive dressing such as moist saline gauze.

When NPWT is used on a split-thickness mesh skin graft, it is placed intraoperatively. A nonadherent dressing must be laid on top of the graft before placement of the sponge. Anything that causes a graft to lose a snug fit against the vascular rich bed of the wound places the graft at risk of failure. Split-thickness skin grafts often fail because of movement or an accumulation of fluid beneath the graft. The placement of a nonadherent dressing protects the fragile graft from trauma and shear during the removal of the foam dressing. NPWT assists with successful take of split-thickness mesh skin grafts by decreasing the ability of the graft to

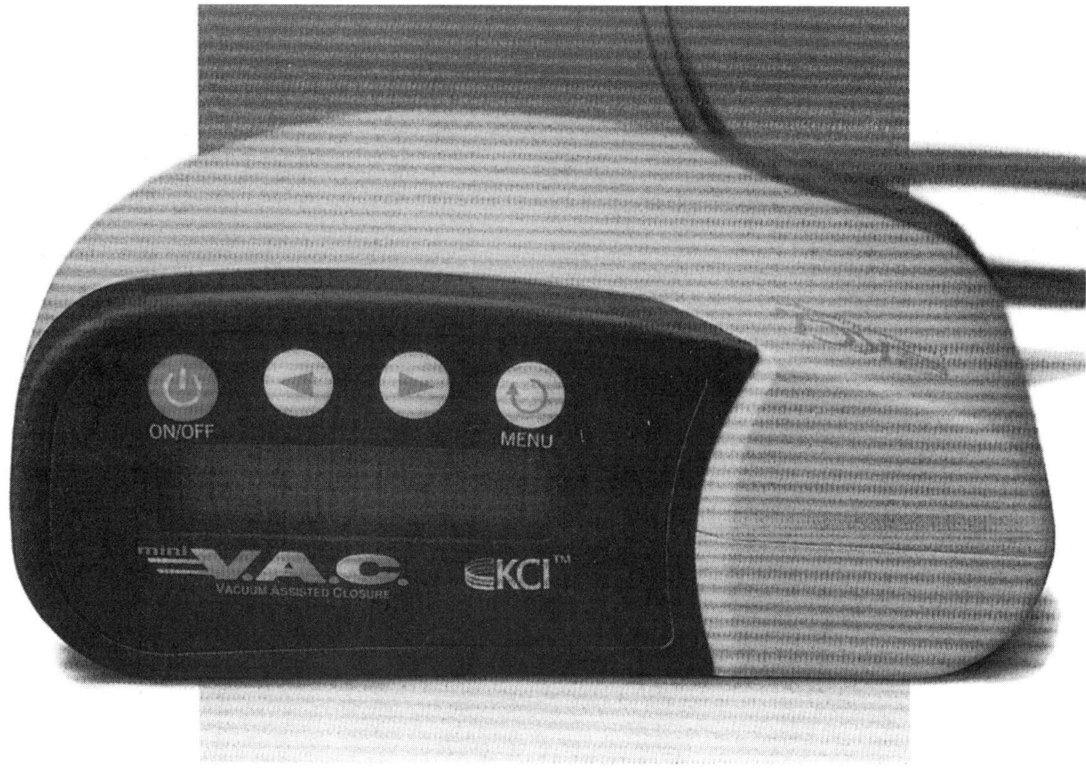

Figure 20-4 The MiniVAC® pump. (Courtesy Kinetic Concepts, Inc. San Antonio, Texas.)

TABLE 20-1 Guidelines for Use of Negative Pressure Wound Therapy (NPWT)

TYPE OF WOUND	NEGATIVE PRESSURE	DRESSING CHANGE REGIMEN	CYCLE	DURATION
Pressure ulcer	125 mm Hg	48 hr after placement Every Monday, Wednesday, and Friday	Continuous Intermittent	Initial 48 hr Throughout remainder of treatment
Vascular ulcer	75 to 125 mm Hg	Every Monday, Wednesday, and Friday	Continuous	Throughout treatment
Neuropathic ulcer	125 mm Hg	Every Monday, Wednesday, and Friday	Continuous	Throughout treatment
Acute wounds	125 mm Hg	48 hr after placement Every Monday, Wednesday, and Friday	Continuous Intermittent	Initial 48 hr Throughout remainder of treatment
Split-thickness mesh skin graft	15 to 100 mm Hg	No scheduled dressing changes	Continuous	Discontinue therapy 5 days postop*

*NPWT is applied intraoperatively and removed on the fifth postoperative day. NPWT may be reapplied for up to 3 additional days if deemed necessary.

NOTE: The parameters for NPWT can be changed if necessary to accommodate excessive drainage or infection in the wound.

BOX 20-3 Negative Pressure Wound Therapy Guidelines for Dressing Application

1. Insert wound drainage canister into side of pump, taking care not to contaminate the distal end.
2. Cleanse wound per routine.
3. Cut dressing to fit wound.
4. Apply skin sealant to adjacent intact skin (optional).
5. Cut packing pieces from dressing to fill only shallow undermined space (so they are retrievable).
6. Insert tube in existing hole in dressing, or create a new hole if dressing size decreases.
7. Cut prepackaged transparent film dressing to conform to body contours; allow for liberal amount of intact periwound skin for dressing to adhere to.
8. While holding dressing in place in wound, apply transparent film over wound as wrinkle-free as possible.
9. Lift tube to pinch transparent film under tube to obtain airtight seal.
10. Remove top plastic liner and perforated edges from transparent film dressing.
11. Reinforce tube or body contour edges as needed with additional transparent film dressing to reinforce seal.
12. Place thin hydrocolloid, gauze, or other types of dressing between tube-skin interface to prevent pressure damage from the tube. Position tube away from bony structures.
13. Connect distal end of tube to canister.
14. Open clamps.
15. Turn pump on at desired settings. Transparent dressing should visibly contract down over wound dressing if an airtight seal has been achieved.

NOTE: This procedure requires universal precautions, clean nonsterile gloves are imperative, and goggles and gown should be worn if splashing during wound cleansing is anticipated.

From Hartnett JM: Use of vacuum-assisted closure in three chronic wounds, *J Wound Ostomy Continence Nurs* 25:281, 1998.

shift and evacuating any fluid that may build up beneath the graft and cause a gap in the interfacing of the graft and vascular matrix of the wound bed.

BOX 20-4 Negative Pressure Wound Therapy Guidelines for Dressing Application

1. Gently remove transparent dressing from skin toward wound. Use water-dampened gauze or cloths to push skin away from adhesive and thus gently break the bond.
2. To facilitate removal of dressing, gently irrigate wound.
3. Remove all pieces of dressing using a forceps or similar type of instrument.
4. Cleanse wound per routine or protocol.
5. Assess wound and condition of periwound skin.

NOTE: This procedure requires universal precautions, nonsterile gloves are imperative, and goggles and gown should be worn if splashing during wound cleansing is anticipated. Clean gloves should be worn to apply a new dressing.

From Hartnett JM: Use of vacuum-assisted closure in three chronic wounds, *J Wound Ostomy Continence Nurs* 25:281, 1998.

NPWT is used on split-thickness mesh skin grafts for 4 to 5 days after the procedure. Upon removal of the dressing, the graft is evaluated for adherence. If the graft has a full "take," the NPWT is removed and discontinued. If there are areas of the graft that have not taken, the NPWT can be replaced for up to 3 additional days. If excess graft was harvested in surgery, it can be applied before NPWT replacement if needed. The addition of banked graft can be done at the bedside without the requirement of an additional surgical procedure.

Monitoring of the periwound site, computerized pump and its parameters, and fluid collection are included in the daily maintenance of NPWT. As with any therapy, the area visible around the dressing must be monitored for changes in character, such as erythema or warmth. The character and the amount of drainage must also be assessed at least daily. Acute changes should be reported to the physician. Wound measurement, tissue and fluid characterization, odor, and the periwound site should be monitored and documented with each dressing change.

Dressing changes for NPWT are completed at the patient bedside using aseptic technique. Boxes 20-3 and 20-4 list guidelines for dressing application and removal. The disposal collection chamber located on the computerized pressure pump is changed weekly or as it is filled. The pump has a digital display and alarm that indicate if the programmed pressure is not being maintained, the canister is full, or the pump is tilted. If the pump is unable to maintain the appropriate pressure, then the dressing should be checked for leaks. Leaks in the transparent dressing can be patched with tape or extra dressing. An airtight seal is necessary to maintain a negative pressure environment.

Pain has been reported in association with NPWT and is triggered by application of the suction and removal of the dressing (Hartnett, 1998). The use of analgesics at dressing changes can reduce the procedural pain (e.g., pain caused by dressing removal). Lowering the initial amount of negative pressure can also be used to decrease pain. Increasing the amount of negative pressure slowly may allow the patient to tolerate the therapy if pain is a factor.

Cost of Treatment

Since NPWT can be used in any health care setting, including the home, it presents the possibility of eliminating delays when transferring patients out of acute care. Cost savings may be realized through decreased healing time, number of dressing changes, and nursing visits. When comparing costs of care, Preslar (1995) reported a 76% decrease in the mean charge for patients receiving NPWT as compared with a mean decrease of just 36% in those who used more traditional wound care therapies. Hartnett (1998) used NPWT in a VA hospital system and reported the direct cost of the treatment to be $100 per day.

Currently, NPWT has not received an official Medicare reimbursement code. Most, but not all, major health insurance providers have also approved reimbursement. It is, however, important to investigate reimbursement criteria for each paient before making the decision to use NPWT because the financial constraints of an uncovered therapy must be considered and discussed with the patient before use.

Summary

Negative pressure therapy is an unusual treatment that has generated interesting results. It has been used in wounds until closure and until the wound has reduced in size or granulated sufficiently in preparation for surgical closure. The wound care nurse should be aware of the appropriate indications for this type of therapy. However, additional randomized clinical trials are needed to confirm findings from previous reports and to determine the quality of healing in these wounds.

ELECTRICAL STIMULATION

The effects of electrical currents on wound healing were first documented in the late 1600s when gold foil applied topically over cutaneous ulcerations was found to promote healing and prevent scarring (Robertson, 1925). However, serious study of the role of electrical current in the wound-recovery process did not occur until 1960 when Becker (1961) discovered that after amputation the regenerating limb of the salamander produced a measurable current and that the polarity of that current varied in a special way during the regeneration process. His hypothesis that the body maintains an electrical current within itself, which is responsible for healthy tissue, provided the impetus for basic and clinical research on its role in all phases of the wound-healing process. These studies constitute the developing body of knowledge related to the role of electrical stimulation and wound healing.

Types of Electrical Stimulation

Several electrotherapy modalities are cited in the literature. Although several terms are used to describe these therapies, only four types of electrical waveforms have been applied to wound healing: 1) low-voltage continuous microamperage direct current, 2) high-voltage pulsed current (HVPC), 3) low-voltage pulsed microamperage current, and 4) low-voltage pulsed milliamperage current. These waveforms are distinguished by the pattern of the current being delivered (Figure 20-5). An alternate type of electrotherapy, pulsed electromagnetic energy, has also been studied as a modality for promotion of wound healing. To understand the basis of

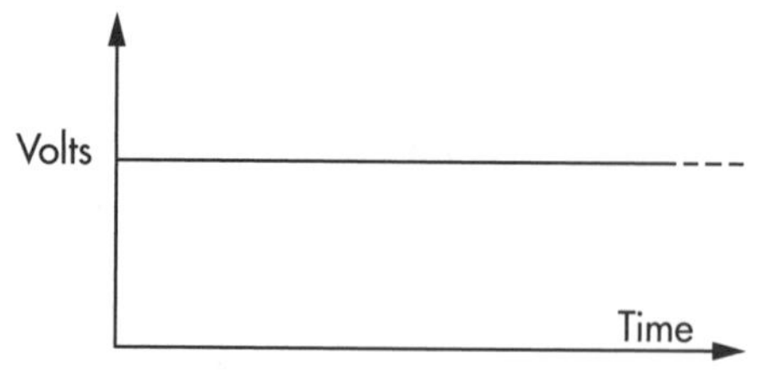

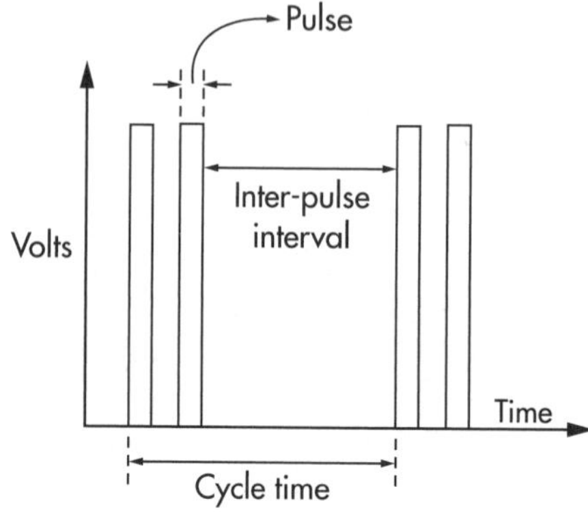

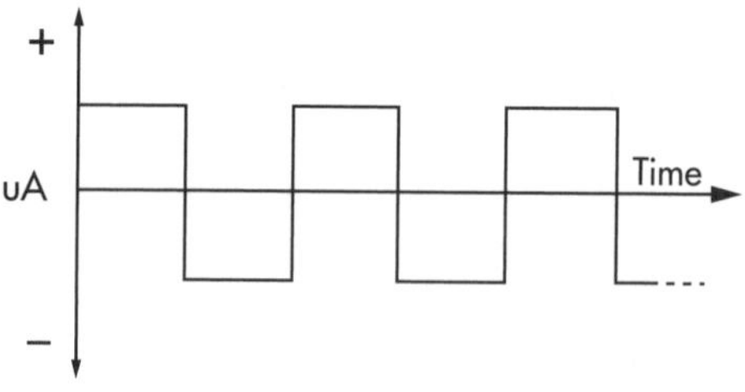

Figure 20-5 Pattern of current for three types of electrical waveforms: low-voltage continuous direct current (*top*), high-voltage pulsed current (*middle*), and low-voltage pulsed current (*bottom*). The low-voltage pulsed current can be with microamperage (μA) or milliamperage (mA).

electrical stimulation, it is important to be familiar with key terms. Box 20-5 provides definitions of terms used to describe the different types of electrical stimulation waveforms.

Low-voltage continuous microamperage direct current is characterized as a continuous, monophasic waveform in which the voltage does not vary with time. This type of current can be delivered to the wound tissue with an electrode that has either a positive (anode) or negative (cathode) charge. Typically, the regimen for applying direct current therapy uses 20 to 200 microamps (μA) of current at low voltage (<8 volts) (Wolcott et al, 1969). Treatment is applied by placing the active electrode on saline-soaked gauze packing in the wound for 2 to 4 hours per day, 5 to 7 days per week. Initially, stimulation is provided with the cathode for 3 to 5 days to reduce bacterial levels in the wound. Once the wound is clean, polarity is reversed to anode stimulation until closure is achieved. Electrochemical reactions with ions in the tissues may create an alkaline enviroment at the cathode or an acid environment at the anode. The alkaline-producing reaction at the cathode may be used for its bactericidal effect or to facilitate debridement in response to sclerolytic activity that breaks up thrombi (Sawyer and Pate, 1957) and necrotic tissue. Local wound care includes cleansing and covering the wound with saline gauze dressings.

High-voltage pulsed current features a waveform of paired short-duration pulses with a long interpulse interval. The pulses may be either positive or negative polarity with respect to the dispersive electrode. When compared with sound waves, high-voltage pulsed current would be characterized by short staccato sounds, whereas low-voltage continuous microamperage direct current would be represented by a continuous hum. Treatment with high-voltage pulsed stimulation is generally delivered at 75 to 200 volts and 50 to 100 pulses per second (pps). The maximum total current reaching the tissue is approximately 2.5 mA when standard size electrodes are used (McCulloch, Kloth, and Feedar, 1995).

Throughout the high-voltage pulsed current therapy, the wound receives routine cleansing and dressing with saline-soaked gauze or other moist wound-healing product. Treatments are delivered by placing the active electrode over saline-soaked gauze on the wound bed for 45 minutes to 1 hour, five to seven times per week. For the first 3 to 5 days of treatment, stimulation is provided with the cathode as the active electrode. As the drainage from the wound becomes more serosanguinous, the polarity is changed to positive current. This polarity is maintained until closure occurs, unless the wound reaches a plateau and fails to progress toward healing. In these instances the polarity would be reversed in an effort to restart the healing trajectory. Although

BOX 20-5 Electrical Stimulation: Definition of Terms

Alternating current	Uninterrupted, bidirectional current flow; also referred to as *biphasic*.
Amplitude	The maximum (peak) excursion of a voltage or current pulse.
Amperage	Measure of the rate of flow of current; expressed as amperes (A), milliamperes (mA), or microamperes (uA).
Direct current	Continuous, uninterrupted, unidirectional current; also referred to as *galvanic*; direction of flow determined by polarity used.
Frequency	Number of pulses delivered per unit of time; also known as *pulse rate*. Frequency is the reciprocal of cycle time. Usually measured as pulses per second (pps), or Hz (Hertz). 0.1 Hz is on for 10 seconds, and a pulse of 1000 Hz is on for 1 millisecond. Typical personal computers have clock speeds of several hundred megahertz (MHz).
Interpulse interval	Time between pulses when there is no voltage applied and no current flowing.
Polarity	By definition, current flows from the positive pole (anode) to the negative pole (cathode).
Pulse duration	Time during which current is flowing.
Voltage	Measure of force of the flow of electrons (V); (Voltage = Current × Resistance*). Can be low-voltage devices (60-100 V) and high-voltage devices (100-500 V).
Waveform	Graphic representation of current flow; may be monophasic (current that deviates from baseline in one direction and then returns to baseline) or biphasic (current that deviates above and below baseline); may be symmetric or asymmetric.

*In wound healing, subcutaneous tissue, edema, necrotic tissue, etc. all provide resistance.

the polar capabilities with this waveform have not been addressed directly in the literature, it has been theorized that the polar effects observed with direct current are equally likely to occur with short-duration pulsed stimulation.

The third type of waveform, low-voltage pulsed microamperage current, is similar to high-voltage pulsed current but is actually an interrupted direct current with a wide rectangular pulse width and a short interpulse interval. Current can be delivered as either constant polarity monophasic pulses or as alternating polarity biphasic pulses through paired carbonized rubber electrodes. Treatment parameters have varied, although amplitudes of 600 μA and a frequency of 0.5 pps have been employed commonly. Moist wound-healing methods are used between the electrical stimulation sessions.

Low-voltage pulsed milliamperage current delivers symmetric biphasic pulses. With most devices, the quantity of charge contained in the two symmetric phases of each pulse is equal, and therefore the accumulation of charge residual in the tissues is zero. Consequently, there is no polarity in the tissue and no electrochemical reaction. The device most commonly associated with this type of current is the transcutaneous electrical nerve stimulator (TENS). When used to augment wound healing, current is delivered at 15 to 20 mA with 150 μs pulse width and 85 Hz (standard low-frequency) (Frantz, 1990). Electrodes are placed at the edges of the ulcer, and in some protocols a second pair of electrodes is placed in the dorsal web space of the hand and ulnar border of the wrist on the ipsilateral extremity. Other devices capable of delivering low-voltage pulsed milliamperage current have been applied to wounds in an effort to promote healing (Feedar, Kloth, and Gentzkow, 1991; Gentzkow et al, 1991). In these applications the cathode and anode were alternately applied directly to the wound in relation to changes in wound appearance. The peak amplitude is maintained at 29.2 mA, and the pulse frequency is adjusted downward from 128 pps as the wound clears of debris and begins to fill with granulation tissue. Regardless of the type of device being used, local treatment to the wound consists of cleansing and dressing with saline-soaked gauze.

Although not a therapy that applies electrical current directly to wound tissue, pulsed electromagnetic energy has been explored as a modality to promote wound healing. Pulsed electromagnetic energy uses pulsed, nonthermal, high-frequency, high peak power electromagnetic energy delivered at 27.12 MHz, with pulse repetitions of 80 to 600 pps and a pulse width of 65 μs, a duty cycle of 0.5% and 3.9%, and a per-pulse power range between 293 and 975 peak watts (Salzberg et al, 1995). Energy is induced at the ulcer site by a 9-inch-diameter, drum-shaped treatment head placed in direct contact with the gauze dressing on the wound surface. Therapy is generally administered for 30 minutes twice daily until the ulcer heals.

Effects of Electrotherapy on Wound Healing

Underlying the physiologic effects of electrotherapy on wound healing is the influence of electrical charge (i.e., positive or negative polarity). All three modalities of electrical stimulation (waveforms) have the capability of delivering current of the same charge to the active electrode. A synthesis of the research literature indicates that certain physiologic changes occur at the tissue and cellular levels in a wound exposed to exogenous electrical stimulation. These changes provide the basis for stimulation of the wound-healing process.

Current of Injury. The concept of the "current of injury" has evolved from experiments demonstrating that the surface of human and animal skin is electronegative with respect to deeper skin layers (Barker, 1981; Barker, Jaffe, and Vanable, 1982; Cunliffe-Barnes, 1945; Foulds and Barker, 1983). As a result, the skin has electrical potentials across it that resemble a battery. This biologic battery is driven by a sodium-ion pump (Jaffe and Vanable, 1984). Current can flow between parts of the skin if the current is completed, as when wounding occurs and ionic fluids are available to transmit electricity between the outer and inner layers (Black, 1984). This effect was demonstrated by Becker (1970), who found that after amputation the regenerating limb of the salamander produces a measurable current and that the polarity of this current varies in a special way during the regeneration process. As healing is completed or arrested, these currents no longer flow. Electrical stimulation may work by mimicking the natural currents of injury, thereby restarting or accelerating the wound-healing process (Foulds and Barker, 1983).

Galvanotaxic Effects. It has been demonstrated that cells move along the path of current, a phenomenon referred to as the *galvanotaxic effect.* When applied to wounded tissue, electrical currents have influenced migration of cells essential to the infammatory process. Fukushima (1953) demonstrated a galvanotaxic effect on neutrophils that were attracted to both the anode and cathode but in the presence of inflammation were attracted to the cathode. Eberhardt, Szczypiorski, and Korytowski (1986) showed that electrical stimulation increased the relative number of neutrophilic granulocytes in human skin exudate. Orida and Feldman (1982) found that macrophages migrate toward the cathode. Given the role of neutrophils and macrophages in the inflammatory phase of wound healing, the capability to enhance cell migration implies that electrotherapy can promote the initial phase of wound healing. Furthermore, Weiss, Eaglstein and Falanga (1989) suggested that mast cells, which are associated with diseases of abnormal fibrotic healing and keloid formation, may be inhibited from migrating into a wounded area when treated with electrical stimulation. Their finding of decreased mast cells and reduced scar-tissue thickness in healing human wounds undergoing electrotherapy substantiates further the potential benefit of electrical stimulation on soft tissue repair.

Stimulatory Effects on Cells. Electrical current has been shown to have a stimulatory effect on fibroblasts, a key cell in wound contraction and collagen synthesis. Cruz, Bayron, and Suarez (1989), using the pig model, demonstrated that there are significantly more fibroblasts in burn wounds treated with electrical stimulation than in controls. Alvarez and colleagues (1983), also employing the pig model, documented more fibroblasts and increased collagen synthesis in partial-thickness wounds. Bourguignon and Bourguignon (1987), who found that fibroblasts in culture increase DNA and protein (including collagen) synthesis in response to electrical stimulation, reported the effect of electrical current on fibroblasts. This effect was most noticeable near the negative electrode.

Blood Flow. Several studies have documented improved blood flow as a result of electrical stimulation. Hecker, Carron, and Schwartz (1985) have shown in normal subjects that negative polarity increased blood flow in the upper extremity as measured by plethysmography. In 1982, Kaada (1982) demonstrated that application of distant, low-frequency transcutaneous electrical nerve stimulation produced pronounced and prolonged cutaneous vasodilatation in patients diagnosed with Raynaud's disease and diabetic polyneuropathy. Using skin temperature as a measurement of peripheral vasodilatation, he found a rise in the temperature of ischemic extremities from 71.6° to 75.2° F (22° to 24° C) to 87.8° to 93.2° F (31° to 34° C). The latency from the stimulus onset to the abrupt rise in temperature averaged 15 to 30 minutes with a duration of response from 4 to 6 hours.

Antibacterial Effects. Preliminary evidence indicates that electrical stimulation has bacteriostatic and bactericidal effects on microorganisms that are known to infect chronic wounds. Rowley, McKenna, and Chase (1974) demonstrated inhibition of *Pseudomonas aeruginosa* in infected ulcers of rabbit skin when negative polarity was used. They hypothesized that the inhibition was the result of electrochemical changes created by the current. In a study of 20 patients with burn wounds that had been unresponsive to conventional therapy for 3 months to 2 years, Fakhri and Amin (1987) showed a quantitatively lower level of organisms after treatment with direct current stimulation for 10-minute intervals twice weekly. This decrease in bacterial count was accompanied by epithelialization of the wound margins within 3 days of beginning electrical stimulation. Although the mechanism underlying the bactericidal or bacteriostatic effect of microamperage direct current remains unclear, the galvanotaxic effect on macrophages and neutrophils has been implicated (Eberhardt, Szczypiorski, and Korytowski, 1986; Fukushima et al, 1953; Orida and Feldman, 1982). These studies suggest that the anodal attraction of phagocytic macrophages and the anodal or cathodal attraction of neutrophils to tissue with high bacterial levels may be a primary mode of action, rather than destruction of pathogens by electrolysis or raising of the tissue pH.

In summary, the literature provides evidence that electrical stimulation is associated with enhanced cellular processes that normally accompany the restoration of injured soft tissue and with inhibition of certain types of bacteria. These studies provide indirect evidence of its potential to enhance wound healing. However, the reliance on small sample sizes and the variability in type and level of electrical stimulation tested supports the need for additional research to identify the optimum treatment protocol to support these physiologic processes.

Efficacy of Electrical Stimulation

The efficacy of electrical stimulation has been evaluated by use of different types of electrical-current waveforms on a variety of chronic wounds, including diabetic ulcers, pressure ulcers, venous ulcers, accidental injuries, and ulcers associated with arteriosclerotic disease. Initial research was conducted with low-voltage continuous microamperage direct current. More recently, other waveforms have been applied to wound healing. When viewed in the aggregate, these studies provide encouraging support of the potential for electrical stimulation to enhance the wound-healing process.

Wolcott and colleagues (1969) conducted one of the earliest clinical trials testing low-voltage continuous microamperage direct current on human subjects with 75 ischemic skin ulcers previously resistant to healing. They reported complete healing of 34 of the lesions with treatment, and the range of improvement in the remaining 41 ranged from 0% to 97%. Gault and Gatens (1976) subsequently reported similiar results with the use of low-voltage continuous microamperage direct current. Using six subjects with contralateral ulcerations as controls, their results showed a mean weekly healing ratio of 30% for the treated group compared with 14.7% for the control group. Mean healing after 4 weeks was 74% in those treated with electrical stimulation and 27.3% in the controls. The beneficial effects of low-voltage continuous microamperage direct current were further substantiated by

Carley and Wainapel (1985), who studied 30 subjects with chronic ulcerations who were paired according to age; diagnosis; and ulcer cause, location, and size. One member of the pair received low-voltage continuous microamperage direct current therapy, whereas the other acted as the control. Results showed a 1.5 to 2.5 times faster healing rate for the treated group as compared with the controls.

More recently, the efficacy of high-voltage pulsed current has been evaluated in randomized controlled trials. Kloth and Feedar (1988) studied 16 subjects with stage 4 pressure ulcers who were randomly assigned to receive either a high-voltage, monophasic, pulsed current or a sham treatment. The ulcers treated with the HVPC had a mean healing rate of 44.8% with 100% healing in a mean period of 8 weeks. Those in the sham treatment group showed an increase in ulcer size of 29% over a period of 7.4 weeks. Similiar acceleration of healing was demonstrated by Griffin and colleagues (1991), who studied high-voltage pulsed current on 17 patients with spinal cord injury who had stage 2, 3, and 4 pressure ulcers. Subjects were randomly assigned to receive either HVPC or a placebo treatment for 1 hour per day for 20 consecutive days. Findings revealed that ulcers treated with electrical stimulation showed a significant decrease in wound surface area as compared with the placebo-treated ulcers at day 5 ($p < 0.05$), day 15 ($p < 0.05$), and day 20 ($p < 0.05$). Alon, Azaria, and Stein (1986) described the benefits of HVPC on healing diabetic foot ulcers in a case series of 15 patients. Anodal stimulation was applied for 1 hour three times a week. Twelve of the fifteen wounds achieved closure in a mean period of 2.6 months.

Pulsed microamperage direct current has been investigated to a more limited extent. Barron Jacobson, and Tidd (1985) reported using low-voltage pulsed microamperage current to treat pressure ulcers in six geriatric patients. Treatment was perfomed three time a week for 1 hour at an amplitude of 600 μA and a frequency of 0.5 pps (Barron, Jacobson, and Tidd, 1985). Metal probe electrodes placed 2 cm from the wound edge were used to deliver the current. Although no control group was described, five of the six ulcers that were treated with the electrical current were reported to have essentially healed within 1 month. More recently, low-voltage pulsed microamperage current was studied in a multicenter trial of 71 patients with 74 stage 2 and 3 pressure ulcers (Wood et al, 1993). Forty-three ulcers were treated with an active device, and 31 ulcers received a placebo treatment, three times a week, for 8 weeks as part of a double-blind protocol. Negative current was delivered initially via probe electrodes at 0.8 pps to three different locations on opposite sides of the ulcer for 1 minute at 300 μA, followed by 3 minutes at each site at 600 μA. Of the 43 ulcers in the active treatment group, 25 had healed by the end of 8 weeks, whereas only one of the 31 ulcers in the placebo group healed.

Initial studies of low-voltage pulsed milliamperage current conducted by Kaada (1982) suggest that remote stimulation by placing the cathode in the webspace between the first and second metacarpals of the ipsilateral hand and the anode on the ulnar border of the ipsilateral wrist improved circulation in peripheral tissues. Others have applied this type of current directly to wound tissue in an effort to augment healing. In a randomized, controlled trial of 50 chronic wounds, Feedar, Kloth, and Gentzkow (1991) treated 26 ulcers twice daily for 30 minutes with pulsed cathodal stimulation at a frequency of 128 pps and a peak amplitude of 29.2 mA. The negative polarity electrode was maintained until the ulcer was debrided and serosanguinous drainage appeared. Thereafter, the polarity was alternated between positive and negative every 3 days until the wound filled with granulation tissue. At this stage of healing, the frequency was decreased to 64 pps while maintaining the same peak amplitude. The polarity of the treatment electrode was changed daily until the wound healed. The remaining 24 ulcers received a placebo control. The weekly rate of healing for the active treatment group was 14% compared with 8.25% for the control group. Using a similar protocol, Gentzkow and colleagues (1991) studied 37 subjects with 40 ulcers that were treated with low-voltage pulsed milliamperage current or a placebo for 30 minutes twice daily. At the end of the 4-week trial, the ulcers treated with electrical stimulation showed a 49.8% decrease in surface area compared with a 23.4%

decrease in size of the placebo treated ulcers ($p = 0.042$). The rate of healing of the actively stimulated group of ulcers was 12.5% per week compared with 5.8% per week for the placebo-treated group.

Randomized double-blind studies of the efficacy of pulsed electromagnetic energy in healing pressure ulcers in humans have been limited to one investigation (Salzberg et al, 1995). Thirty patients with spinal cord injury who had pressure ulcers were treated for 30 minutes twice daily for 12 weeks using nonthermal, pulsed, high-frequency, electromagnetic energy or a placebo. Findings showed that after controlling for baseline status of the ulcer, active pulsed electromagnetic energy was independently associated with a significantly shorter median time to complete healing of the ulcer (13.0 vs. 31.5 days, $p = 0.002$).

Preliminary experimental evidence indicates that application of electrical stimulation has the potential to enhance the healing of chronic, recalcitrant wounds. However, sample sizes have been small in reported studies to date, leaving many questions regarding the optimum treatment protocols, timing of the treatments, and compatibility of electrotherapy with various local wound care regimens. Attempts to evaluate the effect of stimulation waveform and electrode placement on healing have been limited to two studies conducted on different chronic wound populations (Baker et al, 1996, 1997). In the earlier study, a total of 185 pressure ulcers received 30 minutes of stimulation daily with one of four randomly assigned treatment protocols: asymmetric biphasic waveform, symmetric biphasic waveform, microcurrent stimulation, or a sham control. Analysis of the "good response" ulcer ($n = 104$) showed significantly better healing rates for those receiving stimulation with the asymmetric biphasic waveform compared with the control and the microcurrent groups. However, healing rates for the symmetric biphasic-treated ulcers did not differ significantly from the other treatment groups.

The second study applied the same four treatment protocols in random fashion to 80 subjects with diabetic foot ulcers. Consistent with the findings of the earlier study, the healing rate for the asymmetric biphasic waveform group was significantly faster than for the control group (defined as the combined microcurrent stimulation and sham control groups). Healing of the symmetric biphasic-treated group failed to show a significant difference from the other treatment groups. Although these findings suggest that various waveforms may produce different rates of healing, further research is needed to identify the optimal electrotherapy parameters needed to maximize healing outcomes.

Summary

Application of electrical stimulation as a wound-healing modality in routine clinical practice remains limited. Two factors have restricted the transfer of this therapy to mainstream practice. The Food and Drug Administration (FDA) has not approved as yet any type of electrical stimulation device for wound healing. Consequently, devices cannot be marketed for this indication, although they can be marketed for other already approved indications, such as treatment of edema and pain. Approval of an electrical stimulation device by the FDA necessitates submission by a device manufacturer of a product market approval application (PMA) containing sufficient data based on randomized controlled trials to establish safety and efficacy. Reimbursement policies of third-party payers, including the Health Care Financing Administration (HCFA), have created additional obstacles to its use in practice. A well-defined policy for coverage of electrical stimulation for wound healing is slow to be defined because of the absence of rigorous trials employing sufficient sample sizes to substantiate efficacy. Additional controlled clinical trials are needed to delineate the efficacy of electrotherapy as a treatment modality for chronic wound healing before widespread clinical application will be realized.

SUMMARY

By definition, adjuvant wound therapies such as those discussed in this chapter are conducted in conjunction with appropriate topical wound treatments. In most situations, these treatments are not considered first-line interventions for a variety of reasons (e.g., reimbursement, availability, access, extent of research evidence). The wound care nurse should be familiar with the techniques and remain abreast of the growing body of evidence surrounding that particular intervention.

SELF-EVALUATION EXERCISE

1. Define *hyperbaric oxygenation.*
2. Which of the following statements about hyperoxygenation that occurs with hyperbaric treatment is true?
   a. Hyperoxygenation occurs because the hemoglobin molecule is saturated with oxygen molecules
   b. Hyperoxygenation results from increasing the oxygen-carrying capacity of the plasma
   c. It takes several treatments to achieve hyperoxygenation
   d. It is possible for hyperoxygenation to be sustained for 8 to 10 hours after exposure
3. List five complications associated with hyperbaric treatment and one risk-reduction intervention.
4. All of the following personal care items are contraindicated during hyperbaric treatment EXCEPT:
   a. Hairspray
   b. Hearing aides
   c. Contact lenses
   d. Perfume
5. True or False: Wound care dressings with a petrolatum base should be removed during hyperbaric treatment.
6. Which of the following statements is true of high-voltage pulsed current?
   a. Currents of high voltage are delivered with a wide rectangular pulse width
   b. Currents are continuous and have a monophasic waveform
   c. Skin burns are more common under the electrode when using HVPC
   d. HVPC features a waveform of paired short-duration pulses with a long pause between pulses
7. Define *galvanotaxic effects.*
8. List at least four parameters that must be set to deliver pulsed electrical stimulation wound treatments.
9. Which of the following functions does negative pressure therapy support?
   a. Evacuation of third-space fluid
   b. Mechanical stretch
   c. Moist wound environment
   d. All of the above
10. Which of the following situations would be a contraindication for negative pressure wound therapy?
    a. Patient who is paraplegic and has a stage 4 sacral pressure ulcer
    b. Patient with obesity who has a venous stasis ulcer
    c. Patient who developed a dehisced abdominal surgical wound after the removal of a malignant tumor
    d. Patient with diabetes who has a neuropathic foot ulcer and osteomyelitis
11. Which of the following dressing change regimens is appropriate for a patient using negative pressure wound therapy on a vascular ulcer?
    a. Every day
    b. Every other day
    c. Every 48 hours
    d. Every fifth day

REFERENCES

Abramovich A et al: Hyperbaric oxygen for carbon monoxide poisoning, *Harefuah* 132(1):21, 1997.

Alon G, Azaria M, Stein H: Diabetic ulcer healing using high voltage TENS (Abstract). *Phys Ther* 66:775, 1986

Alvarez OM et al: The healing of superficial skin wounds is stimulated by external electrical current, *J Invest Dermatol* 81(2):144, 1983.

Argenta LC, Morykwas M, Rouchard R: *The use of negative pressure to promote healing of pressure ulcers and chronic wounds in 75 consecutive patients* (abstract). Joint Meeting, Wound Healing Society and European Tissue Repair Society, Amsterdam, Aug 22-25, 1993.

Baker L et al: Effect of electrical stimulation waveform on healing of ulcers in human beings with spinal cord injury, *Wound Rep Regen* 4(1):21, 1996.

Baker L et al: Effects of electrical stimulation on wound healing in patients with diabetic ulcers, *Diabetes Care* 20(3):405, 1997.

Barker A: Measurement of direct current in biological fluids, *Med Biol Eng Comput* 19:507, 1981.

Barker A, Jaffe L, Vanable J: The glabrous epidermis of cavies contains a powerful battery, *Am J Physiol* 11:R358, 1982.

Barron J, Jacobson W, Tidd G: Treatment of decubitus ulcers: a new approach, *Minn Med* 68(2):103, 1985.

Becker R: The bioelectric factors in amphibian limb regeneration, *J Bone Joint Surg* 43(5): 643, 1961.

Becker R: The electrical control system regulating factor healing in amphibians, *Clin Orthop* 73:169, 1970.

Black J: Tissue response to exogenous electromagnetic signals, *Orthop Clin North Am* 15(1):15, 1984.

Bourguignon G, Bourguignon L: Electric stimulation of protein and DNA systhesis in human fibroblasts, *FASEB J* 1(5):398, 1987.

Capes JP, Tomaszewski C: Prophylaxis against middle ear barotrauma in US hyperbaric oxygen therapy centers, *Am J Emerg Med* 14(7):645, 1996.

Carl UM et al: Treatment of radiation proctitis with hyperbaric oxygen: what is the optimal number of HBO treatments? *Strahlenther Onkol* 174(9):482, 1998.

Carley PJ, Wainapel SF: Electrotherapy for acceleration of wound healing: low intensity direct current, *Arch Phys Med Rehabil* 66(7):443, 1985.

Cianci P, Sato R: Adjunctive hyperbaric oxygen therapy in the treatment of thermal burns: a review, *Burns* 20(1):5, 1994.

Clark JM: Oxygen toxicity. In Kindwall EP, editor: *Hyperbaric medicine practice*, Flagstaff, Ariz, 1995, Best Publishing Company.

Cruz N, Bayron F, Suarez A: Accelerated healing of full-thickness burns by the use of high-voltage pulsed galvanic stimulation in the pig, *Ann Plast Surg* 23(1):49, 1989.

Cunliffe-Barnes T: Healing rate of human skin determined by measurement of electric potential of experimental abrasions: study of treatment with petrolatum and with petrolatum containing yeast and liver extracts, *Am J Surg* 69(1):82, 1945.

Eberhardt A, Szczypiorski P, Korytowski G: Effect of transcutaneous electrostimulation on the cell composition of skin exudate, *Acta Physiol Pol* 37(1):41, 1986.

Elliott DH: Decompression sickness. In Kindwall EP, editor: *Hyperbaric medicine practice*, Flagstaff, Ariz, 1995, Best Publishing Company.

Fakhri O, Amin M: The effect of low-voltage electric therapy on the healing of resistant skin burns, *J Burn Care Res* 8(1):15, 1987

Feedar J, Kloth L, Gentzkow G: Chronic dermal ulcer healing enhanced with monphasic pulsed electrical stimulation, *Phys Ther* 71(9):639, 1991.

Foster JH: Hyperbaric oxygen treatment contraindications and complications, *J Maxillofac Surg* 50:1081, 1992.

Foulds I, Barker A: Human skin battery potentials and their possible role in wound healing, *Br J Dermatol* 109:515, 1983.

Frantz R: The effectiveness of TENS in healing decubitus ulcers: an ongoing study. In Funk S et al, editors: *Key aspects of recovery: improving mobility, rest and nutrition*, New York, 1990, Springer.

Fukushima K et al: Studies of galvanotaxis of human neutrophilic leukocytes and methods of its measurement, *Med J Osaka Univ* 4:195, 1953.

Gault W, Gatens P: Use of low intensity direct current in management of ischemic skin ulcers, *Phys Ther* 56(3):265, 1976.

Gentzkow G et al: Improved healing of pressure ulcers using Dermapulse®, a new electrical stimulation device, *Wounds* 3(5):158, 1991.

Goad RF et al: Diagnosis and treatment of decompression sickness. In Shilling CW, Carlston CB, Mathias RA, editors: *The physician's guide to diving medicine*, New York, 1984, Plenum Press.

Gottlieb SF, Neubauer RA: Multiple sclerosis: its etiology, pathogenesis, and therapeutics with emphasis on the controversial use of HBO, *J Hyperbaric Med* 3(3):43, 1988.

Griffin J et al: Efficacy of high voltage pulsed current for healing of pressure ulcers in patients with spinal cord injury, *Phys Ther* 71(6):433, 1991.

Hammarlund C: The physiologic effects of hyperbaric oxygen. In Kindwall EP, editor: *Hyperbaric medicine practice*, Flagstaff, Ariz, 1995, Best Publishing Company.

Hart GB: The monoplace chamber. In Kindwall EP, editor: *Hyperbaric medicine practice*, Flagstaff, Ariz, 1995, Best Publishing Company.

Hartnett JM: Use of vacuum-assisted wound closure in three chronic wounds, *J Wound Ostomy Continence Nurs* 25:281, 1998.

Hecker B, Carron H, Schwartz D: Pulsed galvanic stimulation: effects of current frequency and polarity on blood flow in healthy subjects, *Arch Phys Med Rehabil* 66(6):369, 1985.

Heimbach RD: Physiology and pharmacology of HBO_2. In *Jefferson C. Davis Wound Care and Hyperbaric Medicine Center* [Course]. Hyperbaric Medicine Team Training, Southwest Texas Methodist Hospital and Nix Medical Center, March 4, 1998, San Antonio, Tex.

Hirn M: Hyperbaric oxygen in the treatment of gas gangrene and perineal necrotizing fasciitis: a clinical and experimental study, *Eur J Surg* 570(suppl A9D):1, 1993.

Hsu LH, Wang JH: Treatment of carbon monoxide poisoning with hyperbaric oxygen, *Chung Hai I Hsueh Chih* 58(6):407, 1996.

Hughes AJ, Schwarer AP, Miller IL: Hyperbaric oxygen in the treatment of refractory haemorrhagic cystitis, *Bone Marrow Transplantation* 22(6):585, 1998.

Jaffe L, Vanable J: Electric fields and wound healing, *Clin Dermatol* 2(3):34, 1984.

Kaada B: Vasodilation induced by transcutaneous nerve stimulation in peripheral ischemia (Raynaud's phenonenon and diabetic polyneuropathy), *Eur Heart J* 3(4):303, 1982.

Kidder TM: Myringotomy. In Kindwall EP, editor: *Hyperbaric medicine practice*, Flagstaff, Ariz, 1995, Best Publishing Company.

Kindwall EP: A history of hyperbaric medicine. In Kindwall EP, editor: *Hyperbaric medicine practice*, Flagstaff, Ariz, 1995a, Best Publishing Company.

Kindwall EP: *Clinical hyperbaric medicine*. Environmental Tectonics Corporation, Feb 1, 1999. Available at etcusa.com/clinical.htm.

Kindwall EP: Contraindications and side effects to hyperbaric oxygen treatment. In Kindwall EP, editor: *Hyperbaric medicine practice*, Flagstaff, Ariz, 1995b, Best Publishing Company.

Kindwall EP: Gas embolism. In Kindwall EP, editor: *Hyperbaric medicine practice*, Flagstaff, Ariz, 1995c, Best Publishing Company.

Kindwall EP: Management of complications in hyperbaric treatment. In Kindwall EP, editor: *Hyperbaric medicine practice*, Flagstaff, Ariz, 1995d, Best Publishing Company.

Kindwall EP: The multiplace chamber. In Kindwall EP, editor: *Hyperbaric medicine practice*, Flagstaff, Ariz, 1995e, Best Publishing Company.

Kloth L, Feedar J: Acceleration of wound healing with high voltage, monophasic, pulsed current, *Phys Ther* 68(4):503, 1988.

Laden G: HOT MI pilot study: hyperbaric oxygen and thrombolysis in myocardial infarction [Letter], *Am Heart J* 136(4 Pt 1):749, 1998.

Lee HC et al: Hyperbaric oxygen therapy in clinical application: a report of a 12-year experience, *Chung Hua I Hsueh Tsa Chih (CHQ)* 43(5):301, 1989.

Ludwig LM: The role of hyperbaric oxygen in current emergency medical care, *J Emerg Nurs* 15(3):229, 1989.

Mader JT, Ortiz M, Calhoun JH: Update on the diagnosis and management of osteomyelitits, *Clin Podiatr* 13(4):701, 1996.

Maki RD: Ophthalmic side effects of hyperbaric oxygen therapy, *Insight* 21(4):114, 1996.

Marx RE: Radiation injury to tissue. In Kindwall EP, editor: *Hyperbaric medicine practice*, Flagstaff, Ariz, 1995, Best Publishing Company.

McCulloch J, Kloth L, Feedar J: *Wound healing alternatives in management*, ed 2, Philadelphia, 1995, F.A. Davis.

Morykwas MJ et al: Vacuum assisted closure: a new method for wound control and treatment: animal studies and basic foundation, *Ann Plast Surg* 38:553, 1997.

Mullner T et al: The use of negative pressure to promote healing of tissue defects; a clinical trial using the vacuum sealing technique, *Br J Plast Surg* 50:194, 1997.

National Fire Protection Association: *NFPA 99: standard for health care facilities*, Quincy, Mass, 1993, NFPA.

Nighoghossian N, Trouillas P: Hyperbaric oxygen in the treatment of the acute ischemic stroke: an unsettled issue, *J Neurol Sci* 150(1):27, 1997.

Neubauer R: Hyperbaric oxygen therapy beats carbon monoxide poisoning, decompression sickness, broken bones, gangrene, multiple sclerosis, severe burns, *Bottom Line/Health* 12(5):13, 1998.

Orida N, Feldman J: Directional protrusive pseudopodial activity and motility in macrophages induced by extracellular electric fields, *Cell Motil* 2:243, 1982.

Pascual J: Hyperbaric oxygen and relief of migraine and cluster headache, *J Neurosci* 27(4), 261, 1995.

Preslar L: *Annual report of the medical center*, Winston Salem, NC, 1995, Bowman Gray School of Medicine and North Carolina Baptist Hospitals.

Reillo MR, Altieri RJ: HIV antiviral effects of hyperbaric oxygen therapy, *J Assoc Nurses AIDS Care* 7(1):43, 1996.

Robertson W: Digby's receipts, *Ann Med History* 7(3):216, 1925.

Rowley B, McKenna J, Chase G: The influence of electrical current on an infecting microorganism in wounds, *Ann NY Acad Sci* 238:543, 1974.

Ryan T, Barnhill R: Physical factors and angiogenesis. In *Development of the vascular system*, London, 1983, Pitman Books.

Salzberg C et al: The effects of non-thermal pulsed electromagnetic energy (Diapulse®) on wound healing of pressure ulcers in spinal cord-injured patients: a randomized, double-blind study, *Wounds* 7(1):11, 1995.

Sawyer P, Pate J: Bio-electric phenomena as etiological agents in intravascular thrombosis, *Surgery* 34(3):491, 1957.

Sheffield PJ: Hyperbaric medicine: a historical perspective. In *Jefferson C. Davis Wound Care and Hyperbaric Medicine Center* [Course]. Hyperbaric Medicine Team Training, Southwest Texas Methodist Hospital and Nix Medical Center, March 1, 1998b, San Antonio, Tex.

Sheffield PJ: Physics of the hyperbaric environment. In *Jefferson C. Davis Wound Care and Hyperbaric Medicine Center* [Course]. Hyperbaric Medicine Team Training, Southwest Texas Methodist Hospital and Nix Medical Center, March 1, 1998a, San Antonio, Tex.

Shilling CW, Faiman MD: Physics of diving and physical effects on divers. In Shilling CW, Carlston CB, Mathias RA, editors: *The physician's guide to diving medicine*, New York, 1984, Plenum Press.

Siriwanij T, Vattanavongs V, Sitprija V: Hyperbaric oxygen therapy in crush injury [letter], *Nephron* 75(4):484, 1997.

Sparacia B, Sparacia G, Sansone A: *H.B.O. and cerebral investigations in stroke*. University of Palermo Institute of Anesthesiology/Undersea and Hyperbaric Oxygen Therapy Section, Jan 15, 1999. Available at mbox.unipa.it/~ccare/hbo/h_stroke.htm.

Stegmen DJ: Decompression sickness. In *Jefferson C. Davis Wound Care and Hyperbaric Medicine Center* [Course]. Hyperbaric Medicine Team Training, Southwest Texas Methodist Hospital and Nix Medical Center, March 3, 1998, San Antonio, Tex.

Stephens MB: Gas gangrene: potential for hyperbaric oxygen therapy, *Postgrad Med* 99(4):217, 1996.

Swanson K: The role of hyperbaric oxygen therapy in wound healing, *World Council of Enterostomal Therapists Journal*, 18(1):7, 1998.

Tai YJ et al: The use of hyperbaric oxygen for preservation of free flaps, *Ann Plast Surg* 28(3):284, 1992.

Undersea and Hyperbaric Medical Society: *Guidelines for clinical multiplace hyperbaric facilities: report of the Hy-*

perbaric Chamber Safety Committee of the Undersea and Hyperbaric Medical Society, Kensington, Md, 1994, UHMS.

Undersea and Hyperbaric Medical Society: *Hyperbaric oxygen therapy: a committee report*, Kensington, Md, 1996, UHMS.

Undersea and Hyperbaric Medical Society: *Purpose*, Jan 15, 1999. Available at www.uhms.org.

Vrabec JT, Clements KS, Mader JT: Short-term tympanostomy in conjunction with hyperbaric oxygen therapy, *Laryngoscope* 108(8):1124, 1998.

Wallace DJ et al: Use of hyperbaric oxygen in rheumatic diseases: case report and critical analysis, *Lupus* 4(3):172, 1995.

Weaver LK, Straas MB, editors: *Monoplace hyperbaric chamber safety guidelines: report to the Hyperbaric Chamber Safety Committee of the Undersea and Hyperbaric Medical Society*, Kensington, Md, 1991, UHMS.

Weiss D, Eaglstein W, Falanga V: Exogenous electric current can reduce the formation of hypertrophic scars, *J Dermatol Surg Oncol* 15(12):1272, 1989.

Wolcott L et al: Accelerated healing of skin ulcer by electrotherapy: preliminary clinical results, *South Med J* 62(7):795, 1969.

Wood J et al: A multicenter study on the use of pulsed low-intensity direct current for healing chronic stage II and stage III decubitus ulcers, *Arch Dermatol* 129(8):999, 1993.

Zonis Z et al: Salvage of the severely injured limb in children: a multidisciplinary approach, *Pediatr Emerg Care* 11(3):176, 1995.

CHAPTER

21

Principles for Practice Development

RUTH BRYANT

OBJECTIVES

1. Explain the role of the wound care nurse, including examples of how they function as an expert, educator, and researcher.
2. Discriminate among prevalence, cumulative incidence, and incidence rate, addressing the formula for each measure and the use of each measure.
3. Describe the essential elements of a time management database and how they can be used.

A comprehensive wound care program is essential to any organization, agency, or health care system, offering a full scope of services to their clientele. The wound care nurse is essential in facilitating state-of-the-art wound management, conducting education programs, controlling wound-related costs, facilitating quality improvement activities, and heightening staff and patient awareness of the Wound Patient's Bill of Rights (Appendix D). The wound care nurse is instrumental in bringing together many departments to more fully embrace and manage a patient's condition. There are many ways in which a wound care nurse can affect the quality of care in an organization or agency, including administrative activities, collaboration with materials management personnel, establishing a skin/wound care team, and consulting on patient care. Visibility and role clarity are important in building a successful wound care program in any setting.

Regardless of the health care setting in which the wound care nurse plans to practice, role implementation will share many common facets. For example, the wound care nurse often serves as a clinical expert, educator, and researcher. As a clinical expert, the nurse must determine the parameters of their practice and what should be expected of the nursing staff. This clear delineation of roles is important to avoid duplication of efforts, foster an empowering environment, and maximize efficient use of resources, including personnel. Table 21-1 provides some examples of role delineation.

WOUND CARE NURSE AS CLINICAL EXPERT

Fundamental activities of the clinical expert in any practice setting are the development of a wound care formulary and wound care policies and procedures and the implementation of these tools. These activities can pose a formidable task because a gap of 8 to 30 years exists between the reporting of research findings and adoption into clinical practice (MacGuire, 1990; Michel and Sneed, 1995). Furthermore, health care personnel's knowledge and attitudes concerning wound care and pressure ulcer prevention vary. Beitz, Fey, and O'Brien (1999) warn that, ". . . professional staff who perceive little need for additional wound care education may 'tune out' opportunities for increasing their knowledge base because they consider themselves 'competent.'" However, knowledge gaps among nursing staff concerning wound care are wide and unpredictable. Bostrom and Kenneth (1992) surveyed 245 staff registered nurses (RNs) from multiple health care settings about pressure sore prevention and found staff knowledge about pressure ulcer risk factors to be high (91% identified 9 out of 11 risk factors). Surprisingly, however, the staff did not consider promotion of skin integrity to be a priority, and only one third of the nurses had updated their knowledge re-

TABLE 21-1 Examples of Delineation of Roles: Wound Care Nurse and Staff Nurse

WOUND CARE NURSE	STAFF NURSE
1. Facilitate creation and implementation of pressure ulcer risk-assessment protocol.	Conduct risk assessment per protocol.
2. Establish protocol for prevention guidelines to correlate with risk assessment.	Implement appropriate risk-reduction interventions.
3. Establish protocol for management of minor skin lesions (candidiasis, skin tears, stage 1 and 2 pressure ulcers, etc.).	Implement appropriate care of minor skin lesions.
4. Formulate wound care formulary to specify indications and use parameters of wound dressings.	Use wound dressings as per formulary. Notify wound care nurse if product performs poorly or wound fails to respond.
5. Conduct wound assessment, establish plan of care for complex ulcers (i.e., leg ulcers, stage 3 and 4 pressure ulcers), and conduct regular re-evaluation of wound.	Notify wound care nurse of complex wounds. Implement appropriate care as per wound care nurse direction.
6. Provide regular staff education opportunities for updates in procedures, products, assessment, etc.	Identify and recommend topics of interest for staff education and updates.
7. Identify quality-improvement activities concerning wound care and risk assessment (e.g., documentation of interventions, reliability of assessments)	Participate in quality-improvement activities.

garding pressure ulcer treatment in the last 2 years. In a study of 75 experienced critical care nurses' knowledge of pressure ulcer prevention, staging, and description, Pieper and Mattern (1997) found that only a few had read the 1992 *AHCPR Guideline on Pressure Ulcer Prevention*. This is of concern since critical care patients constitute a large proportion of hospitalized patients with pressure ulcers.

Gaps in knowledge are primarily attributed to pressure ulcer risk assessment and prevention. Beitz, Fey, and O'Brien (1999) surveyed a convenience sample of RNs, licensed practical nurses (LPNs), and nurse aides (NAs) (n = 86) and found their greatest knowledge deficits to be in the areas of etiologic factors generating pressure ulcers, support surfaces, staging, and treatment modalities. In a retrospective study of 167 patients using high or low air-loss beds and using documentation as a reflection of nursing knowledge and abilities, Pieper et al (1990) reported that the nursing documentation was lacking critical wound descriptors such as location, stage, size, color, exudate, and odor. These knowledge gaps all underscore the importance of the role of the wound care nurse as educator.

WOUND CARE NURSE AS EDUCATOR

Knowledge about pressure ulcer prevention, appropriate wound care, and comprehensive, accurate documentation is essential to maintaining and restoring skin integrity. By auditing chart documentation or surveying the staff's knowledge about specific areas of wound care, the nurse can identify needs and target educational activities to satisfy those needs. When the staff receives information about pressure ulcer prediction and prevention and wound care on a routine basis, they have more knowledge about these conditions, the incidence of pressure ulcers declines, costs of care decreases, and healing rates improve (Jones et al, 1993; Pieper and Mott, 1995; Specht, Bergquist, and Frantz, 1995).

Although education is an important role and tool for the wound care nurse, it does not guarantee implementation of new policies or procedures or a change in practice patterns. The information could be viewed as a burden rather than an innovation that may decrease work time or improve patient outcomes (Landrum, 1998b). An individual's reaction to and decision about new information, ideas, or practice (i.e., innovations) is something

TABLE 21-2 Five Stages of Rogers' Innovation-Decision Process

STAGE	DESCRIPTION
1. Knowledge stage	An individual becomes aware of an innovation and of how it functions. May occur with reading, reviewing posted flyers, attending lectures, etc.
2. Persuasion stage	Formation of a favorable or unfavorable attitude toward an innovation. To form a favorable attitude, the individual must be convinced that the innovation has greater value than current practice (e.g., identify patients at risk for pressure ulcers or target appropriate interventions).
3. Decision stage	Individual receives enough information to form an opinion about innovation. The individual pursues activities that lead to adoption or rejection of the innovation.
4. Implementation stage	Once a decision to adopt the innovation has been made, barriers (structural, process, or psychic) to implementation must be overcome (e.g., adequate number of forms is available).
5. Confirmation stage	Individuals seek to reinforce their decision. Observable and positive results are critical at this stage to prevent a reversal in decision. Careful monitoring is required, and information validating positive effects is important (e.g., a decrease in the incidence of pressure ulcers after adoption of a new risk assessment tool).

Data from Landrum BJ: Marketing innovations to nurses, Part I. How people adopt innovations, *J Wound Ostomy Continence Nurs* 25:194, 1998.

TABLE 21-3 Attributes that Influence Adoption of Innovation

ATTRIBUTES OF INNOVATION	DESCRIPTION
Relative advantage	Is this better than an existing practice (e.g., potential decrease in costs, decrease in staff time, ease of use)?
Compatibility	Is this consistent with the individual's existing values, experiences, and needs?
Complexity	Is this innovation difficult to understand or use (e.g., when a protocol is developed that links risk-assessment scores with nursing interventions, the decision about which preventive nursing intervention to use may be perceived as less complex than before the protocol; therefore the protocol may be more likely to be adopted)?
Trialability	Can the individual experiment with the innovation on a limited basis?
Observability	Are the results of an innovation visible to others? Subtle outcomes are harder to communicate to others, so the innovation is often slower to be adopted.

Adapted from Landrum BJ: Marketing innovations to nurses, Part I. How people adopt innovations, *J Wound Ostomy Continence Nurs* 25:194, 1998.

that develops over time and is seldom spontaneous. Landrum (1998a) describes how people adopt innovations using five stages as defined by Rogers in *Diffusion of Innovations* (1995). Whether attempting to implement a new product or improve upon an existing product and whether the product is preventive or has immediate observable results, a failure to consider these stages can spell disaster and frustration. Table 21-2 outlines these stages, the definition of each stage, and considerations relative to the specialty of wound care.

Five attributes of the innovation significantly influence the rate at which it is adopted: relative advantage, compatability, complexity, trialability, and observability (Table 21-3). These attributes should be considered before the persuasion stage so that adjustments can be made to enhance the likelihood of success with the education efforts.

WOUND CARE NURSE AS RESEARCHER

The wound care nurse also serves as a researcher. The extent to which the nurse functions in this capacity

BOX 21-1 Formulas for Prevalence, Cumulative Incidence, and Incidence Rate

$$\text{Prevalence} = \frac{\text{Number of existing cases of a disease at a given point in time}}{\text{Total population during that point in time}}$$

$$\text{Cumulative incidence} = \frac{\text{Number of new cases of a disease during a given period of time}}{\text{Number of people considered to be at risk during that period of time}}$$

$$\text{Incidence rate} = \frac{\text{Number of new cases of a disease during a given period of time}}{\text{Total person-time of observation during that period of time}}$$

can vary widely depending on their educational preparation, agency support, and general interests. However, there are three research-based activities in which all wound care nurses should be involved: "mini-studies" that support quality-improvement activities, the critical appraisal and application of research to clinical practice, and data collection.

Quality-Improvement Activities

Quality-improvement activities may involve chart audits in an attempt to ascertain adequacy of documentation of assessment parameters, interventions, and effects or outcomes. Prevalence and incidence studies may also be conducted as part of quality-improvement activities. These types of studies can be an onerous undertaking but yield considerable information if the objective is clear from the onset.

Prevalence, cumulative incidence, and incidence rate are primary epidemiologic measures of disease frequency and are not interchangeable terms. Box 21-1 provides the formula for calculating these measures.

Prevalence. Prevalence is a measurement of the volume or frequency of a particular condition at a specific point in time. It is a proportion (or a ratio, not a rate*) that reflects how many people in a specific population have the condition (such as pressure ulcers) at a point in time. For example, the prevalence of pressure ulcers in the orthopedic unit for the month of July may be 5 out of a unit census of 50 (5/50, or 10%). Prevalence is a cross-sectional measure; it is essentially a snapshot in time and conveys how many pressure ulcers, for example, exist in a setting on a given day or during a specific time period. The issue of whether the condition is "new" or existing is irrelevant when calculating prevalence; all patients with the condition are counted. Generally considered to be stable, prevalence should not vary significantly over time unless changes in practice patterns, referral bases, or marketing have occurred or the average duration of the disease has increased. As a measure of disease frequency (or burden of disease), prevalence is a useful tool for health care planning (Pieper et al, 1999). It provides a means of identifying workload needs, staff needs, or resource allocation needs to meet the demands of that disease burden or volume (Baumgarten, 1998). Prevalence should never be misconstrued as a measure of quality of care or a measure of risk. An institution or agency that specializes in wound care is expected to have a high volume or prevalence of wounds based on the fact that their marketing strategies are geared to the recruitment or enrollment of patients with wounds.

Cumulative Incidence. Cumulative incidence, on the other hand, is a risk measure. It provides an estimate of the probability (risk) of developing a condition or disease over a specific period of time (Kelsey et al, 1996). The formula for calculating cumulative incidence is provided in Box 21-1. Several characteristics of cumulative incidence are important (Gordis, 1996):

1. Cumulative incidence is a measure of *new* cases (not existing cases) of a particular condition.
2. The denominator must include only those individuals at risk for developing the condition.
3. Cumulative incidence always refers to a specific time period (e.g., 1 day, 1 week, 1 month, or 1 year).
4. As with prevalence, cumulative incidence is a proportion (not a rate*) and ranges from 0 to 1 or 0% to 100%.

---

*A *rate* is strictly defined as a ratio in which the numerator and denominator are related (e.g., the numerator is a subset of the denominator) and the denominator contains a measure of time (e.g., number of pressure ulcers per 500 inpatients during a 1-month period) (Hennekens and Buring, 1987).

5. All individuals in the group at risk (represented by the denominator) are followed or observed for the entire time period specified.

To calculate cumulative incidence, consider the following situation. The number of patients with diabetes who have a major operation during July is 50 (the population at risk); 5 are admitted with an existing pressure ulcer, and 5 develop a pressure ulcer during that month. The cumulative incidence of pressure ulcers in the patient with diabetes after major surgery will be as follows: 50 patients minus the 5 patients with an existing pressure ulcer equals a total of 45 patients at risk (the denominator). Five of the 45 patients developed a pressure ulcer, so the cumulative incidence of pressure ulcers in patients with diabetes after a major operation during July is 5/45, or 11%.

An underlying assumption of the cumulative incidence is that all patients are at risk for the condition or disease for the same period of time. Not all patients in the denominator will be followed for the full time period specified; the follow-up period may not be uniform because some patients may be discharged early or die. For example, when calculating the cumulative incidence of pressure ulcers in the postoperative patient with diabetes for the month of July, the length of time that each patient with diabetes remains in the hospital will vary. Some patients may be in the hospital 3 days before discharge, whereas others may be in the hospital for 2 weeks after surgery. Consequently, these individuals will be observed (and at risk) for differing periods of time. The first patient is at risk of pressure ulcer formation for only 3 days, whereas the second patient is at risk for 2 weeks. Gallagher (1997) suggests using the average length of stay as the study time period to avoid the problem of variability in follow-up time. Another option that produces a more specific estimate of risk is to calculate the incidence rate (Baumgarten, 1998; Gordis, 1996; Hennekens and Buring, 1987; Oleske, 1995).

Incidence Rate. Incidence rate, also known as *incidence density*, is the rate at which new cases of disease occur in a specific time period, and is used when the individuals at risk in the study are followed for different lengths of time (Oleske, 1995). The numerator remains the same: the number of new conditions or diseases during a specified time period. However, the denominator, expressed in terms of person-time units, is the sum of the time each individual is observed and remains free of the condition. Relative to pressure ulcers, the person-time unit used is patient-days. *Person-years* is probably the more common term for person-time but is more appropriate for diseases that require a long time (years) between exposure and development of the disease.

Person-time is the sum of all the time that each individual in the study was followed. An example is provided in Table 21-4. Specifically, it is the time until the end of that patient's participation in the study. The patient's participation in the study may end because the specified time has passed, the patient died before the end of the study, or the patient developed the disease or condition being measured.

Conducting Prevalence and Incidence Studies. Various methods have been described for conducting an incidence and prevalence study (Baumgarten, 1998; Gallagher, 1997; Lake, 1999). One of the key decisions in planning the study is to decide what population to study, or the at-risk population. Many studies report incidence for hospital-wide populations, which assumes that all patients who are hospitalized are at risk. It is perhaps more feasible to conduct incidence and prevalence studies on targeted patient populations (Aronovitch, 1999; Grous, Reilly, and Gift, 1997; Hammond et al, 1994; Jacksich, 1997). For example, a study could examine all patients experiencing an operation lasting 3 hours or longer, all patients with a specific diagnosis such as hip fracture, patients who have diabetes and are admitted to home care from Hospital Z, or all patients on a specific hospital unit. Allman and colleagues (1995) reported a 12.9% cumulative incidence of pressure ulcers after a median of 9 days from admission to final skin examination in a very specific patient population: patients were 55 years of age or older, had a hip fracture, or were confined to bed or chair for at least 5 days, and did not have a stage 3 or greater pressure ulcer.

It is also possible to create an ongoing monthly record of incident cases by establishing a policy that all new pressure ulcers are reported to one central location (Figure 21-1), such as the wound care nurse or the infection control nurse (Kartes, 1996). In doing so, the incident pressure ulcer for

TABLE 21-4 Calculation of Person-Time for Incidence Rate in a 30-Day Unit-Based Study

PATIENT	DEVELOPED A PRESSURE ULCER?	EVENT	NUMBER OF DAYS IN STUDY
1	No	Discharged on day 4	4
2	No	Discharged on day 15	15
3	Yes	Still in hospital day 30	30
4	No	Transferred to nursing home on day 22	22
5	Yes	Died on day 10	10
6	Yes	Transferred to different unit on day 12 and discharged from hospital on day 19	12
7	Yes	Discharged on day 5; readmitted 3 days later; discharged on day 7	5
8	No	Discharged on day 9	9
Totals:			
8 new patients	4 new cases		107 patient days

Incidence (density) rate = 4 new pressure ulcers per 107 patient days
= 4 ÷ 107
= 0.037 pressure ulcers per patient day, or 3.7 pressure ulcers per 100 patient days. A factor of 10 may be used to calculate the rate so that the decimal fraction created by dividing a large at-risk population (the denominator) into a small number of events (the numerator) can be eliminated. Generally, it is desirable to use the power of ten (i.e., 10, 100, 1000) that moves at least one digit to the left of the decimal point.

1 month must then be counted only as a prevalent pressure ulcer in the subsequent months. Furthermore, patients will be hospitalized for varying lengths of time so that they are not all at risk for the same time period. Therefore an incidence rate using person-time units in the denominator rather than an average census should be calculated. Because this ongoing monthly record of incident cases relies on staff reports, some incident cases might be missed that would result in an underreporting of pressure ulcer incidence. Strategies such as comparing monthly reports with periodic audits could be conducted to assess reliability of this reporting method.

Generalizability of Incidence and Prevalence Measures. Benchmarking is a common practice for quality-improvement activities. However, comparing one setting's incidence and prevalence data with published incidence and prevalence data can lead to erroneous conclusions (Mark and Burleson, 1995). The key is to look at who was included in the incidence and prevalence study. For example, many studies do not include stage 1 pressure ulcers. Therefore this actually results in an underreporting of the frequency of pressure ulcers. Similarly, it is important to look at how incidence or prevalence was calculated; the choice of denominator will influence the resulting frequency. Patient populations should also be similar to justify comparing incidence from different sources. It is also possible to calculate incidence and prevalence according to severity of risk as determined by the Braden Scale (Lake, 1999). This is a method of "adjusting" or standardizing incidence and prevalence according to risk level as is commonly done for patient acuity.

Although the incidence measures obtained from a narrow or specific at-risk patient population are unlikely to be appropriate to compare or benchmark against national incidence measures, repeated studies within the patient population of interest will provide a baseline and trends. The key advantages to conducting incidence studies on a defined at-risk patient population are twofold:

1. The study suddenly becomes much more feasible and less labor intensive. Implementation is vastly simplified by restricting the types of patient included.
2. In response to the results obtained, an appropriate intervention specific for that patient population can be identified and implemented in a manageable and effective manner.

Critical Appraisal and Application of Research Findings

Research findings must be used to aid decision-making in patient care. Rather than requesting samples of a new dressing or product to trial informally, the wound care nurse should request and expect randomized controlled clinical trials demonstrating efficacy (the product performs as expected), safety (the product does not increase the patient's risk of harm or adverse events), and effectiveness (the product performs as expected in the real world of missed appointments, dressing change delays, etc.).

Although it is easy to be tempted by glossy case series or anecdotal reports, such documents lack the scientific rigor necessary to ensure an unbiased appraisal of the product's performance. Unfortunately, scientific studies on wound care products are sparse. This is largely because wound dressings are considered by the FDA as nonsignificant risk devices and only require safety data and a demonstration of "equivalency to an existing device" (Bolton, 1995). The wound care nurse should review published guidelines such as those published by the Wound, Ostomy and Continence Nurses Society (WOCN, 1992a, 1992b), the Wound Healing Society (WHS), the National Guideline Clearinghouse (www.guideline.gov), the Clinical Practice Guidelines Directory (AMA, 1999), and the Cochrane Collaboration (www.cochrane.org) to remain current. Several textbooks, journal articles, and websites (see Appendix E) are available for further information on clinical trial design, systematic reviews, guidelines, and evidence-based practice (Bolton, 1995; Kelsey et al, 1996; Oleske, 1995; Piantadosi, 1997; Rothman and Greenland, 1998).

Data Collection

Data collection is a critical function for the wound care nurse. This becomes the tool by which workload is measured, trends are identified, outcomes are quantified, and the valuable contribution of the wound care nurse is communicated (WOCN, 1999b). Data measurement (i.e., data collection) and practice improvement are inseparable; improvement requires measurement (Nelson et al, 1998). Data collection should be of two types: a time management program and a clinical practice database.

Time Management Data Collection

When cost containment, efficient use of resources, and managed care dominate discussions, information concerning time use is invaluable. This type of data can validate any subjective perception of an increase or change in workload and communicates a much stronger objective message to management. Data should be recorded daily and tabulated weekly, monthly, quarterly, and annually. Additional sample forms for data collection are provided in Figures 21-1 to 21-6. Summary data (e.g., number of patient referrals, number of visits, average length of visits, average number of visits per patient or wound type, reason for referral, number of projects/activities, and time per project) should be submitted to the wound care nurse's supervisor on a monthly basis with trends highlighted. Plots can graphically display time or volume by month. Data collection can be maintained in paper format, although a computerized time management data collection tool is also available (WOCN, 1999a). The computer-savvy wound care nurse can also enter these data elements into one of the many commercially available computer software packages for data management.

Clinical Practice Data Collection

The clinical practice data collection tool should serve as an information system within which demographic and clinical data can be stored and nursing interventions and outcomes can be documented (Jacobson, 1996). To be most useful, the clinical practice data collection tool should be integrated with the agency or institution information system and computerized. This reduces duplication of data entry, reduces the potential for errors in data entry, and expands the amount of information, correlations, and comparisons that can be extracted. Although several patient care-based data sets exist (e.g., Nursing Minimum Data Set, the OMAHA Intervention

Text continued on p. 469

Unit or Station (Year) ______________

	Jan	Feb	Mar	Apr	May	June	July	Aug	Sept	Oct	Nov	Dec	Average
1. # of patients w/pressure ulcer from previous month													
2. New admits w/pressure ulcer													
3. # of patients w/new pressure ulcer (developed this month at this facility)													
4. Total # patients with pressure ulcer													
5. Total # patient days													
6. Prevalence = item 4/item 5													
7. Incidence rate (density) = item 3/item 5													

8. Source of new admit:													
a. Hospital xyz													
b. Hospital abc													
c. Community													
9. Site of new pressure ulcers													
a. Trochanter													
b. Ischial tuberosity													
c. Heels													
d. Sacrum													

Figure 21-1 Sample pressure ulcer monthly prevalence and incidence documentation. (Modified from Kartes SK: A team approach for risk assessment, prevention, and treatment of pressure ulcers in nursing home patients, *J Nurse Care Qual* 10(3):34, 1996.)

Rm #	Patient name	Adm date	Consult date	Adm diagnosis	Type of wound	MD	Time (15 min = 1 unit)					Total # visits	Total # units
							Mon	Tues	Wed	Thurs	Fri		

Figure 21-2 Sample weekly activity worksheet and patient demographics.

Date ____________

	Monday		Tuesday		Wednesday		Thursday		Friday		Totals	
	Units	Visits	Units	Visits	Units	Visits	Units	Visits	Units	Visits	Units	Visits
Facility A (or unit)												
Facility B (or unit)												
Clinic												
Projects: Research committee												
Forms committee												
Quality improvement												
Activities: Administration												
Staff education												
Grand Totals												

Figure 21-3 Sample weekly time summary form (Units = 15 min).

Month/Year ____________________

Patient name	Age	Facility			Type patient		Wound etiology*	Reason for consultation	Total # visits	Total # units
		Xyz	Abc	Tuv	New	Return				

*Wound etiology codes:

1 = Arterial ulcer
2 = Venous ulcer
3 = Pressure ulcer stage 1
4 = Pressure ulcer stage 2
5 = Pressure ulcer stage 3
6 = Pressure ulcer stage 4
7 = Pressure ulcer unstagable
8 = Diabetic neuropathy
9 = Mixed arterial/venous
10 = Epidermal stripping
11 = Burn
12 = Perianal denudation
13 = Candidiasis
14 = Pyoderma gangrenosum
15 = Fistula
16 = Other

Figure 21-4 Sample demographics record.

(Week) Month/Year ______________

Activity	Total number	# of units	# of visits
Patient Care			
Inpatients			
Clinic patients			
New referrals (inpatients)			
Reason for Referral			
Arterial ulcer			
Venous ulcer			
Mixed arterial/venous			
Pressure ulcer			
Projects			
Activities			

Figure 21-5 Sample weekly/monthly activity summary.

Wound Location:
_____ Sacrum
_____ Ischium L ____ R ____
_____ Trochanter L ____ R ____
_____ Heel L ____ R ____
_____ Medial malleolus L ____ R ____
_____ Lateral malleolus L ____ R ____
_____ Knee L ____ R ____
_____ Other (site: ____________________)

Wound History:
_____ Pressure ulcer stage when first detected
_____ Date wound first detected
_____ Type of wound
Art = Arterial
VSU = Venous ulcer
Mixed = Mixed venous/arterial ulcer
Diab = Diabetic/neuropathic ulcer
PU = Pressure ulcer
Other: please specify etiology

DATE Wound parameter						
Length						
Width						
Depth						
Tunnel or undermining						
% Granulation						
Tissue						
% Eschar						
% Slough						
% Fibrin covering						
Volume of exudate (large, moderate, small, none)						
Type of exudate (serous, sero-sanguinous, purulent)						
Odor (yes, no)						
Surrounding skin:						
• Intact (yes/no)						
• Inflamed (yes/no)						
• Indurated (yes/no)						
• Denuded (yes/no)						
• Maceration (yes/no)						

Figure 21-6 Sample wound documentation.

Classification Scheme, the Minimum Data Set Plus, and OASIS), no standardized minimum database for wound care exists. Bates-Jensen (1995), the WOCN (1999a), and the National Pressure Ulcer Advisory Panel (NPUAP, 1999) have taken steps to create clinical practice data sets.

SUMMARY

Establishing a wound care practice within an institution or home care setting or in private practice requires the skills of an entrepreneur and a strong foundation in pathophysiology and clinical management. The wound care nurse must determine how his or her role will be implemented, how his or her relationship with colleagues will be defined, what quality management processes can be implemented, and what type of data is needed. Data should describe how time is spent and what outcomes are being achieved. The wound care nurse must also stay current in the art and science of wound management by adopting lifelong learning strategies such as regularly attending continuing education programs, critically reading journals, and monitoring select websites (see Appendix E). The time and energy spent in initial and ongoing practice development is critical to a successful, satisfying, and effective wound care practice.

SELF-ASSESSMENT EXERCISE

1. Which of the following activities is reflective of a wound care nurse operating in a consultant capacity within an institution?
   - **a.** Encourage referrals to the wound care nurse for patients with stage I and 2 pressure ulcers
   - **b.** Conduct routine dressing changes for assessment purposes
   - **c.** Establish protocols for pressure ulcer risk reduction based on level of risk
   - **d.** Perform reassessment of pressure ulcer risk twice weekly
2. When implementing a new process for pressure ulcer risk reduction, you plan to meet with several staff nurses to discuss what is currently being done, discuss the current national standards, and present the advantages of the new process. According to Roger's Innovation-Decision Process, which stage does this reflect?
   - **a.** Knowledge stage
   - **b.** Persuasion stage
   - **c.** Decision stage
   - **d.** Confirmation stage
3. Which of the following statements is true of incidence density?
   - **a.** Incidence density is a rate that describes how many people have a particular condition at a specific point in time
   - **b.** Incidence density is a rate expressed in terms of person-time units
   - **c.** Incidence density is a measure used to identify workload or staff needs
   - **d.** Incidence density is calculated with a numerator that includes all the patients at risk for the disease
4. When a long-term care institution specializes in wound management, it can be anticipated that which of the following measures would be higher than the national average?
   - **a.** Cumulative incidence
   - **b.** Incidence rate
   - **c.** Prevalence
   - **d.** Cumulative incidence and prevalence

REFERENCES

Allman RM et al: Pressure ulcer risk factors among hospitalized patients with activity limitation, *JAMA* 273(11):865, 1995.

American Medical Association: *Clinical practice guidelines directory*, Chicago, 1999, AMA.

Aronovitch S: Intraoperatively acquired pressure ulcer prevalence: a national study, *J Wound Ostomy Continence Nurs* 26(3):130, 1999.

Bates-Jensen BM: Toward an intelligent wound assessment system, *Ostomy Wound Manage* 41(suppl 7A):80s, 1995.

Baumgarten M: Designing prevalence and incidence studies, *Adv Wound Care* 11:287, 1998.

Beitz JM, Fey J, O'Brien D: Perceived need for education vs actual knowledge of pressure ulcer care in a hospital nursing staff, *Dermatol Nurs* 11(2):125, 1999.

Bolton L: Clinical studies and product evaluations: how to maximize their value, *Ostomy Wound Manage* 41(suppl 7A): 88S, 1995.

Bostrom J, Kenneth H: Staff nurse knowledge and perceptions about prevention of pressure sores, *Dermatol Nurs* 4(5):365, 1992.

Gallagher SM: Outcomes in clinical practice: pressure ulcer prevalence and incidence studies, *Ostomy Wound Manage* 43(1):28, 1997.

Gordis L: *Epidemiology*, Philadelphia, 1996, W.B. Saunders.

Grous CA, Reilly NJ, Gift AG: Skin integrity in patients undergoing prolonged operations, *J Wound Ostomy Continence Nurs* 24:86, 1997.

Hammond MC et al: Pressure ulcer incidence on a spinal cord injury unit, *Adv Wound Care* 7(6)57, 1994.

Hennekens CH, Buring JE: *Epidemiology in medicine*, Boston, 1987, Little, Brown and Company.

Jacksich BB: Pressure ulcer prevalence and prevention of nosocomial development: one hospital's experience, *Ostomy Wound Manage* 43(3):32, 1997.

Jacobson T: Standardized ET Nursing database: imagine the possibilities, *J Wound Ostomy Continence Nurs* 23:5, 1996.

Jones S et al: A pressure ulcer prevention program, *Ostomy Wound Manage* 39:33, 1993.

Kartes SK: A team approach for risk assessment, prevention, and treatment of pressure ulcers in nursing home patients, *J Nurse Care Qual* 10(3):34, 1996.

Kelsey JL et al: *Methods in observational epidemiology*, ed 2, New York, 1996, Oxford University Press.

Lake NO: Measuring incidence and prevalence of pressure ulcers for intergroup comparison, *Adv Wound Care* 12:31, 1999.

Landrum BJ: Marketing innovations to nurses, Part 1. How people adopt innovations, *J Wound Ostomy Continence Nurs* 25:194, 1998a.

Landrum BJ: Marketing innovations to nurses, Part 2. Marketing's role in the adoption of innovations, *J Wound Ostomy Continence Nurs* 25:227, 1998b.

MacGuire JM: Putting nursing research findings into practice: research utilization as an aspect of the management of change, *J Adv Nurse* 15:614, 1990.

Mark BA, Burleson BL: Measurement of patient outcomes: data availability and consistency across hospitals, *JONA* 25(4):52, 1995.

Michel Y, Sneed N: Dissemination and use of research findings in nursing practice, *J Prof Nurse* 11:306, 1995.

National Pressure Ulcer Advisory Panel: *PUSH tool*, August, 1999. Available at www.npuap.org/pushins.htm.

Nelson EC et al: Building measurement and data collection in to medical practice, *Ann Intern Med* 128:460, 1998.

Oleske DM, editor: *Epidemiology and the delivery of health care services: methods and applications*, New York, 1995, Plenum Press.

Piantadosi S: *Clinical trials: a methodologic perspective*, New York, 1997, John Wiley & Sons.

Pieper B et al: Nurses' documentation about pressure ulcers, *Decubitus* 3:32, 1990.

Pieper B et al: Wound prevalence, types and treatment in home care, *Adv Wound Care* 12:117, 1999.

Pieper B, Mattern JC: Critical care nurses' knowledge of pressure ulcer prevention, staging, and description, *Ostomy Wound Manage* 43(2):22, 1997.

Pieper B, Mott M: Nurses' knowledge of pressure ulcer prevention, staging, and description, *Adv Wound Care* 8:34, 1995.

Rogers EM: *Diffusion of innovations*, ed 4, New York, 1995, Free Press.

Rothman KJ, Greenland S: *Modern epidemiology*, ed 2, Philadelphia, 1998, Lippincott-Raven.

Specht JP, Bergquist S, Frantz R: Adoption of research-based practice for treatment of pressure ulcers, *Nurs Clin North Am* 30:553, 1995.

Wound, Ostomy and Continence Nurses Society: *Standards of care: patients with dermal wounds: lower extremity ulcers*, Laguna Beach, Calif, 1992a, WOCN.

Wound, Ostomy and Continence Nurses Society: *Standards of care: patients with dermal wounds: pressure ulcers*, Laguna Beach, Calif, 1992b, WOCN.

Wound, Ostomy and Continence Nurses Society: *Patient information data base*, Laguna Beach, Calif, 1999a, WOCN.

Wound, Ostomy and Continence Nurses Society: *Professional practice manual*, ed 2, Laguna Beach, Calif, 1999b, WOCN.

CHAPTER 22

Home Environment: Implications for Wound Care Practice Development

KRISTY WRIGHT & LAURIE LOVEJOY McNICHOL

OBJECTIVES

1. Describe how the Outcome and Assessment Information Set (OASIS) database affects the practice of the wound care nurse.
2. Describe how *homebound status* and *home* are defined in terms of qualifying for home care.
3. Explain the strengths that the wound care nurse brings to the home care program.
4. List at least five wound characteristics that Medicare considers sufficient to qualify the patient for a skilled nurse visit.
5. Identify documentation requirements for Medicare reimbursement of home care services.
6. Distinguish among the different methods of reimbursement for home care services.

Essential to the success of service delivery in the home is the basic element of trust. In this setting, home health care providers are entrusted with the privilege of an intimate view of family living that is ordinarily reserved for family members only (Doherty, Hurley, and Perfetti, 1994). Home health care professionals and paraprofessionals become privy to and connected with family dynamics, interactions, lifestyle choices, multigenerational relationships, coping strategies, and financial issues, usually at a time of critical vulnerability for the patient and the family. The nurse, using refined communication skills, must learn what the patient and family's desired goals and outcomes are and accept that they may not be the same as those of the health care professional. It is important to remember that the health care provider is an invited guest in a patient's home.

PHYSICAL CONDITIONS OF THE HOME

The nurse's ability to affect the patient's outcome in the home care setting is influenced by the home environment. For example, without an adequate water supply, wound care programs are affected. Unsanitary conditions and the presence of insects or vermin negatively affect wound care interventions. All home care nurses must be vigilant for personal safety issues for their clients and for themselves because they visit in a variety of home environments. Generally, principles of infection control in home care are the same as in other settings, although adjustments can be made in specific circumstances to accommodate either the facilities or caregiver capabilities. To summarize, those things that affect clinical care affect the outcomes of care.

CAREGIVERS

Inherent to the intermittent nature of home health care is the ability of patients to care for themselves between the nurse's visits, with or without the assistance of a caregiver. Although this sounds reasonable, on closer inspection, it is troublesome. As the elderly population grows, an increasing number of elderly people will have health problems that prevent them from caring for themselves.

Caregivers fall into two broad categories: 1) caregivers working for pay who are part of the formal health care sector (i.e., homecare workers) and 2) unpaid "informal" caregivers (usually family members) who are motivated by a deeper commitment to the patient. (In this section, the term *family caregiver* is used, although it is recognized that often the informal caregiver is not related to the patient.) The ideal picture is one of families caring for seniors or seniors caring for other seniors. In reality, demographic trends suggest that family members may not be available to provide care when needed and that seniors may be suffering from a chronic illness when they are needed as a family caregiver.

Additionally, family caregivers of chronically ill patients have been shown to experience psychosocial, physical, and economic burdens, which negatively affect their quality of life (Covinsky, Goldman, and Cook, 1994). The proportion of caregivers experiencing anxiety and depression is often greater than the proportion of patients experiencing those same symptoms (Shulz, Visintainer, and Williamson, 1990). In many instances, the home health nurse must see to the needs of an entire family system.

OUTCOME-BASED/ EVIDENCE-BASED PRACTICE

Home care nursing research and researchers are entering an exciting era of growth and opportunity. Although the momentum of home care research activities is less than that of the industry in general, interest in practice-based nursing research is expanding. The number, diversity, and sophistication of studies being conducted are increasing. Most importantly, research studies are being developed to address significant practice issues, and findings are being used in the practice setting, a trend that will lead to improved client care (Martin, 1988). Nurses contribute at every level, from study design to data collection, and must continually strive to critically review and selectively apply research study findings to their practice.

Specifically, home care nurses may be expected to contribute to agency standards of care, develop policies and procedures and clinical pathways, participate in competency checks for both new and experienced staff nurses, and/or lead interdisciplinary teams within their specialty. They may be responsible for quarterly data collection and use the information found to develop materials that the agency could use for marketing purposes (e.g., patient or physician satisfaction surveys, decrease in cost per visit data, etc.).

OUTCOME-BASED QUALITY IMPROVEMENT AND OASIS DATA SET

Outcome-based quality improvement (OBQI) resulted from a project that began in 1988 when the Health Care Financing Administration (HCFA) began looking for a way to develop outcome measures for home care on a nationwide basis. Simultaneously, the Robert Wood Johnson Foundation was reviewing home care outcome measures on a more local agency level and was interested in dovetailing their work with the national project to measure home care quality in a comprehensive manner (Crister, 1997). The early discussions resulted in a 5-year project when the HCFA awarded the University of Colorado Center for Health Services and Policy Research a contract to explore the following questions (Shaughnessy et al, 1994):

1. Could valid outcome measures of home care quality be developed?
2. What were the data items necessary to measure patient outcomes in a valid and reliable way?
3. Would outcome measures provide a way to distinguish between home health agencies if quality of care was used as a measure?

Initially the group studied sources of patient level information available in a few agencies to determine if the information needed for outcome measures was already being collected. They also considered if collecting additional information or information in a different format would present an unreasonable burden to home health staff. The group determined a large set of outcome measures for preliminary evaluation and, in 1991, set about to test if the measures were valid and reliable and could determine the quality of home care delivered to patients.

During this phase, researchers considered that the outcomes, once validated as useful for quality improvement activities, could be analyzed in statistical comparisons. Agencies could then acquire an outcome report showing them how they compare with other agencies or with themselves in a prior period (Crister, 1997). Home care organizations could explore how they could improve care that was found less than optimal or reinforce aspects of care delivery that were exemplary. The effect of interventions could be evaluated in the next outcome report.

At the completion of the study in 1994, the branch of HCFA known as the Health Standards and Quality Bureau (HSQB), took the set of data items and established a work group with representatives from different disciplines: a physical, occupational, and speech therapist; a social worker; one physician; and several nurses. Their task was to develop a comprehensive assessment instrument that would also include the items necessary to measure outcomes (Crister, 1997). The group made recommendations of core assessment items that could be used for all patient types. After evaluating the outcome measurement items from the OBQI initial project and agreeing that they were valid, they added 12 general assessment and care data items to the list. Therefore this data collection tool is called an Outcome and Assessment Information Set (OASIS) (Shaughnessy et al, 1994).

The OASIS tool is designed to measure changes in adult clients' health status and to statistically risk-adjust these outcomes. The OASIS data are collected at the initiation of care, at follow-up, and at discharge to determine the effectiveness of interventions and to document outcomes.

After the adoption of this tool, the HCFA requested that the program be tested in a demonstration project that would further test the instrument and the OBQI approach. Currently, organizations receiving Medicare or Medicaid reimbursement must collect OASIS data and implement OBQI. Likewise, ORYX, the name the Joint Commission on Accreditation of Healthcare Organizations (JCAHO) has given to the accreditation requirement pertaining to the collection of OASIS data, states that those agencies failing to collect outcomes data and implement performance improvement will not be in JCAHO compliance.

It is imperative that nurses working in home care understand and become involved with their agencies' plan to interpret OASIS data and in the overall OBQI plan to improve outcomes in targeted problem areas.

QUALIFYING CRITERIA FOR HOME CARE SERVICES

How a patient qualifies for home care services varies with the third-party payer. Medicare, being the largest payer of home care services, has the most comprehensive requirements. These complex, frequently revised, and often controversial guidelines dictate the qualifying criteria for home care services and the type and frequency of care provided. Other payers frequently fashion their criteria as some variation of the Medicare requirements. If the patient is self-pay or the home care provider is under a capitated agreement, however, the type and amount of care provided are ideally determined by patient need and the provider of services.

All types of third party payers cover skilled nursing services provided in the home care setting. Typically, *home* is defined as a patient's place of residence, including his or her own home, an apartment, a relative's home, a personal care home, or another type of nonskilled institution. A patient usually does not qualify for home care services if he or she resides in a skilled nursing or intermediate-care facility.

Depending on the third party payer, the patient may have to meet certain "homebound" criteria. In general, a patient will be considered to be homebound if he or she has a condition caused by an illness or injury that restricts his or her ability to leave the home (except with the assistance of supportive devices such as crutches, canes, walkers, and wheelchairs or the assistance of another person) or if leaving the home is medically contraindicated. The condition of these patients should be such that there exists a normal inability to leave home and, consequently, leaving home would require a considerable effort.

For home care services to be reimbursable, the services provided must be reasonable and medically necessary to the treatment of the patient's illness or injury. The method of reviewing this eligibility criterion is determined in different ways depending on the third party payer. Medicare performs postcare reviews of services provided and retroactively approves or denies reimbursement. In serving Medicare patients, the home care provider is expected to evaluate the need for services, determine eligibility, and provide only those services that meet Medicare guidelines. Most managed care payers require preapproval for services to be reimbursed. Through documentation and discussion with the home care provider, a case manager from the managed care company determines the necessity, frequency, and duration of ongoing home care services.

Usually the availability of a willing and able caregiver does not affect the patient's eligibility to receive home care if there is a documented need for skilled home health services. The trend for all payer sources, however, is to stabilize the patient's condition and teach the patient and caregivers the necessary skills in order to provide self-care with the short-term intermittent intervention of a nurse or other skilled provider. The once permissible long lengths of stay, often spanning several months or even years, are no longer accepted as reasonable home care.

Specifically, skilled nursing care is typically considered reasonable and necessary for a patient with a wound to perform 1) assessment and observation, 2) complex dressing changes and 3) teaching and training of patient and family. The complexity of the dressing change, the overall condition of the patient, and the ability of the caregiver may justify more frequent nursing visits if thorough assessment and documentation clearly substantiate the need.

For example, if a patient has a wound requiring a routine daily dressing change, skilled nursing assessment would be reasonable for a short period to monitor the progress of wound healing. The daily dressing changes would require a skilled nurse to teach the patient or caregiver the procedure and monitor his or her technique. Once wound healing is considered "stable" (e.g., expected healing rate without infection or other complications), nursing management would be reasonable and necessary to periodically assess the wound and revise the plan of care as needed. If the wound was draining or was infected and the caregiver was unable to manage a more complicated dressing change, daily visits by the nurse for a longer period of time may be reasonable.

DOCUMENTATION REQUIREMENTS FOR REIMBURSEMENT

As with qualifying criteria, documentation requirements for home care services specific to reimbursement vary with the third-party payer. All payers require a signed physician's order and plan of treatment for the provision of skilled home care services. The home care nurse usually participates in developing the plan of treatment with the physician. Input from the nurse includes assessment of the patient's condition, environmental factors, and available resources.

Other documentation requirements include a nursing care plan, nursing assessments, and progress notes. These documents are frequently used to determine the patient's eligibility for skilled home care and the ongoing need for services.

Although not a requirement, photographs are helpful when providing care to a patient with a wound. A single picture or a series of pictures can document the condition, progress, or deterioration of a wound and substantiate the need for home care services when written description does not suffice.

MEDICARE REQUIREMENTS FOR WOUND CARE

Medicare specifically addresses coverage for wound care services provided by a home health care nurse. Wounds may include but are not limited to ulcers, burns, pressure sores, open surgical sites, fistulas, tube sites, and tumor erosion. For skilled nursing services to be considered reasonable and necessary to treat the wound, the size, depth, nature of drainage (color, odor, consistency, and quantity), condition, and appearance of the skin surrounding the wound must be documented (HCFA, 1996). Although staging of a pressure ulcer is appropriate for descriptive purposes, coverage of the home care services is not based solely on the stage of the wound.

All clinical findings and the physician's plan of care are considered in determining the reasonableness and necessity of the services provided. Box 22-1 lists the wound characteristics that Medicare considers to usually require the skills of a nurse.

Wounds that show redness, edema, or induration without further documentation of complications are not considered to require direct hands-on care by a skilled nurse but may still require observation and assessment.

REIMBURSEMENT METHODS

Cost Reimbursement

Medicare has reimbursed home care providers under the cost reimbursement method since it began covering this type of health care in the mid-1960s.

BOX 22-1 Wound Characteristics Interpreted by Medicare to Require Skilled Nursing Visits

1. Open wounds that are draining purulent or colored exudate, have a foul odor present, or for which the patient is receiving antibiotic therapy
2. Wounds with a drain or T-tube
3. Wounds that require irrigation or instillation of a sterile cleansing or medicated solution and/or packing with sterile gauze
4. Recently debrided wounds
5. Pressure sores with the following characteristics:
   a. Partial tissue loss with signs of infection
   b. Full-thickness tissue loss that involves exposure of adipose tissue or invasion of other tissue such as muscle or bone
6. Wounds that have a proclivity for hemorrhage, especially with the dressing change
7. Open wounds or widespread skin complications after radiation therapy or as a result of immune deficiency or vascular insufficiency
8. Postoperative wounds where there are complications such as infection or allergic reaction or where there is an underlying disease that has a reasonable potential to adversely affect healing (e.g., diabetes)
9. Second- and third-degree burns where the size of the burn or presence of complications causes skilled nursing care to be needed
10. Skin conditions that require application of nitrogen mustard or other chemotherapeutic medication that presents a significant risk to the patient
11. Other open or complex wounds that require treatment that can only be provided safely and effectively by a licensed nurse
12. Foot care and nail trimming for patients with diabetes or circulatory problems

From Health Care Financing Administration: *Medicare home health agency manual,* Baltimore, Md, 1996, USDHHS, HCFA.

Simplistically, this is a retrospective type of reimbursement method that reimburses the provider whatever it costs to provide the service.

Since there is no incentive to contain costs in this method, Medicare also stipulates certain "caps" on the amount it will pay. Limits are set for each discipline of care (e.g., nursing, physical therapy, home health aide, etc.), and reimbursement is determined by an "aggregate per visit limit or cost cap." Medicare will pay a home care provider an aggregate cost per visit up to this limit. The visit caps vary throughout the country depending on location, wage costs, and other variables. The provider's aggregate cost per visit is determined by adding the total costs for all visits regardless of discipline, certain routine patient care supplies (e.g., gloves, Band-Aids, etc.), and associated overhead costs (also referred to as *general and administrative costs*), and then dividing by the total number of visits billed.

Before the proliferation of managed care, many of the commercial third-party payers had indemnity health plans that also reimbursed on a cost basis, some without caps. Although a few of these plans still exist, they are quickly becoming the exception and not the rule.

Interim Payment System

In late 1997 and early 1998, Medicare implemented a revised cost-reimbursement method that was intended to contain home health care costs in the "interim" until a prospective payment system could be devised as was legislated in the Balanced Budget Act of 1997. This method is referred to as the *Interim Payment System* (IPS). Although the IPS is still a cost-reimbursement method, it contains a per-beneficiary cap in addition to the visit cap. The per-beneficiary cap also varies throughout the country and with each provider. The per-beneficiary cap establishes an aggregate payment limit per patient admitted to a home health provider. The patient can only be counted once per annum; therefore readmissions of the same patient in a fiscal year do not count as an additional patient. Each home health provider determines their exact cap through a complex series of calculations specified by the HCFA.

An example of a per-beneficiary calculation is $3000 per patient per year. To stay under this calculated per-beneficiary cap, a home health provider would have to have average costs per individual patient of no more than $3000.

Under the IPS, a provider must stay under both the visit and per-beneficiary cost caps. This has proven to be difficult for many home health providers, and as a result many have either had to close or make severe cost cuts. Cost-reducing strategies have included staff layoffs, discontinuation of specialty and advanced practice nursing services, and cessation of providing complex wound supplies.

Since patients with complex and/or chronic wounds can be cost intensive in terms of supplies and personnel, some providers have either not accepted these patients or cut resources in caring for them. In overall cuts being made, some providers have discontinued use of wound care specialists and referred patients to retail suppliers for wound dressings.

The IPS is a controversial payment system that, at the time of this writing, is under scrutiny by legislators. Changes have been and may continue to be made in the regulations. The system is slated to be replaced by a prospective payment system.

Prospective Payment System

The Prospective Payment System (PPS) is a Medicare reimbursement methodology that will pay home health providers prospectively per episode of care. The basis of this system is similar to the acute care diagnosis-related group (DRG) payment method by reimbursement of set amounts within which all services must be provided. At the time of this writing, the details of the system are preliminary and subject to change over the next several months. The PPS is to become effective late in the year 2000; however, that timetable is also subject to revision.

Under PPS, a case-mix adjustment is to be a component of the system. The adjustment is intended to explain variations in individual patient care costs and result in appropriate payment level modifications (St. Pierre, 1999). Early reports of case-mix adjusters, which will result in higher cost requirements and therefore higher reimbursement, include the presence of ulcers and wounds. With this in mind, the goal for home health providers will be to provide quality services to wound patients while using a minimum of resources. It will be advantageous for providers to develop cost-effective processes to care for patients with ulcers and wounds. This would include reliable outcome data, efficient use of wound supplies, and staff with clinical wound care expertise.

Fee-for-Service

The fee-for-service methodology is an historically widely used method of reimbursement. A set fee is negotiated between the home health provider and the payer for a designated service. Typically the defined service for a home care patient is a "visit." A visit rate is set for the various types of disciplines that provide direct care to the patient (e.g., nurse, home health aide, physical therapist, etc.). Special fees may also be set for more complex or high-tech patients, such as patients with IVs or complex wounds, and minimum and maximum visit lengths may be determined. Supplies may or may not be included in the fee agreement.

Commercial indemnity types of payers most frequently use this type of reimbursement. It is quickly losing favor since the incentive is to keep individual visit costs (e.g., length of visit) to a minimum but to make as many visits as possible.

A variation of the traditional fee-for-service method is referred to as a *discounted fee-for-service* method. In this method, the payer requests that the providers accept a percentage discount on the normal fee-for-service rate. This may vary from 5% to as much as 25% off the normal fee.

Capitation

Capitation in the home health setting is managed in a similar way in other health care settings. It is not a prevalent reimbursement method and is used only in certain areas of the country. The difficulty in determining a capitated rate for a specific population's home care needs is the lack of available data for the provider or the payer to determine a fair per-month, per-life rate.

ROLE OF COMMUNICATION TECHNOLOGY IN HOME CARE

Advanced communications technology will play a vital role in the future of home health care. Concepts such as "tele-health" and "tele-medicine" are likely to become a crucial component of providing cost-efficient home care. As the reimbursement for home health services decreases and with the advent of PPS methods, the need for monitoring a patient's condition and educating the patient and caregiver without a costly nursing visit will become paramount to the financial viability of the home care provider. These technologies already exist, but their application to the home health setting is in its infancy. As the demand increases, the technology will no doubt keep pace.

Another area of communication technology that has advanced in the home health setting is computerization of the clinical process. Many providers are already partially or fully clinically computerized. It is not uncommon for each service provider to have a laptop or palm computer for use in the patient's home. This technology allows for rapid communication of patients' clinical status, resource use, and outcome results. These types of systems also can provide access to Internet sites for education purposes and for intraorganization communication (e.g., e-mail, shared bulletin boards, etc.). Direct communication with physicians, third-party payer case managers, and other members of the health care team also becomes possible.

IMPLICATIONS FOR PRACTICE AND PATIENT CARE

The rapid changes occurring in home health care present numerous implications for nursing practice and the care of patients. Home care is being forced to measure and substantiate the outcomes of the services provided. Traditionally this was not an expectation for a home care provider. The opportunity exists for wound care nurses to be instrumental in designing outcome measures to validate the effectiveness of wound care protocols.

Another tremendous opportunity will present with the advent of the PPS, especially if the case-mix adjusters include wounds, which it is likely to do. Since caring for patients with wounds can be financially prohibitive for a home care provider, it will be essential that care is designed, implemented, and monitored in the most cost-efficient way possible. Wound care nurses will be in an ideal position to offer services that will accomplish just that. Initial assessment and periodic reassessments, patient and family teaching, staff education, policy and procedure development, case management, quality improvement, and utilization review are a few services that the wound care nurse can provide the home care agency (WOCN, 1999).

In conclusion, the future presents the dual challenge of substantiating through outcomes the quality of the wound care given and providing that care in the most cost-efficient way possible. The wound care nurse is likely to play a pivotal role in helping home care providers meet the challenges. To be recognized, however, the wound care nurse must be knowledgeable about not only the clinical aspects of care but also the financial and business considerations of home care (WOCN, 1997, 1998, 1999).

SELF-ASSESSMENT EXERCISE

1. OASIS is a tool used to:
   a. Evaluate a patient's eligibility for home care
   b. Determine a patient's wound care needs in the home environment
   c. Measure a patient's response to wound care interventions
   d. Document outcomes of home care patients
2. Which of the following statements about qualifying criteria for home care is accurate?
   a. All Medicare patients qualify for home care
   b. Qualifying criteria are set by the third-party payer
   c. Patients can qualify only if they reside in their own home or apartment
   d. A patient with a willing and able caregiver does not qualify for home care
3. Define the homebound status criteria.
4. True or False: An infected thigh incision in a patient with diabetes after coronary artery bypass surgery is a wound that would be interpreted by Medicare as requiring skilled nursing visits.
5. The design, implementation, and monitoring of cost-efficient wound care is most important in which of the following reimbursement systems?
   a. Cost reimbursement
   b. Interim Payment System
   c. Fee-for-service
   d. Prospective Payment System

REFERENCES

Covinsky KE, Goldman L, Cook EF: The impact of serious illness on patients' families, *JAMA* 272:1839, 1994.

Crister KS: Outcome-based quality improvement and the OASIS data set, *Home Healthc Nurse* 15(3):203, 1997.

Doherty M, Hurley SJ, Perfetti CB: Suburban home care: cost, financing, and delivery, *Nurs Clin North Am* 29(3):483, 1994.

Health Care Financing Administration: *Medicare home health agency manual,* Baltimore, Md, 1996, USDHHS, HCFA.

Martin K: Research in home care, *Nurs Clin North Am* 23(2):373, 1988.

Shaughnessy PW et al: *A study to develop outcome-based quality measures for home health services,* Denver, 1994, Center for Health Policy Research and Center for Health Services Research, University of Colorado Health Sciences Center.

Shulz R, Visintainer P, Williamson GM: Psychiatric and physical morbidity effects of caregiving, *J Gerontol* 45:181, 1990.

St. Pierre M: A look to the future: home health PPS, *Caring,* p 16, March, 1999.

Wound, Ostomy, and Continence Nurses Society: *Professional practice fact sheet: contractural services: establishing contractural services for WOC (ET) nurse services,* Laguna Beach, Calif, 1997, WOCN. Available at www.wocn.org under Resources, Fact Sheets.

Wound, Ostomy, and Continence Nurses Society: *Professional practice fact sheet: Medicare Part B coverage for support surfaces in the home health setting,* Laguna Beach, Calif, 1998, WOCN. Available at www.wocn.org under Resources, Fact Sheets.

Wound, Ostomy, and Continence Nurses Society: *Professional practice fact sheet: reimbursement/home health: reimbursement options for WOC (ET) nurses in home health,* Laguna Beach, Calif, 1999, WOCN. Available at www.wocn.org under Resources, Fact Sheets.

CHAPTER 23

Practice Development in Acute and Long-Term Care Settings

MONICA BESHARA, GAYLE JAMESON, & BARBARA BARR

OBJECTIVES

1. Describe how the Resident Assessment Protocol (RAP) and the Minimum Data Set (MDS) databases are used, and correlate this with the practice of the wound care nurse in the long-term care setting.
2. List two opportunities for the wound care nurse to influence cost-effectiveness within an acute or long-term care center.
3. Name at least four departments that may influence the effectiveness of a wound care program.
4. List at least three departments or groups to whom the wound care nurse should specifically approach to describe the role of the wound care nurse.
5. Cite three examples of how the wound care nurse can influence cost savings within an institution.
6. Describe how the wound care program may be able to classify services for billing purposes within the acute and long-term care settings.
7. Describe environmental and cultural differences between the acute and long-term care settings.

There are many steps that must be taken to establish an effective wound care practice within an institution. These steps are not related to specific wound care interventions; they deal with the nonclinical aspects such as marketing and financial considerations. This chapter discusses these aspects of practice development in the acute and long-term care settings.

ACUTE CARE SETTING

Many factors influence the success of a wound care nurse's practice in the acute care setting. One key factor is credibility, which must be earned and is done so by demonstrating clinical competence and critical thinking. A strong knowledge base in wound care and in the relevant pathologies that are pertinent to wound care is essential. The wound care nurse should also be self-confident and eager to share information with colleagues. These behaviors are empowering to others and foster a positive learning environment.

Communication and Marketing

Another key factor to a successful wound care practice is effective communication with colleagues, such as physicians and nurses. This communication is a form of marketing and serves to 1) clarify and describe the role of the wound care nurse and 2) establish how to access the wound care nurse.

Role Development. Participation in staff orientation programs is a key strategy. This offers an opportunity to orient new staff members to *their* role in wound care and in pressure ulcer prevention, as well as how the wound care nurse can be used and accessed. It is important to emphasize the role of the wound care nurse as a consultant. The wound care nurse is not responsible to conduct every wound assessment or dressing application. Goals of this orientation process should be to increase the staff's familiarity with the role of the wound care nurse as a resource and to empower the staff to feel more confident of their own skills and abilities. The role of the wound care nurse is to provide support, recommend treatment, and follow up on problems identified by them. The wound care nurse should provide a specialized service, not basic assessments or simple dressing changes. The nursing staff is often a key contact for obtaining appropriate referrals because they are so closely involved with the patient's entire plan of care.

Key physicians should be approached, and the role of the wound care nurse should be discussed and clarified. As with all discussions, it is important to emphasize the benefits to their practice. The support and confidence of key physicians is so critical that the extra effort and time it takes to nurture this relationship is time well spent. Ultimately, however, the wound care nurse will need to demonstrate competence and confidence in his or her practice. Allies within the nursing staff can be a source of positive influence with physicians.

The availability of many ancillary services can maximize the effectiveness of a wound care nurse. These services may include, but are not limited to, diabetes educators, dietitians, physical therapists, occupational therapy, pedorthy, discharge planners/home health care staff, radiology/vascular laboratory, billing, materials management, and central supply.

With the expertise of diabetes educators and dietitians, the wound care nurse is at an advantage regarding care for patients with diabetes in that the wound care nurse can be confident that the complex daily maintenance and education issues are being adequately addressed. Physical therapists can provide a different perspective related to wound care (e.g., pulse lavage, whirlpool, electrical stimulation, ultrasound), off-loading, and seating equipment. A close relationship with the radiology department will enhance the ability to obtain definitive diagnoses (e.g., vascular studies, x-ray procedures to rule out osteomyelitis, and/or the presence or absence of foreign bodies in wounds). A professional relationship with materials management is important to ensure an adequate and appropriate hospital formulary, access to products that are off-formulary, and involvement in relevant discussions concerning new wound care products or problems. The wound care nurse must work closely with discharge planners to facilitate a smooth transfer and plan for needs such as the frequency of home care visits, products, and procedures.

Patient referrals are the signpost of successful marketing and can come from a variety of sources. It should be expected that the nursing staff provide the majority of referrals. Working closely with medical/surgical clinical specialists and critical care nurses will also heighten their awareness of skin- and wound care needs within their patient population, which ultimately results in increased referrals to the wound care nurse.

Policy Development. The wound care nurse must work through and with the nursing staff. It is impossible for the wound care nurse, for example, to see all patients with skin care needs or who are at risk for pressure ulcer development. For these reasons, it is critical that certain policies and procedures be established to guide select skin– and wound–care-related activities. For example, a policy is needed addressing pressure ulcer risk assessment (such as the Braden scale) on admission and then routine reassessments. Incorporation of this assessment data into the nursing admission form is critical to ensure that the data are collected (Figures 23-1 to 23-3). Such data can also be incorporated into the daily documentation flow sheets. Flow sheets that are dedicated to wound assessment and interventions are particularly useful because they will best reflect changes in wound status over time. A policy should exist to delineate appropriate interventions for different risk levels as well as for the referral of high-risk patients (Box 23-1 on p. 484) to the wound care specialist.

Documentation. Documentation by the wound care nurse should be in a consistent location in the chart. Preferably, documentation should be in the progress notes so that all physicians and ancillary services involved in the patient's care are kept informed. Documentation should be direct, concise, and objective. The documentation should include a thorough assessment, including pertinent quantitative information, interventions, education, and the plan for follow-up. A wound documentation form may also be used to record the initial consultation assessment and plan (Figure 23-4 on p. 486). A flowchart can also be developed to record wound assessments so that a trend in the status of the wound can be conveyed (Figure 23-5 on p. 488). The Pressure Ulcer Scale for Healing (PUSH) tool or the Pressure

SECTION IV: RN: Complete all shaded areas for all adult patients; other sections as appropriate for patient.

ASSESSMENT ON ADMISSION:

BRADEN CHART ☐ Examined ☐ Verbal

Note any identifying marks on figures

SKIN: Surface Intact ☐ Y ☐ N ☐ Warm ☐ Dry ☐ Pink ☐ Pale
☐ Cool ☐ Moist ☐ Mottled ☐ Cyanosis

A - Abrasion | Br - Bruises | D - PU | Lc - Lice | P - Pin
Amp - Amputation | R - Rash | E - Erythema | L - Laceration | S - Scar
B - Burn | I - Incision | W - Wound | O - Ostomy | V - Vascular access
J - Jaundice | Dr - Drain

RISK:
15-16 Low
13-14 Mod
<11 High

Score:

Sensory Perceptions	1 Completely Limited	2 Very Limited	3 Slightly Limited	4 No Impairment	
Moisture	1 Completely Moist	2 Very Moist	3 Occasionally Moist	4 Rarely Moist	
Activity	1 Bedfast	2 Chairfast	3 Walks Occasionally	4 Walks Frequently	
Mobility	1 Completely Immobile	2 Very Limited	3 Slightly Impaired	4 No Limitations	
Nutrition	1 Very Poor	2 Probably Inadequate	3 Adequate	4 Excellent	
Friction and Shear	1 Problem	2 Potential Problem	3 No Apparent Problem	W Score <16	Total Score

SIGNATURE: DATE TIME:

Figure 23-1 Nursing admission form with Braden Scale incorporated adult assessment section. (Reprinted with permission, Wound Ostomy Continence Nursing Department, Wellstar Health System, Marietta, Ga.)

SECTION VI: REFERRALS: RN/LPN/Tech/Sec. Complete on all adult patients.

Notify: By computer or phone within 24 hours of admission to unit.

	Initiated By	Date/ Time	Referral Accept. By		Initiated By	Date/ Time	Referral Accept. By
Wnd Ostomy Continence Nurse (W)		/		Pastoral Care (C)		/	
Food and Nutrition (N)		/		Social Services (S)		/	
Diabetic Education (D)		/		Pharmacy (P)		/	
Respiratory Therapy (R)		/				/	
Discharge Planning (DP)		/		*Rehab Services (RS)		/	
Care Coordinator (CC)		/		*MD order PT, OT, ST		/	

Figure 23-2 Referral section of nursing admission form includes referral to wound nurse. (Reprinted with permission, Wound Ostomy Continence Nursing Department, Wellstar Health System, Marietta, Ga.)

Sore Status Tool (PSST) reflect change in status over time and may be used instead of creating a flowchart (Bates-Jensen, 1995; NPUAP, 1999).

Financial Considerations

From a financial standpoint, the wound care nurse must become astute to cost savings and cost-effectiveness. Information concerning the cost implications of the wound care practice or cost savings that have been generated must be gathered and specifically communicated to the supervisor routinely. Wound management is costly; in most situations more costly than prevention (Lapsley and Vogels, 1996). Effective wound management reduces costs by using fewer supplies and providing more efficient and effective use of dressings. In addition, cost savings can be realized when preventive interventions are linked to risk level (Richardson, Gardner, and Frantz, 1998). This could result in a significant decrease in annual expenditures for materials used. Cost-effectiveness is a positive way of acquiring the support of the nursing administration (Kuhn and Coulter, 1992), which is essential to obtain institutional support.

The wound care nurse also must get involved with the establishment of supply contracts. This can help materials management and administration see the wound care nurse as a valuable colleague in

Section VIII: Multidisciplinary Action Plan

PHYSICIAN DOCUMENTATION REVIEWED BY ALL DISCIPLINES AS FOUNDATION OF PATIENT PLAN OF CARE.

Discipline	Date	Learning/Discharge Need:	Plan and/or Action	Signature
Nursing				
Nutrition				
Respiratory				
Pharmacy				
Rehab Services OT, PT, ST				
Diabetic Education				
Wnd/ Ostomy Continence				
Discharge Planning				
Social Services				
Other				
Other				

MDC Dates: Attended by:

1. ______
2. ______
3. ______
4. ______

Figure 23-3 Multidisciplinary action plan section of nursing admission form. (Reprinted with permission, Wound Ostomy Continence Nursing Department, Wellstar Health System, Marietta, Ga.)

sorting through the maze of different products and indications. A successful means of proven cost-effectiveness is to limit the number of similar supplies stocked by the facility. By creating a wound care product formulary, product use can be standardized. Furthermore, the wound care nurse can serve as a resource to materials management, providing clarification on product use and distinctions between clinical use of products. Collaboration with materials management can also increase the success of contractual arrangements with manufacturers and increase the ability to maintain compliance with the contract.

Another area of potential for cost savings is by standardizing use of support surfaces. A policy should be developed that describes patient indicators for the use of specialty beds, and compliance with contracts for these specialty beds should be supported. It is also important to set up a procedure for "stepping down" from the specialty bed as the patient's condition warrants. In addition, units with a high prevalence of at-risk patient populations might benefit from the implementation of replacement mattresses. By standardizing products used and providing indicators or patient characteristics to guide use, overuse can be reduced and appropriate use can be enhanced.

The wound care nurse has the opportunity to prove clinical effectiveness and cost-effectiveness. Through ongoing continuing education opportunities, the wound care nurse can foster state-of-the-art patient care and evidence-based practice by using products that have scientific evidence of their effectiveness. Again, not only do the patients benefit from this expertise, but the facility benefits financially by cutting expenditures. The wound care nurse can work with quality improvement team members to identify select aspects of care that could be monitored and tracked over time and thus obtain outcome data and clinical effectiveness information.

The wound care program, like all departments, must have a means to track productivity. With the assistance of the billing department, a mechanism to document visits and referrals could be formulated (WOCN, 1999). One method could be to establish a "charge code" for the wound care services that are based on increments of time or services provided (Box 23-2 on p. 489). This is an excellent way to track, document, and justify the value of a wound care nurse. However, it is important that the wound care nurse avoid providing services that are considered basic nursing care to inflate the number of charges. This charging system may also assist with the compilation of workload and time management data for the department. It is important to avoid focusing solely on the number of patients or charges, and to focus instead on the types of patients and services provided. Also to be considered is whether the wound care nurse's interventions are affecting outcomes.

Depending on payer sources, the services that are provided through the wound care program might be billable. If the services are classified as a therapy rather than a nursing service, the services may be billable (WOCN, 1997a, 1997b, 1997c). The availability of wound care services may also enable the institution to market itself for managed care contracts. This again defines the value of a wound care program. However, inpatient wound care services will seldom, if ever, be a revenue-producing area. Working closely with the billing department and fiscal intermediaries may be productive regarding revenues.

The value of a wound care program is not just limited to providing care to inpatients. The wound care nurse can serve as a link to community programs and outreach programs and provide education that can draw attention to the wound care program and the facility. The wound care nurse can provide education within his or her facility in collaboration with colleagues, such as physical therapists and occupational therapists. Grants may be available from manufacturers to conduct some of these programs. The manufacturers often have established programs that have been approved by licensing boards for continuing education hours. These may be a cost-effective way to provide continuing education to staff. Continuing medical education programs may also be attractive. Well-recognized speakers can be invited to conduct an educational session at a dinner program.

The role of the wound care nurse in an acute care facility is not predetermined, and there are many opportunities for the program to become successful and invaluable. When initially starting the wound care program, the wound care nurse may want to conduct a series of chart audits or perform a prevalence and incidence study. These activities will provide information that is helpful to determine if a certain problem (e.g., pressure ulcers, inadequate documentation) exists. From this information, the continuous improvement process can be initiated with involved departments and personnel so that problems can be discussed and possible solutions can be identified. As the wound care nurse begins an inpatient practice, it is essential to

Text continued on p. 489

BOX 23-1 Sample Policy and Procedure for Prediction and Prevention of Pressure Ulcers

Purpose

To identify patients at risk for developing a pressure ulcer and to institute appropriate preventive interventions tailored to their level of risk.

Definition

Pressure ulcers are localized areas of tissue necrosis that develop when soft tissue is compressed between a bony prominence and an external surface (e.g., a bed, cast, or nasal oxygen tubing) for a prolonged period of time.

Policy

1. The Braden Scale will be used on admission and every Monday, Wednesday, and Friday to identify patients at risk for developing pressure ulcers.
2. Patients with a Braden Score of 13 to 14 will be considered at MODERATE RISK for pressure ulcer development.
3. Patients with a Braden Score of less than 11 will be considered at HIGH RISK for pressure ulcer development.
4. Staff nurses will institute appropriate prevention interventions when a patient has a Braden Score of 14 or less.
5. Patients with a HIGH RISK score (<11) will be referred to the wound care nurse for additional HIGH RISK prevention plans.

Procedure

1. The Braden Score will be calculated on all patients admitted to this facility within 24 hours.
2. Reassessment of the Braden Score will be obtained on all patients on Monday, Wednesday, and Friday and documented in the nursing notes.
3. Preventive interventions for patients with a Braden Score of 14 or less include the following:
   a. Observe skin daily for redness that does not disappear within 30 minutes of turning, poor blanching, and/or breaks in skin integrity, such as over bony prominences and skin folds.
   b. Assess for skin discoloration, blanching, induration, pallor or mottling, and absence of superficial skin layers.
   c. Identify factors contributing to skin breakdown (such as infection, dehydration, edema, and compromised perfusion) and institute corrective measures.
   d. Request nutritional screenings on all patients identified as moderate to high risk.

e. Turn patient at least every 2 hours, more frequently if necessary. Avoid positioning patients directly on their trochanters. Patient should be positioned at 30 degrees (a lateral position). Patient confined to a wheelchair may use wheelchair cushions to reduce pressure when sitting. Maintain the head of the bed at the lowest degree of elevation consistent with medical conditions and other restrictions to decrease friction and shear. Limit the amount of time the head of the bed is elevated.
f. Pad areas where skin touches skin; use blankets and pillows, especially between the knees and ankles. Heels should be protected and elevated from the mattress.
g. Keep patient and linens clean. Consider the use of noninvasive devices (e.g., fecal incontinence collectors, male external catheters) to manage incontinent patients. Patients with a foley catheter should avoid use of diapers.
h. Avoid shear by using draw sheets (to lift and position patient), socks, and lightly sprinkled powder on sheets. Inspect linen frequently to be sure that they are clean and dry.
i. Limit or avoid use of tape on fragile skin. Use skin sealants under tape. Use adhesive solvents or removers to assist in removal of adhesives.
j. Skin cleansing should occur at the time of soiling and at routine intervals. Minimize skin exposure to moisture caused by incontinence, perspiration, or wound drainage. Avoid hot water, and use a mild cleansing agent that minimizes irritation and dryness of the skin. Use moisturizers or emollient lotions for dry skin. Apply moisturizers or emollients immediately after bathing. Use moisture-barrier creams for incontinence.
k. Teach patient and significant others relevant preventive care.
l. Eliminate anything that may increase ischemic damage, such as massaging areas of redness and the use of donut devices.
m. Monitor patient every shift for additional sites of pressure: endotracheal tube, the external ear, drain sites, and catheters.
n. Remove antiembolism stockings every 8 hours to assess skin integrity.

4. Heel wounds and blisters should remain intact and protected. Heels should be suspended off of the bed surface. Foot protectors may be implemented for HIGH RISK patients.
5. When the reddened area is not resolving within 24 to 48 hours after initial preventive interventions, contact wound care specialist.

Modified and reprinted with permission, Wound Ostomy Continence Nursing Department, Wellstar Health System, Marietta, Ga.

Skilled Nursing Visit Report
Wound Care

Client: ______________________
Last First

SS#: ______________________

Date:	Time In:	Time Out:

T	PA ☐Reg ☐Irreg	PR ☐Reg ☐Irreg	R	BP	WT

Wound Location: ☐ Resolving ☐ Partial Thickness ☐ Full Thickness Stage ☐ I ☐ II ☐ III ☐ IV ☐ Unstageable

SIZE ☐ See Wound Diagram	WOUND BASE	PERIWOUND TISSUE	EXUDATE		WOUND PAIN
Measure Weekly	☐ Granulation %	☐Intact	☐None ☐Moderate	Color: ☐ NA	☐Yes ☐No
Width cm	☐ Eschar %	☐Macerated	☐Scant ☐Large	☐Sero-Sang	Describe:
Length cm	☐ Slough %	☐Edematous	☐Small ☐Copius	☐Purulent	
Depth cm	☐ Not Visible %	☐Erythema	Type, Amt, Number Dressings Removed:	☐Serous	Lower Extremities:
Sinus Tract: ☐Yes ☐No		☐Warm		☐Bloody	☐NA
Location:	Color: ☐ NA	☐Denuded		Odor: ☐Yes ☐No	☐Edema:
	☐Red ☐Yellow	Comments:		Describe:	
Undermining☐Yes ☐No	☐Pink ☐Black				☐Pulse:
Location:	☐White		Comments:		

Functional Limitations: Client ☐Unwilling ☐Unable Due To: ____________
Caregiver ☐NA ☐Unwilling ☐Unable Due To: ____________

Other Systems Assessed:

Nursing Diagnosis	Nursing Interventions	Client Outcome	Plan
Alteration in Skin Integrity	☐O/E wound status as above	☐No change in wound	☐No change in wound care
	☐O/E S/S of infection as above	☐Wound improving	☐See updated wound care plan
	☐Wound care done per care plan	☐Wound deteriorating	☐See updated medication profile
	☐See Wound Teaching Flowsheet for instructions given	☐No S/S of infeciton present	☐Call MD ☐New MD orders
		☐S/S of infection ☐local ☐systemic	☐If new infection: Call Infection Control VM -- 672-7855
		☐See Wound Teaching Flowsheet	Consult: ☐ Nutrition Support
			☐ WOC Nurse

WOC Nurse Recommendation:

Care Coordination: ☐Nurse ☐MD ☐Rehab ☐SW ☐HHA/HMKR

Homebound Due to: ☐Poor endurance ☐Medical contraindication ☐Other/Comments:

HHA Supervision: ☐Indirect
☐Plan meets needs
☐Care plan changes

Signature/Title

White: Medical Record Yellow: Case Manager Pink: Home File

Figure 23-4 Sample wound care documentation form designed for use in home care but can be adapted for initial visit in hospital. (Reprinted with permission, Fairview Home Care and Hospice, Fairview Health Systems, Minneapolis, Minn.)

Pressure Ulcer Staging

Stage I: Non-blanchable erthemia not resolving within 30 min. of pressure relief. Epidermis remains intact. Darker skin tones: persistent red, blue, or purple hues.

Stage II: Epidermis lost, dermis present. Maybe blister. Free of necrotic tissue. Painful.

Stage III: Tissue loss through dermis into subcutaneous layer. Presents as shallow crater unless covered by eschar. May include necrotic tissue, undermining sinus tracts exudate and/or infection. Wound base is usually not painful.

Stage IV: Tissue loss through subcutaneous tissue exposing fascia, muscle, bone. Presents as a deep crater wound base is usually not painful.

If wound involves necrotic tissue, staging cannot be confirmed until wound base is visible.

Anatomical Terms

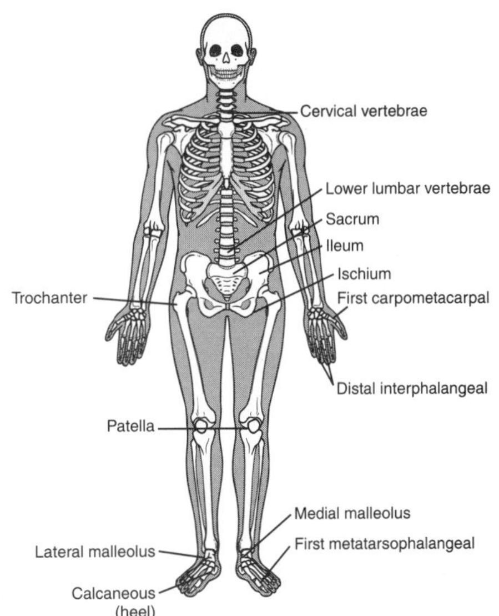

Assessment of Pitting Edema.

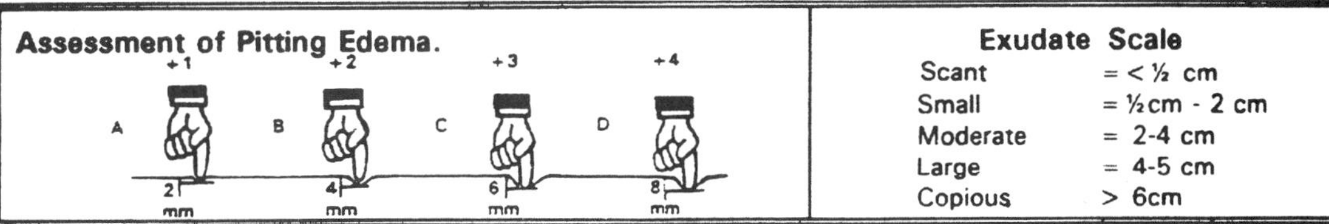

Exudate Scale

Scant	= < ½ cm
Small	= ½cm - 2 cm
Moderate	= 2-4 cm
Large	= 4-5 cm
Copious	> 6cm

Terminology

Distal .... Furthest point of attachment.
Erythema .... Diffuse redness of skin.
- **Blanchable:** .... Reddened area which turns white with application of pressure.
- **Non-blanchable**..... Redness of skin that does not pale when gentle pressure is applies. (**Stage I**)

Eschar .... Scab.
Exudate .... Drainage.
Granulation .... "beefy red" fragile connective tissue in a wound base.
Induration .... An area of hardened tissue.
Ischemia .... Decreased blood supply as a result of constriction of a blood vessel.
Lateral .... Away from the midline.
Maceration .... Softening of connective tissue by soaking in fluids resulting in degerative changes giving the tissue a whitish appearance which can be easily teased apart.
Medial .... Toward the midline.
Necrotic .... Dead, avascular tissue.
Proximal .... Nearest point of attachment (ie wrist is proximal to the fingers).
Purulent .... Containing or forming pus.
Serous .... Clear drainage.
Serosanguinous........................ A pink tinged drainage
Sinus tract .... A tunnel, leaving space which can potentially become infected and cause an abscess.
Slough .... Non viable tissue characterized loose string like, moist, often yellow, green or gray in color.
Undermining .... (Ledge) skin edges of a wound that have lost supporting tissue, tender intact skin.
Wound base .... Uppermost viable tissue layer of wound; may be covered with slough or eschar.

Figure 23-4, cont'd.

WOUND DOCUMENTATION FORM

Baseline Assessment **DATE** ____________

Type of Wound: Pressure ___; Venous ___; Arterial ___; Neuropathic ___; Surgical___; Burn ___; Skin Tear ___; other ___

Location: ____________________

Date first noted: ________

If pressure ulcer, stage at baseline: Stage _____

Size (in cm): (L×W×D) __________

Wound bed: % G____; % LS______; % AS______; % E______

Tunnels or undermining __________

Drainage: ____________________

Odor: ______________________

Periwound skin: ____________________

Was wound present upon admission? Yes____ No____

Brief review of past wound treatments and patient's level of participation:

____

KEY:

Status: NC=no change; I=improving; D=deteriorating

Wound base: G=granular; LS=loose slough; AS=adherent slough; E=eschar

Drainage: S=scant; M=moderate; C=copious

Odor: Y=yes; N=none

Periwound skin: I=intact; M=macerated; E=erythematous; IND=indurated

Pressure relief measures: 1=seating cushion; 2=mattress overlay; 3=pressure reduction mattress; 4=low air loss bed; 5=air-fluidized bed; 6=heels elevated; 7=elbow protectors; 8=patient teaching done; 9=other, see careplan. List all interventions used.

Stage 1: Nonblanchable erythema of intact skin; in darkly pigmented skin, persistent red, blue, or purple hues present.

Stage 2: Partial thickness skin loss involving epidermis, dermis, or both (includes blister and abrasion).

Stage 3: Full-thickness skin loss involving damage to or necrosis of subcutaneous tissue that may extend down to, but not through, underlying fascia. A deep crater with or without undermining.

Stage 4: Full-thickness skin loss with extensive destruction, tissue necrosis, or damage to muscle, bone, or supporting structures. May have undermining or sinus tracts.

Wound Parameter	Date	Date	Date	Date	Date	Date	Date
Size (L×W×D)							
Tunnels							
Undermining							
Wound bed: % G							
% LS							
% AS							
% E							
Drainage							
Odor							
Periwound skin condition							
Risk-reduction interventions							

Figure 23-5 Sample flowchart for documentation of wound assessments.

BOX 23-2 Wound-Related Codes

Inpatient Charge Codes

45525	G-tube change
67059	Wound care nurse consult—30 min
67028	Skin care—30 min
67047	Fistula care/management—30 min
67024	Pressure ulcer care—30 min
67040	Ulcer/wound care—30 min
67042	Tube care/replacement—30 min
67053	Nail/foot care—30 min
67054	Wound irrigation—30 min
67175	Surgical wound—30min

Outpatient Treatment Room Codes

67049	**Level I**: Follow-up evaluation to assess the patient's progress related to implemented plan of care (< 15 minutes)
67050	**Level II**: Treatment of stage 1 to stage 2 pressure ulcers, management of simple wound foot/nail care (15-30 minutes)
67051	**Level III**: Treatment of stage 3 to stage 4 pressure ulcers, tunneling wound, venous ulcers, and wound/tube pouching (30-60 minutes)
67052	**Level IV**: Complicated wound involving conservative debridement and extensive wound care modalities, such as evaluation and management of difficult fistula pouching situations

Reprinted with permission, Wound Ostomy Continence Nursing Department, Wellstar Health System, Marietta, Ga.

be visible. Being open to new ideas and opportunities will assist the wound care nurse in creating and maintaining a successful program. Maintaining visibility and an alliance with physicians and staff will reinforce the message that the wound care program is an indispensable service.

LONG-TERM CARE PRACTICE DEVELOPMENT

The 17,000 long-term care facilities in the United States represent 1.5 million people (American Health Care Association, 1999a). Close to 90% of this population is over 65 years of age, and 75% of them are females (American Health Care Association, 1999a). Most people will spend 3 or more years in the long-term care facility once admitted. The primary payment source used by 68% of the long-term care population is Medicaid, Medicare funds pay for 9%, and other insurance plans plus private funds account for approximately 23% of the currently used funding sources (American Health Care Association, 1999b). As the population ages and lives longer, the number of long-term care facilities can be expected to increase along with the acuity level of the people they serve.

Residents

Patients in long-term care facilities are usually referred to as *residents* since the facility is their residence for an extended period of time. Most residents present with at least two to three chronic health conditions, such as cardiovascular diseases, respiratory ailments, and endocrine disorders; 42% of nursing facility residents suffer from some level of dementia, and 25% have documented symptoms of depression (American Health Care Association, 1999c). Most residents will need help with four of five activities of daily living (eating, transferring, toiletting, dressing, and bathing) (American Health Care Association, 1999a). In some instances, the decision to seek placement in the long-term care facility is precipitated by an exacerbation of a chronic condition requiring hospitalization and prolonged treatment or a traumatic event, such as a fall with a hip fracture, that necessitates extensive rehabilitative services. In other cases, the admission to long-term care may follow an extended period of care by family members and their reluctant realization that they can no longer provide for the needs of their loved one in the home care setting. Urinary incontinence is often the problem that families providing care in the home find the most difficult to manage and that causes them to seek long-term care placement. Management of percutaneous feeding tubes and problematic ostomies, in conjunction with other health management issues, may also necessitate long-term care admission.

Long-term care facilities strive to foster a different environment and culture compared with acute care hospitals. They emphasize a caring, home-like atmosphere, offering structured activities and services while meeting the medical needs of the resident.

Residents and family members are actively involved in all care and treatment decisions affecting the individual resident, and a resident advisory board has input into decisions about daily life in the facility. Ensuring quality of life and the highest practical functional level for each resident is the goal of the long-term care facility.

Staff

In the long-term care setting, resident care is usually coordinated by a registered nurse (RN), but the majority of direct, bedside care is delivered by a licensed practical/vocational nurse (LPN) and certified nurse assistants (CNAs). In one study, 76% of institutions reported using RNs as the highest professional level of care providers responsible for pressure ulcer care; 14% reported LPNs as the highest professional level (Pase and Hoffman, 1998). Therefore although the RN may coordinate or be responsible for wound care, it cannot be assumed that the RN actually delivers the wound care. It is important to understand that the LPN/LVN and CNA are prepared to deliver basic nursing and personal hygiene care to the resident but often lack well-developed assessment and problem-solving skills that would give them insight into the causes of and solutions to resident care problems.

In contrast to the acute care setting, access to consultants for the long-term care staff is usually limited to consultation ordered by a primary physician to direct care for an individual resident. Many times this consultation occurs outside the facility, and communication between the consultant and the long-term care staff consists of progress notes and written directives only, with an occasional follow-up telephone call, usually initiated by the long-term care staff, to monitor resident progress or to clarify written orders.

The average nursing facility in 1997 had a daily census of 88 residents and an average facility bed size of 107. A facility of this size has an average of 54 direct care staff personnel (36 CNAs, 11 LPNs, and 7 RNs). They have a staff-to-bed ratio of 0.5 to 1 and an average of 3.5 total direct care staff hours per resident day (American Health Care Association, 1999c).

Reimbursement Issues

There are numerous federal and individual state regulations that mandate how long-term care facilities operate and how they receive funding for their services. These regulations directly affect the delivery of resident care by prescribing the Resident Assessment Instrument (RAI) as the assessment tool that must be used to identify resident problems and formulate the resident's care plan.

The RAI consists of the Minimum Data Set (MDS) and the Resident Assessment Protocol (RAP), both of which must be completed by the facility staff at specified intervals during the resident's length of stay. The issues identified through this assessment process are then incorporated into an interdisciplinary care plan that is individualized for each resident. Specific goals with timeframes for completion are detailed, and approaches are formulated to assist the resident and staff in meeting the stated goals.

On July 1, 1998, the Health Care Financing Administration (HCFA) began implementation of the Medicare Prospective Payment System (PPS) for long-term care facilities. The PPS uses the MDS assessment data to determine the level of care that the resident requires and bases payment rates on the MDS assessment for a Part A Medicare covered stay. The PPS requires more frequent MDS documentation and makes facilities totally dependent on accurate and timely completion of the MDS to secure appropriate Medicare funding for care delivered to Part A Medicare residents. Long-term care facilities are also required to electronically transmit all MDS data collected to the state agency, which in turn forwards some data to the HFCA, to assist in establishing a national database for long-term care.

Obtaining and maintaining the necessary supplies to meet the needs of the varied population of a typical long-term care facility can present a significant challenge. The facility may have limited access to a variety of vendors for product selection because of restrictive contracts or consignment systems. The necessary space to maintain an adequate stock supply is often an issue and dictates limiting choices to tried and true product categories. Reimbursement coverage for supply costs must be considered when treatment decisions are made because it will affect facility revenues.

Wound Care Nurse in Long-Term Care

Resident Assessment. Resident assessment skills have gained new importance in the long-term care industry now that reimbursement is directly linked to accurate and timely resident assessment. The wound care nurse can emphasize and reinforce the essential nature of accurate and extensive documentation for optimal reimbursement. Long-term care facilities must often view resident admission in terms of how much revenue the resident will generate versus how expensive the delivery of care will be for the resident. The wound care nurse is qualified to assist long-term care staff in this process by assessing risk factors for wound development and identifying the potential for healing in each resident.

The MDS is used to assess the long-term care resident's functional capacities (Brandeis et al, 1995). Eighteen specific conditions (such as pressure ulcer) are addressed with the RAPs. Unfortunately, the items in the pressure ulcer RAP may not adequately assess key risk factors for pressure ulcer development, such as friction, shear, sensory perception, and nutritional status (Zulkowsky, 1998a). In an earlier study, Zulkowsky (1998b) revealed that the pressure ulcer RAP predicted pressure ulcer prevalence in 19.76% of subjects. Pressure ulcer risk in long-term care residents may be best estimated by considering MDS items from Section H (Physical Functioning and Structural Problems) in conjunction with the RAP for pressure ulcers (Zulkowsky, 1999).

The wound care nurse can also provide direction in determining appropriate staffing needs for prevention of skin breakdown, appropriate indications for prevention interventions, and appropriate wound treatment. A correlation between level of pressure ulcer risk and prevention intervention, such as repositioning, can have a significant affect on the daily cost of care per patient (Richardson, Gardner, and Frantz, 1998; Xakellis, Frantz, and Lewis, 1995). The wound care nurse can ascertain the need for specialty beds or advanced support surfaces so that efficient, appropriate use can be promoted. It is critical that the wound care nurse streamline processes in the long-term care setting so that early intervention (prevention) is provided in a timely fashion and is linked to the resident's level of risk. The key to securing an employment position or contractural relationship with a long-term care facility will be the ability of the wound care nurse to articulate the ways in which he or she can improve the facility's "bottom line" and clinical outcomes (WOCN, 1997d).

Surprisingly several pressure ulcer risk assessment tools and treatment protocols are used in long-term care settings; some are derivations of the Norton or Braden Scales, whereas some facilities have no risk-assessment process in place (Pase and Hoffman, 1998). Less than half of the institutions surveyed by Pase and Hoffman (1998) reported using a pressure ulcer treatment protocol. This low number is disturbing because without protocols, the resulting care is inconsistent, is incomplete, or consists of outdated treatments. Recommendations cited by these researchers for the wound care nurse in the long-term care setting include 1) developing pressure ulcer treatment protocols and 2) integrating routine and regular risk assessment into documentation and daily activities. In addition, the wound care nurse should train care providers on the use of protocols (including administration of risk-assessment tools and treatment methods), promote multidisciplinary collaboration for protocol development, and conduct periodic updates to the protocols (Pase and Hoffman, 1998). It would also be advantageous to institute a data management system that would support the quality improvement process so that nosocomial pressure ulcers are monitored and wound outcomes are tracked.

Wound Management Issues. The management of acute and chronic wounds in the long-term care facility presents many complex issues that support the need for the skills of the wound care nurse. The wound care nurse has the expertise to holistically evaluate the wound treatment plan, review the facility supplies and practices, and creatively formulate a wound management plan that will meet the medical needs of the resident, as well as promote the best quality of life for the individual. Facility staff, especially when dealing with chronic wounds, may need assistance with recognition of reasonable goals for wound care management. Often, quality of life for the resident can be greatly enhanced by using innovative containment and pouching techniques that may be unfamiliar to long-term care staff. Odor control related to wound sites and drainage is another area where the wound care nurse can have a major influence with positive results.

Foot Care. Foot care for the resident of the long-term care facility is an underserved area. The wound care nurse possesses assessment and intervention skills that may reduce, in some cases, the need for surgical amputation of diabetic extremities. The wound care nurse may also provide routine toenail hygiene. Long-term care staff and residents often need additional information to guide decision making for selection of proper footwear and when seeking podiatry care (Sussman, 1996). The knowledge and skills of the wound care nurse can fill a pivotal role in providing foot care to long-term care residents, thereby reducing pain, suffering, and loss of mobility.

Staff Support. The educational needs of long-term care staff are as varied as the residents they serve. Residents and their family members need information to make informed decisions about issues that affect their treatment and quality of life. The wound care nurse practicing in the long-term care arena is presented with numerous opportunities for conducting formal and informal educational sessions. Techniques common to the wound care nurse may be unfamiliar to long-term staff and residents. New knowledge and skills introduced to long-term care staff by the wound care nurse are usually well-received if the staff is convinced that the wound care nurse recognizes and values their contribution to resident care. Many long-term care facilities are involved in community education programs in areas such as foot care and prevention of skin problems that are of particular interest to the wound care nurse.

The recognition of successful practices and the remedying of unsuccessful ones is as important in long-term care facilities as it is in other medical care settings. Collecting and analyzing data to recognize and improve practice is a valuable service of the wound care nurse in long-term care. Data analysis by the wound care nurse can lead to positive outcomes in reducing skin breakdown, promoting cost-efficient wound healing, and appropriately using specialty beds and support surfaces. The wound care nurse can also assist the long-term care facility staff in evaluating new products using sound research principles to guide practice and purchase decisions.

As new knowledge, techniques, and products are introduced into the facility, the need for revised or new policies and procedures arises. The wound care nurse is well-versed in national standards such as Joint Commission on Accreditation of Healthcare Organizations (JCAHO) and Agency for Healthcare Research Quality (AHRQ, formerly the Agency for Health Care Policy and Research [AHCPR]) guidelines. This expertise can be used to ensure that facility policy and procedure are in compliance with the industry standard so that the facility remains current in its resident care practices.

Long-term care today encompasses a community of facilities that provide a wide range of services. Facilities include subacute care centers, rehabilitation centers, intermediate care centers, residential care facilities, and assisted-living centers. Services include subacute medical care, ongoing skilled nursing care, adult day care, and care for the developmentally disabled (American Health Care Association, 1999c). However, the focus of care in all of the long-term care arenas is to provide the best possible quality of life for all residents while meeting their medical needs. This must be accomplished in a manner that balances medical and psychosocial needs to sustain the whole person. The wound care nurse can implement interventions that contribute to normalizing life for the resident and assist the staff to recognize when interventions need to be revised. The staff of the long-term care facility often feels that their best efforts are not good enough. More often than not, their residents do not get well and go home; they expire because of complex health problems compounded by the frailties of advanced age. The wound care nurse can play a significant role in validating staff efforts as being medically appropriate and sensitive to resident needs.

SUMMARY

The wound care nurse has numerous opportunities in the area of health care today. Issues such as reimbursement commonly influence the parameters of practice. Many similarities exist in creating a practice in the different health care settings. For example, policies and procedures should be in place for use of support surfaces; the role should be from a consultative perspective rather than direct care provider; and extensive, accurate documentation is critical.

SELF-ASSESSMENT EXERCISE

1. List three ways in which a wound care specialist can influence costs within an institution.
2. Name one strategy that the wound care nurse can use to communicate his or her role to staff nurses.
3. True or false: With a consultation model, the wound care nurse should be certain to assess the healing status of wounds directly by conducting dressing changes.
4. Which of the following sources best reflects trends in wound status?
   a. Progress (or physician) notes
   b. Nursing admission form
   c. 24-hour flow sheet
   d. Wound flow sheet

REFERENCES

American Health Care Association: *The looming crisis: profile: nursing facility resident*, accessed March 3, 1999a. Available at www.ahca.org/secure/nfres.htm.

American Health Care Association: *Today's nursing facilities and the people they serve, 1998,* accessed March 3, 1999b. Available at www.ahca.org/who/profile3.htm.

American Health Care Association: *Research and data: the nursing facility sourcebook*, accessed March 3, 1999c. Available at www.ahca.org/research/nftoc.htm.

Bates-Jensen BM: Indices to include in wound healing assessment, *Adv Wound Care* 8(4):28, 1995.

Brandeis GH et al: Pressure ulcers: the Minimum Data Set and the Resident Assessment Protocol, *Adv Wound Care* 8(6):18, 1995.

Kuhn BA, Coulter SJ: Balancing the pressure ulcer cost and quality equation, *Nurs Econ* 10:353, 1992.

Lapsley HM, Vogels R: Cost and prevention of pressure ulcers in an acute teaching hospital, *Int J Qual Health Care* 8(1):61, 1996.

National Pressure Ulcer Advisory Panel: *Stage I assessment in darkly pigmented skin*, August, 1999. Available at www.npuap.org/positn4.htm.

Pase MN, Hoffman RG: Selection and use of pressure ulcer risk-assessment tools and treatment protocols in extended-care facilities in the southwest, *J Wound Ostomy Continence Nurse* 25:44, 1998.

Richardson GM, Gardner S, Frantz RA: Nursing assessment: impact on type and cost of interventions to prevent pressure ulcers, *J Wound Ostomy Continence Nurs* 25:273, 1998.

Sussman C: Whirlpool in wound care, *Advancement of Wound Healing and Diabetic Foot Pathology* 1(2):1, 1996.

Wound, Ostomy, and Continence Nurses Society: *Professional practice fact sheet: reimbursement for WOC (ET) nurse services in the acute care setting*, Laguna Beach, Calif, 1997a, WOCN. Available at www.wocn.org under Resources, Fact Sheets.

Wound, Ostomy, and Continence Nurses Society: *Professional practice fact sheet: contractural services: establishing contractural services for WOC (ET) nurse services*, Laguna Beach, Calif, 1997b, WOCN. Available at www.wocn.org under Resources, Fact Sheets.

Wound, Ostomy, and Continence Nurses Society: *Professional practice fact sheet: establishment of wound ostomy continence clinics*, Laguna Beach, Calif, 1997c, WOCN. Available at www.wocn.org under Resources, Fact Sheets.

Wound, Ostomy, and Continence Nurses Society: *Professional practice fact sheet: reimbursement for WOC (ET) nurse services in the long-term care setting*, Laguna Beach, Calif, 1997d, WOCN. Available at www.wocn.org under Resources, Fact Sheets.

Wound, Ostomy, and Continence Nurses Society: *Professional practice fact sheet: reimbursement options for WOC (ET) nurses in ambulatory care*, Laguna Beach, Calif, 1999, WOCN. Available at www.wocn.org under Resources, Fact Sheets.

Xakellis GC, Frantz RA, Lewis A: Cost of pressure ulcer prevention in long-term care, *J Am Geriatri Assoc* 43:496, 1995.

Zulkowski K: Construct validity of minimum data set items within the context of the Braden Conceptual Schema, *Ostomy Wound Manage* 44(10):36, 1998a.

Zulkowski K: MDS+RAP items associated with pressure ulcer prevalence in newly institutionalized elderly, *Ostomy Wound Manage* 44(11):40, 1998b.

Zulkowski K: MDS+items not contained in the pressure ulcer RAP associated with pressure ulcer prevalence in newly institutionalized elderly, *Ostomy Wound Manage* 45(1):24, 1999.

CHAPTER

24 Team Approach to a Wound Care Program

NANCY TOMASELLI & MARK S. GRANICK

OBJECTIVES

1. Distinguish between the patient population focus of an inpatient wound care program and an outpatient wound care program.
2. Describe the rationale for a multidisciplinary team in a wound care program.
3. List the activities in which the inpatient wound care team should participate.
4. Compare and contrast the potential constituents of a wound care team for hospitalized patients and for an outpatient care setting.

The delivery of health care is being restructured by the managed care system. Research-based outcomes and standards of care will ultimately govern reimbursement rates and influence the way in which nurses will practice. Managed care's influence on wound care has coerced practitioners into defining outcomes, healing rates, and paradigms of care. It is estimated that in 1998, $2.5 billion will be spent annually on wound care and pressure-reducing products in the United States. However, this cost does not cover the associated medical, financial, and psychologic effects of chronic ulcers on afflicted patients and families. Rather than allowing the managed care industry to arbitrarily dictate economically derived pathways of care, sufficient research data must be amassed to provide a more scientific approach to streamlining treatment strategies. Consequently, clinical decision making for wound care management must shift from the traditional roots to a more scientific, research-based paradigm across the continuum of care (Baharestani, 1995).

Chronic, nonhealing wounds often result in exorbitant health care costs, increased length of stay, increased mortality rates, increased litigious potential, and the imposition of multiple limitations on lifestyle and psychologic well-being (Baharestani, 1995). Cost containment is the driving force that is shifting wound care from inpatient to outpatient settings. However, the care of chronic wounds in the outpatient population is fragmented among several disciplines, none of which specialize in the prevention and treatment of chronic, nonhealing wounds (Ratliff and Rodeheaver, 1995).

ECONOMIC EFFECT OF CHRONIC WOUNDS

Pressure ulcers are a serious problem among hospitalized patients and are presently one of the most serious challenges to the current health care market. The prevalence of stage 2 or greater pressure ulcers in acute care hospitals is between 3.5% and 29.5% with an incidence of 2.7% to 29.5%. Specific populations present an even higher risk, including patients with quadriplegia who have a 60% prevalence, elderly patients admitted for femoral fracture with a 66% incidence, and critical care patients with a 33% incidence and a 41% prevalence (AHCPR, 1994).

Pressure ulcers may require debridement or definitive surgical treatment and may be complicated by sepsis, fasciitis, cellulitis, or osteomyelitis. Development of a progressive pressure ulceration is associated with a several-fold increased risk of in-hospital death, as well as prolonged and expensive hospitalizations (Allman, 1988). Malpractice settlements of up to $65 million have also been awarded to patients with pressure ulcers (Baharestani, 1995).

Wound care in the acute care setting has become a multibillion dollar industry with 14% to 20% of all patients at risk for developing pressure ulcers (Allman et al, 1986; Barbanel et al, 1977; Ek and Boman, 1982). During hospitalization, 1.2% to 2.7% of all patients have a stage 2 or greater pressure ulcer (Anderson and Kvorning, 1982; Gerson, 1975; Gosnell, Johannsen, and Ayres, 1992). About 5.4% of all patients admitted without an ulcer develop a stage 1 ulcer (Gosnell, Johannsen, and Ayres, 1992). In 1992, Medicare costs for treatment of pressure ulcers in acute care were estimated at $836 million with a mean hospital cost per patient with an admitting diagnosis of a pressure ulcer of $21,675 (Bergstrom et al, 1994; Miller and Delozier, 1994). The total cost for all settings was $1.335 billion. A significant decrease in patient morbidity and health care costs could be significantly decreased if patients at risk were identified and aggressive interventions take place before development or progression of wounds (Granick, McGowan, and Long, 1998; Long and Granick, 1998).

The Agency for Health Care Policy and Research (AHCPR; currently known as the Agency for Healthcare Research and Quality [AHRQ]) anticipates that its guideline for *Pressure Ulcers in Adults: Prediction and Prevention* will stimulate the development of effective prevention programs, which will reduce the incidence of pressure ulcers (AHCPR, 1992). The implementation of the AHCPR Clinical Practice Guideline #15, *Treatment of Pressure Ulcers*, is estimated to reduce the cost of pressure ulcer treatment by 3%, or $40 million (Bergstrom et al, 1994). The cost in terms of patient morbidity is inestimable. Increased awareness of risk factors associated with pressure ulcers is essential to establishing effective prevention and treatment of such ulcers.

The number of documented cutaneous lower-extremity ulcers, primarily venous ulcers and diabetic ulcers, has also reached staggering proportions. In 1989, approximately 3 million patients in the United States were diagnosed with diabetic foot ulcers. In the United States, 25% of the population have peripheral vascular occlusive disease or venous insufficiency, resulting in more than 500,000 leg ulcers each year. Within this group of patients with leg ulcers, 60,000 amputations were performed. The growing number of patients with underlying medical conditions, such as diabetes mellitus, venous or arterial insufficiency, and confinement to a wheelchair or bed, has resulted in the increasing incidence of chronic soft tissue wounds (Barharestani, 1995; Glover et al, 1997).

RATIONALE FOR THE WOUND CARE TEAM

Hospitals across the nation are faced with many of the same challenges, including a changing reimbursement picture, labor shortages, and increased patient acuity. To maintain and improve the level of care in the face of these changes, one must have the vision and commitment to pay special attention to wound care since wound care represents a significant drain on already limited resources. A failure to do so may result in deterioration in quality of care (The Gaymar TEAM Program, 1989).

The team approach for wound care can be implemented in inpatient and outpatient settings. In the inpatient setting, the focus is on prevention of iatrogenic wounds, primarily pressure ulcers. Recognition of patients at risk for skin breakdown and early aggressive intervention are the emphases in the hospital setting (Granick, McGowan, and Long, 1998; Long and Granick, 1998). The focus in the outpatient setting mainly concerns chronic lower-extremity ulcers. Treatment programs revolve around maintenance of chronic diseases.

In many acute care institutions, wound and skin care are fragmented and there is inconsistent adherence to state-of-the-art standards. There is not always systematic risk assessment at the time of admission. Pressure sore identification in early stages of development must be the standard. There should be a consistent and logical approach to treatment of identified wounds according to the etiology of the wound. To accomplish this, coordination between nursing, medicine, surgery, nutrition, and rehabilitation must occur. Identification of prevention and treatment protocols is necessary to provide cost-effective and realistic treatment for patients and caregivers in terms of accessibility, affordability, and ease of use. Appropriate data collection and statistical analyses are needed to demonstrate clinical outcomes for various wound-healing and tissue-repair programs. Toward this end, a holistic, collaborative approach by a multidisciplinary team who diligently monitors the patient's health status across care settings is essential to facilitate state-of-the-art care (Granick et al, 1996; Tomaselli and Oxler, 1997).

GOALS FOR THE WOUND CARE TEAM

The etiology of wounds is multidimensional, and the solution demands an aggressive multidisciplinary approach. A multidisciplinary prevention-based program standardizes pressure ulcer and wound care (AHCPR, 1992; Bergstrom et al, 1994; WOCN, 1992a, 1992b). Therefore the goals of a comprehensive skin care program are to provide protocols and programs and to educate the health care team in prevention and treatment measures. The program should improve quality of care at all levels of providers, including medical staff, professional and paraprofessional staff, and lay caregivers. Standardization occurs based on outcome findings, cost savings, and appropriate and efficient use of supplies. These goals may be accomplished through a consistent approach to collaborative decision making.

The anticipated outcome is a comprehensive, research-based skin care program that is standardized within and across care settings. This would provide professionals with a better understanding of care provided by other disciplines. Referrals can be made based on decision trees. Appropriate use of resources facilitates a decrease in nosocomial pressure ulcers, shortened wound healing time, appropriate referral of unresponsive chronic wounds, and decreased length of stay. In addition, there are decreased discrepancies in wound documentation, improved financial outcomes, and increased patient knowledge and participation (Granick, McGowan, and Long, 1998; Tomaselli and Oxler, 1997).

TEAM CONSTITUENTS AND RESPONSIBILITIES

The charge of the wound and skin care team ideally is to act as the health care team for prevention and treatment of wounds (Moody et al, 1988). Ongoing data collection and evaluation of research findings will focus the team to identify hospital trends through clinical rounds and statistical analysis that affect cost effectiveness, reimbursement, and clinical care issues (Bolton, Van Rijswijk, and Shaffer, 1996; Phillips, 1996). Interdisciplinary collaboration should occur to ensure quality patient outcomes (AHCPR, 1992; Bergstrom et al, 1994; The Gaymar TEAM Program, 1989). Recommendations for standardization of skin care protocols should be made in concert with Joint Commission on Accreditation of Healthcare Organizations (JCAHO) guidelines and the AHCPR guidelines for prevention and treatment of pressure ulcers (Suntken et al, 1996; WOCN, 1992a, 1992b). Opportunities should be identified to reduce liability (Miller and Delozier, 1994). The team fosters a consistent approach of documenting and communicating clinical findings (Motta, Thimsen-Whitaker, and Demoor, 1995) and recommends changes and/or revisions to policies, procedures, and patient care standards (Baharestani, 1995; Knight, 1996). Standardized protocols for risk assessment must be supported (Hunter et al, 1995; Kresevic and Naylor, 1995). The team can also direct clinical trials of products using standard evaluation protocols (Turnbull, 1996). The team reviews quality assurance findings, patient care outcomes, and support initiatives to improve quality scores (Gates, 1996; Lessner, 1996). A link with the patient education department should occur to support development of patient education materials. Finally, the team evaluates and communicates the results of outcome analysis (Tomaselli and Oxler, 1997).

The wound care committee structure includes a multidisciplinary group to formalize and standardize operation and clinical, financial and biomedical issues related to prevention and treatment of wounds (Granick et al, 1996). The team serves as the final reviewing body for such issues and makes recommendations to other committees as appropriate. The multidisciplinary group includes administration, geriatrics, plastic surgery, vascular surgery, a wound care nurse, nursing, nutrition, pharmacy, materials management, purchasing, infection control, quality assurance, physical and occupational therapy, finance, biomedical, and home care. Ad-hoc members include trauma, risk management, and staff development. Consultants include dermatology, podiatry, orthotic specialists, diabetology, social service, and rehabilitation.

The wound care committee may also interface with clinical working groups such as a specialty bed committee, practice and procedure committee, quality review committee, and a research committee. These groups can meet periodically to coordinate and implement advisory group recommendations.

ACTIVITIES AND COMPONENTS OF THE WOUND CARE PROGRAM

A mechanism must be developed to fully implement and provide continuing evaluation of the skin and wound care program. Key elements include organizing the multidisciplinary committee, planning a comprehensive program, and evaluating and selecting products. Specific components of the comprehensive program are risk assessment, prevention and treatment strategies, clinical pathways, product selection guidelines and recommendations, data collection guidelines, staff development guidelines and tools, and an ongoing evaluation process. None of these processes are effective without an intensive educational program with ongoing reinforcement. It is also necessary to obtain medical staff approval. Without the support of the admitting physicians, this endeavor is doomed.

All patients should be initially screened for skin breakdown. There are several risk-assessment tools available. A scale should be selected according to its usefulness in a particular setting. However, the Braden Scale and the Norton Scale have been tested extensively and are recommended by the AHCPR (1992). These tools serve as guidelines to ensure systematic evaluation of individual risk factors. From this assessment, proactive interventions can be developed to treat patients with different degrees of risk to prevent or keep current ulcers from getting worse (Bergstrom et al, 1995, 1996). Risk assessment needs to be performed at periodic intervals with documentation of all assessments (AHCPR, 1992).

Prevention and treatment strategies, wound care, and documentation guidelines are imperative to ensure effective and appropriate care. The AHCPR (AHCPR, 1992; Bergstrom et al, 1994) and the Wound, Ostomy, and Continence Nurses Society (WOCN, 1992a, 1992b, 1996, 1997, 1999a; Tomaselli, 1994a) have guidelines and fact sheets to assist the team with developing such strategies.

Product selection guidelines and recommendations are another necessary component of the comprehensive skin care program. There are several categories for wound care products. One product from each category can be selected for use. Once the objective for wound care is determined, a product can be selected for use from the appropriate category (Granick et al, 1996). The creation of a formulary is also discussed in Chapter 5. If other products are needed, the wound care team can select them as deemed necessary for individual cases.

Educational programs should be designed to facilitate the development and implementation of effective treatment strategies and should be updated on an ongoing basis to integrate new knowledge, techniques, or technologies. The AHCPR (Bergstrom et al, 1994) recommends an educational program that includes prevention and treatment, assessing tissue damage, and monitoring outcomes (see Appendix C).

The prevention and treatment program includes a comprehensive approach to prevention and effective treatment protocols that promote healing and prevent recurrence. This program should be for patients, caregivers, and health care providers across the continuum of care. Principles of adult learning should be used to maximize retention and ensure a carryover into practice. The patient and caregiver should be encouraged to participate in and comply with decisions regarding prevention and treatment strategies. Those responsible for the treatment should be identified, and roles should be defined.

The program for assessing tissue damage should emphasize the importance of accuracy and consistency in assessing and documenting the extent of tissue injury. There are multiple facets of wound healing that should be understood before any treatment interventions. Clearly, the risk factors for a particular patient and the etiology need to be clarified. The protocol for staging (Bergstrom et al, 1994, Tomaselli, 1994b) should be used for consistency and compatibility to treatments described in the literature. Coordinating the medical and nutritional management of the patient is a priority before any direct wound treatments are prescribed. Specific treatment of the wound itself incorporates a thorough understanding of the principles of wound cleansing and infection control, available dressings, and manipulation of the mechanical environment of the wound, and recognizing when surgery is indicated. Patient positioning and support surfaces are critical in this patient population (Wind, Tomaselli, and Goldberg, 1993).

Data collection and analysis are inextricably linked to a quality wound care program because this is the only way to determine the effect of the program. The nursing assessment form completed upon admission to the hospital should be reviewed and revised to include pertinent baseline skin/wound care parameters. If possible, the twice-weekly wound assessments should be computerized to facilitate the development of a minimum data set that can be abstracted and analyzed easily (Werley et al, 1991; WOCN, 1999c).

Treatment outcomes should be monitored periodically, and the data collection should include implementing guideline recommendations, healing existing wounds, reducing the incidence of new or recurrent wounds, and preventing deterioration of existing wounds. Information from these surveys serves to identify deficiencies, evaluate effectiveness of care, and determine the need for education and policy changes. Staff education will then focus on identified deficiencies (Bergstrom et al, 1994).

Quality improvement is an integral part of the skin care program. The goal of quality improvement is provide a feedback mechanism to evaluate the effectiveness of the program. Continuous or intermittent monitoring of all aspects of the program is necessary so that the team can evolve as an effective force. Incidence and prevalence studies provide baseline data from which the team can extract information about the effectiveness of the protocols. A responsive wound care team will regularly use this information to modify their protocols. This information will similarly influence the focus of the ongoing educational program (Bergstrom et al, 1994).

Granick and Ladin (1998) have described the differing approaches that can be used to implement such a team in different hospitals. The greatest barrier to a wound care team is lack of understanding of what it can accomplish and how it can influence hospital savings and lower patient morbidity (Granick, McGowan, and Long, 1998). Nevertheless, economic factors, concerns over patient control, legal responsibility for patient care, administrative issues, organization of nursing services, educational infrastructure, and hospital politics are all potential yet major impediments in the development of an effective wound care team.

Comprehensive approaches to wound care management in acute care have been previously reported (Granick and Ladin, 1998, Granick et al, 1996, Klingel, 1996, Suntken et al, 1996). Prevalence and incidence studies establish a database for tracking policy effectiveness and compliance. The wound care team can then assess areas that need improvement and monitor the effect of changes in health care, including downsizing of staff, cost cutting, equipment changes, and new wound care products. Wound care teams can also improve cost-effectiveness in product and specialty bed use and become indispensable for the delivery of optimal patient care (Long and Granick, 1998).

WOUND CARE PROGRAMS IN THE CLINIC SETTING

In the outpatient setting, the team deals with a different spectrum of diseases. Approximately 70% to 75% of wounds are chronic leg ulcers, including venous and diabetic ulcers, post-radiation wounds, skin disorders, and wounds related to other disease processes. The focus of the team is to improve and standardize wound care in the home, long-term, and subacute care settings. Medical problems need to be optimized before wounds will heal. Administrative approval is necessary to develop protocols for treatment of various wounds. This team could be an extension of the acute care team.

The team optimally consists of a nurse coordinator, wound care nurse, vascular surgeon, plastic surgeon, orthopedic surgeon, general surgeon, endocrinologist, podiatrist, and an insurance coordinator. Any health care professional with an interest in wound care should be encouraged to participate. Good communications with the primary care physicians are essential. Patient access is needed for noninvasive vascular studies, physical therapy, and nutritional consultation. Nonclinical staff such as the receptionist or scheduling clerk are also valued members of the team. Wound healing and efficiency of the clinic can be influenced by nonattendance or failed appointments (Pieper and DiNardo, 1998). The receptionist may be instrumental in minimizing missed appointments by calling the patient to remind him or her of scheduled appointments.

Implementation of the program occurs through a program of marketing and education of referring physicians, health care providers, and caregivers. The WOCN (1997, 1999a) has developed fact sheets for establishing clinics and for reimbursement for services in an ambulatory setting.

Services provided by the multidisciplinary team include assessment of the patient's wound and his or her medical and nutritional status. Recommendations can then be made for correction of etiologic factors. Compression therapy is instituted for patients with venous stasis ulcers. Recommendations for nutritional support and topical therapy are also instituted along with conservative sharp debridement and chemical cauterization of excessive granulation tissue. Education of the patient, family, and caregiver is imperative. Prophylactic foot and nail care for patients with diabetes and lower-extremity arterial ulcers includes nail debridement, paring of corns and calluses, and patient education for foot care and appropriate footwear.

The team can coordinate referrals for problems that cannot be addressed in the outpatient wound care setting and provide ongoing evaluation, treatment, and long-term follow-up care. Outcome data are imperative to demonstrate wound healing, overall awareness, and appropriate allocation of resources. The goals should include not only a healed wound but also overall adjustment of patients to the outpatient environment and to coping with these wounds. The result of treating patients in an outpatient setting is that it contributes to fewer costly emergency room visits and hospital admissions. More patients will be treated on an outpatient basis as the acuity of hospital admissions rises. Ultimately, patients will receive expert care at a significantly reduced price in a timely fashion.

SUMMARY

Wound and skin care needs are pervasive in any health care setting. Wounds need to be assessed, skin needs to be monitored, documentation needs to be accurate, wound and skin management needs to be consistent, and implementation of prevention interventions needs to be routine. An organized formal wound and skin care program is essential for all hospital-based wound care nurses. The need for an outpatient program quickly becomes apparent once the inpatient program is operational. Resources such as data collection forms, job descriptions, and position statements are available (WOCN, 1999b, 1999c). The types of wounds that may be dominant in an outpatient clinic versus the inpatient setting may differ. Therefore the constituents of a wound care team and the emphasis of care may be different. Because wounds are multifactorial in nature, a multidisciplinary team approach to wound management is critical to ensure efficient, effective realization of positive outcomes.

SELF-ASSESSMENT EXERCISE

1. All of the following statements about an outpatient wound care program is true EXCEPT:
   a. A pressure ulcer risk assessment protocol is essential
   b. A variety of chronic lower leg wounds should be anticipated
   c. An insurance coordinator should be a member of the wound care team
   d. Nutritional assessment is a key activity of the wound care team
2. Provide two arguments for implementing a wound and skin care team in an acute care setting.
3. List at least five activities of the wound and skin care team in the acute care setting.

REFERENCES

Agency for Health Care Policy and Research: *Pressure ulcers in adults: prediction and prevention*, Rockville, Md, 1992, USDHHS, AHCPR Pub. No. 92-0047.

Allman R: The use of specialized beds and mattresses for the prevention and treatment of pressure ulcers. In Como J, Farringer J, editors: *Drug information bulletin*, Birmingham, 1988, University of Alabama.

Allman R et al: Pressure sores among hospitalized patients, *Ann Intern Med* 105:337, 1986.

Anderson K, Kvorning S: Medical aspects of the decubitus ulcer, *Int J Dermatol* 21:265, 1982.

Baharestani M: Clinical decision making in wound care management: the need for a paradigmatic shift, *Wounds: A Compendium of Clinical Research and Practice* 7(suppl A):84A, 1995.

Barbanel J et al: Incidence of pressure sores in the Greater Glasgow Health Board Area, *Lancet* 2:548, 1977.

Bergstrom N et al: Multi-site study of incidence of pressure ulcers and the relationship between risk level, demographic characteristics, diagnoses, and prescription of preventive interventions, *J Am Geriatr Soc* 44:22, 1996.

Bergstrom N et al: *Treatment of pressure ulcers*, Clinical Practice Guideline #15, Rockville, Md, 1994, USDHHS, PHS, AHCPR Pub. No. 95-0652.

Bergstrom N et al: Using a research-based assessment scale in clinical practice, *Nurs Clin North Am* 30(3):539, 1995.

Bolton L, Van Rijswijk L, Shaffer F: Quality wound care equals cost-effective wound care, *Nurs Manage* 27(7):30, 1996.

Ek A, Boman G: A descriptive study of pressure sores: the prevalence of pressure sores and the characteristics of patients, *J Adv Nurs* 7:51, 1982.

Gates J: Total quality management: pressure ulcer prevention, *Nurs Manage* 27(4):48E, 1996.

Gerson LW: The incidence of pressure sores in active treatment hospitals, *Int J Nurs Stud* 12(4):201, 1975.

Glover JL et al: A 4-year outcome-based retrospective study of wound healing and limb salvage in patients with chronic wounds, *Adv Wound Care* 10:33, 1997.

Gosnell D, Johannsen J, Ayres M: Pressure ulcer incidence and severity in a community hospital, *Decubitus* 5:56, 1992.

Granick MS et al: Wound management and wound care. In Habal HB, editor: *Advances in plastic and reconstructive surgery*, vol 12, St Louis, 1996, Mosby.

Granick MS, Ladin DA: The multidisciplinary wound care team: two models, *Adv Wound Care* 11(2):80, 1998.

Granick MS, McGowan E, Long CD: Outcome assessment of an in-hospital cross-functional wound care team, *Plast Reconstr Surg* 101(5):1243, 1998.

Hunter SM et al: The effectiveness of skin care protocols for pressure ulcers, *Rehabil Nurs* 20(5):250, 1995.

Klingel P: Exploring the process of a skin care team, *Ostomy Wound Manage* (42):30, 1996.

Knight C: The chronic wound management decision tree: a tool for long-term care nurses, *J Wound Ostomy Continence Nurs* 23(2):92, 1996.

Kresevic D, Naylor M: Preventing pressure ulcers through the use of protocols in a mentoring nursing model, *Geriatr Nurs* 16(5):225, 1995.

Lessner W: Small but successful changes prepare MDs for advent of decubitus protocol, *Quality Improvement/Total Quality Management* 6(1):1, 1996.

Long C, Granick M: A multidisciplinary approach to wound care in the hospitalized patient, *Clin Plast Surg* 25(3):425, 1998.

Miller H, Delozier J: *Cost implications of the pressure ulcer treatment guideline*, Columbia, Md, Center for Health Policy Studies, Contract No. 282-91-0070, p. 17, 1994. Sponsored by the AHCPR.

Moody B et al: Impact of staff education on pressure sore development in elderly hospitalized patients, *Arch Intern Med* 10:2241, 1988.

Motta GJ, Thimsen-Whitaker K, Demoor MA: Documenting outcomes of wound care, *Contin Care* 14(8):16, 1995.

Phillips T: Cost-effectiveness in wound care, *Ostomy Wound Manage* 42(1):56, 1996.

Pieper B, DiNardo E: Reasons for nonattendance for the treatment of venous ulcers in an inner-city clinic, *J Wound Ostomy Continence Nurs* 25:180, 1998.

Ratliff C, Rodeheaver G: The chronic wound care clinic: "one-stop shopping," *J Wound Ostomy Continence Nurs* 22(2):77, 1995.

Suntken G et al: Implementation of a comprehensive skin care program across care settings using the AHCPR pressure ulcer prevention and treatment guidelines, *Ostomy Wound Manage* 42(2):20, 1996.

The Gaymar TEAM Program: *A step by step approach to pressure ulcer management*, Lourdes, France, 1989, Hospital/Gaymar Industries, Inc.

Tomaselli N: WOCN position statement for conservative sharp wound debridement for registered nurses, *WOCN News*, p 13, Aug/Sept, 1994a.

Tomaselli N: Wound staging alert, *WOCN News*, p 11, Oct/Nov, 1994b.

Tomaselli N, Oxler K: *Thomas Jefferson University Hospital comprehensive skin care program*, Philadelphia, 1997, Thomas Jefferson University Hospital.

Turnbull G: The international committee on wound management (ICWM) statement on cost-effective wound care: evaluating your supply use to prepare for managed care, *Ostomy Wound Manage* 42(2):72, 1996.

Werley JJ et al: The nursing minimum data set: abstraction tool for standardized, comparable, essential data, *Am J Public Health* 81(4):421, 1991.

Wind S, Tomaselli N, Goldberg ME: Pressure-relieving and pressure-reducing devices. In Boggs RL, Wooldridge-King M, editors: *AACN procedure manual for critical care*, ed 3, Philadelphia, 1993, W.B. Saunders.

Wound, Ostomy, and Continence Nurses Society: *Standards of care: patients with dermal wounds: pressure ulcers*, Laguna Beach, Calif, 1992a, WOCN.

Wound, Ostomy, and Continence Nurses Society: *Standards of care: patients with dermal wounds: lower extremity ulcers*, Laguna Beach, Calif, 1992b, WOCN.

Wound, Ostomy, and Continence Nurses Society: *Clinical practice fact sheets: quick assessment of leg ulcers, venous insufficiency (stasis), peripheral neuropathy, arterial insufficiency*, Laguna Beach, Calif, 1996, WOCN. Available at www.wocn.org under Resources, Fact Sheets.

Wound, Ostomy, and Continence Nurses Society: *Professional practice fact sheet: establishment of wound ostomy continence clinics*, Laguna Beach, Calif, 1997, WOCN. Available at www.wocn.org under Resources, Fact Sheets.

Wound, Ostomy, and Continence Nurses Society: *Professional practice fact sheet: reimbursement options for WOC (ET) nurses in ambulatory care*, Laguna Beach, Calif, 1999a, WOCN. Available at www.wocn.org under Resources, Fact Sheets.

Wound, Ostomy, and Continence Nurses Society: *Professional practice manual*, ed 2, Laguna Beach, Calif, 1999b, WOCN.

Wound, Ostomy, and Continence Nurses Society: *Clinical practice data management system*, Laguna Beach, Calif, 1999c, WOCN.

APPENDIX

A SELF-ASSESSMENT ANSWERS

CHAPTER 1

1. The skin serves as a protective barrier against the external environment and contributes to maintenance of a homeostatic internal environment.
2. Epidermis, basement membrane, dermis, and hypodermis.
3. Cells in the stratum corneum are primarily epithelial cells, which are referred to as *keratinocytes* because they are almost completely filled with keratin, a fibrous protein.
4. c
5. Rete ridges are the epidermal protrusions of the basal layer that point downward into the dermis. They help to anchor the epidermis, thus providing structural integrity.
6. b
7. The two dermal proteins are collagen and elastin. *Collagen* is the protein that gives skin its tensile strength; key constituents are proline, glycine, hydroxyproline, and hydroxylysine. Collagen is secreted by dermal fibroblasts. *Elastin* provides the skin with elastic recoil; key constituents are proline and glycine (not hydroxyproline).
8. Protection, thermoregulation, sensation, metabolism, and communication
9. • The keratinocytes of an intact stratum corneum provide a resistant barrier; the constant shedding of squames prevents entrenchment of microorganisms.
   - The sebum secreted by the sebaceous glands maintains an acid pH (4.0 to 6.8), which inhibits growth of microorganisms.
   - The normal skin flora provides bacterial interference to pathogens.
   - The skin has an immune system: Langerhans' cells in the epidermis; macrophages and mast cells in the dermis. Langerhans' cells are antigen-presenting cells, macrophages phagocytize bacteria; mast cells contribute to the inflammatory response by release of histamine.
10. c
11. c
12. *Premature infant skin* is thin, poorly keratinized, and functions weakly as a barrier. Transepidermal water loss is high as are evaporative heat losses. *Newborn skin* and nails are thinner than those in the adult; with aging they will gradually increase in thickness. Newborn skin is not an effective barrier to transcutaneous water loss. Newborn dermis is 60% as thick as adult dermis; dermal fibers are finer than adult dermal fibers. Newborn dermis has a higher cellular component than adult skin. Rete ridges are weakly developed at birth. Capillary beds in the newborn dermis are disorganized.
13. *Adolescent skin.* Hormonal stimulation increases the activity of sebaceous glands and hair follicles. *Adult skin.* Dermis thickens; epidermal turnover time is increased; barrier function is reduced; number of active melanocytes is decreased; skin is dry; wrinkles diminished sensory receptors, vitamin D production is decreased.
14. b
15. True
16. c

CHAPTER 2

1. Wounds involving only the epidermis and dermis heal relatively quickly because epithelial, endothelial, and connective tissue can be reproduced. Wounds extending through the dermis and involving deeper structures must

heal by scar formation because the deep dermal structures, subcutaneous tissue, and muscle do not regenerate.

2. Wounds that are well approximated with minimal tissue defect are said to heal by *primary intention.* Wounds that are left open and allowed to heal by production of granulation tissue are said to heal by *secondary intention.* Wound are described as healing be *tertiary intention* when there is a delay between injury and reapproximation of the wound edges.
3. Inflammatory response, epithelial proliferation and migration, and reestablishment and differentiation of epidermal layers. If dermis is involved, connective tissue repair proceeds concurrently with reepithelialization.
4. A moist wound surface facilitates epidermal migration because epidermal cells can migrate only across a moist surface. In a dry wound, epidermal cells must tunnel down to a moist level and secrete collagenase to lift the scab away from the wound surface in order to migrate. Connective tissue repair begins earlier when the wound surface is kept moist because new connective tissue forms only in the presence of suitable exudate.
5. *Inflammatory phase.* Hemostasis and inflammation. *Proliferative phase.* Neoangiogenesis, matrix deposition/collagen synthesis, epithelialization, and when a full-thickness wound is left to heal by secondary intention, contraction of wound edges. *Maturation phase.* Matrix deposition and collagen lysis.
6. d
7. Key events are 1) hemostasis, mediated by clotting factors and platelets, and 2) inflammation, mediated by neutrophils and macrophages. The overall result of this phase is control of bleeding and establishment of a clean wound bed. Characteristics of wounds in the inflammatory phase are erythema, edema, pain, and exudate.
8. *Granulation* refers to the formation of new connective tissue (scar formation) to *fill* a defect and involves neoangiogenesis and collagen synthesis. Granulation tissue appears very red, moist, and granular. *Epithelialization* refers to the migration of epithelial cells to *resurface* a defect. New epithelial tissue initially appears pink and dry and then gradually repigments to match the person's skin tone.
9. The fibroblast synthesizes the new connective tissue that fills the defect; wound healing cannot take place without normal fibroblast function.
10. The hypoxia resulting from disruption of vascular pathways creates an oxygen "gradient" between the vascularized periphery of the wound and its hypoxic center. Macrophages thrive in this hypoxic environment and release growth factors that "attract" vascular endothelial cells, which stimulate capillary regrowth. Hypoxia also results in lactate production, which stimulates fibroblasts to synthesize collagen. Thus hypoxia in the wound center helps to drive tissue repair. Oxygen is required for cellular proliferation and migration and for immune system function. Therefore the ability to respond to the hypoxic stimulus with capillary proliferation, the ability to synthesize collagen, and the ability to control bacterial proliferation are all dependent on adequate oxygen levels at the advancing wound edge.
11. b
12. There is a limit to epidermal cell migration, and in full-thickness wounds epidermal cells are present only at the wound margins. In partial-thickness wounds, epidermal cells are present in the lining of hair follicles and sweat glands as well as the wound periphery.
13. The two components are extracellular matrix breakdown and matrix production, otherwise referred to as *collagen lysis* and *collagen synthesis.* The desired outcome is a well-organized scar with maximum tensile strength (80% that of nonwounded tissue).
14. Chronic wounds are likely to begin with circulatory compromise as opposed to injury. Injury initiates hemostasis, which triggers the wound-healing cascade; circulatory compromise does not trigger the wound-healing cascade. Chronic wounds also contain increased levels of protease produced by the prolonged

presence and increased volume of proinflammatory cells.

15. Tissue perfusion and oxygenation, nutritional status, infection, diabetes mellitus, corticosteroid administration, immunosuppression, aging. Systemic factors include renal or hepatic disease, malignancy, sepsis, hematopoietic abnormalities, sleep, and stress.

16. d

17. b

CHAPTER 3

1. a

2. d

3. b

4. c

5. d

6. c

7. b

8. d

9. b

10. e

CHAPTER 4

1. • *Measurement of existing wound.* The focus of measurement is to determine the size of the wound either with linear measurements, fluid instillation, wound molds, photographs, planimetry, or foam. Measurement captures only one aspect of the wound.

• *Assessment of wound healing status.* The focus is to delineate the subtle changes within the wound that indicate that healing is occurring. Known markers would be used as barometers of the wound's health status. Ideally, repeated assessment of wound status would also reveal the wound's healing trajectory. For example, the Wound Characteristics Instrument (WCI) contains 17 items that provide a framework to complete a systematic evaluation of the status of an open, soft tissue, postsurgical wound.

2. c

3. b

4. *Partial thickness.* Tissue loss that is limited to the epidermal or dermal layers of the skin; damage does not penetrate below the dermis.

Full thickness. Tissue loss that extends below the dermis. Unfortunately the exposed tissue may be subcutaneous tissue, muscle, tendon, or bone. The phrase does not indicate the extent of the full-thickness damage.

5. **a.** Reliability of the measurements obtained can be varied, so inconsistent linear measures may be reported.

b. Quality of the tissue in the wound or presence of granulation, epithelial tissue, or nonviable tissue is not reflected in the measurement.

c. Condition of the surrounding skin (such as erythema, induration, maceration) is not captured by the terminology.

d. The presence of odor or exudate is not indicated.

e. The fact that wounds are irregularly shaped makes it difficult to get an accurate reflection of the size; most commonly, the clinician measures each axis only by the widest dimension.

6. Size, extent of wound, presence of undermining or tracts, anatomic location, type of tissue in wound base, color, exudate (amount, consistency, odor), edge of open wound, presence of foreign bodies, condition of the surrounding skin, and duration of the wound

7. **a.** *Nonviable.* Tissue that is not healthy or living; may also be more specific to state that it is eschar, adherent, slough, or other descriptive terms.

b. *Eschar.* Thick, leathery, black necrotic tissue.

c. *Granulation.* Establishment of capillaries and collagen in a full-thickness wound; appearance is beefy red, granular, and moist.

d. *Epithelialization.* Process of epithelial cells resurfacing in a full- or partial-thickness wound.

CHAPTER 5

1. d

2. d

3. a

4. c

5. b

6. d
7. b
8. d
9. b
10. c
11. Tissue hydration is one of the functions of the stratum corneum. Dressings serve as a surrogate stratum corneum in wounded skin. Moisture vapor transmission rate (MVTR) is a measure of moisture vapor per area of material per time period. If the dressing transmits less moisture vapor than the wound loses, the wound will remain moist. For example, skin damaged by tape stripping has an approximate MVTR of over 7000 g/m^2/day, whereas most transparent dressings have an MVTR of 400 to 800 g/m^2/day.
12. **a.** *Prevent/manage infection.* Can use a semi-occlusive dressing such as a hydrocolloid or transparent dressing to prevent contamination from fecal incontinence or a fistula.
    b. *Cleanse wound.* Use a normal saline applied with correct amount of pressure such as with a 35-ml syringe and 19-gauge angiocatheter.
    c. *Remove nonviable tissue.* Many dressings provide autolysis by creating a moist environment; could select an enzyme and gauze dressing.
    d. *Manage exudate.* May use a hydrocolloid or wound fillers for small to moderate amount of exudate; alginate for large amount of exudate. Change dressing at appropriate time intervals.
    e. *Eliminate dead space.* Use wound fillers, amorphous hydrogels, or alginates, for example, depending upon extent of dead space.
    f. *Control odor.* Change dressings at appropriate time intervals.
    g. *Protect wounds.* Use skin sealants as needed around wound edges to protect from maceration.
13. Wound is packed to fill dead space to avoid potential abscess formation or premature wound closure and to ascertain that the entire wound bed surface is contacted by a moisture-retentive dressing. Packing is placed loosely into the wound, often with a cotton-tipped applicator so that the entire wound bed is in contact with the dressing. Overpacking is to be avoided

CHAPTER 6

1. Mechanical, chemical, vascular, allergic, infectious, immunologic, burn, and disease-related
2. b
3. a
4. *Ulcers* involve the loss of epidermis and dermis. Healing occurs by scar formation. *Erosion* involves partial loss of epidermis; tissue loss does not extend below the epidermis. Healing occurs without scarring.
5. Do not apply tape under tension; remove tape slowly by peeling skin away; use porous adhesives; use skin sealants, thin hydrocolloids, or solid-wafer barriers under adhesives; avoid use of tapes by using roll gauze or self-adherent tape; use Montgomery straps.
6. Apply moisture barrier ointments after each stool, apply rectal pouch if stooling more than three times per 8 hours, apply ointment pastes if moisture-barrier ointment is ineffective.
7. b
8. d
9. Sensitization phase and elicitation phase
10. c
11. d
12. TEN, SSSS, GVHD

CHAPTER 7

1. d
2. c
3. Inactivated by heavy metal ions: chlorine, silver, and mercury; slow method of debridement; requires once to three times daily dressing changes; little evidence or criteria available to guide selection of debriding enzyme; primarily based on clinician preference, cost, availability, and ease of use; transient erythema and irritation on intact skin with papain/urea agents.

4. a
5. b

CHAPTER 8

1. b
2. d
3. a
4. d
5. a
6. c
7. d
8. d
9. e

CHAPTER 9

1. Oxidative killing, effective phagocytosis, collagen production by fibroblasts
2. Lack of drainage, erythema, dehiscence, excessive pain; well-approximated edges
3. False
4. False
5. Actively re-warm patient postoperatively, replace fluid, adequately control pain with medications and positioning, decrease exposure to cold, and reduce anxiety with patient education and/or medications
6. Palpable incisional induration is indicative of new collagen at postop days 4 to 8 and beyond
7. Pain, cutting of afferent nerves, cold, hypovolemia, fear, and surprise
8. d

CHAPTER 10

1. All three phases: inflammatory, proliferative, and maturation. The inflammatory response is seen with the vasodilatation and increased capillary permeability, epidermal cells proliferate between the mesh grafts and with partial-thickness wounds, and scar tissue formation and remodeling occur during the maturation phase.
2. Thermal burns occur in the home with cooking, scalds from hot water, and electrical malfunctions.
3. The zone of coagulation is the area closest to the heat source.
4. **(b)** The zone of stasis is an area of ischemia; restoration of circulation, prevention of desiccation, and infection will prevent further damage.
5. Amount of injury, depth, and severity.
6. **(a)** The Lund and Bower chart takes into consideration the degree and surface area of the burn.
7. **(b)** The inflammatory response releases various vasoactive and chemotactic agents that affect vasoconstriction, fluid balance, and metabolism.
8. **(c)** The most accurate method to assess fluid resuscitation adequacy is a urine output of at least 50 ml/hr in an adult.
9. **(b)** Early excision should occur after the fluid resuscitation, before wounds can become colonized.
10. **(b)** Sheet grafts are more cosmetically pleasing.
11. **(a)** Prevention of contractures, which should begin with admission
12. **(a)** Gram-positive bacteria
13. **(d)** All the above are considered minor burns.

CHAPTER 11

1. *Prevalence* is the number of patients with an existing pressure ulcer on a specific day. It is a cross-sectional measure that reflects the day-to-day baseline burden of a condition. Prevalence includes the patients who have the existing problem as well as new developments of the problem. *Incidence* is the number of new patients with a pressure ulcer that develops during a specific period of time in a population of patients who are at risk for developing a pressure ulcer. It is measured prospectively over a specified period of time. Incidence provides an indication of quality of care since it measures only new occurances.
2. Differences in the range within similar settings and between settings exist because 1) the data collector's ability to recognize damaged skin varies, 2) a standardized classification system is lacking (i.e., some studies define pressure ulcers as always having breaks in the skin, thus overlooking the potential for

pressure damage with intact skin), 3) some institutions have a concentrated population of patients shown to be at increased risk for pressure development, and 4) studies vary in population, design, and expertise of researchers. According to the NPUAP, the prevalence of pressure ulcers in acute care hospitals is 3% to 14% and in nursing homes is 15% to 25%. The literature reports a prevalence range of 25% to 40.4% for patients with spinal cord injury and 11.6% to 27.7% in the elderly.

3. A localized area of tissue necrosis that develops when soft tissue is compressed between a bony prominence and an external surface for a period of time

4. a

5. Intensity of pressure, duration of pressure, and tissue tolerance

6. b

7. c

8. It is difficult to accurately assign a numerical value to capillary closing pressure because 1) capillary blood pressure is influenced by values such as arterial blood pressure and venous pressure, which vary from individual to individual, from one bony prominence to another, and from time to time; and 2) capillary closing pressure, which is commonly reported as 25 to 31 mm Hg is based on studies in healthy adult males, whereas recent studies report capillary closing pressures as low as 12 mm Hg in the elderly.

9. c

10. When tissue interface pressures exceed capillary pressures, capillaries close and tissue hypoxia ensues; tissue hypoxia is tolerable for short periods of time, but prolonged ischemia results in tissue necrosis.

11. Amount and duration share an inverse relationship in producing tissue ischemia. It takes a long time for low pressure to create ischemia, whereas it takes a short time for high pressure to cause tissue ischemia.

12. d

13. b

14. Venous thrombus formation, endothelial cell damage, redistribution of blood supply in ischemic tissue, altered lymphatic fluid flow in the area of pressure

15. Occlusion of capillaries, imparied perfusion through edematous tissue, accumulation of metabolic wastes

16. Pressure is highest at the point of contact between soft tissue and bone; thus tissue necrosis initially occurs at the bone-soft tissue interface. Once a pressure ulcer manifests itself cutaneously, deeper tissue damage has already occurred.

17. a

18. *Specificity* measures "true negatives," the percentage of patients who did not develop pressure sores and were identified as being not at risk. *Sensitivity* measures "true positives," the percentage of patients who did develop pressure sores and were identifed as being at risk.

19. *Norton Scale*
- **a.** Five parameters
- **b.** Scale for parameters is from 1 to 4
- **c.** One- and two-word descriptors are given per rating of parameter
- **d.** Lower scores indicate increased risk

Gosnell Scale
- **a.** Five parameters
- **b.** Two- and three-sentence descriptive statements for each rating of parameter
- **c.** High scores denote increased risk

Braden Scale
- **a.** Six parameters
- **b.** Scale for parameters is from 1 to 4 (except for friction or shear category)
- **c.** Brief descriptions accompany each parameter
- **d.** Lower scores denote increased risk

20. Pressure reduction, pressure relief, control of moisture and maceration, kinetic therapy

21. Transducer size and shape, load shape and its interaction with the support material, method of equilibrium detection, uniformity of measurement technique, skill of person doing the test

22.
- **a.** *Overlay*. Device that is placed on top of a standard hospital mattress.
- **b.** *Replacement mattress*. Mattress that is used in place of the standard hospital mattress

and provides pressure reduction as well as the features of a standard mattress (long-term use, terminal cleaning).

c. *Specialty bed.* Bed used in place of standard hospital bed to provide pressure relief, relief of shear and friction, or kinetic therapy, or all three.

23. Thickness of 3 to 4 inches, density of 1.3 to 1.6 lb/ft^3, indentation load deflection (ILD; 25% ILD of about 30 pounds; ratio of 60% ILD to 25% ILD of 2.5 or greater)

24. Water overlays effectively reduce interface pressure by flotation therapy. However, water overlays have several disadvantages that make them less appropriate for acute care settings: potential for water leaks, which can create safety hazards; weight; requirement for personnel to set up and maintain overlay; potential for water displacement resulting in higher pressure in the heel area; limitations on patient positioning; difficulties with temperature regulation; potential for underfilling or overfilling; difficulty performing procedures (such as CPR) because of fluid motion.

25. Air overlays provide high-level pressure reduction, and some may provide pressure relief. Air overlays can be classified as either static or dynamic. *Static devices* are composed of interconnecting air cells that are inflated before patient use. They are called static devices because they reduce interface pressure by maintaining a constant inflation. Many static devices require daily monitoring for loss of air, with reinflation provided as needed; these are most effective in settings with adequate staff. Some static devices (low-air-loss overlays) are connected to pumps to maintain constant inflation and provide air flow to control moisture. *Dynamic devices* use electrical currents to create alternating currents of air for weight redistribution. In addition to weight redistribution, this change of air is believed to enhance blood flow by creating high and low pressure areas. Some dynamic devices also provide low levels of air flow to reduce maceration.

26. a

27. *Pressure relief* is indicated for patients who are unable to turn or be turned and for patients who have breakdown involving multiple turning surfaces. The rationale is that these patients need a surface that maintains continuous blood flow to the tissues. *Pressure reduction* is indicated for patients who can turn or be turned and whose breakdown (if present) is limited to one turning surface. The rationale is that these patients have at least two turning surfaces and can thus be maintained effectively with pressure reduction and a turning schedule.

28. **a.** Therapeutic considerations. Need for pressure relief versus pressure reduction, relief of shear and friction, moisture control, kinetic therapy (in determining need for pressure relief versus pressure reduction, one must consider caregiver compliance with turning).

b. Duration of therapy

c. Independence issues. Support surface should be selected so that it does not compromise patient's mobility and independence.

d. Setup and maintenance required and availability of such surfaces

e. Environmental issues, such as requirement for electricity in the home, disposal, and cost of disposal

f. Financial feasibility

CHAPTER 12

1. c
2. b
3. c
4. d
5. Small craters with well-defined borders, wound bed is pale or necrotic, there is minimal exudate from the wound, wound pain is present, and the wound is located distally on pressure points of the feet or in the area of trauma.
6. d
7. Venous blood in the lower leg creates a column of hydrostatic pressure (equal to about 90 mm Hg while standing). For venous blood to return to the heart, it must flow uphill

against this pressure. The deep veins, intact one-way valves within the veins, and the contraction of skeletal muscles facilitate venous blood return. During ambulation, the calf muscle contracts and pumps blood out of the deep veins, the one-way valves in the perforator system close to prevent backflow into the superficial veins, the calf muscle relaxes, and the valves in the perforator open to permit blood flow into the deep veins.

8. b
9. Elastic compression devices deliver a sustained pressure regardless of the patient's activity level (ambulatory or sedentary). Inelastic compression devices work by compressing the calf muscle during ambulation.
10. b
11. Compression devices provide a constant compression to the tissues and superfical veins; they also support the calf during ambulation. This constant compression increases interstitial tissue pressure to reduce leakage of fluid from capillaries. By supporting superficial dilated veins, the diameter of vessels is decreased so that blood velocity is increased and sluggishness of blood flow is decreased, which diminishes the tendency for leukocyte margination and extravasation.

CHAPTER 13

1. *Sensory neuropathy*. Reduced sensitivity to pain and temperature changes results in increased susceptibility to injury. *Motor neuropathy*. Loss of innervation to the muscles causes foot deformities and changes in gait, which alter weight bearing and result in repetitive stress. These predispose the patient to callus formation and ulceration, unless weight is properly redistributed. *Autonomic neuropathy*. Loss of sweating, which leads to chronically dry skin and predisposes the skin to cracking.
2. True
3. d
4. Causative factors, vascular status, presence of infection, presence of foreign body, degree of neuropathy, presence of necrotic tissue, presence of callus formation, glycemic control, nutritional status, contributing systemic factors (e.g., smoking, obesity, visual impairment).
5. Daily washing with a mild soap, lubrication/moisturizing after bathing, daily skin inspection and prompt reporting of any skin lesion or callus formation, shoes must fit properly, going barefoot is never appropriate, and professional care of toenails, corns, and callus.
6. Many disciplines may be involved in delivering care to the individual with neuropathy. The members of the team may include, but are not limited to, nurses, dietitian, social worker, podiatrist, diabetologist/internist, orthopedic surgeon, vascular surgeon, physical therapist, orthotist, and others as driven by patient need and regional variability.

CHAPTER 14

1. Presence of foreign body close to suture line, tension on suture line, improper suturing technique, distal obstruction, hematoma or abscess formation in mesentery at anastomotic site, presence of tumor or disease in area of anastomosis, inadequate blood supply to anastomosis
2. d
3. Fluid and electrolyte imbalances, malnutrition, sepsis
4. An abnormal passage between two or more structures or spaces.
5. b
6. **a.** Fistula between small bowel and skin
   b. Fistula between colon and skin
   c. Fistula between bladder and vagina
   d. Fistula between rectum and vagina
   e. Fistula between colon and bladder
7. Stabilization, investigation, conservative treatment, and definitive therapy
8. c
9. Complete disruption of bowel continuity, distal obstruction, foreign body in fistula tract, epithelium-lined tract contiguous with the skin, cancer in site, previous irradiation to site, Crohn's disease in site, presence of large abscess
10. Skin protection, containment of drainage,

odor control, patient comfort, accurate measurement of effluent, patient mobility, ease of use, cost containment

11. c

12. c

13. The bridging procedure should be used when it is helpful to isolate one area of a wound from another area of the wound. This may be needed for very large wounds or for wounds that have two distinct areas of "needs."

14. *Wounds managed with dressings.* Charcoal dressings can be secured over wound dressings; charcoal dressings must be kept dry. *Wound managed with pouches.* Meticulous pouch hygiene, pouch deodorants, and room deodorants. Oral deodorants may be an option in either situation.

15. c

16. d

CHAPTER 15

1. Drainage and decompression, nutritional support when the patient is at risk for aspiration pneumonia

2. Name and purpose of procedure, characteristics of normal tube function, why tube stabilization is important and how to ensure adequate stabilization, routine site care, signs and symptoms of complications (leakage, hyperplasia) and appropriate response, tube feeding schedule and procedure (when applicable), what to do if the tube falls out

3. **a.** *Janeway.* Gastrostomy intended for long-term use, surgically constructed to provide mucosa-lined stoma, which can be intubated as needed. *Stamm.* Gastrostomy intended for short-term use; surgically placed; tube remains in place and must be stabilized with internal bolster or balloon and external stabilization device.

b. *PEG.* Nonsurgical endoscopic placement of gastrostomy tube; important to seat gastrostomy tube against gastric mucosa and externally against abdominal wall. Has a lower complication rate than with surgery. *Gastrostomy button.* Short silicone tube with flip-top opening and one-way valve, which prevents external reflux of stomach contents. Feedings are administered after an adapter is passed through the one-way valve. Insertion can be done as outpatient.

c. *Foley catheter.* Latex tube with balloon port; must be inflated to designated balloon size internally and have external tube stabilization device to properly anchor tube and prevent migration; balloon is degraded by gastric contents and needs to be replaced monthly. *Gastrostomy replacement catheter.* Silastic catheter with balloon for internal anchoring against stomach wall and external bumper or flange for external stabilization.

4. Radiologic approach to enteral feeding is appropriate when patient is not a surgical candidate and cannot have endoscopy safely performed because of obesity, ascites, difficulty transilluminating the abdomen, etc.

5. *Advantages.* Low profile, prevents many complications associated with gastrostomy tubes (migration, leakage, inadvertent removal, tissue reaction), one-way valve allows feeding but provides continence
Disadvantages. Potential dysfunction of antireflux valve with leakage, need for replacement approximately every 3 to 4 months

6. Using a surgical marking pen, highlight on the abdomen any scars, the costal margin, hernias, beltline, creases, folds, etc.

7. Tube stabilization reduces tube migration, which can cause gastric outlet obstruction (with gastrostomy tubes), compromised tube function, and tract erosion, resulting in leakage and skin breakdown.

8. Use of commercial tube-stabilization devices, use of baby-bottle nipple placed around tube and secured to skin-barrier wafer, use of baby-bottle nipple placed around tube and secured with convex insert snapped over nipple and inside flange of skin-barrier wafer with flange, use of a gastrostomy replacement catheter that has attached external flange and internal balloon or bumper.

9. a
10. c
11. b
12. b

CHAPTER 16

1. b
2. b
3. d
4. b
5. c
6. d
7. a

CHAPTER 17

1. d
2. a
3. Eliminate the cause of the pain by avoiding cytotoxic topical agents, avoiding dressings that adhere to the wound bed, positioning the patient off the wound, and using lift sheets to reposition the patient; protect wound margins with skin sealants or ointments; use topical anesthetic agents before conservative sharp debridement; control inflammation and edema by using compression bandages and sequential compression pumps and by elevating swollen extremities; stabilize the wound with body positioners and splints, especially when mobilizing the patient; "BE WITH the patient"
4. a
5. False
6. (d) All of these are procedures (e.g., a dressing change or debridement) that may result in wound pain.
7. c
8. c
9. True
10. The patient can rate the intensity of wound pain by using a simple descriptive Pain Intensity Scale, a Numeric Pain Intensity Scale, a Visual Analog Scale (VAS), or the Wong-Baker Faces Pain Rating Scale.

CHAPTER 18

1. a
2. **a.** Spasticity must be controlled, either surgically or pharmacologically.
   b. Infection must be eliminated.
   c. The cause of the lesion must be identified and corrected.
   d. Nutritional status must be optimized; in general, flap closure should not be done if the patient's serum albumin is less than 3.0 g/dl.
3. **a.** Intraoperative positioning should provide maximal "stretch" on the flap; this reduces the risk of postoperative dehiscence resulting from tension on the flap.
   b. Perioperative antibiotic coverage should be provided based on culture results.
   c. The bony prominence should be partially excised to remove any infected bone and to increase the surface area upon which the patient rests.
   d. The entire ulcer and any granulation tissue should be excised so that only healthy unscarred tissue is left as a wound base.
   e. Incisions should be made with possible recurrences in mind.
   f. Incisions should be made so as to avoid suture lines over bony prominences.
   g. The defect should be filled with healthy, unscarred, well-vascularized tissue.
   h. Gradually increase mobility postoperatively and observe skin and suture lines.
   i. Skin grafts are not indicated because they lack durability.
4. a
5. d
6. d
7. d

CHAPTER 19

1. Selectins, integrins, and cell adhesion molecules
2. False
3. d

CHAPTER 20

1. Hyperbaric oxygenation is the administration of 100% oxygen at pressures 2 to 2.4 times that of normal atmospheric pressure. Hyper-

baric oxygenation requires immersion in a monochamber or multiperson chamber and cannot be applied locally to an extremity alone.

2. b
3. • *Aural or sinus barotrauma*. Instruct patient on air equalization techniques.
   • *Pneumothorax*. Instruct patient to *not* hold breath during ascent.
   • *Hypoglycemia*. Obtain a random serum glucose level before treatment.
   • *Pulmonary compromise*. Assess for adequacy of breath sounds before treatment.
   • *Hypertension crisis*. Check vital signs for hypertension before treatment.
   • *Oxygen toxicity*. Check vital signs for oral temperature greater than 102° F.
4. b
5. True
6. d
7. Galvanotaxic effects describe the movement of cells along the path of current. For example, with the presence of inflammation, neutrophils are attracted to the cathode. Macrophages migrate toward the cathode.
8. Placement of cathode and anode, duration of pulse, frequency of pulses, pulse width, length of interpulse interval, amperage
9. d
10. d
11. c

CHAPTER 21

1. c
2. b
3. b
4. c

CHAPTER 22

1. d
2. b
3. Patient who has a condition due to an illness or injury that restricts his or her ability to leave home unless he or she has the assistance of devices (such as crutches or canes) or the assistance of another person or when leaving the home is medically contraindicated.
4. True
5. d

CHAPTER 23

1. Establish a policy for use and discontinuation of support surfaces, collaborate with materials management to establish a formulary of wound care products, provide guidelines to staff to standardize appropriate use of wound care dressings, provide guidelines to staff that address pressure ulcer prevention interventions that are based on level of risk.
2. Participate in new staff orientation programs.
3. False
4. d

CHAPTER 24

1. a
2. **a.** Chronic nonhealing wounds are costly in terms of increased length of stay, increased mortality rates, and increased litigious potential. Implementation of guidelines or protocols for prevention and management can reduce these liabilities.
   b. Care of chronic wounds is fragmented among several disciplines that do not have expertise in prevention and treatment of chronic wounds. Wounds are multifaceted in etiology and require multidisciplinary interventions.
3. Implement standardized protocols for risk assessment, establish standardized skin care and wound care protocols, foster standardized approach to documentation of wound status, conduct clinical trials of wound-related products, institute continuous quality-improvement activities, link with patient education department to provide and develop patient education materials, collaborate with materials management concerning wound care product formulary, conduct staff development programs for non-team members, provide opportunities for wound care team members to further develop professionally and remain current in wound care.

APPENDIX

B RISK ASSESSMENT SCALES

BRADEN SCALE FOR PREDICTING PRESSURE SORE RISK

Patient's Name ______________________ Evaluator's Name ______________________

					Date of Assessment			
SENSORY PERCEPTION Ability to respond meaningfully to pressure-related discomfort	**1. Completely limited:** Unresponsive (does not moan, flinch, or grasp) to painful stimuli, due to diminished level of consciousness or sedation, OR limited ability to feel pain over most of body surface.	**2. Very Limited:** Responds only to painful stimuli. Cannot communicate discomfort except by moaning or restlessness, OR has a sensory impairment which limits the ability to feel pain or discomfort over 1/2 of body.	**3. Slightly Limited:** Responds to verbal commands but cannot always communicate discomfort or need to be turned, OR has some sensory impairment which limits ability to feel pain or discomfort in 1 or 2 extremities.	**4. No Impairment:** Responds to verbal commands. Has no sensory deficit which would limit ability to feel or voice pain or discomfort.				
MOISTURE Degree to which skin is exposed to moisture	**1. Constantly Moist:** Skin is kept moist almost constantly by perspiration, urine, etc. Dampness is detected every time patient is moved or turned.	**2. Moist:** Skin is often but not always moist. Linen must be changed at least once a shift.	**3. Occasionally Moist:** Skin is occasionally moist, requiring an extra linen change approximately once a day.	**4. Rarely Moist:** Skin is usually dry; linen requires changing only at routine intervals.				
ACTIVITY Degree of physical activity	**1. Bedfast:** Confined to bed	**2. Chairfast:** Ability to walk severely limited or nonexistent. Cannot bear own weight and/or must be assisted into chair or wheelchair.	**3. Walks Occasionally:** Walks occasionally during day but for very short distances, with or without assistance. Spends majority of each shift in bed or chair.	**4. Walks Frequently:** Walks outside the room at least twice a day and inside room at least once every 2 hours during waking hours.				
MOBILITY Ability to change and control body position	**1. Completely Immobile:** Does not make even slight changes in body or extremity position without assistance.	**2. Very Limited:** Makes occasional slight changes in body or extremity position but unable to make frequent or significant changes independently.	**3. Slightly Limited:** Makes frequent though slight changes in body or extremity position independently.	**4. No Limitations:** Makes major and frequent changes in position without assistance.				
NUTRITION Usual food intake pattern	**1. Very Poor:** Never eats a complete meal. Rarely eats more than 1/3 of any food offered. Eats 2 servings or less of protein (meat or dairy products) per day. Takes fluids poorly. Does not take a liquid dietary supplement, OR is NPO and/or maintained on clear liquids or IV's for more than 5 days.	**2. Probably Inadequate:** Rarely eats a complete meal and generally eats only about 1/2 of any food offered. Protein intake includes only 3 servings of meat or dairy products per day. Occasionally will take a dietary supplement, OR receives less than optimum amount of liquid diet or tube feeding.	**3. Adequate:** Eats over half of most meals. Eats a total of 4 servings of protein (meat, dairy products) each day. Occasionally will refuse a meal, but will usually take a supplement if offered, OR is on a tube feeding or TPN regimen, which probably meets most of nutritional needs.	**4. Excellent:** Eats most of every meal. Never refuses a meal. Usually eats a total of 4 or more servings of meat and dairy products. Occasionally eats between meals. Does not require supplementation.				
FRICTION AND SHEAR	**1. Problem:** Requires moderate to maximum assistance in moving. Complete lifting without sliding against sheets is impossible. Frequently slides down in bed or chair, requiring frequent repositioning with maximum assistance. Spasticity, contractures, or agitation leads to almost constant friction.	**2. Potential Problem:** Moves feebly or requires minimum assistance. During a move skin probably slides to some extent against sheets, chair, restraints, or other devices. Maintains relatively good position in chair or bed most of the time but occasionally slides down.	**3. No Apparent Problem:** Moves in bed and in chair independently and has sufficient muscle strength to lift up completely during move. Maintains good position in bed or chair at all times.					
				Total Score				

NORTON SCALE

NORTON RISK ASSESSMENT SCALE

		Physical Condition	Mental Condition	Activity	Mobility	Incontinent	TOTAL SCORE
		Good 4 Fair 3 Poor 2 Very Bad 1	Alert 4 Apathetic 3 Confused 2 Stupor 1	Ambulant 4 Walk/help 3 Chairbound 2 Bed 1	Full 4 Sl. limited 3 V. limited 2 Immobile 1	Not 4 Occasional 3 Usually/Urine 2 Doubly 1	
Name	Date						

From Norton D, McLaren R, Exton-Smith AN: *An investigation of geriatric nursing problems in hospital,* Churchill Livingstone, 1975, Edinburgh.

GOSNELL SCALE*

PRESSURE SORE RISK ASSESSMENT

I.D. ______________________
Age ______________ Sex ________
Height __________ Weight ________
Date of Admission ______________
Date of Discharge ______________

Medical Diagnosis:
Primary ______________
Secondary ______________
Nursing Diagnosis:
____
____

Instructions: Complete all categories within 24 hours of admission and every other day thereafter. Refer to the accompanying guidelines for specific rating details.

DATE	**Mental Status:** 1. Alert 2. Apathetic 3. Confused 4. Stuporous 5. Unconscious	**Continence:** 1. Fully controlled 2. Usually controlled 3. Minimally controlled 4. Absence of control	**Mobility:** 1. Full 2. Slightly limited 3. Very limited 4. Immobile	**Activity:** 1. Ambulatory 2. Walks with assistance 3. Chairfast 4. Bedfast	**Nutrition:** 1. Good 2. Fair 3. Poor	TOTAL SCORE

Date	Vital Signs				Diet	24-Hour Fluid Balance		COLOR	GENERAL SKIN APPEARANCE			Interventions		
								1. Pallor 2. Mottled 3. Pink 4. Ashen 5. Ruddy 6. Cyanotic 7. Jaundice 8. Other	**Moisture** 1. Dry 2. Damp 3. Oily 4. Other	**Temperature** 1. Cold 2. Cool 3. Warm 4. Hot	**Texture** 1. Smooth 2. Rough 3. Thin/Transp 4. Scaly 5. Crusty 6. Other			
	T	P	R	BP		Intake	Output					No	Yes	Describe

PRESSURE SORE RISK ASSESSMENT MEDICATION PROFILE

Medication	Dosage	*Frequency	Route	Date Begun	Date Discon.

*Suggested flow sheets for monitoring data.

GOSNELL SCALE

GUIDELINES FOR NUMERICAL RATING OF THE DEFINED CATEGORIES

Rating	1	2	3	4	5
Mental Status: An assessment of one's level of response to his environment.	**Alert:** Oriented to time, place, and person. Responsive to all stimuli, and understands explanations.	**Apathetic:** Lethargic, forgetful, drowsy, passive and dull. Sluggish, depressed. Able to obey simple commands. Possibly disoriented to time.	**Confused:** Partial and/or intermittent disorientation to transpulmonary pressure. Purposeless response to stimuli. Restless, aggressive, irritable, anxious and may require tranqualizers or sedatives.	**Stuporous:** Total disorientation. Does not respond to name, simple commands, or verbal stimuli.	**Unconscious:** Nonresponsive to painful stimuli
Continence: The amount of bodily control of urination and defecation.	**Fully Controlled:** Total control of urine and feces.	**Usually Controlled:** Incontinent of urine and/or of feces not more often than once. q 48 hrs. OR has Foley catheter and is incontinent of feces.	**Minimally Controlled:** Incontinent of urine or feces at least once q 24 hrs.	**Absence of Control:** Consistently incontinent of both urine and feces.	
Mobility: The amount and control of movement of one's body.	**Full:** Able to control and move all extremities at will. May require the use of a device but turns, lifts, pulls, balances, and attains sitting position at will.	**Slightly Limited:** Able to control and move all extremeties but a degree of limitation is present. Requires assistance of another person to turn, pull, balance, and/or attain a sitting position at will but self-initiates movement or request for help to move.	**Very Limited:** Can assist another person who must initiate movement via turning, lifting, pulling, balancing, and/or attaining a sitting position (contractures, paralysis may be present.)	**Immobile:** Does not assist self in any way to change position. Is unable to change position without assistance. Is completely dependent on others for movement.	
Activity: The ability of an individual to ambulate.	**Ambulatory:** Is able to walk unassisted. Rises from bed unassisted. With the use of a device such as cane or walker is able to ambulate without the assistance of another person.	**Walks with Help:** Able to ambulate with assistance of another person, braces, or crutches. May have limitation of stairs.	**Chairfast** Ambulates only to a chair, requires assistance to do so OR is confined to a wheelchair.	**Bedfast:** Is confined to bed during entire 24 hours of the day.	
Nutrition The process of food intake.	Eats some food from each basic food category every day and the majority of each meal served OR is on tube feeding.	Occasionally refuses a meal or frequently leaves at least half of a meal.	Seldom eats a complete meal and only a few bites of food at a meal.		

Vital Signs:	The temperature, pulse, respiration, and blood pressure to be taken and recorded at the time of every assessment rating.
Skin appearance:	A description of observed skin characteristics: color, moisture, temperature, and texture.
Diet:	Record the specific diet order.
24-hour fluid balance:	The amount of fluid intake and output during the previous 24-hour period should be recorded.
Interventions:	List all devices, measures and/or nursing care activity being used for the purpose of pressure sore prevention.
Medications:	List name, dosage, frequency, and route for all prescribed medications. If a PRN order, list the pattern for the period since last assessment.
Comments:	Use this space to add explanation or further detail regarding any of the previously recorded data, patient condition, etc. OR Describe anything which you believe to be of importance but not accounted for previously.

APPENDIX C GUIDELINES

Guidelines are statements or recommendations to assist or guide the care of patients with specific clinical conditions and are prepared by a team of reviewers. The team develops these statements by conducting a rigorous, comprehensive, and systematic review of the scientific literature. Reviewers are individuals who have expertise in the content area or in the scientific review methodology. Final recommendations are peer reviewed within the team; often a public review is also solicited prior to release of the final document. Updates to published guidelines must follow the most current scientific methodology for systematic reviews. Additional information about guideline development or the systematic review process is available at many of the websites listed in Appendix E.

PRESSURE ULCERS IN ADULTS: PREDICTION AND PREVENTION*

This guideline was made available in 1992 and reflects the state of current knowledge at that time regarding the effectiveness and appropriateness of procedures and practices designed to predict and prevent pressure ulcers. The strength of evidence supporting each recommendation within this guideline is based on the following criteria:

(A) There is good research-based evidence to support the recommendation.

(B) There is fair research-based evidence to support the recommendation.

(C) The recommendation is based on expert opinion and panel consensus.

The level of evidence rating assigned each recommendation follows each recommendation statement in parenthesis. The reader is encouraged to search the available literature for updates and revision to this guideline relative to the specific recommendation as well as the evidence rating.

A. Risk Assessment Tools and Risk Factors. Bed- and chair-bound individuals or those with impaired ability to reposition should be assessed for additional factors that increase risk for developing pressure ulcers. These factors include immobility, incontinence, nutritional factors such as inadequate dietary intake and impaired nutritional status, and altered level of consciousness. Individuals should be assessed on admission to acute care and rehabilitation hospitals, nursing homes, home care programs, and other health care facilities. A systematic risk assessment can be accomplished by using a validated risk assessment tool such as the Braden Scale or Norton Scale. Pressure ulcer risk should be reassessed at periodic intervals. **(A)** All assessment of risk should be documented. **(C)**

B. Skin Care and Early Treatment

1. All individuals at risk should have a systematic skin inspection at least once a day, paying particular attention to the bony prominences. Results of skin inspection should be documented. **(C)**
2. Skin cleansing should occur at the time of soiling and at routine intervals. The frequency of skin cleansing should be individualized according to need and/or patient preference. Avoid hot water, and use a mild cleansing agent that minimizes irritation and dryness of the skin. During the cleansing process, care should be taken to

* Panel for the Prediction and Prevention of Pressure Ulcers in Adults: *Pressure ulcers in adults: prediction and prevention*, Clinical Practice Guideline #3, Rockville, Md, 1992, USDHHS, PHS, AHCPR Pub. No. 92-0047.

minimize the force and friction applied to the skin. **(C)**

3. Minimize environmental factors leading to skin drying, such as low humidity (less than 40%) and exposure to cold. Dry skin should be treated with moisturizers. **(C)**
4. Avoid massage over bony prominences. **(B)**
5. Minimize skin exposure to moisture caused by incontinence, perspiration, or wound drainage. When these sources of moisture cannot be controlled, underpads or briefs can be used that are made of materials that absorb moisture and present a quick-drying surface to the skin. For information about assessing and managing urinary incontinence, refer to *Urinary Incontinence in Adults: Clinical Practice Guideline* (available from the AHRQ [formerly known as the AHCPR]) Topical agents that act as barriers to moisture can also be used. **(C)**
6. Skin injury caused by friction and shear forces should be minimized through proper positioning, transferring, and turning techniques. In addition, friction injuries may be reduced by the use of lubricants (such as corn starch and creams), protective films (such as transparent film dressings and skin sealants), protective dressings (such as hydrocolloids), and protective padding. **(C)**
7. When apparently well-nourished individuals develop an inadequate dietary intake of protein or calories, caregivers should first attempt to discover the factors compromising intake and offer support with eating. Other nutritional supplements or support may be needed. If dietary intake remains inadequate and if consistent with overall goals of therapy, more aggressive nutritional intervention such as enteral or parenteral feedings should be considered. **(C)** For nutritionally compromised individuals, a plan of nutritional support and/or supplementation should be implemented that meets individual needs and is consistent with the overall goals of therapy. **(C)**
8. If potential for improving mobility and activity status exists, rehabilitation efforts should be instituted if consistent with the overall goals of therapy. Maintaining current activity level, mobility, and range of motion is an appropriate goal for most individuals. **(C)**
9. Interventions and outcomes should be monitored and documented. **(C)**

C. Mechanical Loading and Support Surfaces

1. Any individual in bed who is assessed to be at risk for developing pressure ulcers should be repositioned at least every 2 hours if consistent with overall patient goals. A written schedule for systematically turning and repositioning the individual should be used. **(B)**
2. For individuals in bed, positioning devices such as pillows or foam wedges should be used to keep bony prominences (e.g., knees or ankles) from direct contact with one another, according to a written plan. **(C)**
3. Individuals in bed who are completely immobile should have a care plan that includes the use of devices that totally relieve pressure on the heels, most commonly by raising the heels off the bed. Do not use donut-type devices. **(C)**
4. When the side-lying position is used in bed, avoid positioning directly on the trochanter. **(C)**
5. Maintain the head of the bed at the lowest degree of elevation consistent with medical conditions and other restrictions. Limit the amount of time the head of the bed is elevated. **(C)**
6. Use lifting devices such as a trapeze or bed linen to move (rather than drag) individuals in bed who cannot assist during transfers and position changes. **(C)**
7. Any individual assessed to be at risk for developing pressure ulcers should be placed when lying in bed on a pressure-

reducing device, such as foam, static air, alternating air, gel, or water mattresses. **(B)**

8. Any person at risk for developing a pressure ulcer should avoid uninterrupted sitting in a chair or wheelchair. The individual should be repositioned, shifting the points under pressure at least every hour or be put back to bed if consistent with overall patient management goals. Individuals who are able should be taught to shift weight every 15 minutes. **(C)**
9. For chair-bound individuals, the use of a pressure-reducing device such as those made of foam, gel, air, or a combination is indicated. Do not use donut-type devices. **(C)**
10. Positioning of chair-bound individuals in chairs or wheelchairs should include consideration of postural alignment, distribution of weight, balance and stability, and pressure relief. **(C)**
11. A written plan for the use of positioning devices and schedules may be helpful for chair-bound individuals. **(C)**

D. Education

1. Educational programs for the prevention of pressure ulcers should be structured, organized, and comprehensive and directed at all levels of health care providers, patients, and family or caregivers. **(A)**
2. The educational program for prevention of pressure ulcers should include information on the following items: **(B)**
   - **a.** Etiology and risk factors for pressure ulcers
   - **b.** Risk assessment tools and their application
   - **c.** Skin assessment
   - **d.** Selection and/or use of support surfaces
   - **e.** Development and implementation of an individualized program of skin care
   - **f.** Demonstration of positioning to decrease risk of tissue breakdown
   - **g.** Instruction on accurate documentation of pertinent data
3. The educational program should identify those responsible for pressure ulcer prevention, describe each person's role, and be appropriate to the audience in terms of level of information presented and expected participation. The educational program should be updated on a regular basis to incorporate new and existing techniques or technologies. **(C)**
4. Educational programs should be developed, implemented, and evaluated using principles of adult learning. **(C)**

TREATMENT OF PRESSURE ULCERS: CLINICAL PRACTICE GUIDELINE #15*

This guideline was made available by the panel in 1994 and is based on current scientific evidence and professional judgment. The purpose of the guideline is to offer recommendations for the treatment of pressure ulcers. These recommendations are not intended to address any other types of wounds, acute or chronic or those caused by vascular disease, neuropathy, neoplasm, primary skin disease, or thermal or chemical injury. The strength of evidence supporting each recommendation within this guideline is based on the following criteria:

(A) Results of two or more randomized controlled clinical trials on pressure ulcers in humans provide support.

(B) Results of two or more controlled clinical trials on pressure ulcers in humans provide support, or when appropriate, results of two or more controlled trials in an animal model provide indirect support.

(C) This rating requires one or more of the following: 1) results of one controlled trial, 2) results of at least two case series or descriptive studies on pressure ulcers in humans, or 3) expert opinion.

The level of evidence rating assigned each recommendation follows each recommendation statement in parenthesis. The reader is encouraged to search the available literature for updates and

* Bergstrom N et al: *Treatment of pressure ulcers.* Clinical Practice Guideline #15, Rockville, Md, 1994, USDHHS, PHS, AHCPR Pub. No. 95-0652.

revision to this guideline relative to the specific recommendation as well as the evidence rating.

I. Assessment

A. Assessing the Pressure Ulcer

1. Assess the pressure ulcer initially for location, stage (NPUAP, 1989*), size, sinus tracts, undermining, tunneling, exudate, necrotic tissue, and the presence or absence of granulation tissue and epithelialization. **(C)**

2. Reassess pressure ulcers at least weekly. If the condition of the patient or of the wound deteriorates, reevaluate the treatment plan as soon as any evidence of deterioration is noted. **(C)**

3. A clean pressure ulcer should show evidence of some healing within 2 to 4 weeks. If no progress can be demonstrated, reevaluate the adequacy of the overall treatment plan as well as adherence to this plan, making modifications as necessary. **(C)**

B. Assessing the Individual with a Pressure Ulcer

1. History and physical examination. Perform a complete history and physical examination, because a pressure ulcer should be assessed in the context of the patient's overall physical and psychosocial health. **(C)**

2. Assessing complications. Clinicians should be alert to the potential complications associated with pressure ulcers. **(C)**

3. Nutritional assessment and management

a. Ensure adequate dietary intake to prevent malnutrition to the extent that this is compatible with the individual's wishes. **(B)**

b. Perform an abbreviated nutritional assessment, as defined by the Nutrition Screening Initiative, at least every 3 months for individuals at risk for malnutrition. These include individuals who are unable to take food by mouth or who experience an involuntary change in weight. **(C)**

c. Encourage dietary intake or supplementation if an individual with a pressure ulcer is malnourished. If dietary intake continues to be inadequate, impractical, or impossible, nutritional support (usually tube feeding) should be used to place the patient into positive nitrogen balance (approximately 30 to 35 calories/kg/day and 1.25 to 1.50 grams of protein/kg/day) according to the goals of care. **(C)**

d. Give vitamin and mineral supplements if deficiencies are confirmed or suspected. **(C)**

4. Pain assessment and management

a. Assess all patients for pain related to the pressure ulcer or its treatment. **(C)**

b. Manage pain by eliminating or controlling the source of pain (e.g., covering wounds, adjusting support surface, repositioning). Provide analgesia as needed and appropriate. **(C)**

5. Psychosocial assessment and management

a. All individuals being treated for pressure ulcer should undergo a psychosocial assessment to determine their ability and motivation to comprehend and adhere to the treatment program. The assessment should include but not be limited to the following:

(1) Mental status, learning ability, depression
(2) Social support
(3) Polypharmacy or overmedication
(4) Alcohol and/or drug abuse
(5) Goals, values, and lifestyle
(6) Sexuality
(7) Culture and ethnicity
(8) Stressors

* National Pressure Ulcer Advisory Panel: Pressure ulcer prevalence, cost and risk assessment: consensus development conference statement, *Decubitus* 2(2):24, 1989.

Periodic reassessment is recommended. **(C)**

b. Assess resources (e.g., availability and skill of caregivers, finances, equipment) of individuals being treated for pressure ulcers in the home. **(C)**

c. Set treatment goals consistent with the values and lifestyle of the individual, family, and caregiver. **(C)**

d. Arrange interventions to meet identified psychosocial needs and goals. Follow-up should be planned in cooperation with the individual and caregiver. **(C)**

II. Managing Tissue Loads

A. While in Bed

1. Positioning techniques

a. Avoid positioning patients on a pressure ulcer. **(C)**

b. Use positioning devices to raise a pressure ulcer off the support surface. If the patient is no longer at risk for developing pressure ulcers, these devices may reduce the need for pressure-reducing overlays, mattresses, and beds. Avoid using donut-type devices. **(C)**

c. Establish a written repositioning schedule. **(C)**

d. Assess all patients with existing pressure ulcers to determine their risk for developing additional pressure ulcers. For those individuals who remain at risk, institute the following measures:

(1) Avoid positioning immobile individuals directly on their trochanters, and use devices such as pillows and form wedges that totally relieve pressure on the heels, most commonly by raising the heels off the bed. **(C)**

(2) Use positioning devices such as pillows or foam to prevent direct contact between bony prominences (such as knees or ankles). **(C)**

(3) Maintain the head of the bed at the lowest degree of elevation consistent with medical conditions and other restrictions. Limit the amount of time the head of the bed is elevated. **(C)**

2. Support surfaces

a. Assess all patients with existing pressure ulcers to determine their risk for developing additional pressure ulcers. If the patient remains at risk, use a pressure-reducing surface. **(C)**

b. Use a static support surface if a patient can assume a variety of positions without bearing weight on a pressure ulcer and without "bottoming out." **(B)**

c. Use a dynamic support surface if the patient cannot assume a variety of positions without bearing weight on a pressure ulcer, if the patient fully compresses the static support surface, or if the pressure ulcer does not show evidence of healing. **(B)**

d. If a patient has large stage 3 or 4 pressure ulcers on multiple turning surfaces, a low-air-loss bed or an air-fluidized bed may be indicated. **(C)**

e. When excess moisture on intact skin is a potential source of maceration and skin breakdown, a support surface that provides airflow can be important in drying the skin and preventing additional pressure ulcers. **(C)**

B. While Sitting

1. Positioning techniques

a. A patient who has a pressure ulcer on a sitting surface should avoid sitting. If pressure on the ulcer can be relieved, limited sitting may be allowed. **(C)**

b. Consider postural alignment, distribution of weight, balance, stability, and pressure relief when positioning sitting individuals. **(C)**

c. Reposition the sitting individual so that the points under pressure are shifted at least every hour. If this schedule cannot be kept or is inconsistent with overall treatment goals, return the patient to the bed. Individuals who are able should be taught to shift their weight every 15 minutes. **(C)**

2. Support surfaces
   a. Select a cushion based on the specific needs of the individual who requires pressure reduction in a sitting position. Avoid donut-type devices. **(C)**
   b. Develop a written plan for the use of positioning devices. **(C)**

III. Ulcer Care

A. Debridement

1. Remove devitalized tissue in pressure ulcers when appropriate for the patient's condition and consistent with patient goals. **(C)**
2. Select the method of debridement most appropriate to the patient's condition and goals. Sharp, mechanical, enzymatic, and/or autolytic debridement techniques may be used when there is no urgent clinical need for drainage or removal of devitalized tissue. If there is urgent need for debridement, as with advancing cellulitis or sepsis, sharp debridement should be used. **(C)**
3. Use clean, dry dressings for 8 to 24 hours after sharp debridement associated with bleeding; then reinstitute moist dressings. Clean dressings may be used in conjunction with mechanical or enzymatic debridement techniques. **(C)**
4. Heel ulcers with dry eschar need not be debrided if they do not have edema, erythema, fluctuance, or drainage. Assess these wounds daily to monitor for pressure ulcer complications that would require debridement (e.g., edema, erythema, fluctuance, drainage). **(C)**
5. Prevent or manage pain associate with debridement as needed. **(C)**

B. Wound Cleansing

1. Cleanse wounds initially and at each dressing change. **(C)**
2. Use minimal mechanical force when cleansing the ulcer with gauze, cloth, or sponges. **(C)**
3. Do not clean ulcer wounds with skin cleansers or antiseptic agents (e.g., povidone iodine, iodophor, sodium hypochlorite solution [Dakin's solution], hydrogen peroxide, acetic acid). **(B)**
4. Use normal saline for cleansing most pressure ulcers. **(C)**
5. Use enough irrigation pressure to enhance wound cleansing without causing trauma to the wound bed. Safe and effective ulcer irrigation pressures range from 4 to 15 psi. **(B)**
6. Consider whirlpool treatment for cleansing pressure ulcers that contain thick exudate, slough, or necrotic tissue. Discontinue whirlpool when the ulcer is clean. **(C)**

C. Dressings

1. Use a dressing that will keep the ulcer bed continuously moist. Wet to dry dressings should be used only for debridement and are not considered continuously moist saline dressings. **(B)**
2. Use clinical judgement to select a type of moist wound dressing suitable for the ulcer. Studies of different types of moist wound dressings show no difference in pressure ulcer healing outcomes. **(B)**
3. Choose a dressing that keeps the surrounding intact (periulcer) skin dry while keeping the ulcer bed moist. **(C)**
4. Choose a dressing that controls exudate but does not desiccate the ulcer bed. **(C)**

5. Consider caregiver time when selecting a dressing. **(B)**
6. Eliminate wound dead space by loosely filling all cavities with dressing material. Avoid overpacking the wound. **(C)**
7. Monitor dressings applied near the anus because they are difficult to keep intact. **(C)**

D. Adjunctive Therapies
1. Consider a course of treatment with electrotherapy for stage 3 and 4 pressure ulcers that have proved unresponsive to conventional therapy. Electrical stimulation may also be useful for recalcitrant stage 2 ulcers. **(B)**
2. The therapeutic efficacy of hyperbaric oxygenation; infrared, ultraviolet, and low-energy laser irradiation; and ultrasound has not be sufficiently established to permit recommendation of these therapies for the treatment of pressure ulcers. **(C)**
3. The therapeutic efficacy of miscellaneous topical agents (e.g., sugar, vitamins, elements, hormone, other agents), growth factors, and skin equivalents has not yet been sufficiently established to warrant recommendation of these agents. **(C)**
4. The therapeutic efficacy of systemic agents other than antibiotics has not been sufficiently established to permit their recommendation for the treatment of pressure ulcers. **(C)**

IV. Managing Bacterial Colonization and Infection

A. Pressure Ulcer Colonization and Infection
1. Minimize pressure ulcer colonization and enhance wound healing by effective wound cleansing and debridement. If purulence or foul odor is present, more frequent cleansing and possibly debridement are required. **(C)**
2. Do not use swab cultures to diagnose wound infection because all pressure ulcers are colonized. **(C)**
3. Consider initiating a 2-week trial of topical antibiotics for clean pressure ulcers that are not healing or are continuing to produce exudate after 2 to 4 weeks of optimal patient care (as defined in this guideline). The antibiotic should be effective against gram-negative, gram-positive, and anaerobic organisms (e.g., silver sulfadiazine, triple antibiotic). **(A)**
4. Perform quantitative bacterial cultures of the soft tissue and evaluate the patient for osteomyelitis when the ulcer does not respond to topical antibiotic therapy. **(C)**
5. Do not use topical antiseptics (e.g., povidone iodine, iodophor, sodium hypochlorite [Dakin's solution], hydrogen peroxide, acetic acid) to reduce bacteria in wound tissue. **(B)**
6. Institute appropriate systemic antibiotic therapy for patients with bacteremia, sepsis, advancing cellulitis, or osteomyelitis. **(A)** Systemic antibiotics are not required for pressure ulcers with only clinical sign of local infection. **(C)**
7. Protect pressure ulcers from exogenous sources of contamination (e.g., feces). **(C)**

B. Infection Control
1. Follow body substance isolation (BSI) precautions or an equivalent system appropriate for the health care setting and the patient's condition when treating pressure ulcers. **(C)**
2. Use clean gloves for each patient. When treating multiple ulcers on the same patient, attend to the most contaminated ulcer last (e.g., in the perianal region). Remove gloves and wash hands between patients. **(C)**
3. Use sterile instruments to debride pressure ulcers. **(C)**
4. Use clean dressings, rather than sterile ones, to treat pressure ulcers, as long as dressing procedures comply with

institutional infection-control guidelines. **(C)**

5. Clean dressings may also be used in the home setting. Disposal of contaminated dressings in the home should be done in a manner consistent with local regulations. **(C)**

V. Operative Repair of Pressure Ulcers

A. Patient Selection. Determine patient need and suitability for operative repair when clean stage 3 or 4 pressure ulcers do not respond to optimal patient care. Possible candidates are medically stable and adequately nourished and can tolerate operative blood loss and postoperative immobility. Quality of life, patient preferences, treatment goals, risk of recurrence, and expected rehabilitative outcome are additional considerations. **(C)**

B. Controlling Factors that Impair Healing. Promote successful surgical closure by controlling or correcting factors that may be associated with impaired healing, such as smoking, spasticity, levels of bacterial colonization, incontinence, and urinary tract infection. **(C)**

C. Operative Procedures

1. Use the most effective and least traumatic method to repair the ulcer defect. Wounds can be closed by direct closure, skin grafting, skin flaps, musculocutaneous flaps, and free flaps. To minimize recurrence, the choice of operative technique is based on the individual patient's needs and overall goals. **(C)**
2. Prophylactic ischiectomy is not recommended because it often results in perineal ulcers and urethral fistulas, which are more threatening problems than ischial ulcers. **(C)**

D. Postoperative Care

1. Minimize pressure to the operative site by use of an air-fluidized bed, a low-air-loss bed, or a Stryker frame for a minimum of 2 weeks. Assess postoperative viability of the surgical site as clinically indicated. Have the patient slowly increase periods of time sitting or lying on the flap to increase its tolerance to pressure. To determine the degree of tolerance, monitor the flap for pallor, redness, or both that do not resolve after 10 minutes of pressure relief. Ongoing patient education is imperative to reduce the risk of recurrence. **(C)**
2. Assess for recurrence of pressure ulcers as an ongoing component of care. Caregivers should provide education and encourage adherence to measures for pressure reduction, daily skin examination, and intermittent relief techniques. **(A)**

VI. Education and Quality Improvement

A. Education

1. Prevention and treatment: a continuum

   a. Design, develop, and implement educational programs for patients, caregivers, and health care providers that reflect a continuum of care. The program should begin with a structured, comprehensive, and organized approach to prevention and should culminate in effective treatment protocols that promote healing and prevent recurrence. **(C)**

   b. Develop educational programs that target appropriate health care providers, patient, family members, and caregivers. Present information at an appropriate level for the target audience to maximize retention and ensure a carryover into practice. Use principles of adult learning (e.g., explanation, demonstration, questioning, group discussion, drills). **(C)**

   c. Involve the patient and caregiver, when possible, in pressure ulcer treatment and prevention strategies and options. Include information on pain, discomfort, possible outcomes, and duration of treatment, if known. Encourage the patient to actively participate in and comply with decisions regarding pressure ulcer prevention and treatment. **(C)**

d. Educational programs should identify those responsible for pressure ulcer treatment and describe each person's role. The information presented and the degree of participation expected should be appropriate to the audience. **(C)**

2. Assessing tissue damage

a. Educational programs should emphasize the need for accurate, consistent, and uniform assessment, description, and documentation of the extent of tissue damage. **(C)**

b. Include the following information when developing an educational program on the treatment of pressure ulcers: **(C)**

(1) Etiology and pathology

(2) Risk factors

(3) Uniform terminology for stages of tissue damage based on specific classification

(4) Principles of wound healing

(5) Principles of nutritional support with regard to tissue integrity

(6) Individualized program of skin care

(7) Principles of cleansing and infection control

(8) Principles of postoperative care including positioning and support surfaces

(9) Principles of prevention to reduce recurrence

(10) Product selection (i.e., categories and uses of support surface, dressings, topical antibiotics, or other agents)

(11) Effects or influence of the physical and mechanical environment on the pressure ulcer, and strategies for management

(12) Mechanisms for accurate documentation and monitoring of pertinent data, including treatment interventions and healing progress

c. Update educational programs on an ongoing and regular basis to integrate new knowledge, techniques, or technologies. **(C)**

3. Monitoring outcomes

a. Evaluate the effectiveness of an educational program in terms of measurable outcomes: implementing guideline recommendations, healing existing ulcers, reducing the incidence of new or recurrent ulcers, and preventing the deterioration of existing ulcers. **(C)**

b. Include a structured, comprehensive, and organized educational program as an integral part of quality improvement monitoring. Use information from quality assurance/improvement surveys to identify deficiencies, to evaluate the effectiveness of care, and to determine the need for education and policy changes. Focus inservice training on identified deficiencies. **(C)**

4. Quality improvement

a. Obtain intradepartmental and interdepartmental quality improvement support of pressure ulcer management as a major aspect of care. **(C)**

b. Convene an interdisciplinary committee of interested and knowledgeable persons to address quality improvement in pressure ulcer management. **(C)**

c. Identify and monitor the occurrence of pressure ulcers to determine their incidence and prevalence. This information will serve as a baseline to the development, implementation, and evaluation of treatment protocols. **(C)**

d. Monitor the incidence and prevalence of pressure ulcers on a regular basis. **(C)**

e. Develop, implement, and evaluate educational programs based on the data obtained from quality improvement monitoring. **(C)**

APPENDIX

D WOUND PATIENT'S BILL OF RIGHTS

You have a right to:

- Actively participate as a member of your wound care team if you are able and willing.
- Have your wound assessed and monitored by trained health care personnel.
- Have your questions about wound care answered openly and completely.
- Know what wound treatment options are available to you.
- Know the benefits, risks, and side-effects of your wound care treatments.
- Participate in the development of your treatment plan with your wound care team.
- Receive timely and cost-effective wound treatment.
- Have your wound treated appropriately with safe and effective products.
- Have your pain adequately controlled.
- Seek other opinions about your wound treatment plan if you so desire and consult a specialist as necessary.
- Consult other health care professionals for advice about diet, exercise, therapy, or products.

Used with permission of the Association for the Advancement of Wound Care (AAWC), 950 West Valley Rd, Suite 2800, Wayne, Penn, 19087.

APPENDIX

E WEBSITES

www.wocn.org	Website for the Wound, Ostomy, and Continence Nurses Society (WOCN); provides discussion forums, online journals, and access to professional resources
www.guidelines.gov/index.asp	Provides a national clearinghouse for guidelines in cooperation with the AHRQ, the American Medical Association, and the American Association of Health Plans
www.amda.com	Website for American Medical Directors Association (AMDA), which has released a clinical practice guideline for pressure ulcer therapy
www.woundsource.com	Provides access to the Wound Product Sourcebook Online and includes a monthly newsletter and a professional resource center
www.smtl.co.uk/World-Wide-Wounds	An electronic journal of wound management practice that provides a newsletter and offers an online discussion forum
www.woundcarenet.com	Online resource of the Wound Care Communication Network (WCCN) at Springhouse Corporation
www.medicaledu.com/wndguide.htm	The Wound Care Information Network provides educational information for professionals as well as updates and discussion forum
www.ncbi.nlm.nih.gov/PubMed	National Library of Medicine (NLM) search service to access MEDLINE and other related databases
www.hcfa.gov	Website for the Heath Care Financing Administration (HCFA) to access the latest on coverage policies on wound care products and support surfaces
www. npuap.org	Website for the National Pressure Ulcer Advisory Panel (NPUAP); provides latest version of the Pressure Ulcer Scale for Healing (PUSH) tool
www.woundcare.org	The Wound Care Institute, Inc.(WCI), a tax exempt, non-profit organization for the advancement of wound care, publishes articles online
www.ahrq.gov	Website for the Agency for Healthcare Research and Quality (AHRQ; formerly the Agency for Healthcare Policy and Research [AHCPR]); provides guidelines, technology assessment, and outcomes
www.woundheal.org	Website for the Wound Healing Society (WHS), a non-profit organization of clinical and basic scientific investigators interested in wound healing

www.cinahl.com	Cinahl Information Systems provides access to valuable databases and publications and the ability to order full text articles
www.shef.ac.uk/uni/academic/R-Z/scharr/ir/netting.html	Provides a list of websites pertaining to evidence-based practice
www.evidence.org	The online journal of *Clinical Evidence* (produced jointly by BMJ Publishing Group and the American College of Physicians–American Society of Internal Medicine; a compendium of best available research findings on common and important clinical questions
http://hiru.mcmaster.ca/ebm	A workshop on how to teach evidence-based clinical practice assembled by McMaster University Department of Clinical Epidemiology and Biostatistics
www.mls.cps.bc.ca/cites/index.htm	The Medical Library Services of the College of Physicians and Surgeons of British Columbia; produces newsletters *Cites and Bytes* and *Evidence Based Medicine Cites and Bytes*
www.cochrane.org	The Cochrane Collaboration, whose mission is preparing, maintaining, and promoting accessibility of systematic reviews of the effects of health care interventions; the Cochrane News is available online, and guidelines for conducting systematic reviews are available
www.york.ac.uk/depts/hstd/centres/evidence/ev-intro.htm	The University of York, Department of Health Studies; Centre for Evidence-Based Nursing

GLOSSARY

abscess Localized collection of pus in any part of the body.

advanced wound care dressings Refers to any of the newer dressings that are semiocclusive.

aerobe Microorganism that lives and grows in the presence of free oxygen.

altered tissue perfusion Condition when oxygenated blood does not flow freely through the vessels to the tissue.

anaerobe Microorganism that lives and grows in the absence of free oxygen.

antibacterial Agent that inhibits the growth of bacteria.

antimicrobial Agent that inhibits the growth of microbes.

apoptosis Programmed cell death initiated when activating molecules bind to their specific receptors on target cells; a mechanism to delete unwanted cells from the body.

arterial Pertaining to one or more arteries, which are vessels that carry oxygenated blood to the tissue.

arteriosclerosis Term applied to several pathologic conditions in which there is thickening, hardening, and loss of elasticity of the walls of blood vessels, especially arteries.

autocrine stimulation The process of one cell acting on or stimulating specific cellular activities within itself.

autologous skin graft Graft of patient's own skin; also known as autograft.

autolysis Disintegration or liquefaction of tissue or of cells by the body's own mechanisms, such as leukocytes and enzymes.

bactericidal Agent that destoys bacteria.

bacteriostatic Agent that is capable of inhibiting the growth or multiplication of bacteria.

blanching Becoming white; maximum pallor.

cell migration Movement of cells in the repair process.

cellulitis Inflammation of tissue around a lesion, characterized by redness, swelling, and tenderness. Signifies a spreading infectious process.

claudication Inadequate blood supply that produces severe pain in calf muscles during walking; subsides with rest.

collagen Main supportive protein of skin, tendon, bone, cartilage, and connective tissue.

colonized Presence of bacteria that cause no local or systemic signs or symptoms.

contamination The soiling by contact or introduction of organisms into a wound.

contraction The pulling together of wound edges in the healing process.

crater Tissue defect extending at least to the subcutaneous layer.

crusted Dried secretions.

cytokine Substances other than growth factors that contribute to the regulation of cellular function and wound repair; examples include tumor necrosis factor-alpha and interferons.

debridement Removal of devitalized tissue.

debris Remains of broken down or damaged cells or tissue.

decubitus A Latin word referring to the reclining position; a misnomer for a pressure sore; its plural is "decubitus ulcers."

demarcation Line of separation between viable and nonviable tissue.

denude Loss of epidermis.

dependent pain Pain occurring when extremity is lower than the heart.

dermal Related to skin or derma; synonym "integumentary."

dermal wound Loss of skin integrity, which may be superficial or deep.

dermis Inner layer of skin in which hair follicles and sweat glands originate; involved in grade 2 to 4 pressure sores.

edema Presence of abnormally large amounts of fluid in the interstitial space.

endocrine stimulation The process of one cell acting on or stimulating specific cellular activities in distant cells.

enzymes Biochemical substances that are capable of breaking down necrotic tissue.

epibole Edges of top layers of epidermis have rolled down to cover lower edges of epidermis, including basement membrane, so that epithelial cells cannot migrate from wound edges; also described as closed wound edges.

epidermis Outer cellular layer of skin.

epithelialization Regeneration of the epidermis across a wound surface.

erythema Redness of the skin surface produced by vasodilatation.

eschar Thick, leathery necrotic tissue; devitalized tissue.

excoriation Linear scratches on skin.

exudate Acuumulation of fluids in a wound; may contain serum, cellular debris, bacteria, and leukocytes.

fibroblast A cell or corpuscle from which connective tissue is developed.

friction Surface damage caused by skin rubbing against another surface.

full-thickness wound Tissue destruction extending through the dermis to involve the subcutaneous layer and possibly muscle and bone.

granulation Formation or growth of small blood vessels and connective tissue in a full-thickness wound.

growth factors Polypeptides that control growth and differentiation of cells (e.g., platelet-derived growth factor [PDGF], fibroblast growth factor [FGF] and epidermal growth factor [EGF])

hydrophilic Attracting moisture.

hydrophobic Repelling moisture.

hyperemia Presence of excess blood in the vessels; engorgement.

induration Abnormal firmness of tissue with a definite margin.

infection Overgrowth of microorganisms capable of tissue destruction and invasion, accompanied by local or systemic symptoms.

inflammation Defensive reaction to tissue injury; involves increased blood flow and capillary permeability and facilitates physiologic cleanup of the wound; accompanied by increased heat, redness, swelling, and pain in the affected area.

insulation Maintenance of wound temperature close to body temperature.

ischemia Deficiency of blood caused by functional constriction or obstruction of a blood vessel to a part.

lesion A broad term referring to wounds or sores.

leukocytosis Increase in the number of leukocytes ($>10{,}000/mm^3$) in the blood.

maceration Softening of tissue by soaking in fluids.

macrophage Cell that has the ability to destroy bacteria and devitalized tissue.

MMP Matrix metalloproteinase; enzymatic compound capable of connective tissue degradation; classified as collagenases, gelatinases, and stromelysins.

moisture-retentive wound dressings General term that refers to any dressing that is capable of consistently retaining moisture at the wound site by interfering with the natural evaporative loss of moisture vapor.

MVTR Moisture vapor transmission rate; measured in units of weight of moisture vapor per area of material per time period (e.g., $g/m^2/day$).

necrotic Dead; avascular.

occlusive wound dressings No liquids or gases can be transmitted through the dressing material.

paracrine stimulation The process of one cell acting on or stimulating specific cellular activities within a neighboring cell.

partial-thickness wound Loss of epidermis and possible partial loss of dermis.

pathogen Any disease-producing agent or microorganism.

phlebitis Inflammation of a vein.

physiologic wound environment In a wound, the presence of the physical, chemical, and biotic (living) factors that are characteristic of healthy intact skin; desirable to facilitate the natural process of wound healing.

pliable Supple; flexible.

pressure sore Area of localized tissue damage caused by ischemia because of pressure.

pus Thick fluid indicative of infection containing leukocytes, bacteria, and cellular debris.

pyogenic Producing pus.

reactive, hyperemia Extra blood in vessels in response to a period of blocked blood flow.

scab Dried exudate covering superficial wounds.

semiocclusive wound dressings No liquids are transmitted through dressing naturally; variable levels of gases can be transmitted through dressing material; most dressings are semiocclusive.

shear Trauma caused by tissue layers sliding against each other; results in disruption or angulation of blood vessels.

sinus tract Course or pathway that can extend in any direction from the wound surface; results in dead space with potential for abscess formation.

slough Loose, stringy necrotic tissue.

stasis Stagnation of blood caused by venous congestion.

strip Remove epidermis by mechanical means; denude.

synthetic wound dressings Dressings that are composed of man-made materials, such as polymers, as opposed to naturally occurring materials, such as cotton.

TIMP Tissue inhibitor of matrix metalloproteinases; binds to the MMPs to render the MMP inactive.

trophic Changes that occur as a result of inadequate circulation, such as loss of hair, thinning of skin, and ridging of nails.

ulcer Open sore.

undermine Tissue destruction to underlying intact skin along wound margins.

varicosities Dilated tortuous superficial veins.

vasoconstriction Constriction of the blood vessels.

vasodilatation Dilatation of blood vessels, especially small arteries and arterioles; preferred spelling rather than "vasodilation."

venous Pertaining to the veins.

wound base Uppermost viable tissue layer of the wound; may be covered with slough or eschar.

wound margin Rim or border of wound.

wound repair Healing process; partial-thickness healing involves epithelialization; full-thickness healing involves contraction, granulation, and epithelialization.

xenograft Another species (such as a pig) serves as donor for the tissue; also known as heterograft.

INDEX

Page numbers in italics indicate boxes and illustrations. Page numbers followed by *t* indicate tables

J